An Aid to the MRCP PACES
VOLUME 2
STATIONS 2 AND 4

D1427114

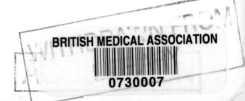

'MRCP; Member of the Royal College of Physicians . . .
They only give that to crowned heads of Europe.'
From *The Citadel* by A.J. Cronin

Dear Reader of *An Aid to the MRCP PACES*,

Please help us with the next edition of these books by filling in the survey on our website for every sitting of PACES that you attend. It does not matter if you pass or fail or pass well or fail badly. We need information from all these situations. These books are only as they are because of candidates in the past who filled in the surveys. Please do your bit for the candidates of the future. The website where you can fill in the survey is **www.ryder-mrcp.org.uk**

Good luck on the day.

Best wishes,
Bob Ryder
Afzal Mir
Anne Freeman

An Aid to the MRCP PACES

FOURTH EDITION
VOLUME 2
STATIONS 2 AND 4

**D. Banerjee, N. Sukumar,
R.E.J. Ryder, M.A. Mir and
E.A. Freeman**

*Departments of Medicine,
Birmingham Heartland Hospital, Heart of England NHS Foundation Trust and
City Hospital, Birmingham,
University Hospital of Wales and
University of Wales College of Medicine, Cardiff
and Department of Integrated Medicine,
Royal Gwent Hospital, Newport*

WILEY-BLACKWELL

A John Wiley & Sons, Ltd., Publication

This edition first published 2013, © 1986, 1999, 2003 by Blackwell Publishing Ltd, 2013 by John Wiley & Sons Ltd.

Wiley-Blackwell is an imprint of John Wiley & Sons, formed by the merger of Wiley's global Scientific, Technical and Medical business with Blackwell Publishing.

Registered office: John Wiley & Sons, Ltd, The Atrium, Southern Gate, Chichester, West Sussex, PO19 8SQ, UK

Editorial offices: 9600 Garsington Road, Oxford, OX4 2DQ, UK
              The Atrium, Southern Gate, Chichester, West Sussex, PO19 8SQ, UK
              111 River Street, Hoboken, NJ 07030-5774, USA

For details of our global editorial offices, for customer services and for information about how to apply for permission to reuse the copyright material in this book please see our website at www.wiley.com/wiley-blackwell
The right of the author to be identified as the author of this work has been asserted in accordance with the UK Copyright, Designs and Patents Act 1988.

Library of Congress Cataloging-in-Publication Data
An aid to the MRCP PACES. – 4th ed. p. ; cm. Aid to the Membership of the Royal College of Physicians Practical Assessment of Clinical Examination Skills includes bibliographical references and index. Summary: "The first volume in this revised suite of the best-selling MRCP PACES revision guides is now fully updated. It reflects both feedback from PACES candidates as to which cases frequently appear in each station. Also taken into account is the new marking system introduced in which the former four-point marking scale has been changed to a three-point scale and candidates are now marked explicitly on between four and seven separate clinical skills"–Provided by publisher. ISBN 978-0-470-65509-2 (v. 1 : pbk. : alk. paper) – ISBN 978-0-470-65518-4 (v. 2 : pbk. : alk. paper) – ISBN 978-1-118- 34805-5 (v. 3 : pbk. : alk. paper)   I. Wiley-Blackwell (Firm)   II. Title: Aid to the Membership of the Royal College of Physicians Practical Assessment of Clinical Examination Skills. [DNLM: 1. Physical Examination–Great Britain–Examination Questions.   2. Ethics, Clinical–Great Britain–Examination Questions. WB 18.2]610.76–dc232012020848

A catalogue record for this book is available from the British Library.

Wiley also publishes its books in a variety of electronic formats. Some content that appears in print may not be available in electronic books.

Cover image: © Wiley-Blackwell
Cover design by Sarah Dickinson

Set in 8.75/11.5pt Minion by Toppan Best-set Premedia Limited
Printed and bound in Malaysia by Vivar Printing Sdn Bhd

1   2013

Contents

Preface

'MRCP; Member of the Royal College of Physicians . . . They only give that to crowned heads of Europe.'*

A short history of *An Aid to the MRCP PACES*

'Remember when you were young, you shone like the sun . . . '†

At the beginning of the 1980s, Bob Ryder, an SHO working in South Wales, failed the MRCP short cases three times.‡ On each occasion I passed the long case and the viva which constituted the other parts of the MRCP clinical exam in those days but each time failed the short cases. Colleagues from the year below who had been house physicians, with me the SHO, came through and passed§ while I was left humiliated and without this essential qualification for progression in hospital medicine.

The battle to overcome this obstacle became a two or more year epic that took over my life. I transformed from green and inexperienced¶ to complete expert in everything to do with the MRCP short cases as viewed from the point of view of the candidate. I experienced every manifestation of disaster (and eventually triumph) recorded by others in Section F of this volume. By the time of the third attempt, I was so knowledgeable that I was out of tune with the examiner on a neurology case simply because I was thinking so widely on the case concerned.‖ I believed at the time that I came close to passing at that attempt, although one never really knows and it was, after all, the occasion where I failed to feel for a collapsing pulse!** This was an important moment in the story because it was from this failure, along with the experience in the neurology case in my second attempt¶, that the examination *routines* and *checklists,* which are so central to this book, emerged. I finally passed on the fourth attempt whilst working as a registrar.†† During the journey, various consultants, senior registrars and colleague registrars tried to help in their various ways and amongst these, one of the consultants in my hospital, Afzal Mir, offered the advice that I should make a list of all the likely short cases and make notes on each and learn them off by heart. His exact advice was to 'put them on your shaving mirror'. An important point should be made at this juncture. In order to be able to achieve this, one needed to attain the insight that it was indeed possible to do this. In those days there was no textbook for the exam, like the one you are reading, and there was no syllabus. Things had perhaps improved a little since the quote at the top of this Preface from A.J. Cronin* but nevertheless, the MRCP did carry with it an awe, a high failure rate and an aura that the exam was indeed one consisting of cases you had not seen before and questions you did not know the answer to. Indeed, many of us sitting it at the time would have found this a reasonable definition of the MRCP short cases.

A crucial part of my two or more years' journey that formed the seed that eventually grew into the first edition of this book was the realization that, in fact, behind the mystique, the reality was that the same old cases were indeed appearing in the exam over and over again, that there was a finite list and, indeed, from that list some cases occurred very frequently indeed.‡‡ The realization of this led me to do exactly what Afzal Mir had advised (without the shaving mirror bit!). At the time there was a free, monthly journal that we all received called *Hospital Update* and it had a regular feature dedicated to helping candidates with the MRCP. In one issue the writer listed 70 cases which he reckoned were the likely short cases to appear in the exam and an eye-balling of this suggested it was fairly comprehensive.

And so I studied each of these 70 cases in the textbooks and made notes which were distilled into their classic features and other things that seemed important to remember and I wrote out an index card for each of the 70. Thus, the original drafts of the main short case *records* were penned whilst I was still sitting the MRCP.

Another major contributor to my final success with the exam was junior doctor colleague Anne Freeman. She had been on the Whipps Cross MRCP course with me prior to our first sittings of the exam and she passed where I had failed. Until that point, I think we would have considered ourselves equals in knowledge, ability and likelihood of passing.‡ I would describe Anne as being like Hermione Granger.§§ In her highly organized manner, she had written down the likely instructions that might be given in the short cases exam and under each had recorded exactly what she would do and in what order, should she get that instruction. She then practised over and over again on her spouse (Dr Peter Williams, to whom she is especially grateful) until she could do it perfectly without thought or mistake or missing something out, even in the stress of the exam.** I, on the other hand, was not like Hermione Granger. I could examine a whole patient perfectly in ordinary clinical life but had not actually thought through exactly what I would do, and in what order, when confronted with an instruction such as 'examine this patient's legs' until it actually occurred in the exam.¶ And so eventually I did what Anne Freeman had done and the first versions of the *checklists* (for which I am especially grateful to my wife, Anne Ryder, who wrote them out tidily and then ticked off each point as I practised the examining, pointing out whenever I missed something out!) and primitive versions of the examination *routines* were born, again whilst I was still sitting the MRCP.

Having finally passed the exam, it seemed a shame to waste all the insights into the exam and the experience I had gained, and all the work creating the 70 short case index cards and the examination *routine checklists* I had created and practised and honed so laboriously – and so I conceived the idea of putting them in a book for others to have the benefit without having to do so much of the work or, perhaps, to go through the ordeal of failing through poor preparation as I had done. I short-listed what seemed to be the four major publishers of the moment and on a day in 1982 was sitting in the library of the University Hospital of Wales penning a draft letter to them. At a certain moment I got stuck over something – I have long since forgotten what – and on an impulse went down to Afzal Mir's office to ask him something to do with whatever it was I was stuck over. It was a defining moment in the history of these volumes. When I left Afzal Mir's office, the project had changed irrevocably. I was a registrar, he was a consultant. He was extremely interested in the subject himself and my consultation with him ended up with the project being one with both of us involved and me with a list of instructions (consultant to registrar!) as to what to do next!

And so an extremely forceful and creative relationship began, which led to *An Aid to the MRCP Short Cases*. It was not that we worked as a peaceful collaborative team – rather the thing came into existence through creativity on a battleground occupied by two equally creative and forceful (in very different ways) people

with very different talents and approaches. There are famous examples of this type of creative force, e.g. Lennon and McCartney or Waters and Gilmour.¶¶ Looking back, there is no doubt that without the involvement of myself and Afzal working together, an entirely different and inferior book would have emerged (probably the short 100-page pocket book desired by Churchill Livingstone – see below) but at the time I did not realize this and only thought that I was losing control of my project through the consultant–registrar hierarchy! My response was to bring in Anne Freeman, who I am sure would be very happy to be thought of as the Harrison/Starr or the Wright/Mason of the band!¶¶

Anne and I, in fact, also became a highly creative force through the development of the idea of surveying successful MRCP candidates to find out exactly what happened in the exam. It started off with me interviewing colleagues and this led to the development of a questionnaire to find out what instruction they had been given, what their findings were, what they thought the diagnosis was and their confidence in this, what supplementary questions they were asked, and their comments on the experience of that sitting. I distributed it to everyone I could find in my own and neighbouring hospitals, whilst Anne took on, with tremendous response, the immense task of tracking down every successful candidate at one MRCP sitting and getting a questionnaire to them! We asked all to report on both their pass and previous fail experiences.

Our overture to the publishers resulted in offers to publish from Churchill Livingstone (now owned by Elsevier Ltd) and Blackwell Scientific Publications (now owned by John Wiley & Sons) with the former coming in first and so we signed up with them. They were thinking of a 100-page small pocket book (70 brief short cases, a few examination routines, hardly any illustrations) sold at a price that would mean the purchaser would buy without thinking. The actual book, however, created itself once we got down to it and its size could not be controlled by our initial thoughts or the publisher's aspirations. We based the book on the, by now, extensive surveys of candidates who had sat the exam and told us exactly what happened in it – the length and the breadth. This information turned the list of 70 cases into 150 and from the surveys also emerged the 20 examination *routines* required to cover most of the short cases which occurred. As to what should be included with each short case, that was determined by ensuring that we gave everything that the candidate might need to know according to what they told us in the surveys. We were determined to cover everything that the surveys dictated might occur or be asked. It was also clear that pictures would help. We battled obsessively over every word and checked and polished it until it was as near perfect as possible. By the time it was finished three years later, the 100-page pocket book had turned into a monster manuscript full of pictures.

I took it to Churchill Livingstone who demanded that it be shrunk down to the size in the original agreement or at least some sort of compromise size. We were absolutely certain that what we had created was what the MRCP short case-sitting candidates wanted and we refused to be persuaded. And so we were rejected by Churchill Livingstone. This was a very depressing eventuality! I resurrected the original three-year-old offer letter from Blackwell Scientific Publications and made an appointment to see the Editorial Director – Peter Saugman. I turned up at his office carrying the massive manuscript and told him the tale. Wearing his very experienced publisher hat, he instantly and completely understood the Churchill Livingstone reaction but also understood something from my passion and certainty about the market for the book. He explained that he was breaking every publishing rule but that he was senior enough to do that and that he would go ahead and publish it in full on a hunch. In 1986, he was rewarded by the appearance of a 400-page textbook-sized book, which rapidly became one bought and studied by almost every MRCP candidate. Indeed, that original red and blue edition can be found on the bookshelves either at home or in the offices of nearly every medical specialty consultant in the UK.

After this, our first and best, we all pursued solo careers, with Afzal making clinical videos of patients depicting how to examine them, and writing other books such as *An Atlas of Clinical Diagnosis* (Saunders Ltd, second edition, 2003), Anne developing services for the elderly and people with stroke in Gwent, and me pursuing diabetes clinical research in various areas. Meanwhile, Anne in particular continued to accumulate survey data and in the second half of the 1990s we came together again to make the second, blue and yellow, edition of the book (1999). The surveys (which by this stage were very extensive indeed) had uncovered a further 50 short cases that needed to be included and the original material all needed updating.

Then, in 2001, the Royal Colleges changed the clinical exam to PACES. Until then the short cases exam had been a room full of patients of all different kinds with the candidate being led round them at random – according to the examiner's whim – for exactly 30 minutes. Anything from four to 11 patients might be seen. This was now transformed into Stations 1, 3 and 5 of the PACES exam, each 20 minutes long, thus doubling the time spent with short cases and ensuring that patients from all the main medical specialty areas were seen by every candidate. Hence, *An Aid to the MRCP Short Cases* was transformed into *An Aid to the MRCP PACES Volume 1*, with the short cases divided into sections according to the Stations. Specialists helped us more than ever with the updating and by now surveys had revealed that there were 20 respiratory cases that might occur, 19 abdominal cases, 27 cardiovascular cases, 52 central nervous system cases, 51 skin cases, 19 locomotor cases, 18 endocrine cases, 21 eye cases and eight 'other' cases. The long case and viva sections of the old clinical exam were replaced by Stations 2 (History taking) and 4 (Communication skills and ethics). To help us with these we recruited new blood – a bright and enthusiastic young physician who had recently passed the MRCP – Dev Banerjee, and he led on the Volume 2 project. Dev now confesses that 'one of the hardest aspects of writing Volume 2 back then before 2003 was coming up with enough surnames. You can not believe how hard it was. Should I refer to the Bible? Should I refer to the Domesday Book? I decided in the end, as I had grown up in Leeds and supported Leeds United all my life, to use the 1970s Leeds United team sheet for surnames. It's not obvious, but if you look carefully, it is there!'. Finally, in 2003, the third edition was published in silver and gold.

After many years intending to do this, we also created a medical student version of the short cases book on the grounds that medical student short cases exams are essentially the same as the MRCP in that it is the same pool of patients and the examiners are all MRCP trained so that is how they think. However, whilst most MRCP candidates continue to use our books, most medical students have not discovered their version – it has the wrong title because medical students no longer have short cases exams – they have OSCEs! Those who have discovered it report that they have found it useful for their OSCEs.

And now the Royal Colleges have changed the exam again. And so *An Aid to the MRCP PACES* has become a trilogy. Stations 1 and 3 remain roughly the same and hence Volume 1 covers Stations 1 and 3 and Volume 3 has been created to deal with the new style of Station 5. Each short case has been checked and updated by one or more specialist(s) and these are now acknowledged at the start of the station concerned against the short case they have taken responsibility for. The same applies to the short cases in Station 5. Nevertheless, I have personally checked every suggestion and update and took final editorial responsibility, changing and amending as I thought fit. The order of short cases was again changed according to new surveys (now done online) and yet again a few more new short cases were found from surveys: only four for Volume 1 – kyphoscoliosis and collapsed lung for Respiratory, PEG tube for Abdominal and Ebstein's anomaly for Cardiovascular. New young blood has again been recruited – a further two bright, young and enthusiastic physicians. The updating of Volume 2 covering Stations 2 (History taking) and 4 (Communication skills and ethics) has been led by Nithya Sukumar. For Volume 3, covering the new Station 5, Ed Fogden has created the new Section H (Integrated clinical assessment).

We are grateful to the specialists, now listed in the appropriate sections, who have checked and updated the short cases in their specialties in Volumes 1 and 3, and who helped Ed Fogden with the scenarios in Section H, Volume 3; and we are especially grateful for the enthusiasm with which they have done this despite the considerable workload involved. We are grateful to Mrs Jane Price, Lead Nurse for Patient Experience, Aneurin Bevan Health Board, for her significant input to the section on Station 4. Her knowledge/experience in communication skills and medical ethics and her years of experience in dealing with these situations in clinical practice and guiding doctors in real-life scenarios have given great insight into the needs of PACES candidates. She has, therefore, contributed significantly to the development of the new cases included in this edition, and she also updated and enhanced the Introduction to Section E. Our surveys have always dictated the content of the books and so we are especially grateful to all the PACES candidates who have taken the trouble to fill in the online MRCP PACES survey at www.ryder-mrcp.org.uk. Finally, we are particularly grateful to our colleagues for their support in the ongoing project, which is a considerable undertaking, and we reiterate the deep thanks to our families expressed in the previous prefaces to Volume 1.

Bob Ryder
2012

---

*From *The Citadel* by A.J. Cronin.

†From the song *Shine on You Crazy Diamond* by Pink Floyd from the album *Wish You Were Here*.

‡'The result comes as a particular shock when you have been sitting exams for many years *without* failing them.' Section F, Quotation 374.

§Section F, Experience 108.

¶Section F, Experience 109.

‖Section F, Experience 145.

**Section F, Experience 144.

††Section F, Experience 175. I measured my pulse just before going in to start this, my final attempt at the MRCP clinical, and the rate I remember is 140 beats/minute, but in retrospect I feel it must have magnified in my mind through the years – nevertheless whatever it was, it was very high. It is clear, though, that stress remains a major component of the exam – see Section F, Experience 15.

‡‡Section F, Useful tip 328 and Quotations 349 and 411–415.

§§A prominent character in the Harry Potter books by J.K. Rowling. Highly organized; expert at preparing for and passing exams.

¶¶Lennon and McCartney were the writing partnership of the Beatles with Harrison and Starr as the other members of the band. Similarly Waters and Gilmore for Pink Floyd with Wright and Mason as the other band members. In both cases it is believed that there was a special creativity through the coming together of the different talents of the individuals concerned, though the relationship was sometimes adversarial.

Introduction

Do not be tempted to skip the introduction here or at the start of each section!!
It will give you valuable pointers to help you through the book and the exams.

'I would have definitely benefited from more practice in history taking and in communication skills before the exam.' *

'Both the history section and the communication/ethics section are very rushed in the exam. It will feel very artificial because you will find there is too much to cover in 14 minutes (plus 1 minute thinking time and then 5 minutes questions) but persevere and be empathic.' †

'I finished the history taking very quickly so had to sit in silence until time was up. That was awful!' ‡

From June 2001, the Royal College of Physicians replaced the traditional MRCP 'clinical' examination, consisting of 30 minutes of short cases, a long case lasting 1 hour and 20 minutes and a viva lasting 20 minutes, with the MRCP PACES exam (Practical Assessment of Clinical Examination Skills). In Autumn 2009, the College changed the format of Station 5 of this exam. The candidate who reaches the MRCP PACES examination has already demonstrated considerable knowledge of medicine by passing the MRCP Part I and MRCP Part II written examinations. The PACES exam is divided into five stations, each of which is timed for precise periods of 20 minutes. Stations 1, 3 and 5 are divided into two substations of 10 minutes each. The stations are:

Station 1	Respiratory system
	Abdominal system
Station 2	History-taking skills
Station 3	Cardiovascular system
	Central nervous system
Station 4	Communication skills and ethics
Station 5	Integrated clinical assessment

This volume deals with Station 2 (History-taking skills) and Station 4 (Communication skills and ethics). Stations 1 and 3 are dealt with in Volume 1 of *An Aid*

*See comment on Section F, Experience 32.
†See comment on Section F, Experience 39.
‡See comment on Section F, Experience 33.

to the MRCP PACES. For this new edition of *An Aid to the MRCP PACES*, a third volume has been added to deal with the new Station 5.

The marking system for PACES is subject to change and you should study it at www.mrcpuk.org. At the time of writing, marking was being done in the skills of:

- Physical examination
- Identifying physical signs
- Clinical communication
- Differential diagnosis
- Clinical judgement
- Managing patient concerns
- Managing patient welfare.

The table on the following page shows, at the time of writing, the stations at which each of these skills are tested.

At the time of writing, the system is such that, on the mark sheet, the examiner in the station concerned gives for each skill being tested in that station one of the following marks:

Satisfactory	mark = 2
Borderline	mark = 1
Unsatisfactory	mark = 0

If you study the marking system and you can be bothered to do the analysis, you will be able to work out the minimum number of scores of 2 that you need, assuming all other scores are 1. However, in practice, this is probably of limited use because undoubtedly you will be trying to get a score of 2 in everything regardless. Two things are important, however.

1. At the time of writing, the College states on its website that:

'The onus is on the candidate to demonstrate each of the skills noted on the marksheet for each encounter (see table) and, in the event that any one examiner decides that a skill was not demonstrated by a candidate in any one particular task, an unsatisfactory mark (score = 0) will be awarded for this skill'.

Skill	Station 1: Respiratory	Station 1: Abdominal	Station 2	Station 3: Cardiovascular	Station 3: Neurological	Station 4	Station 5: Brief clinical consultation 1	Station 5: Brief clinical consultation 2
Physical examination	✓	✓	✗	✓	✓	✗	✓	✓
Identifying physical signs	✓	✓	✗	✓	✓	✗	✓	✓
Clinical communication	✗	✗	✓	✗	✗	✓	✓	✓
Differential diagnosis	✓	✓	✓	✓	✓	✗	✓	✓
Clinical judgement	✓	✓	✓	✓	✓	✓	✓	✓
Managing patient concerns	✗	✗	✓	✗	✗	✓	✓	✓
Managing patient welfare	✓	✓	✓	✓	✓	✓	✓	✓

Thus, it is important to always be aware of the station that you are in and to be proactive, in as far as you can, in ensuring that you attempt to demonstrate your abilities in each of the headings concerned – the ones that are relevant to that station according to the above table.

2. It is important to remember as you move from station to station that all 10 examiners mark independently and as you go into the next station, the examiners have no idea how you did in the station you have just left so essentially you start with a blank sheet with them. If you have done badly in a station and fear you have scored some 0s, these can be compensated for by scoring an excess of 2s in another station. In the 5 minutes between stations it is crucial to recharge yourself psychologically, forget what has just happened in the station you have left and give yourself a complete fresh start – see 'Getting psyched up' in Section A in Volume 1.

The exam is a practical test which assesses various facets of clinical competence in many subtle ways. Although it is generally accepted that clinical competence and communication skills cannot be acquired from textbooks, a book such as this can provide indirect help towards that objective.

Stations 2 and 4 of the PACES examination are designed to be a comprehensive test of a candidate's ability to obtain an in-depth history, provide information to patients, and other relevant people, about sensitive issues such as malignant and sexually transmitted diseases, and their ability to discuss management and care plans with patients and other clinical staff.

Station 2 will assess your history-taking skills. Two examiners will observe how you gather the appropriate and relevant facts from a patient, assimilate that information into either a diagnosis and/or a management plan, and then assess your discussion with them. During the 5-minute interval before you enter this Station, you will be given written instructions for the case you are going to see. This is often in the form of a letter from the patient's GP; thus, the Station simulates an outpatient clinic except that you will have two examiners, instead of two students, silently observing you. You will have 14 minutes with the patient and then 1 minute for reflection during which you must decide how you are going to present the crucial part of the history, which issues you will need to discuss with the examiners, and how you will suggest that you would respond to the referring letter.

Station 4 tests communication and ethics and your ability to guide and organize an interview with the subject (mostly an actor masquerading as a patient, relative or a healthcare worker). During the 5-minute interval preceding this Station, you will receive written instructions summarizing the problem you will have to deal with. As for Station 2, you will have 14 minutes with the subject, in the presence of the examiners, during which you must explore and deal with the problem while providing emotional support whenever necessary, and discuss further management. As the subject leaves the Station, you will have just 1 minute to crystallize your thoughts for the 5-minute discussion with the examiners.

All three parties – the patient/actor, the examiners and you – will each have a preprinted sheet at both

Stations. The patient/actor will respond to your questions according to their brief from the examiners, their required verbal and non-verbal interactions will also be indicated on their sheet as well as the clinical details of the condition that they are role-playing; the examiners will assess you according to their guidance notes; and you will have your briefing of either the GP letter for the history taking or the scenario for the communications station. All this is done to ensure a level playing field for each candidate.

Take note of ALL written and verbal instruction given as the words used are important. They will give you clues about the emphasis of the scenario case.

We have presented here 50 scenarios for Station 2 and 68 scenarios for Station 4 which cover a diverse range of problems seen in clinical practice. For each scenario, we have given the information which you would have outside the exam room (the candidate's information), the information that might be written on the patient/actor's sheet, and what the examiners' guidelines may look like which they will use to assess your interaction with the subject. We have also given some helpful hints before each Section but these will only prove useful if you have thoroughly prepared yourself for these tasks.

Doctors taking this exam need to have practised these skills and should have knowledge not only of the various clinical conditions likely to be encountered, but also of the myriad ethical and legal issues which may arise. Doctors approaching the PACES exam should make a purposeful preparation for it from the outset and, in the process, learn about structured clinical methods and good bedside behaviour.

Preparation

'I would suggest that candidates need to have thought of the answers before they are asked, as the questions were really quite predictable.' *

It is a well-known fact that the best preparation for passing the membership examination is to work on the firm of a good clinical teacher. In the real world of today, there are very few such teachers who would regard teaching as a worthwhile and rewarding pursuit, and those who do hold these beliefs are usually too busy to teach because of the increasing clinical and administrative demands. As one clinical tutor once ruefully remarked, 'In the past we used to teach students and now, in the current environment of political correct-

ness and proper documentation, we spend our time talking about it!'. More than ever, the onus lies with the students to take due care of their learning programme and to make use of any learning opportunity (teaching sessions, clinical meetings, symposia, grand rounds, etc.) during their clinical duties.

History taking

'The candidate mistimed the whole station; he raced through the history of the presenting complaint in about 1 minute, proceeded to briefly take the rest of the history, and then realized he had 9 minutes left. The silence was broken by 'OK then, tell me about those palpitations again'. †

History taking is an art and cannot be acquired simply by reading books. Nonetheless, a book such as this can help you organize your approach to each symptom, select a battery of appropriate questions, interpret the information received, and narrow down the diagnostic hypotheses. It is important that students learn a structured approach from the very beginning during their clinical attachments, but it is never too late for postgraduate students to adapt and develop it.

There are 6–8 principal symptoms in each system and students should consult a book on clinical skills and master a battery of questions for each symptom, and then practise the art of asking these questions at every opportunity during their clinical training. Remembering the questions is easier than the art of asking them, which can be improved by constant practice, self-criticism and helpful comments from a good teacher. A famous neurologist once said, during a teaching session, that diagnosing the cause of headache, the most common symptom in medicine, is like completing a jigsaw puzzle of asking 13 questions. Those who can only count 12 questions should consider asking the final question to the patient as to what he or she thinks is the cause of the headache. The same can be said about any other symptom such as chest pain or palpitations.

It is important to explore the presenting symptoms fully before going on to other aspects of the history taking. The examiners take a dim view of any candidate who skates back and forth from the presenting complaints to past or family history. It becomes easier to identify the chief areas of concern in other parts of the history, and the possible risk factors, only after adequately exploring the presenting complaint(s). Besides, it is imperative to let the patient ventilate fully his or her

---

*See comment on Section F, Experience 20.

†See Section F, Invigilators' diaries, Stations 2 and 4.

major concerns both in clinical practice and in the exam. A systems review will be necessary to find out if the patient has any other complaint which he or she has not mentioned.

During your clinical attachments, foundation programme and core training appointments, you should get into the habit of going over your notes each time you take a history, and judging whether you have covered all aspects of the history and then assembled the appropriate differential diagnoses. Once you have done that you should then prepare a summary of the problem(s) and the possible management plan and articulate it vocally to yourself. This habit will serve you well for any examination. As you prepare for the PACES exam, you should act out each history scenario from this book with a fellow candidate and discuss the conclusions and management plans. This will tighten up your history-taking technique and your presentation skills. Remember, the examiners do not know you are clever; you have to demonstrate it. The exercise will also help to make you a methodical and articulate clinician.

Communication skills and medical ethics

The patient said to the candidate, 'I'm worried this may be something serious'. The candidate replied 'That doesn't surprise me'. *

Unlike the history-taking techniques, which are now taught from the very first year of medical training, guidance and instruction on communication skills are still in their infancy. In the past, young doctors acquired these skills by osmosis from their senior colleagues whom they observed during their discussions with patients and relatives. Since 1995, communication skills have been incorporated in the new undergraduate curricula that have been adopted by most medical schools in the UK. The Royal Colleges of the UK and the General Medical Council have all focused their attention on communication skills, and so their assessment is now part of all major clinical examinations. As a result of this increasing emphasis on good communication, appropriate counselling skills and knowledge of ethics, Station 4 has now been devoted to their assessment in the PACES examination. Most candidates approach this Station with some foreboding.

There are three main reasons why a candidate's heart may sink before entering the communication and ethics station. First, unlike history taking, which has a long-established structure with subsets, communica-

tion skills are fluid and elastic and vary from problem to problem and from person to person. Although there are some recognized basic principles of a counselling interview as outlined at the beginning of Section E, each problem, with its inherently unique circumstances, can impose its own constraints, all of which can differ from patient/actor to patient/actor.

Secondly, the multiangled assimilative exercise of communication skills involves learning from tutors, talking to patients, relatives and other healthcare professionals, and studying the diverse range of ethical and legal issues that surround these problems. Unlike a clinical skill, which can be demonstrated by a tutor, communication skills cannot be imparted by a single demonstration or learned by one useful interview with a patient. It is a continuing learning process and most candidates are conscious that their technique and knowledge have some gaps.

Thirdly, even an apparently straightforward counselling scenario may present an unexpected hurdle, either because of its unique circumstances or because the interviewer forgot some simple principle. We know of a real-life incident when a consultant, during his round in a coronary care unit, was a witness to an unsuccessful cardiopulmonary resuscitation on one of his patients. As he and his entourage emerged from the door, the deceased patient's wife, who had just arrived, asked him about her husband. The consultant told her, as sympathetically as he could, that her husband had passed away. On hearing this the lady fainted, fell on the concrete floor before anyone could catch her and sustained a nasty cut to her forehead. Sometime later, she charitably remarked, 'It was my own fault. I should have been sitting!'. During a busy and eventful round, the consultant had forgotten to observe the basic principles of privacy and comfort which should be afforded to all recipients of bad news. He did not take the lady into a side room, get a nurse to sit with her to offer support and coffee, and then give her the bad news.

These considerations, apart from highlighting the concerns of the candidates, clearly reinforce a well-known fact that there is no shortcut to experience in acquiring communication skills. Medical students should grasp the fundamentals of communication, learn from personal and video demonstrations, and observe intently as many consultations as possible during their rotation through general practice and hospital placements when senior doctors speak to patients and relatives. They should seek permission to sit in on any interview between a senior clinician and a patient

*See Section F, Invigilators' diaries, Stations 2 and 4.

or a relative. As their training advances, and during their junior appointments, they should practise their own communication skills.

Candidates approaching this exam should have already gained some experience and they should use this book in developing it further and improving upon it. There are 68 scenarios on communication skills and ethics, subdivided into seven sections/categories, and we would suggest that two candidates should play out each scenario, one acting as the subject and the other the doctor, and then discuss the problem and the performance in the light of the examiner's information. After playing out each scenario, they should discuss the various ethical and legal issues arising from it. We have provided relevant references to our sources of such information and candidates should look up these for themselves. Possession of adequate knowledge about the various aspects of each problem is essential in order to spare some thought and time to decide on the proper and appropriate kinetic behaviour (body language) in tune with that scenario. It is difficult to be thoughtful of a patient's sensitivities if you are struggling to recall information from distant and faded memory lacunae. Remember that even if all the points raised are addressed, the candidate will still fail if the overall impression of the examiners is of poor empathy and a hesitant interaction with the subject.

To sum up, those candidates who have acquired some personal experience of communication skills, who have studied and gained a thorough knowledge of these 68 scenarios, and who have been through them with fellow candidates would be leaving very little to chance. From our accumulated experience, we have come to believe that no candidate passes the MRCP examination by pure luck, and a candidate who leaves gaps on the chance that the examiners may not explore them may be unsuccessful.

The examination

'They (the examiners) are stone cold in expression and that often makes you think that you are doing badly but that's not always true.' *

By the time you seriously consider taking the PACES examination, you should have gained enough experience in taking a history on almost any presenting complaint, obtained some instruction and experience in counselling and communication, studied several times a standard textbook on medicine and one on clinical skills, and have had many opportunities to summarize and present case histories in various forums. If, in addition, you were blessed with some critical appraisal of your presentations from senior colleagues and, in turn, you have constantly improved your performance by taking a comprehensive account of history and counselling scenarios, including preparing a succinct summary for presentation, then you have made the adequate preliminary preparation to study this book for your final preparation.

Study this book thoroughly; grasp the details of each scenario in the two main sections, play out each scenario with your fellow candidates and polish up your presentation. Get into the habit of summarizing the chief points in each scenario and practise presenting them to anyone who is prepared to listen and provide some helpful criticism. Practise speaking clearly and fluently in front of a mirror and into a tape recorder and play it back. When you have done all of this then you should feel confident and self-assured to enter the PACES exam.

*See comment on Section F, Experience 21.

Section D
History-Taking Skills

'A candidate, after seeing a patient with funny turns, gave no indication of any tests to be performed, any follow-up or any thoughts about the causes for the funny turns, and ended the consultation by saying "Thanks, we've finished now".'*

*Section F, Invigilators' diaries – Stations 2 and 4.

These books exist as they are because of many previous candidates who, over the years, have completed our surveys and given us invaluable insight into the candidate experience. Please give something back by doing the same for the candidates of the future. For all of your sittings, whether they be a triumphant pass or a disastrous fail . . .

Remember to fill in the survey at www.ryder-mrcp.org.uk

THANK YOU

The history-taking station in the PACES examination tests the candidates' ability to explore and probe the presenting complaint(s), gather and interpret information, formulate a plan of action, communicate it to the patient and then discuss the conclusions and management plan with the examiners. The cases presented in the exam, and in this book, are the ones that doctors encounter in their everyday clinical practice and the ones that all candidates should be familiar with. Yet there is strong anecdotal evidence from reliable sources that since the PACES examination was introduced, many candidates have performed poorly both in this station as well as in Station 4. It seems perverse that doctors, trained in the basic skill of medicine from the very first year of medical school and experienced in taking histories from their patients every day, should perform badly. Looking at the reports we have received from our surveys, there seem to be four main reasons for this.

1. The clinician under scrutiny. It is not usual for clinicians to have two senior doctors sitting with them while they are taking a history. Under examination conditions, many candidates become self-conscious to the point of distraction in the presence of the pair of examiners. This can have a detrimental effect on their interview technique and one of two results generally follows. Either a 'machine-gun' approach which results in asking a string of questions about a symptom without pausing for breath, for reflection or allowing the patient to answer any of them properly. The patient/actor can feel as if they are under interrogation and may become panicky and forgetful or agitated and cross. Or, there is the 'butterfly effect' where the candidate flits in an apparently random fashion from one aspect of the history to another in an effort to demonstrate their ability to focus on important issues. Candidates may unwittingly stray into the areas that are not covered in the patient's information sheet. The patient/actor then falls on his or her own resources to manufacture some quick answers and both lose their way.

Whether the candidate is a 'machine-gunner' or a 'butterfly', both of these unfortunate techniques create a bad impression for both the patient and the examiners. By now, the candidate is losing their grip on the situation, their anxiety increases and all is lost.

2. The clinician as logician. Many candidates fail to satisfy the examiners because they have badly handled the presenting complaints. Instead of approaching the problem logically and creating a list of possible diagnoses from the given complaints, they fail to probe each complaint in order to narrow down to a more probable diagnosis.

3. The speedy clinician. Candidates who forget to adopt a systematic approach are most likely to find themselves in this unfortunate position. Pace yourself. You have 14 minutes which should allow you to cover all aspects of the history. Do not rush through the consultation and find that you have 7 minutes of silence to endure, which will seem like an eternity. Also, 'tacking on' additional questions about past history, social history, etc. because you forgot to do it as part of your interview and you now have time on your hands is not impressive. The exam is not a test of whether you can see 10 new patients in one clinic session!

4. And finally . . . the forgetful clinician. Many candidates who fail in this exam have made a bad job of their presentation. In the heat of the moment, some forget that in a history-taking station there are three agencies to answer to:

(a) the patient, who needs to know what is wrong with him/her and what the doctor proposes to do about it

(b) the examiners, who have to be satisfied about a plan of action

(c) the referring doctor, who needs an answer to the problem posed in the letter.

However, there is plenty of hope and you can prepare yourself to negotiate this station successfully. Here are some principles which will help you to succeed.

Preparation, preparation, preparation

As a candidate, you have to be thoroughly prepared for this encounter by studying and acting out the scenarios in this book with your colleagues. These scenarios, presented by very experienced clinicians, have been written in a form similar to the PACES exam. For the purposes of practising each of the scenarios, we have included:

- a GP letter (which you will be given outside the room on the examination day)
- a patient information sheet (which you will not see in the exam) which gives the patient/actor all the necessary information to allow them to respond to your questions
- an examiners' information sheet (which you will not see on the examination day) which gives you a good idea about the main points that the examiners will be looking for and how they will assess you.

We suggest that you study each scenario carefully and then act them out with a fellow candidate and if possible an observer (who can use the examiners' sheet to evaluate your performance).

As you practise, keep in mind the following important guidelines.

- Read the letter carefully and ascertain who is making the referral and the exact nature of their concern. At the end, you will have to answer this by offering a plan of action.
- Note the exact presenting complaints and write them down to remind yourself as you progress through the history taking.
- From the presenting complaint(s), consider the possible differential diagnoses that will need to be explored during the consultation. Based on this, formulate an approach as to how the consultation should be carried out, what relevant questions should be asked and in what order, and what issues should be tackled.
- Be polite and courteous to the patient throughout the interview. If you need to refer to any notes or have to ask what may seem to be irrelevant or very personal questions, ask for their permission before proceeding.
- Introduce yourself to the patient and explain the purpose of the interview, e.g. 'Your GP has written to me explaining that you are having some trouble with your breathing. I would like to ask you some questions, if I may, so that we can then discuss how to investigate and manage this problem'.
- The first question about the presenting complaint(s) is the most important one; it should allow the patient to talk freely, e.g. 'Tell me about it' or 'Tell me all about your breathing difficulty and how it started'. This approach avoids leading the patient and allows him some space and time to say what concerns him the most. This information is vital as it identifies the patient's main problem and allows the candidate to focus accurately on the task set.
  - Open-ended questions are extremely useful when descriptive information is required. This style of questioning enables the patient/actor to volunteer more

about themselves. We know of one incident when an actor/patient (who was either inadequately briefed or just very kind!) regurgitated all that was on the information sheet in answer to this one open-ended question!

 – Closed questions are appropriate when you need to keep the interview on track and when focused factual information is required – for example, 'Have you ever had any of the following: heart problems, epilepsy, etc.?'

- Probe each complaint sequentially (logician) and get an idea of the impact of the symptoms on the patient and the family. Do not 'flit' (butterfly) from one complaint to another without getting a good idea of the nature of each.
- Be attentive and do not lose eye contact with the patient. It is acceptable for you to take brief notes, but do not overdo it and do not appear to be taking dictation.
- Verify and expand on any incidents that the patient may mention. For example, if the patient has uncontrolled asthma and says that he was admitted to the ICU last year, find out what the symptoms were at the time, what was the cause of the exacerbation, how long he was in the ICU, and what treatment was given.
- Complete a brief systems review to ensure that you get the full picture and that you do not miss any symptom that the patient may not have considered important enough to mention.
- Do not appear to be taking the patient's past history, drug history and social history only because you have some time left; make them an essential part of your consultation. In particular, the social history may have an important bearing on the patient's illness, especially if they are elderly.
- As you complete the consultation, ask the patient if there is anything which they want to discuss with you that has not been mentioned already.
- Finally, make sure the concerns in the referral letter have been addressed. Formulate a management plan and explain it to the patient in simple terms. Reassure him that a letter will go to the GP. Tell the patient about the follow-up arrangements that will be made. You will have to explain all this to the examiners during your discussion with them.

Station 2
History-Taking Skills

Case 1 | Abdominal swelling

Candidate information

You are the doctor in a general medical clinic. Mr David Brian has been referred to you by the general practitioner (GP).

Please read this letter and then continue with the consultation.

Dear Doctor

Re: Mr David Brian, age 53

Thank you for seeing Mr Brian urgently in your clinic. He gives a 4-week history of abdominal swelling. There is some discomfort from the swelling but no specific pain and he rarely drinks alcohol. On examination, he is thin, looks unwell but is not jaundiced. However, I suspect that he has ascites.

Please see and advise.

Yours sincerely

Dr G. Practitioner

You have 14 min until the patient leaves the room, followed by 1 min for reflection, before the discussion with the examiners. Be prepared to discuss the solutions to the problems posed by the case and how you might reply to the GP's letter.

Patient information

Mr David Brian is a 53-year-old musician who presents with a 4-week history of progressive abdominal swelling. He has noticed his abdominal wall to be tight and as a result he has some generalized discomfort. He has no specific pain. He has noticed loss of appetite, malaise and some wasting of the muscles of his limbs. He has no associated symptoms of jaundice, ankle swelling, haematemesis, melaena, change in bowel habit or vomiting. He has no other respiratory, cardiovascular or urinary symptoms. He has an unremarkable past medical history. He rarely drinks alcohol and has never had any liver disease previously. He takes no medication except for occasional paracetamol for headaches. He has no risk factors for human immunodeficiency virus (HIV) or viral hepatitis. He has not been abroad recently and he lives with a partner. He has never smoked. He is concerned that he may have cancer.

Examiner information

1. Data gathering in the interview

A good candidate would be able to elicit:
- the details of the abdominal swelling, particularly regarding the time span, if the swelling was progressing, whether the swelling is generalized or focal and any associated pain or discomfort
- other gastrointestinal symptoms which may indicate liver cirrhosis or abdominal malignancy, e.g. haematemesis, melaena, jaundice, change in bowel habit, inguinal lymphadenopathy

- systemic symptoms, e.g. loss of weight and appetite, fever, breathlessness as a result of the ascites and other clues to a malignancy elsewhere
- risk factors for liver cirrhosis, e.g. excessive alcohol consumption, viral hepatitis, drug induced, autoimmune
- other causes of ascites, e.g. symptoms suggestive of acute or chronic pancreatitis, intra-abdominal sepsis/ infection, congestive cardiac failure, hepatic vein thrombosis, nephrotic syndrome and tuberculosis
- any exposure to asbestos (peritoneal mesothelioma is a rare cause of malignant ascites)
- the impact of the illness on him and his work
- the concerns of the patient – if the patient is particularly concerned that he may have a malignancy then this must be addressed appropriately by the candidate (i.e. do not be evasive)
- why he thinks he might have a malignancy – is there a family history? Did his GP mention the possibility? Tell him in an honest and sensitive manner that cancer is part of the differential diagnosis but his abdominal swelling could also be due to one of many other causes. The way to find out for sure would be to admit him and carry out the necessary tests without delay.

Reassure him that you will let him (and his family) know as soon as any of the test results are back.

2. Identification and use of information gathered

The candidate should be able to interpret the history and create a problem list. The objectives for the candidate are to:
- develop a list of possible differential diagnoses
- have a list of investigations
- explain the possible causes of the illness to the patient and explain the need to admit.

3. Discussion related to the case

- Causes of abdominal swelling include obesity, gaseous distension, pregnancy in females, intra-abdominal masses, e.g. ovarian in females, and fluid, i.e. ascites.
- In liver disease, ascites indicates a chronic or subacute disorder and does not occur in acute conditions (e.g. uncomplicated viral hepatitis, drug reactions, biliary obstruction). The most common cause is cirrhosis, especially from alcoholism. Other hepatic causes include chronic hepatitis, severe alcoholic hepatitis without cirrhosis and hepatic vein obstruction (Budd–Chiari syndrome). Portal vein thrombosis does not usually cause ascites unless hepatocellular damage is also present.
- Non-hepatic causes of ascites include generalized fluid retention associated with systemic disease (e.g. heart failure, nephrotic syndrome, severe hypoalbuminaemia, constrictive pericarditis) and intra-abdominal disorders (e.g. carcinomatosis, tuberculous peritonitis). Hypothyroidism occasionally causes marked ascites and pancreatitis rarely causes large amounts of fluid (pancreatic ascites). Patients with renal failure, especially those on haemodialysis, occasionally develop unexplained intra-abdominal fluid.
- A diagnostic tap of 50 mL should be obtained and sent for cytology, microscopy, alcohol- and acid-fast bacilli (AAFB) and amylase. The presence of haemorrhagic ascites is in favour of malignancy, acute pancreatitis and abdominal trauma. Straw-coloured ascites is more commonly found in cirrhosis, infective causes, congestive cardiac failure, nephrotic syndrome and hepatic vein obstruction.
- A neutrophil count of over 250 cells per cubic millimetre is indicative of an underlying bacterial peritonitis, justifying broad-spectrum intravenous antibiotic therapy in the presence of a fever.
- This case favours a diagnosis of a malignancy and the investigation of choice would be a computed tomography (CT) scan of the abdomen.
- Treatment of ascites in a patient with liver cirrhosis aims to reduce sodium intake and increase the renal excretion of sodium with a careful combination of diuretics and fluid restriction.

Comments on the case

This case tests the candidate's ability to generate a list of differential diagnoses for ascites. The patient is unwell and must be admitted for tests.

Case 2 | **Ankle swelling**

Candidate information

You are the doctor in a cardiology clinic. Miss Vicky Daniels is referred to you by her GP.

Please read this letter and then continue with the consultation.

Dear Doctor

Re: Miss Vicky Daniels, aged 29

Thank you for seeing Vicky Daniels who works as a domestic at the local law courts. She has had asthma for 2 years, treated with budesonide and bricanyl inhalers, and also a similar length history of chest pain. However, her breathlessness and pain have worsened over the last 2 months and she now has ankle swelling. I would appreciate your help.

Yours sincerely

Dr G. Practitioner

You have 14 min until the patient leaves the room, followed by 1 min for reflection, before the discussion with the examiners. Be prepared to discuss the solutions to the problems posed by the case and how you might reply to the GP's letter.

Patient information

Vicky Daniels is a 29-year-old domestic cleaner at the local law courts who has had a 2-year history of breathlessness and chest pain. Up to 2 years ago she was reasonably fit and well but she remembers that, after a lower respiratory chest infection, she began to get more breathless with a feeling of tightness in the chest. At that time it was felt she may have asthma and, as there is a strong family history, she was started on budesonide 200 µg bd and bricanyl (prn) turbohalers. Unfortunately, her dyspnoea has progressed, so much so that walking upstairs or up a slight incline is a real effort. The chest pain is usually central, non-pleuritic, without radiation and is occasionally exertional. It usually eases with resting. She also complains of extreme tiredness and ankle swelling up to the lower ends of the tibiae over the last 2 months. She has had to stop working. There are no obvious relieving or precipitating factors or any known allergies to the common household allergens. She has no orthopnoea, syncope, palpitations, cough, sputum, haemoptysis, rash or arthropathy and there are no gastroenterological or neurological symptoms. There is no previous history of pulmonary emboli, congenital heart disease, chronic lung disease, scleroderma, systemic lupus erythematosus (SLE) or HIV infection. She takes no medication apart from the inhalers. She has never smoked and she drinks on occasions. She lives with her mother who also has asthma. There are no pets in the house. She is obviously very worried about her progressive breathlessness and is desperate for help.

Examiner information

1. Data gathering in the interview

A good candidate would be able to elicit:
- the chronology of the symptoms
- the exact features of the dyspnoea and the chest pain with particular reference to her exercise ability. Does the chest pain sound anginal or pleuritic (pulmonary emboli)?
- the recent onset of ankle swelling; which leg or both legs, how far up the leg(s), and whether putting on shoes is difficult
- other respiratory symptoms, e.g. haemoptysis (chronic pulmonary emboli), chronic cough and sputum (chronic lung disease, e.g. bronchiectasis), cardiovascular symptoms, e.g. syncope and palpitations (congenital heart disease, mitral valve disease)
- a full asthma history – is this really asthma? Whether there is any evidence of diurnal symptoms of cough and wheeze, allergy to common household allergens (e.g. cats, house dust mite, pollen), if the inhalers have helped the symptoms, and on what basis did the GP diagnose asthma (serial peak flows versus clinical history)
- any past medical history of congenital heart disease, mitral valve disease, chronic lung disease, thrombotic disease, collagen vascular disease such as scleroderma and SLE
- drug history, e.g. appetite suppressants such as fenfluramine
- family history of primary pulmonary hypertension
- the impact of the illness on her life and her work
- any recent air flights which may have exacerbated symptoms (pregnancy does as well in primary pulmonary hypertension)
- her ideas as to what may be going on, any particular concerns she has and what her expectations are from this consultation.

2. Identification and use of information gathered

The candidate should be able to interpret the history and create a problem list. The objectives for the candidate are to:
- assemble a list of differential diagnoses
- have a list of investigations to be arranged urgently and explain these to the patient
- address any concerns
- arrange follow-up as soon as possible to discuss the results.

3. Discussion related to the case

- This case tests the ability of the candidate to have a list of differential diagnoses for ankle oedema, breathlessness and chest pain in a young, non-smoking, previously fit woman. The possibilities are primary pulmonary hypertension or secondary pulmonary hypertension, e.g. recurrent pulmonary embolism, chronic lung disease, e.g. bronchiectasis, congenital heart disease, collagen vascular disease, e.g. scleroderma or SLE, HIV infection, drug induced, especially from weight-reducing appetite suppressants, or other rarer causes, e.g. veno-occlusive disease.
- In the absence of any secondary causes, this case is most likely to be primary pulmonary hypertension. Investigations would include chest X-ray showing enlarged central pulmonary arteries and clear lung fields, electrocardiogram (ECG) revealing right axis deviation and right ventricular hypertrophy, an echocardiogram demonstrating right ventricular enlargement, a reduction in left ventricular cavity size, and abnormal septal configuration consistent with right ventricular pressure overload, full lung function testing for impaired diffusion and hypoxaemia, ventilation–perfusion scan to rule out pulmonary emboli and cardiac catheterization (with care) to characterize the disease and to exclude an underlying cardiac shunt as the cause.
- A definitive diagnosis of pulmonary hypertension requires right heart catheterization to measure the pulmonary artery pressure – a pressure more than 25 mmHg at rest confirms the presence of pulmonary hypertension. Additionally, patients with idiopathic pulmonary arterial hypertension will have a pulmonary capillary wedge pressure (PCWP) less than 15 mmHg.
- The management is challenging and the patient should be looked after by a cardiologist with a specialist interest. Reduction in pulmonary vascular resistance with short-acting vasodilators, e.g. nitric oxide, intravenous adenosine or intravenous prostacyclin may determine who will respond better to high-dose oral calcium channel blockers, e.g. nifedipine and diltiazem (known as a vasoreactivity test).
- Treatment options for patients with pulmonary hypertension consist predominantly of vasodilatory drugs. Examples of these are prostacyclins (e.g. epoprostenol, treprostinil), endothelin receptor antagonists (e.g. bosentan) or phosphodiesterase 5 inhibitors (e.g. sildenafil, vardenafil or tadalafil). In those who

do not respond, heart and lung transplantation may need to be considered.

- Anticoagulation is also indicated in patients with idiopathic pulmonary hypertension in addition to that due to chronic thromboembolism.

Comments on the case

This lady presents with three symptoms, i.e. dyspnoea, chest pain and ankle swelling. Hence the candidate must be prepared to take *three* clear histories.

Case 3 | Asymptomatic hypertension

Candidate information

You are the doctor in a general medical clinic. Mr Tom Walker is referred to you by his GP.

Please read this letter and then continue with the consultation.

Dear Doctor

Re: Mr Tom Walker, aged 49

Thank you for seeing Mr Walker whom I found to have a blood pressure of 180/95 mmHg. I started him on bendroflumethiazide 2.5 mg od but his BP continues to be elevated. He smokes 15 cigarettes a day and drinks 16 pints at the weekends. Past medical history includes anxiety attacks and mild asthma for which he takes a salbutamol inhaler on a prn basis. He is a self-employed painter and decorator. Please see and advise.

Yours sincerely

Dr G. Practitioner

You have 14 min until the patient leaves the room, followed by 1 min for reflection, before the discussion with the examiners. Be prepared to discuss the solutions to the problems posed by the case and how you might reply to the GP's letter.

Patient information

Mr Tom Walker is a 49-year-old, slightly overweight painter and decorator who is currently asymptomatic with no relevant symptoms such as chest pains, palpitations, headache, dyspnoea, blurred vision, sweating, tremors, weight change or urinary problems. On a recent visit to the GP for a Well-Man clinic appointment, a blood pressure (BP) of 180/95 mmHg was recorded and he was started on bendroflumethiazide 2.5 mg od. Subsequent BP measurements by the GP have shown no improvement. Mr Walker, however, does admit to poor compliance with the bendroflumethiazide due to impotence being a side-effect. He does occasionally have episodes of anxiety that may manifest as irritability, difficulty in sleeping and worry. These have been amplified by a recent reduction in contractual painting and decorating work. He does also admit to high levels of anxiety when visiting his GP. Other past medical history includes mild asthma usually triggered by coryzal illnesses but at present this is stable without any nocturnal symptoms and he rarely needs to take his inhaler. He tends to lead a sedentary lifestyle, smokes 15 cigarettes a day and drinks heavily, particularly at the weekends, about 8 pints of beer a day. He lives with his wife and has two children who have left home. He does admit that the impotence persists even when the bendroflumethiazide is not taken and that this has caused some marital strife.

Examiner information

1. Data gathering in the interview

A good candidate would be able to elicit:

- whether a raised blood pressure has been found before. (If a young woman presents with a history like this, do not forget to ask about pregnancy-induced hypertension)
- any relevant symptoms, e.g. headache, chest pains, palpitations, dyspnoea, ankle oedema, blurred vision, sweating, tremors, weight change, urinary symptoms
- symptoms of an anxiety disorder and obvious triggers, e.g. anxiety when meeting doctors
- previous medical history including ischaemic heart disease, hypercholesterolaemia, renal disease, peripheral vascular disease, diabetes mellitus, endocrine and thyroid disorders
- family history of hypertension, heart disease, hyperlipidaemia and endocrine disorders
- drug history, especially the bendroflumethiazide with particular reference to side-effects (ask about the impotence and its impact), corticosteroids, sympathomimetics, liquorice
- the use of the salbutamol inhaler – overusage causing shakes and tremors
- detailed smoking and alcohol history
- lifestyle, i.e. physical exercise, diet
- work history
- social history, particularly any marital problems.

2. Identification and use of information gathered

The candidate should be able to interpret the history and create a problem list. The objectives for the candidate are to:

- be aware of the possible causes of the hypertension
- decide if anxiety or non-compliance with antihypertensives or the 'white coat' effect may be contributing to the hypertension
- appreciate the reasons for non-compliance, particularly the side-effects of the bendroflumethiazide
- have an understanding of any marital strife and work problems that may be exacerbating the anxiety.

3. Discussion related to the case

- This case tests the ability of the candidate to judge the possible causes of raised blood pressure, i.e. 'white coat' induced, anxiety provoked, essential or secondary causes, e.g. renal (diabetic nephropathy, chronic glomerulonephritis, adult polycystic disease, renovascular disease and chronic tubulointerstitial nephritis), endocrine (Conn's syndrome, adrenal hyperplasia, phaeochromocytoma, Cushing's syndrome and acromegaly), cardiovascular (coarctation of the aorta) and drug induced (oral contraceptive pill, steroids).
- The candidate must be able to (a) address the issues of compliance, (b) assess other cardiovascular risk factors, (c) discuss moderating alcohol consumption with smoking cessation and improving health, e.g. diet and exercise, (d) probe sensitively into the circumstances generating the anxiety and (e) discuss the importance of blood pressure control; this should encourage improved compliance.
- The candidate must have a plan for investigations such as urea and electrolytes (U&E), lipids, urine dipstick, fundoscopy, chest X-ray, ECG and 24-h ambulatory blood pressure monitoring.
- There may be no relevant symptoms unless hypertension has resulted in end-organ damage.
- The candidate must be able to discuss with the examiners (a) the interpretation of 24-h ambulatory BP monitoring, (b) the World Health Organization (WHO) criteria for defining hypertension with or without the presence of diabetes, (c) the impact of the Framingham USA study on outcomes, (d) the causes of secondary hypertension, e.g. renal, endocrine, drug induced and pregnancy induced, (e) the complications of hypertension, (f) relevant retinal changes seen on fundoscopy, (g) drug treatment including side-effects, and (h) the management of malignant hypertension.
- Follow-up will have to be arranged to discuss the results of the 24-h ambulatory measurements. Anxiety control, e.g. relaxation training from a psychologist, may be considered.

The National Institute for Health and Clinical Excellence (NICE) and the British Hypertension Society have produced joint guidelines: 'Hypertension: management of hypertension in adults in primary care' (Clinical Guideline 34, August 2011: www.nice.org.uk/nicemedia/pdf/cg034quickrefguide.pdf). Key points from these guidelines and, specifically, changes from earlier guidelines are as follows.

- More importance should be given to ambulatory blood pressure monitoring (ABPM) or home readings in the diagnosis and monitoring of patients with hypertension.
- If the BP in clinic is >140/90, offer the patient ABPM before confirming the diagnosis. The ABPM readings should consist of the average of 14 readings, taken

twice a day during the patient's waking hours for 7 days.

- The categories of hypertension are defined as follows:
  - Stage 1: clinic BP >140/90 mmHg **and** ABPM average >135/85 mmHg
  - Stage 2: clinic BP >160/100 mmHg **and** ABPM average >150/95 mmHg
  - Severe: clinic systolic BP >180 mmHg **or** clinic diastolic BP >110 mmHg.
- Treatment should be advised for patients under 80 years with stage 1 hypertension and any evidence of end-organ damage or other cardiovascular risk factors. Patients of any age with stage 2 hypertension should be offered treatment.
- Patients <55 years: offer an angiotensin-converting enzyme (ACE) inhibitor (or angiotensin II receptor blocker [ARB] if ACE inhibitor is poorly tolerated). If additional treatment is required, add in a calcium channel blocker (CCB) or, if not tolerated, a thiazide-like diuretic.
- Patients >55 years or of Afro-Caribbean origin of any age: CCB or thiazide-like diuretic (if CCB not tolerated). If additional treatment is required, add in an ACE inhibitor (or ARB if Afro-Caribbean).
- Step 3 treatment should be an ACE inhibitor (or ARB), CCB and thiazide-like diuretic for all patients. If further treatment required above this, consider low-dose spironolactone (keep a close eye on potassium levels) or an α-blocker.
- β-Blockers are not recommended as first-line treatment but if β-blockers are started and additional treatment is required, choose a CCB rather than a thiazide diuretic (to reduce risk of developing diabetes mellitus).
- If a thiazide-like diuretic is being started, chlorthalidone (12.5–25 mg od) or indapamide (1.5 mg slow release od or 2.5 mg od) is preferred over bendroflumethiazide or hydrochlorthiazide.
- In patients under 40 years, consider investigation for secondary causes of hypertension and careful assessment for target end-organ damage (e.g. retinopathy, nephropathy).
- Lifestyle advice should be offered at initial diagnosis and periodically reviewed during subsequent visits.
- The targets to aim for on treatment are:
  - <80 years: <140/90 mmHg (or <135/85 on home BP monitor)
  - >80 years: <150/90 (or <145/85 on home BP monitor).

Comments on the case

This is a common case where a patient may not have a specific symptom. 'Hypertension' is not a presenting complaint, and the candidate must state that the patient is asymptomatic when presenting the case to the examiners. A lot of patients attend specialized clinics after an objective measurement finding, e.g. raised blood pressure, abnormal urine analysis or an abnormal chest X-ray. However, this case tests the candidate's ability to scrutinize and explore more deeply into the history and particularly about hidden problems, i.e. the impotence, the psychology of non-compliance (commonly neglected by candidates), the complex social background and other health issues that would facilitate a primary prevention programme.

Case 4 | Back pain

Candidate information

You are the doctor in a general medical clinic. Mrs Janet Reardon is referred to you by her GP.

Please read this letter and then continue with the consultation.

Dear Doctor

Re: Mrs Janet Reardon, aged 63

Thank you for seeing this lady. She has complained of continuous backache for the last 6 weeks. She is otherwise well. I have tried her with co-codamol without much success. I wonder if she has osteoporosis.

Please see and advise.

Yours sincerely

Dr G. Practitioner

You have 14 min until the patient leaves the room, followed by 1 min for reflection, before the discussion with the examiners. Be prepared to discuss the solutions to the problems posed by the case and how you might reply to the GP's letter.

Patient information

Mrs Janet Reardon is a 63-year-old divorcée who previously worked as a bank clerk. She gives a 6-week history of backache. There was no obvious precipitant to this pain, e.g. falls, trauma, lifting a heavy weight, etc. The pain is localized to the mid-thoracic area and radiates circumferentially along one of the ribs on the right side and around to the front. The pain is sharp and constant and worse on coughing, sneezing and twisting. The pain interrupts her sleep if she twists in bed and there has been minimal relief from co-codamol. There are no pains in her joints, especially the neck, hands and hips. There is no history of any sciatic pain. There are no other symptoms such as fever, malaise, weight loss or any respiratory or abdominal symptoms although she does feel more tired than usual. She has no past history of note apart from one admission for a lower respiratory tract infection 5 years ago. She has not had an oophorectomy. She smokes 20 cigarettes a day and does not drink alcohol. She does not take any medication and in particular has never taken oral corticosteroids. She has been postmenopausal for 14 years and never took hormone replacement therapy (HRT). She lives alone in a bungalow. She is concerned that she may have osteoporosis as there is a strong family history of this (mother and elder sister).

Examiner information

1. Data gathering in the interview

A good candidate would be able to elicit:

- the full details of the backache, especially the site of the pain, nature and character, radiation, precipitating and relieving features and any history of trauma or falls
- if the pain is worse after coughing, sneezing or movement
- if there are any pains in the other joints or evidence of sciatica, claudication or neck pain
- other symptoms, e.g. fever, malaise, weight loss, respiratory or abdominal symptoms
- any symptoms suggestive of neoplasia
- any history of trauma
- any details in the history suggesting the possibility of risk factors for osteoporosis, e.g. early menopause, history of oophorectomy, family history of osteoporosis, smoking, nutrition, corticosteroid therapy and other possible endocrine or rheumatological diseases
- drug history including HRT
- smoking history
- a detailed account of the impact of the pain on her life
- particular concerns, especially the possibility of a diagnosis of osteoporosis.

2. Identification and use of information gathered

The candidate should be able to interpret the history and create a problem list. The objectives for the candidate are to:

- determine a diagnosis of osteoporosis with or without vertebral body collapse/compression, and discuss differentials such as intervertebral disc disease (e.g. herniation), metastatic bone disease, myeloma, Paget's disease, infection (e.g. septic arthritis or chronic brucellosis)
- confirm the diagnosis by arranging the appropriate investigations as mentioned below
- address the pain control
- discuss the possibilities of osteoporosis and the therapeutic options (pharmacological and non-pharmacological)
- discuss smoking cessation, diet and general exercise.

3. Discussion related to the case

- This case tests the ability of the candidate to take a detailed history, to consider the possibility of osteoporosis and to guide the history around the risk factors for osteoporosis. Another possibility, which may commonly present this way, is intervertebral disc disease. It is important to explore the possibility of metastatic disease, especially from a pulmonary or breast malignancy; this patient is a heavy smoker. Myeloma is probably unlikely but still must be acknowledged as a possibility.
- A plan of investigations should include biochemical markers, e.g. bone profile, serum immunoglobulins, full blood count (FBC), liver function tests (LFTs) and X-rays of the thoracic and lumbar spine which may show fractures (though unreliable to evaluate bone density). Bone densitometry such as dual-energy X-ray absorptiometry (DEXA) scanning can be used to investigate osteoporosis and determine its severity. An isotope bone scan may be considered to look for fractures and metastatic deposits. If bone densitometry is normal, a magnetic resonance imaging (MRI) scan of the thoracic and lumbar spine should be considered to look for intervertebral disc disease.
- For discussion, the candidate must be able to define osteoporosis as a bone density of more than 2.5 standard deviations below the young adult mean value for individuals matched for sex and race (known as the T-score). For premenopausal women, the risk of fractures is lower, in the absence of other risk factors, so it is more appropriate to use the term 'low bone mineral density (BMD)' instead of osteopenia or osteoporosis. The former is defined as a BMD more than 2.0 standard deviations below the mean for age-, sex- and ethnicity-matched controls (known as a Z-score).
- Although measurement of BMD is the gold standard to diagnose osteoporosis, it may also be diagnosed clinically when a patient presents with a fragility fracture in the presence of other risk factors.
- The candidate must be able to discuss the risk factors, investigations and management, especially pain control, lifestyle factors (i.e. diet, exercise, smoking cessation) and the role of oestrogen therapy and bisphosphonates.
- The decision on whether or not to treat a woman with osteoporosis should be made after determining if she is at high risk of a fracture. There are tools such as the Fracture Risk Assessment Tool (FRAX) which will give the probability of an individual sustaining an osteoporosis-related fracture in the next 10 years using the femoral neck BMD and other clinical risk factors.

- Management of osteoporosis includes risk factor reduction, particularly reviewing corticosteroid therapy, and prevention of falls. A large body of clinical trial data indicates that various types of oestrogens reduce bone turnover, prevent bone loss and induce small increases in bone mass of the spine, hip and total body. The effects of oestrogen are seen in women with natural or surgical menopause and in late postmenopausal women with or without established osteoporosis.
- The effect of oestrogens on fracture frequency is less well determined. Studies have shown that women taking oestrogen replacement have a 30% decreased risk of hip fracture and 30–50% decreased risk of spine fracture. The beneficial effect of oestrogen is greatest among those who start replacement early and continue the treatment; the benefit wanes after discontinuation such that there is no residual protective effect against fracture by 10 years after discontinuation.
- Recently, a large randomized controlled trial involving over 16,000 postmenopausal women (the Women's Health Initiative trial) showed that, compared to placebo, combined oestrogen-progesterone hormone replacement therapy reduced the risk of hip fractures and colonic cancer but increased the risks of coronary heart disease, stroke, breast cancer and dementia.
- Bisphosphonates, often together with calcium and vitamin D supplementation, remain the first-line treatment for osteoporosis. Bisphosphonates reduce bone resorption, increase bone mass and reduce the incidence of osteoporosis-related fractures.
- Other treatments for osteoporosis include selective oestrogen receptor modulators (e.g. raloxifene), recombinant parathyroid hormone, RANK ligand antibodies (e.g. denosumab) and calcitonin. The candidate should be familiar with the mechanisms of action and indications for the above-mentioned drugs.

Comments on the case

In this case the examiners will expect the candidate to take a detailed history of the backache, including the impact of the symptoms on the patient's life, to discuss osteoporosis (investigations, management, etc.) whilst acknowledging the possibility of other diagnoses. Do not assume the patient has osteoporosis just because this is what the GP is considering as most likely; keep an open mind and do not forget about pathological fractures. The candidate also needs to explore the patient's fears about osteoporosis and so the consultation will involve discussing a plan of management with some counselling on the subject.

Case 5 | Breathlessness

Candidate information

You are the doctor in a respiratory clinic. Mr Alan Smith is referred to you by his GP.

Please read this letter and then continue with the consultation.

Dear Doctor

Re: Mr Alan Smith, aged 76

Thank you for seeing this ex-smoker who has had asthma for 5 years. Recently he has been complaining of increasing breathlessness and wheeze. His peak flow was 150 L/min in the surgery. He is on beclomethasone and salbutamol inhalers. Please see and advise.

Yours sincerely

Dr G. Practitioner

You have 14 min until the patient leaves the room, followed by 1 min for reflection, before the discussion with the examiners. Be prepared to discuss the solutions to the problems posed by the case and how you might reply to the GP's letter.

Patient information

Mr Smith is a 76-year-old man who first presented to his GP 5 years ago after a lower respiratory tract infection manifesting as wheeze, purulent sputum and breathlessness. Then, his peak flow rate was 170 L/min. He continued to complain of breathlessness and wheeze and he was started on regular salbutamol and beclomethasone inhalers by the GP after he suspected asthma. He had not been seen again at the practice until 4 weeks ago but now he is complaining of breathlessness after 50 yards, difficulty with stairs, and inability to walk to the Post Office to collect his pension. Other symptoms include wheezing on exertion, mucoid sputum every day and fatigue. The symptoms of wheeze and breathlessness do not vary during the day. He gets woken twice at night due to the cough. He has no chest pain or ankle swelling. There are no obvious triggers such as pollen, house dust mite, cat dander, pollution, smoke or cold air. He had one infective exacerbation last year but he did not visit his GP for help. His past medical history includes a duodenal ulcer 15 years ago. He has no known drug allergies and he has no pets at home. He lives with his wife in a terraced house and she does most of the housework and shopping. He has previously worked as a welder and smoked 20 cigarettes a day from the age of 15 until 5 years ago. He does not drink alcohol. His main concerns are that he is getting more and more breathless without much relief from the inhalers and that he is unable to go out to meet his family and friends for social events.

Examiner information

1. Data gathering in the interview

A good candidate would be able to elicit:
- how his chest complaints first presented 5 years ago
- his premorbid state before this, i.e. exercise tolerance, symptoms of cough/wheeze/sputum, activities of daily living
- how rapidly his symptoms have deteriorated
- a detailed account of the present symptoms, i.e. breathlessness (over what distance on the flat before he stops, up an incline), ability to do stairs, cough/wheeze/sputum and their variability during the day
- an idea of the number of exacerbations per year, winter exacerbations, ?worse after coryzal illnesses
- any allergic factors, e.g. triggers such as pollen, exercise, smoke, pets, house dust mite; history of allergic rhinitis and/or eczema
- inhaler history; type (i.e. multidose inhaler versus turbohaler versus accuhaler) and technique. Previous use of prednisolone and, if so, any improvements in symptoms and any side-effects
- occupational history, any exposure to agents at work, e.g. isocyanates, platinum salts, hardening agents, soldering fluxes
- smoking history (calculate the pack-years, i.e. one pack of 20 cigarettes per day for 1 year is one pack-year), age when started
- drug history, e.g. use of non-steroidal anti-inflammatory drugs (NSAIDs), diuretics, etc.
- impact of disease both physical and psychosocial, i.e. on dressing, washing, housework, sleep, how often he gets out of the house, ability to attend social events, the impact on the family, embarrassment of using inhalers, especially in public
- his concerns, e.g. does he panic when he cannot get his breath, does he expect his chest to get worse, does he feel embarrassed by having to use inhalers in public?

2. Identification and use of information gathered

The candidate should be able to interpret the history and create a problem list. The objectives for the candidate are to:
- explain what chronic obstructive pulmonary disease (COPD) and asthma are
- address the worsening symptoms
- confirm the correct diagnosis by arranging the appropriate investigations

- consider different inhaler devices if the inhaler technique is poor
- advise on general health such as exercise, nutrition and vaccination (influenza and pneumococcal).

3. Discussion related to the case

- This case tests the ability of the candidate to differentiate the diagnosis of asthma from that of COPD. COPD typically presents with progressive symptoms (usually in the presence of a smoking history) without variable daily symptoms and with no obvious allergen allergy, i.e. triggers that are typical in asthma. A proportion of patients may have both COPD and asthma. The suboptimal peak flow on its own should not lead to the diagnosis of asthma.
- The candidate should have a plan of investigations, e.g. chest X-ray, full blood count, ECG, full lung function tests including spirometry, lung volumes, diffusion, flow volume loops, reversibility of forced expiratory volume in 1 sec (FEV_1) to salbutamol, oxygen saturation on air, serial peak flows and follow-up to discuss these results.
- The previous British Thoracic Guidelines on COPD were recently superseded by the NICE COPD Guidelines (2010; www.nice.org.uk/nicemedia/pdf/CG012_niceguideline.pdf). The reader is advised to be familiar with the complete guidelines. Summary points from it include the following.
  - A diagnosis of COPD should be considered in people over 35 years, with a history of smoking who present with dyspnoea on exertion, chronic cough with sputum production and recurrent wheeze or 'bronchitis' episodes, especially during winter time.
  - Airflow obstruction, which is usually **not** fully reversible in COPD, should be confirmed on post-bronchodilator spirometry. The postbronchodilator FEV_1 (% predicted) can also be used to classify the severity of COPD.
  - Patients with COPD would be expected to have a FEV_1/forced vital capacity (FVC) ratio <0.7.
  - All patients with COPD should be advised to stop smoking and the necessary advice and support provided at every stage.
  - First-line treatment is a short-acting bronchodilator inhaler to be used as required.
  - If the patient still remains breathless or has exacerbations despite the above, second-line treatment is as follows.

(a) FEV_1 ≥50% predicted: either long-acting β2-agonist inhaler (e.g. salmeterol) **or** long-acting muscarinic antagonist inhaler (e.g. tiotropium).

(b) FEV_1 <50% predicted: either long-acting β2-agonist inhaler in combination with an inhaled corticosteroid (i.e. combined preparations) **or** long-acting muscarinic antagonist inhaler.

(c) The long-acting muscarinic antagonist inhaler can be offered **in addition** to a combination inhaler if they remain breathless on the above, regardless of their FEV_1.

- Markers like the BODE Index can be used to assess prognosis. This consists of: Body Mass Index (BMI), airflow Obstruction (using FEV_1 measurement), Dyspnoea (using MRC Dyspnoea Scale) and Exercise tolerance.
- COPD patients who should be considered for long-term oxygen therapy include those with very severe airways obstruction (FEV_1 <30%), oxygen saturation levels <92% on air, cyanosis, peripheral oedema, raised jugular venous pulse, polycythaemia.
- Assessment should be done on arterial blood gases, taken at least 3 weeks apart, on patients with stable COPD already on maximum medical treatment.
- Long-term oxygen therapy (LTOT) should be offered to those with (1) PO_2 <7.3 kPa or (2) PO_2 7.3–8.0 kPa and the presence of pulmonary hypertension, secondary polycythaemia, nocturnal hypoxia or peripheral oedema (regardless of PCO_2 levels).
- Patients on LTOT are usually given it for at least 15 h a day at an oxygen flow rate set between 2 and 4 L/min.
- The presence of hypercapnia is not a contraindication to providing LTOT in a patient who fulfils the criteria for it. However, the patient should be encouraged to remain on the prescribed flow rate.
- Short-burst oxygen therapy for breathlessness in the absence of any hypoxia is not recommended.
- Assessments for LTOT should be carried out by trained respiratory practitioners and not prescribed without any evidence of oxygen measurements. Follow-up reassessments are advised as some patients do not require life-long therapy in the presence of a clinical improvement in their respiratory long-term condition.
- In deciding whether to treat a patient at home or in hospital during an exacerbation, one should ask if the patient is unable to cope at home, whether there is cyanosis, reduced consciousness, moderate breathlessness, poor level of activity and poor social circumstances (all of which should favour hospital admission). If necessary, supplementary oxygen should be given to keep the SpO_2 within the individualized target range. Nebulized bronchodilators and oral prednisolone 30 mg for 7–14 days should be given. Antibiotics should be considered in the presence of two or more of increased breathlessness, increased sputum volume or purulent sputum.

- Asthma may be differentiated from COPD if the following are present (although there may be an overlap of both conditions in some patients): FEV_1 improves by more than 400 mL after bronchodilators or 30 mg prednisolone daily for 2 weeks; serial peak flow measurements show ≥20% diurnal or day-to-day variability.
- Patients with stable asthma are treated according to the five-step guidelines (British Thoracic Society). Essentially, step 1 is the occasional use of relief bronchodilators, step 2 is the addition of a low-dose corticosteroid inhaler, step 3 is the addition of a long-acting β-agonist **and/or** increasing the dose of the corticosteroid inhaler, step 4 is high-dose corticosteroid inhalers and consideration of other drugs like a leukotriene receptor antagonist or sustained-release theophylline and step 5 is starting oral steroids. The best possible results aimed for are reduction in the symptoms, reduced need for relieving bronchodilators and reduced limitation in activity, and an improvement of the peak flow rate with minimal side-effects from medication.
- More recently, the British Thoracic Society and the Scottish Intercollegiate Guidelines Network (SIGN) have updated their asthma guidelines (May 2011) with latest evidence on the monitoring of asthma and pharmacological management, which should be referred to for a full description of the step-wise treatment approach to asthma.
- Checking inhaler technique is essential in the management of patients with COPD and asthma. Typically the most common inhaler, the metered dose inhaler (MDI), has the following instructions: (1) remove cap and shake inhaler, (2) breathe out gently, (3) put mouthpiece in mouth (with the inhaler upright) and at the start of inspiration (slow and deep), press the canister down and continue to inhale deeply, (4) hold breath for 10 seconds, then breathe out and (5) wait about 30 sec before taking another inhalation. Other inhalers include the turbohaler, autohaler and

accuhaler. The candidate will be expected to acknowledge the importance of chlorofluorocarbon (CFC)
versus non-CFC inhalers.

Comments on the case

The candidate will be expected to take a full
history to decide if the patient is describing
asthma or COPD. It is not uncommon for a
patient to be labelled as asthmatic when in
fact he has COPD. Do not be swayed by the
GP's previous diagnosis of asthma – keep an
open mind. Patients with COPD often have a
wheeze and this patient really presented 5
years ago with an exacerbation of COPD
rather than asthma. The candidate will be
expected to address the patient's concerns
and to have a clear idea about management.

Case 6 | Burning of the feet

Candidate information

You are the doctor in the diabetes clinic. Mr Jeremy Duncunson is referred to you by his GP.

Please read this letter and then continue with the consultation.

Dear Doctor

Re: Mr Jeremy Duncunson, aged 52

This man complains of burning pains in his legs which stop him from sleeping. He has type 2 diabetes mellitus and his last HbA1c was high at 8.5%. Recently, he has been found to have hypertension with a BP of 176/78 mmHg, proteinuria and a raised cholesterol (6.5 mmol/L with HDL-cholesterol 2.2 mmol/L and triglycerides 2.33 mmol/L). His current medication is metformin 500 mg tds and aspirin od. I have started him on lisinopril and simvastatin. Unfortunately he drinks excessively.

Please advise on diagnosis and management.

Yours sincerely

Dr G. Practitioner

You have 14 min until the patient leaves the room, followed by 1 min for reflection, before the discussion with the examiners. Be prepared to discuss the solutions to the problems posed by the case and how you might reply to the GP's letter.

Patient information

Mr Jeremy Duncunson is a 52-year-old unemployed previous car attendant who has had diabetes mellitus for the last 8 years. His most recent problem is a 4-month history of pains in both feet and shins. These pains are burning and stabbing in nature and are at their worst at night whilst in bed. He finds sleeping quite irksome with his legs covered, the pressure of the bedclothes and the heat of the bed. Recently, this has been keeping him awake for half the night. During the day he is aware of the burning but, if he is occupied, he manages to ignore it. Tight socks and shoes also aggravate the pain. The pain is not exacerbated by walking and he has found no comfort from simple analgesics. He has no weakness in his legs and no obvious feeling of 'walking on cotton wool' or losing his balance if walking in the dark. He has no ulcers on his feet. He does not have any other systemic symptoms of note. He attempts to follow a diabetic diet and he tests his own glucose levels at home which have been around 9 mmol/L. He is treated with metformin 500 mg three times a day and additionally he takes aspirin. He does not have any past history of coronary artery disease but recently the GP has found a raised blood pressure, a high blood cholesterol level and protein in the urine. For these he has been started on lisinopril and simvastatin. He attends the eye clinic but has not needed laser therapy. He lives alone and stopped smoking 5 years ago (15 cigarettes a day) but he does drink on average about 4 pints a night at the local public house. His excessive alcohol intake does not compromise his diet and he is not malnourished. He is concerned about the feet, particularly about the possibility of vascular disease. He is also concerned about the protein in the urine as the GP has told him that this may be a sign of diabetic kidney disease.

Examiner information

1. Data gathering in the interview

A good candidate would be able to elicit:

- the exact details of the burning pains in the feet; which foot, which part, shins, calves
- when the pains are worse, i.e. night time, walking, tight shoes/socks; whether he has to pull away the bed sheets to relieve the pain and is there a pressure effect from the bed clothes. ?any relief from simple analgesics
- other symptoms such as muscle weakness, wasting, sensory problems, e.g. a feeling of walking on cotton wool, losing balance when walking in the dark or when he has his eyes closed
- impact on life, e.g. sleep quality
- other neurological symptoms, any backache
- any history of peripheral vascular disease. Any suggestion of leg claudication?
- the diabetic history; has control worsened or improved?
- smoking, alcohol and nutrition history (vitamin deficiencies)
- other systemic symptoms suggestive of a neoplasm
- drug history, including those that can cause peripheral neuropathy, e.g. isoniazid, chemotherapy drugs
- social history
- the concerns of the patient. especially with regard to the proteinuria.

2. Identification and use of information gathered

The candidate should be able to interpret the history and create a problem list. The objectives for the candidate are to:

- give a differential diagnosis including neuropathic pain (probably in this case due to poorly controlled diabetes)
- stress the importance of treating the blood pressure and cholesterol levels as a primary prevention measure and to discuss possible targets

- discuss with the patient possible medical treatments for the neuropathy, including improved glycaemic control, foot care
- advise on strategies to cut down his alcohol consumption.

3. Discussion related to the case

- A clinical diagnosis of neuropathy is usually sufficient but if in doubt then nerve conduction studies could be considered. Investigations for other non-diabetic causes of neuropathy should be considered, e.g. alcohol, vitamin deficiency, pernicious anaemia, myeloma, drugs, uraemia, carcinoma, infections (syphilis). Other causes of leg pain include peripheral vascular disease and spinal or nerve root problems.
- It is important to understand the risks of future sensory loss and diabetic foot ulceration.
- Discussion of alcohol abstinence is necessary as alcohol may also be contributing to his neuropathy.
- Discuss treatment for the neuropathy including improved glycaemic control, simple analgesia and possible use of other pain control options such as serotonin and noradrenaline reuptake inhibitors (e.g. duloxetine), anticonvulsants (e.g. pregabalin or gabapentin). Tricyclic antidepressants (e.g. amitryptyline, imipramine) were used in the past and are efficacious but patients are often troubled by side-effects. If pain persists then referral to the pain management team to consider transcutaneous electrical nerve stimulation (TENS), lignocaine or mexiletine injections or spinal stimulation.
- The discussion should focus on the management of peripheral neuropathy as requested in the GP's letter. He does, however, also mention cholesterol and blood pressure levels. Targets for BP control in a patient with uncomplicated type 2 diabetes mellitus would be to treat above 140/90 but in the presence of proteinuria targets would be lower, i.e. <130/75. Cholesterol should not be treated in isolation but here as part of cardiovascular event prevention. Previously, a risk of myocardial infarction (MI) above

30% over 10 years would have been set as a target; however, as the cost of statins falls, this target is expected to reduce to 20% or even 15%.

- Other causes of diabetic neuropathy include symmetrical sensory polyneuropathy which is characterized by loss of vibration sense and temperature sensation. Unrecognized trauma due to ill-fitting footwear is a common problem leading to ulceration. Neuropathic arthropathy (Charcot's joints) sometimes occurs in the diabetic foot.
- Other neuropathies include a painful neuropathy, such as in this case. These typically present as a burning sensation, worse at night, and the pressure from bedclothes may be extremely distressing. Good long-term glycaemic control is essential for its management but, in some patients, the neuropathy is resistant to therapy. Mononeuritis multiplex, diabetic amyotrophy (asymmetrical wasting of quadriceps) and autonomic neuropathy are other neuropathies seen in diabetes mellitus.

Comments on the case

This case tests the ability of the candidate to differentiate diabetic neuropathies (of which there is more than one) with other non-diabetic causes. The candidate must have a list of differential diagnoses thought out before starting the consultation so that the history taking can be guided appropriately. In this case, the diabetes is most likely the principal cause but alcohol may be making an important contribution.

Case 7 | Chest pain

Candidate information

You are the doctor in a cardiology clinic and you are seeing Mr Brian Daniels who has been referred to you by his GP.

Please read this letter and then continue with the consultation.

> Dear Doctor
>
> **Re: Mr Brian Daniels, aged 61 years**
>
> Thank you for seeing Mr Daniels who had a coronary angioplasty with stenting of his right coronary artery 3 years ago. Since then he has been fine and was discharged from your care 9 months ago. For the last 4 months, however, he has been suffering again from chest pain. This does not necessarily occur on exertion but can occur at rest. I have increased his nitrates but his pains persist. I wonder if his stent is not functioning adequately. Please see and advise. His medication includes: aspirin 75 mg, ISMN 60 mg bd, atenolol 50mg od and simvastatin 20 mg.
>
> Yours sincerely
>
> Dr G. Practitioner

You have 14 min until the patient leaves the room, followed by 1 min for reflection, before the discussion with the examiners. Be prepared to discuss the solutions to the problems posed by the case and how you might reply to the GP's letter.

Patient information

Mr Brian Daniels is a 90 kg, 61-year-old, retired HGV driver who previously suffered from angina that would occur on exertion, especially when going up stairs. The chest pain at that time was typically dull in nature and central with radiation to the shoulder. He did not take much notice of it until one day 3 years ago when he developed a non-ST elevation inferior myocardial infarction (MI). An angiogram soon after revealed a right coronary artery occlusion that was subsequently stented. He has been pain free since then and has been leading an active, independent life until 4 months ago when the pain recurred. This pain radiates to the throat but is different from the previous angina in that it is burning and worse after meals. It occurs more at night time and not during exertion. The pain may last for up to 2 h at a time. There is occasional nausea associated with the pain and he has been woken up in the night with a feeling of choking. There are no other symptoms of note, e.g. orthopnoea, dyspnoea, cough, sputum, haemoptysis, ankle oedema, loss of weight or other abdominal symptoms. He used to smoke 10 cigarettes a day until his MI and he drinks approximately 5 pints per week. There are no other cardiovascular risk factors apart from a raised cholesterol of 6.8 which was found 3 years ago. He lives with his wife who has rheumatoid arthritis and he is the main carer for her. He stopped

life-long passion. Her main concerns are her painful fingers and that the work precipitates this. She is also worried that she may lose her fingers.

Examiner information

1. Data gathering in the interview
A good candidate would be able to elicit:
- which fingers are affected, the colour changes and the presence of pain, numbness and burning. Whether the toes, earlobes or tip of the nose are affected and are the thumbs spared?
- frequency of the attacks
- precipitating factors, especially the cold. Are the attacks more frequent during winter?
- whether wearing gloves helps?
- whether the fingers are normal between attacks?
- any other associated symptoms, especially peripheral vascular disease, e.g. claudication or symptoms suggestive of connective tissue disorders, e.g. scleroderma, SLE, dermatomyositis, rheumatoid arthritis such as dyspnoea, dry cough, dysphagia, reflux, arthralgia, rashes
- history suggestive of cervical spine problems, neurological disease such as syringomyelia, carpal tunnel syndrome, or blood dyscrasias, e.g. cryoglobulinaemia, myeloproliferative disorders, Waldenström's macroglobulinaemia
- past history of trauma, e.g. vibrational injury, electric shocks, cold injury
- past history of chronic bronchitis and exacerbation, ischaemic heart disease
- full medication history, e.g. β-blockers and chemotherapy drugs such as bleomycin, vinblastine and cisplatin
- full smoking history
- working history and precipitating factors at work
- family history of Raynaud's disease
- concerns of the patient, particularly the worry of losing any of the fingers.

2. Identification and use of information gathered
The candidate should be able to interpret the history and create a problem list. The objectives for the candidate are to:

- identify the possibilities of a secondary cause for her symptoms. If not, the patient most likely has Raynaud's disease (idiopathic)
- identify the precipitating features, particularly at work
- discuss smoking cessation with the patient
- explain general measures for avoiding attacks such as wearing gloves at work (keeping fingers warm)
- reassure that in idiopathic cases, there is no long-term damage and it is rare for finger tips to be amputated for gangrene.

3. Discussion related to the case
- This case tests the ability of the candidate to differentiate secondary causes of Raynaud's phenomenon from idiopathic (Raynaud's disease).
- Common secondary causes include connective tissue disorders, peripheral vascular disease, drug induced, neurological, trauma induced and blood dyscrasias.
- If there is no suggestion of a secondary cause, there is no specific investigation; angiography of the digits is not indicated.
- Management is smoking cessation, keeping hands warm, and occasionally nifedipine 10 mg tds may be helpful.

Comments on the case
This case stresses the importance of taking a history, particularly of precipitating factors at work, possible secondary causes and a smoking history. The candidate will be expected to provide smoking cessation advice to this patient.

Case 9 | Collapse? cause

Candidate information

You are the doctor in a general medical clinic and Mr John Weston is referred to you by his GP. Mr Weston is accompanied by his wife.

Please read this letter and then continue with the consultation.

Dear Doctor

Re: Mr John Weston, aged 53

Thank you for seeing Mr Weston so soon. He was found by his wife unconsciousness in a chair after a meal last week. The wife was the only witness and tells me that he was unconscious for at least 3 minutes. He has type 2 diabetes mellitus and takes Novomix 30 insulin 34 units am and 36 units pm. He is not on any other medication. Please see and advise.

Yours sincerely

Dr G. Practitioner

You have 14 min until the patient leaves the room, followed by 1 min for reflection, before the discussion with the examiners. Be prepared to discuss the solutions to the problems posed by the case and how you might reply to the GP's letter.

Patient information

Mr John Weston is a 53-year-old unemployed man who had an episode of collapse last week that was witnessed only by his wife. He is normally fit and well and leads an independent life. During this acute episode, he had sat down in the armchair after an evening meal and, according to the wife, he went grey, became unconscious and was unrousable for about 3 minutes. The meal was uneventful, i.e. no choking, etc. There were no obvious limb movements, aura, tongue biting or incontinence. After about 2 minutes he became flushed and it was another 5 minutes before he regained full consciousness. The wife did a blood sugar during the recovery phase and this was 11 mmol/L. He was alert and orientated by this time but had a slight headache. There was no limb weakness or dysphasia. Mr Weston declined to go to casualty but did agree to see the GP the next day. Presently, Mr Weston feels fine with no further episodes and no current history of chest pain, palpitations, dyspnoea, limb weakness or numbness. He has had diabetes for 12 years, initially presenting with polyuria and polydipsia. Despite initial oral medication (full tolerable doses of gliclazide and metformin), he was switched over to insulin after 1 year. He regularly visits the hospital diabetic clinic and has had one episode of laser therapy to both eyes. His last hypoglycaemic attack was 2 months ago. These normally present with a feeling of faintness and dizziness but rarely with any loss of consciousness. He had taken the correct dose of insulin before the meal and his blood sugars are normally between

6 and 10. There is no other previous history of cardiovascular or neurological disease or head trauma. Apart from the insulin, he takes no other medications or illicit drugs. He drinks 3 pints a day and occasionally has spirits at the weekend. There is no family history of seizures. He lives with his wife who is obviously concerned that Mr Weston may have had a fit. He does not drive.

Examiner information

1. Data gathering in the interview

A good candidate would be able to elicit:
- at what time of day the collapse occurred
- if he felt light-headed, nauseated or sweaty just before collapsing. Was the episode preceded by any chest pain, palpitations or sudden onset of headache?
- whether the patient was sitting down at the moment of the collapse. If so, this would point away from a vasovagal cause
- if unconscious, for how long
- if he went a particular colour, e.g. white, blue, grey
- his colour on recovery
- if there were any jerking movements of his limbs or face? If so, which limbs and which part of the face? Where did the jerking movements start and where did they spread?
- whether he bit his tongue. Was he incontinent of urine? Did he injure himself?
- whether he regained consciousness gradually. Was he confused or alert? Did he have a headache, difficulty in speaking, weakness or aches in his limbs?
- if he has had any previous similar episodes
- a detailed history of the diabetes, especially the insulin treatment, any previous hypoglycaemic episodes and their characteristics
- a detailed cardiovascular and neurological history, ascertaining the possibility of a neurological or cardiovascular cause of the collapse, e.g. dysrhythmia
- full alcohol and drug (including illicit) history
- past history of trauma
- a family history of seizures
- the concerns expressed by Mr and Mrs Weston.

2. Identification and use of information gathered

The candidate should be able to interpret the history and create a problem list. The objectives for the candidate are to:
- differentiate the possible causes of the collapse, e.g. cardiac dysrhythmia, seizure, alcohol-related collapse, transient ischaemic attack, hypoglycaemia, vasovagal or intracranial lesion
- explain the possible reasons for the collapse
- explain that the cause is not totally clear
- give a list of investigations needed to determine the cause
- address any concerns the couple may express.

3. Discussion related to the case

- This case tests the candidate's ability to differentiate between the above stated causes. A plan of investigations would include routine FBC, U&E, LFT, γ-glutamyl transferase (GGT), calcium, glycated haemoglobin (HbA1c), and blood glucose. This should be followed by a resting ECG, chest X-ray, 24-h ECG recording, echocardiogram, electroencephalogram (EEG) and CT scan of the head.
- The candidate should be able to discuss the strengths and weaknesses of each diagnosis. This case, on balance, suggests a cardiac cause for the collapse.
- The candidate should be able to discuss with the patient a management plan if the results of tests are normal, i.e. consideration of exercise ECG test.
- The candidate should be able to discuss further management if a cardiovascular or neurological cause is found.

Comments on the case

This case illustrates how important it is to have a witness when the patient has passed out. There may well be a partner giving a history in the exam. Be sure to obtain a thorough description of the events and to make sure you consider in detail each possible diagnosis. Do not assume this was a seizure. It is important to have an idea of the nature of any previous hypoglycaemic attacks. Be sure to have a plan of management as the couple are understandably concerned.

Case 10 | Confusion

Candidate information

You are the doctor in a care of the elderly clinic. Mr George Watkins is referred to you by his GP and is accompanied by his daughter.

Please read this letter and then continue with the consultation.

Dear Doctor

Re: Mr George Watkins, aged 82 years

Thank you for seeing this elderly man who has been getting progressively more confused and forgetful over the last year. He lives alone and his past medical history includes a CVA 7 years ago. His present medication is aspirin only. His daughter is concerned that this may be Alzheimer's disease. Please see and advise.

Yours sincerely

Dr G. Practitioner

You have 14 min until the patient leaves the room, followed by 1 min for reflection, before the discussion with the examiners. Be prepared to discuss the solutions to the problems posed by the case and how you might reply to the GP's letter.

Patient information

Mr George Watkins is an 82-year-old retired tool mechanic who presents with increasing confusion and forgetfulness over the last year. The daughter, who lives four houses away, accompanies him. She tells you that her father has been slightly frail since his CVA 7 years ago. This affected his right arm and leg but he made a good recovery, so much so that he has managed to live alone. He manages most of his own affairs (with shopping help from the daughter) and he walks with a stick. He has had a tendency to forget certain things since the CVA but for the last year Mr Watkins has had difficulty in knowing what day or month it is and, more worryingly, has left the gas cooker on by mistake on two separate occasions. Occasionally, he gets the names of his daughters the wrong way round. There have been two occasions when the neighbour found him wandering outside the house at midnight. The confusion and forgetfulness have deteriorated rapidly during the last 6 months but he remains continent with appropriate emotions. There has been no recent history of falls, strokes, decreased consciousness or tremor. He does not take any other medication apart from aspirin (although he does forget to take this now and again) and he does not drink alcohol. He lives alone (widowed for 5 years) in a two-storey house and normally does his own cooking on a gas cooker. Until recently, the daughter only did the shopping but, during the last 3 weeks, she has had to do all the cooking and most of the household chores.

Examiner information

1. Data gathering in the interview

A good candidate would be able to elicit:

- how long ago the symptoms were first noticed and how these symptoms have progressed – gradually or with sudden, worsening episodes?
- if the patient has any insight into the symptoms
- a few examples of the confusion and forgetfulness
- whether he forgets what day or time it is
- whether he forgets where he is or loses his way around his house
- whether he forgets who his daughter is
- quality of long-term and short-term memory, i.e. remote versus recent events
- problems in concentrating, personal hygiene, emotions, continence
- history of possible head trauma, seizures, vascular symptoms, e.g. diplopia, vertigo and neurological symptoms, e.g. abnormal gait, decreased consciousness, ataxia, peripheral neuropathy, tremor
- history of the stroke, recovery and any physical, psychological and social problems as a result of that
- drug history, e.g. benzodiazepines and barbiturates, and alcohol history
- psychiatric illnesses, particularly depression
- social history with risk assessment, e.g. boiling water, cooking (gas), heating
- the input from the daughter and how the situation has affected their lives, e.g. family, work, etc.
- what the daughter thinks is going on or if she has any particular concerns that she wishes to address.

2. Identification and use of information gathered

The candidate should be able to interpret the history and create a problem list. The objectives for the candidate are to:

- decide if the symptoms fit clinically with Alzheimer's dementia
- have a plan of investigations, i.e. dementia screen (see below)
- explain in depth the possible diagnoses and their impact

- address the concerns of the family
- offer possible referral to a specialist with a specific interest in dementia (e.g. at a memory clinic) who may be able to offer a multidisciplinary care package.

3. Discussion related to the case

- This case tests the candidate's ability to take a detailed history from a relative. The presence of dementia is diagnosed clinically but can be aided by using psychometric testing. The historian has to be someone who knows the patient well. Clinical features such as disturbance of higher cortical function including memory, comprehension, learning capacity, language, orientation, apraxia, agnosia and an inability to plan and organize must be looked for. Behavioural changes such as wandering, agitation and aggression are common as well, as is depression.
- Investigations would include FBC, U&E, LFT, glucose, calcium, vitamin B12, thyroid-stimulating hormone (TSH), thyroxine (T4), syphilis serology (if indicated), chest X-ray and CT scan of the head to confirm cerebral atrophy or exclude other intracranial pathology, e.g. tumour, multi-infarct dementia, chronic subdural haematoma.
- A formal cognitive test should be performed such as the 30-point Mini-Mental State Examination (MMSE) or the General Practitioner Assessment of Cognition Score (GPCOG).
- The candidate should be able to discuss the pathophysiology of Alzheimer's disease, the other types of dementia such as multi-infarct dementia, Parkinson's disease-related dementia, Lewy body dementia, Creutzfeldt–Jakob disease, Pick's disease (frontotemporal dementia) and others, e.g. toxic (alcohol), post-trauma, endocrine (e.g. hypothyroidism) and vitamin deficiency (e.g. vitamin B12).
- The candidate should be able to discuss the pharmacological management of Alzheimer's disease, particularly acetylcholinesterase inhibitors such as donepezil, rivastigmine and galantamine. Memantine (an NMDA receptor antagonist) is an option for moderate or severe Alzheimer's dementia in patients who are unable to take an acetylcholinesterase inhibitor.

Comments on the case

This case highlights the importance of taking a detailed history from the relative, particularly with regard to the impact of the disease on the family. As dementia is a clinical diagnosis, the importance of looking for features of Alzheimer's disease in the history cannot be overemphasized. There has to be a plan of management addressing the disease, treating any associated behavioural disturbances and caring for the family, without which the candidate will be failing both the patient and the family. The relative may ask for a prognosis and future management; if you feel this will put you out of your depth then it will be wise to refer to a specialist who has a multidisciplinary approach to managing such patients.

Case 11 | Cough

Candidate information

You are the doctor in a chest clinic. Mrs Indira Shah is referred to you by her GP.
Please read this letter and then continue with the consultation.

> Dear Doctor
>
> **Re: Mrs Indira Shah, aged 42**
>
> Thank you for seeing this lady who has recently returned from visiting relatives in India. She has been complaining of a cough for nearly 9 months. She is otherwise fit and well. She has hypertension for which I started ramipril a year ago. This was stopped soon after the cough started and she was then given amlodipine 10 mg od instead. I have tried her on a salbutamol inhaler for the last 2 months but her cough persists. A recent chest X-ray has been reported as showing normal lung fields. Please see and advise.
>
> Yours sincerely
>
> Dr G. Practitioner

You have 14 min until the patient leaves the room, followed by 1 min for reflection, before the discussion with the examiners. Be prepared to discuss the solutions to the problems posed by the case and how you might reply to the GP's letter.

Patient information

Mrs Shah is a 42-year-old lady of Indian origin who has lived in the UK for 25 years. She returned back from a 2-week holiday in India 4 weeks ago. Until 9 months ago she was fit and well, leading an active, independent life as a shop assistant. However, she developed a cough which is worse at night and is increasing in severity, so much so that now she has occasional episodes of urinary incontinence and poor sleep quality. The cough persisted during her trip to India. The cough is associated with occasional mucoid phlegm (never purulent) and there is no evidence of blood. There is no wheeze or breathlessness but she does feel tired if she walks up an incline. Her only other symptom is occasional heartburn, particularly after a large meal, which is relieved by Gaviscon. There is no loss of weight or appetite, ankle swelling, chest pain or fever. She is a known hypertensive and was started on ramipril 1 year ago. The cough started 3 months after this but, despite discontinuing the ramipril, the cough has persisted. There is no contact or family history of tuberculosis. There is no other past medical history of note such as allergic rhinitis or any history suggestive of an inhaled foreign body. There are no pets at home and she has never smoked. Her husband does not smoke either. There are no obvious allergic triggers at home or work. Her medication now includes amlodipine 10 mg od and a salbutamol inhaler which has not been of any help though her inhaler technique is good. She lives with her two sons and husband who owns a shop. She is particularly concerned with the poor sleep quality and the incontinence and together these are causing family strife.

Examiner information

1. Data gathering in the interview

A good candidate would be able to:

- obtain a detailed history of the cough with particular reference to the start of treatment with an ACE inhibitor
- confirm when the cough is worse, e.g. at night, morning
- confirm any associated sputum, haemoptysis, dyspnoea, orthopnoea, wheeze and fever and pay particular attention to any history of heartburn
- look for any other possible cause of cough such as allergic rhinitis/sinusitis (postnasal drip), asthma, tuberculosis (contact history in the UK and India?)
- elicit a smoking and occupational history
- elicit any allergic history, especially common household allergens, e.g. cats, dogs, pollen, house dust mite, mould
- elicit a detailed drug history including ACE inhibitors and any other drugs which may cause a pneumonitis, e.g. amiodarone
- determine the impact of the cough on the patient and the family, with particular attention paid to the poor sleep pattern and urinary incontinence.

2. Identification and use of information gathered

The candidate should be able to interpret the history and create a problem list. The objectives for the candidate are to:

- decide a possible cause for this cough
- explain the possible differential diagnoses of a cough with a normal chest X-ray and to reassure that there is no evidence of lung cancer, pneumonia or tuberculosis on the X-ray
- sympathize with the patient with regard to the impact of the symptoms on her and the family
- have a plan of investigations
- stress that there will be no immediate curative treatment for the cough until the results of all the investigations are available.

3. Discussion related to the case

- This case is a common dilemma presenting to respiratory physicians and it tests the ability of the candidate to structure the history towards finding an aetiological cause for the cough. This patient probably has gastro-oesophageal reflux to explain the night-time cough, particularly with a history of heartburn. Other possibilities include (a) asthma which may not necessarily manifest with wheeze, (b) postnasal drip as a result of allergic rhinitis or sinusitis, (c) ACE inhibitor induced – it is still possible for symptoms to persist beyond 9 months after discontinuation of treatment, and (d) chronic bronchitis which again is doubtful as she has never smoked and there is no obvious strong occupational history such as working with coal fires. Tuberculosis must always be considered as a cause of a chronic cough but there are no typical symptoms suggestive of this and reassuringly the chest X-ray was normal. An inhaled foreign body (e.g. a pea) should also be considered but the chest X-ray in such a case would be expected to show some radiological changes such as collapse, consolidation or effusion.
- Investigations should always start with a chest X-ray to rule out other obvious causes of a cough (associated with radiological abnormalities) such as pneumonia, lung neoplasm, sarcoidosis and heart failure. Simple investigations such as serial peak flow monitoring should be the next line of investigation, looking for any diurnal variation which would be suggestive of asthma. If sinusitis is strongly suspected then a CT scan of the sinuses may be useful. Other invasive investigations such as 24-h intraluminal oesophageal pH monitoring or bronchoscopy may be reserved until trials of corticosteroid inhalers for asthma, proton pump inhibition for oesophageal reflux or nasal corticosteroid sprays for allergic rhinitis have failed to achieve any symptomatic improvement.

Comments on the case

This case tests the ability of the candidate to think about the possible differential diagnoses before commencing the consultation, otherwise important aspects of the history will be missed. Again, it is a typical case where investigations may be normal and a clinical diagnosis is made purely on the history. It is also a typical case of where no obvious immediate cure may be available and this has to be communicated to the patient; she may be expecting an answer to all her symptoms that day. Chronic cough is a symptom that can have an immense impact on the rest of the family and hence the candidate must show sympathy and have an understanding rapport throughout the consultation.

Case 12 | Diabetic feet

Candidate information

You are the medical doctor in the diabetes clinic. Mr Gordon Wright is referred to you by his GP.

Please read this letter and then continue with the consultation.

Dear Doctor

Re: Mr Gordon Wright, aged 67

Thank you for seeing this man urgently in clinic. He has a long history of diabetes and, when seen by the local chiropodist last week, a small ulcer over his left fourth toe was seen. I saw him in my surgery today and I found that the toe had turned black. Mr Wright has a long history of a sensory neuropathy and I could not detect any pulses in the left foot.

Current medication: Novomix 30 40 units am and 26 units pm, simvastatin 10 mg od, imdur 60 mg od, aspirin 150 mg od, amlodipine 5 mg od, ramipril 5 mg od.

Please advise on diagnosis and management.

Yours sincerely

Dr G. Practitioner

You have 14 min until the patient leaves the room, followed by 1 min for reflection, before the discussion with the examiners. Be prepared to discuss the solutions to the problems posed by the case and how you might reply to the GP's letter.

Patient information

Mr Gordon Wright is a 67-year-old retired salesman. He has had diabetes mellitus for 12 years and has been on insulin for 4 years. Last week, after wearing some new shoes, he noticed an ulcer over the fourth toe on his left foot. He booked an emergency appointment with the chiropodist as he had been advised to do so if this ever happened. The ulcer was dressed and the chiropodist said that he did not need antibiotics as it was very superficial. Today he went back to have it redressed. He had been worried, even before the dressing came off, because the toe had been throbbing all night and he was horrified to see that it had turned black. He was seen straight away by the GP, who could not detect any pulses in the left foot. He has had a bilateral sensory neuropathy (characterized by numbness) for 3 years and laser therapy for retinopathy 2 years ago. He was converted to insulin 4 years ago although this was delayed as long as possible due to a phobia of self-injection. Previous history includes an MI in 1992 when he presented with central, crushing chest pain. He remembers being given streptokinase. He made a good recovery but does get occasional angina when walking uphill against a cold wind. He does not suffer from calf claudication.

He also has hypertension for which he takes amlodipine and lisinopril. Otherwise, he is reasonably well, ambulant and self-caring. He smokes five cigarettes a day and is trying hard to give up. He does not drink and lives with his wife who needs help with washing and dressing as she has severe rheumatoid arthritis. He is obviously concerned about the state of his toe, with fears of an imminent amputation, and any admission will mean arranging care for his wife. He also believes that delaying the conversion to insulin may have caused this.

Examiner information

1. Data gathering in the interview

A good candidate would be able to elicit:
- a detailed history of the events surrounding the development of the gangrenous toe
- a detailed history of the diabetes, especially any past history of microvascular (retinopathy, neuropathy) and macrovascular complications (previous MI, and absent left foot pulses)
- history of the MI and any current angina. Any history of peripheral vascular disease
- other past medical history and cardiovascular risk factors, e.g. hypertension, hyperlipidaemia, family history of coronary artery disease
- drug history, including insulin and diabetic diet
- smoking history
- social circumstances, especially care needed for the wife
- concerns of the patient.

2. Identification and use of information gathered

The candidate should be able to interpret the history and create a problem list. The objectives for the candidate are to:
- speculate on the contribution of the micro- and macrovascular disease to the ischaemic toe and to his neuropathy
- explain to the patient that he will need an urgent assessment by the vascular surgeons and that management will be jointly shared by the diabetologists and the surgeons
- explain that vascular studies will determine whether he will need surgery to his arteries to improve the blood supply or just local treatment for his toe
- consider whether this patient needs admission or close follow-up in a diabetes foot clinic. Enquire whether arrangements need to be made for his wife's care

- explain the importance of good blood pressure and glycaemic control
- advise on stopping smoking
- explain that diabetic complications are usually due to a long period of poor control and are made worse by smoking, but at least reassure him that he has been right in seeking urgent advice for the toe.

3. Discussion related to the case

- This gentleman has both macro- and microvascular complications of diabetes. He has type 2 diabetes mellitus which is now treated with insulin, and from the history we note that contributory risk factors have been poor glycaemic control and smoking.
- Foot ulcers occur in as many as 25% of individuals with diabetes during their lifetime, and a significant subset of those individuals will at some time undergo amputation (14–24% risk with that ulcer or subsequent ulceration). Diabetes mellitus is the most common cause of non-traumatic lower limb amputations in the western world. Risk factors for foot ulcers or amputation include male sex, diabetes >10 years duration, peripheral neuropathy, abnormal structure of foot (bony abnormalities, callus, thickened nails), peripheral vascular disease, smoking, and a history of previous ulcer or amputation. Bad glycaemic control is also a risk factor – each 2% increase in the HbA1c increases the risk of a lower extremity ulcer by 1.6 times and the risk of lower extremity amputation by 1.5 times.
- This gentleman was at risk of foot ulceration because of established neuropathy and additionally he probably has macrovascular disease affecting the legs in view of the missing foot pulses, although he does not have a history of intermittent claudication. He will also have a contribution from microvascular disease and superimposed infection is a distinct possibility. The need for inpatient or outpatient treatment will depend on the extent of the ulceration/gangrene and the findings of the vascular surgeons. He may get

away without admission as the vascular surgeons can arrange urgent outpatient angiography, and he can be managed in a multidisciplinary foot clinic with an admission if there is a need for angioplasty or bypass. If this arrangement is not possible, and with the high likelihood of infection and the need for intravenous antibiotic treatment, the patient will need to be admitted with arrangements made for the wife. Subcutaneous low molecular weight heparin and a pressure-relieving mattress should be included in the management plan. Activity should be restricted and temporary footwear provided. Intensive control of blood glucose will be important. The toe may need amputation but if the arterial supply can be improved, it may dry up and autoamputate.

- Distinguishing ischaemia and neuropathy is a basic assessment need for the patient. Both may coexist. Ischaemia is characterized by rest pain, claudication, cold feet, poor pulses with painful ulceration, especially heels, ankles and toes; and sensory neuropathy is usually painless with warm feet and bounding pulses.

- Patient education should emphasize: (1) careful selection of footwear, (2) daily inspection of the feet to detect early signs of poor-fitting footwear or minor trauma, (3) daily foot hygiene to keep the skin clean and moist, (4) avoidance of self-treatment of foot abnormalities and high-risk behaviour (e.g. walking barefoot) and (5) prompt consultation with a health-care provider if an abnormality arises.

- Discussion with the examiners may include the incidence of vascular disease in patients with diabetes, the contributing causes for diabetic foot disease and the importance of a multidisciplinary care team in the management of the diabetic foot, including the early identification and treatment of coexisting osteomyelitis.

Comments on the case

This case tests the candidate's ability to take a diabetic foot history. The patient, like many other such patients, has several complications as a result of the diabetes, and hence it is essential for the candidate to really explore deeply into these problems in order to be able to manage the patient optimally.

Case 13 | Difficulty in walking

Candidate information

You are the doctor in a neurology clinic. Mrs Sheila Harrison is referred to you by her GP.

Please read this letter and then continue with the consultation.

Dear Doctor

Re: Mrs Sheila Harrison, aged 63

Thank you for seeing Mrs Harrison so quickly. She has been complaining of a gradual progression of difficulty in walking for 5 months with some numbness in her feet. She has chest pain and a long-standing cough from her chronic bronchitis. She smokes 40 cigarettes a day. She uses a salbutamol inhaler and needs paracetamol for the pain. Please see and advise.

Yours sincerely

Dr G. Practitioner

You have 14 min until the patient leaves the room, followed by 1 min for reflection, before the discussion with the examiners. Be prepared to discuss the solutions to the problems posed by the case and how you might reply to the GP's letter.

Patient information

Mrs Sheila Harrison is a 63-year-old retired hospital domestic who complains of a gradual, progressive weakness affecting both legs and leading to difficulty in walking over the last 5 months. Her symptoms have deteriorated significantly in the last 4 weeks. At the onset, 5 months ago, she remembers tripping over whilst shopping one day. During the last 6 weeks she has found walking up stairs much harder and indeed has had two falls at home last week. She has global weakness in both legs and finds getting out of a chair difficult without using her arms. She has noticed a progressive loss of sensation initially in the feet and now up to around the middle of her chest. The symptoms are constant throughout the day and she has no headache, diplopia, muscle wasting or tremor. She has recently noticed difficulty in micturating and occasional urinary incontinence (bowel control is presently intact). Her general systemic symptoms include constant dull central chest pain with a band-like radiation bilaterally, which is worse on sneezing, coughing and straining. The pain is worsening and now keeps her awake at night. She has had a productive cough for more than 4 years and this is due to her chronic bronchitis. She smokes 40 cigarettes a day and has done so for over 40 years. There is no haemoptysis, gastrointestinal or gynaecological symptoms, loss of weight or loss of appetite. There is no past history of diabetes mellitus, spinal injury/trauma, intervertebral disc disease, sciatica, arthritis, neuromuscular disorder, e.g. myasthenia, metabolic history, e.g. hyperthyroidism,

Cushing's syndrome, or electrolyte disturbance. She takes a salbutamol inhaler for her bronchitis and regular paracetamol for her pain. She has had a lot of break-through pain in the chest recently. There is no previous history of taking cortico-steroids or diuretics and she does not drink alcohol. She has no family history of neuromuscular disorders. She is widowed and lives alone and is naturally worried about her progressive symptoms. She has found that she is relying on her neighbour to do the shopping and now does not go out of the house. She lives in a big four-bedroom house with stairs and is finding the general maintenance of the house difficult.

Examiner information

1. Data gathering in the interview

A good candidate would be able to elicit:
- how long the symptoms have persisted and whether they are worsening
- if there is weakness in both legs and where (distal versus proximal versus global)
- if she is having any falls or trips
- if she can get out of a chair without using her arms. Can she walk up stairs?
- if the symptoms are worse towards the end of the day (myasthenia gravis)
- if there are any other neurological symptoms, e.g. headache, diplopia, muscle wasting, sphincter prob-lems, tremor of hands, backache and paraesthesia (if so, to what level?)
- other respiratory, abdominal and gynaecological symptoms that could be suggestive of a neoplasm (primary)
- the band-like chest pain worse on coughing, sneezing and straining that may suggest a level of spinal cord compression. Is there adequate pain relief?
- a history of diabetes mellitus, spinal injury/trauma, disc disease, sciatica, arthritis, neuromuscular disor-der, e.g. myasthenia gravis, metabolic history, e.g. hyperthyroidism, Cushing's syndrome or electrolyte disturbance
- drug history, especially corticosteroids (proximal myopathy), diuretics
- alcohol and smoking history
- the impact of her symptoms on activities of daily living
- the concerns of the patient.

2. Identification and use of information gathered

The candidate should be able to interpret the history and create a problem list. The objectives for the candi-date are to:
- assemble a differential diagnosis list
- discuss these possibilities with the patient
- discuss the investigations to be arranged
- consider admission as she lives alone and her social circumstances are deteriorating
- address the concerns of the patient, especially regard-ing cancer and admitting that you are not sure if the diagnosis is definitely cancer but that this has to be a possibility.

3. Discussion related to the case

- This case illustrates how spinal cord compression in the thoracic region may present. Causes of neo-plastic spinal cord compression include extradural (e.g. metastatic spread particularly from lung and breast – although onset is usually more acute), extramedullary (e.g. meningioma, neurofibroma and ependydoma) and intramedullary (e.g. glioma, which usually presents over many years). This case illustrates that radicular pain at the site of the com-pression (thoracic band-like pain worse on coughing, straining and sneezing), spastic paraparesis and sensory loss up to the level of the compression are typical in a case such as an extradural meningioma. Other possibilities include vertebral disc protrusion especially in the cervical spine, inflammatory causes such as tuberculous and epidural abscess and, rarely, epidural haemorrhage and haematoma.

- The candidate must have a plan of investigations to relay to the patient. Time wasted cannot be tolerated. A routine chest X-ray may detect an unsuspected lung cancer, and plain spinal X-ray films may show destruction of a vertebral body but the investigation of choice is an *urgent* MRI scan.

Comments on the case

This is a case where the symptoms are classic and the candidate really should have an idea of exactly what he/she is dealing with. The patient is obviously anxious that this may be cancer and although the candidate cannot say whether it is or not, he/she must be seen to share the patient's worry and urgency.

Case 14 | Dizziness and feeling faint

Candidate information

You are the doctor in a care of the elderly clinic. Mrs Edna Richards is referred to you by her GP.

Please read this letter and then continue with the consultation.

Dear Doctor

Re: Mrs Edna Richards, aged 83

Thank you for seeing Mrs Richards who has complained of several episodes of feeling faint and dizzy over the last few months. On examination, I heard a carotid bruit on the left and I wonder if this may be a reason for her symptoms. She has a past history of hypertension and takes bendroflumethiazide 2.5 mg od. She has never smoked. Her BP is 155/88 mmHg. I am concerned as she lives alone and has no family. Please see and advise.

Yours sincerely

Dr G. Practitioner

You have 14 min until the patient leaves the room, followed by 1 min for reflection, before the discussion with the examiners. Be prepared to discuss the solutions to the problems posed by the case and how you might reply to the GP's letter.

Patient information

Mrs Edna Richards is an 83-year-old retired secondary school headmistress who has had several episodes of dizziness and of feeling faint with transient disturbance of consciousness during the last 6 months. These are occurring about once a fortnight, and on the last three occasions she has fallen and had difficulty in getting up again. The symptoms come on suddenly and unexpectedly, usually when she is at home. Once, it occurred when she was hanging out the washing. The dizziness lasts for about 1–2 min. Normally she has to sit down to rest and by 10 min she is back to her normal self. She cannot remember much else about the symptoms. There are no obvious sensations of 'spinning of her head', palpitations, chest pain, dyspnoea, tinnitus, vomiting, headache, weakness or numbness in the arms or legs or urinary incontinence. The symptoms do not occur during micturition nor if she gets up quickly from the chair. Her past medical history includes hypertension for the last 12 years for which she takes bendroflumethiazide 2.5 mg and the GP is reasonably happy with the blood pressure. She is otherwise fit and well, living on her own (widowed for 3 years) and doing her own shopping and cooking. She has no other family. She has never smoked and does not drink alcohol.

Examiner information

1. Data gathering in the interview

A good candidate would be able to elicit:

- a full description of the symptoms, especially whether the symptoms are a sensation of imbalance or faintness, or does she mean vertigo, e.g. sensation of revolving in space or the surroundings revolving around her?
- how often the symptoms occur
- how long each episode lasts for
- what triggers the dizzy spells, e.g. stooping, standing up quickly from a sitting position, turning her head sharply, etc.
- whether the dizzy spells abate spontaneously, e.g. by lying down, or do they lead to unconsciousness?
- if there is any associated nausea, vomiting, nystagmus, tinnitus (vertigo)
- if there are any associated palpitations or syncope (cardiac dysrhythmias)
- if there are any associated diplopia, paresis, confusion, dysphasia or numbness (transient ischaemic attacks)
- details regarding the falls, if she has difficulty in getting up or whether she has had any injuries
- a drug history, especially antihypertensives, diuretics
- any past medical history of diabetes mellitus, ischaemic heart disease, hyperlipidaemia, hypertension
- any obvious blood loss leading to anaemia
- a social history, particularly about the house and especially an accident risk assessment, e.g. steepness of stairs, etc.
- impact of the symptoms on the patient.

2. Identification and use of information gathered

The candidate should be able to interpret the history and create a problem list. The objectives for the candidate are to:

- understand the exact circumstances surrounding the case and that there may not be a witness available to give more details of the episodes
- explain the possible causes for her symptoms
- have a plan of investigations
- explain in simple terms that the GP has found a carotid bruit and that this may or may not be related to the symptoms

- explain what a carotid ultrasound involves, stressing that the test is non-invasive.

3. Discussion related to the case

- This case tests the candidate's ability to take a detailed history and to differentiate the possible causes such as carotid artery stenosis, carotid sinus hypersensitivity, orthostatic hypotension, cardiac dysrhythmias, transient ischaemic attack, drug induced and anaemia.
- This scenario suggests carotid sinus hypersensitivity due to excessive sensitivity of the carotid sinus commonly found in the elderly. She describes symptoms when she moves her neck, especially when hanging up the washing.
- Investigations should include routine tests looking for anaemia and disturbance of the urea and electrolytes as a result of the bendroflumethiazide, resting ECG, 24-h ECG tape, sitting and standing blood pressure and carotid Doppler ultrasound. Tilt table assessment may be useful in cases of impaired autonomic reflexes as a cause of postural hypotension, particularly in the elderly.
- As she lives alone, it would be prudent to admit her for investigations and for an occupational therapy assessment of her safety at home; the GP has expressed concern as well.

Comments on the case

This is a typical case where the candidate has a patient who (a) may not remember too many details of the symptoms, (b) may use terms such as 'dizziness' to mean something completely different to what the candidate understands. Hence it is vitally important to ask exactly what the patient means by 'dizziness' or feeling 'faint', etc. Do not assume that you and the patient are talking about the same thing! It is important to read the GP's letter carefully to make a judgement about his concerns. Do not dismiss these concerns; the GP knows the patient better than you do so you must respect his anxieties.

Case 15 | **Double vision**

Candidate information

You are the doctor in a general medical clinic. Mr Alfred Lee is referred to you by his GP.

Please read this letter and then continue with the consultation.

> Dear Doctor
>
> **Re: Mr Alfred Lee, aged 50**
>
> Thank you for seeing Mr Lee who gives a 12-month history of diplopia. He felt this was due to fatigue when working late but now he finds it difficult to keep his eyes open in the evenings. Routine blood tests including FBC, U/E, LFT, calcium and a chest X-ray are all normal. Please see and advise.
>
> Yours sincerely
>
> Dr G. Practitioner

You have 14 min until the patient leaves the room, followed by 1 min for reflection, before the discussion with the examiners. Be prepared to discuss the solutions to the problems posed by the case and how you might reply to the GP's letter.

Patient information

Mr Lee is a 50-year-old lawyer who has had diplopia for the last 12 months. The diplopia is worse towards the end of the day. He has also recently noticed, when he is at his desk, that when looking up at someone for a prolonged time, his eyelids close. Initially he put all this down to general fatigue which he has had over the last year. The fatigue has become worse over the last 3 months and he finds that walking home from the train station, which includes climbing two flights of steps, in the evenings is particularly arduous; walking to the station in the morning is not such a problem. He has also noticed that he has some weakness in his limbs. When his son asked him to help assemble a set of shelves, he could not hold these up for more than a minute. He has not had any problems with chewing, swallowing, speech production or breathing. He does not have any other symptoms of cardiovascular or gastrointestinal disease, hyperthyroidism or neurological symptoms such as headache, loss of consciousness or ataxia. There have been no obvious precipitants causing an acute deterioration of his symptoms. He has always been well with no significant past medical history. There is no past history of note or any family history of autoimmune disorders such as pernicious anaemia, rheumatoid disease, hyperthyroidism or SLE. He has never smoked and drinks wine occasionally at home. He lives with his wife and his main concerns are about the effect of these symptoms on his work. He is particularly worried that this may all be due to motor neurone disease.

Examiner information

1. Data gathering in the interview

A good candidate would be able to elicit:

- the details of the diplopia, when and how first noticed (usually early sign of myasthenia), which direction and which part of the day he can read print (visual acuity). Whether there is ptosis and if so is this complete and which eye(s) is/are involved. Is the ptosis worse after looking upwards for a prolonged time?
- history of tiredness, weakness and fatigability – whether it is worse after repetitive usage of muscle groups and improves with rest or sleep. Which limbs and which muscle groups, e.g. proximal, distal or both muscle groups? Seek examples of when he has had particular problems with limb weakness
- history of weakness of other muscle groups, e.g. facial (myasthenic 'snarl' when attempting to smile), bulbar involvement (difficulty in chewing and swallowing, dysarthria at the end of sentences), respiratory muscle weakness
- other neurological symptoms suggestive of an intracranial lesion, or other systemic symptoms suggestive of a neoplasm (e.g. Lambert–Eaton syndrome secondary to small cell lung cancer)
- any past history of autoimmune disorders (associated with myasthenia gravis), e.g. hyperthyroidism, thyroiditis, SLE, rheumatoid disease and pernicious anaemia
- a drug history, e.g. D-penicillamine for rheumatoid arthritis, aminoglycosides in large doses, procainamide
- smoking and alcohol history
- impact of symptoms on family and work
- concerns of the patient.

2. Identification and use of information gathered

The candidate should be able to interpret the history and create a problem list. The objectives for the candidate are to:

- explain the possible differential diagnoses to the patient
- have a list of investigations and explain this to the patient
- concede that it is a disabling disorder and will need treatment
- outline the main principles of management
- address the concerns of the patient and reassure him that this is not motor neurone disease.

3. Discussion related to the case

- This scenario illustrates myasthenia gravis (IgG antibodies to acetylcholine receptor protein), particularly as the patient describes fatigability when looking up at someone or holding up shelves. He also describes extraocular muscle weakness and diplopia as a result.
- Investigations to confirm diagnosis are important, e.g. anti-acetylcholine receptor (AChR) radioimmunoassay: 90% positive in generalized myasthenia gravis, 50% in ocular myasthenia and 25% in those in remission. A negative result does not exclude myasthenia and patients with pure ocular myasthenia are more likely to be seronegative.
- In patients with negative anti-AChR antibodies, antibodies to muscle-specific receptor tyrosine kinase (MuSK) can be tested. This is positive in 40–50% of patients with generalized myasthenia who are AChR antibody negative.
- Edrophonium chloride (Tensilon) 2 mg test dose, then 8 mg intravenous (IV) (an acetylcholinesterase inhibitor); highly probable diagnosis if unequivocally positive (an immediate improvement in weakness). Repetitive nerve stimulation shows a decrement of muscle-evoked muscle action potential >15% at 3 Hz.
- In patients with ptosis, the ice pack test has a sensitivity of around 80% and is a simple bedside test that can be done. It is based on the principle that neuromuscular transmission improves at lower temperatures and is performed by placing an ice pack on a closed eyelid for 2 min. An improvement of the ptosis constitutes a positive result.
- The candidate will be expected to discuss other relevant diagnoses. Other conditions that cause weakness of the cranial and/or somatic musculature include drug-induced myasthenia (e.g. anaesthetic agent, aminoglycosides, penicillamine, phenytoin), Lambert–Eaton myasthenic syndrome (LEMS), myotonic dystrophy, hyperthyroidism, botulism, intracranial mass lesions (if suspected, e.g. sphenoid ridge meningioma, must have MRI), non-organic cause of apathy and tiredness, and progressive external ophthalmoplegia with mitochondrial disorders.
- The candidate would also be expected to discuss the importance of a thymoma in the general outcome, the management of myasthenia gravis (oral pyridostigmine, steroids/other immunosuppressive drugs, plasmapheresis/IV immunoglobulin) and of myasthenic crises.

Comments on the case

In this case the candidate must ask the patient for examples of his weakness and fatigue to get a feel of the history and to make sure that this is not motor neurone disease, which is the patient's foremost worry.

Case 16 | Dysphagia

Candidate information

You are the doctor in a gastroenterology clinic. Mr Fred Williams is referred to you by his GP for an urgent consultation.

Please read this letter and then continue with the consultation.

Dear Doctor

Re: Mr Fred Williams, aged 63

Thank you for seeing Mr Williams who complains of difficulty in swallowing for the last 12 weeks. As a consequence he has lost 2 kg in weight. He is naturally concerned about the possibility of a cancer. In the past he has had arthritis of the right knee for which he takes paracetamol. He has had heartburn for many years for which he takes ranitidine.

Yours sincerely

Dr G. Practitioner

You have 14 min until the patient leaves the room, followed by 1 min for reflection, before the discussion with the examiners. Be prepared to discuss the solutions to the problems posed by the case and how you might reply to the GP's letter.

Patient information

Mr Fred Williams is a 63-year-old former accountant for the city council. He has had difficulty in swallowing for the last 12 weeks. This has gradually progressed from an inability to eat large meals to having to cut up meat into small pieces, and to now finding that these meat pieces intermittently stick in the lower part of the chest and are associated with some pain. He has no pain between meals. He also suffers from heartburn which he has had for many years. He has had two recent episodes of waking up in the middle of the night choking and with a feeling of acid in his mouth. There has been a 2 kg loss of weight but no other symptoms of vomiting, haematemesis, loss of appetite, dyspnoea or hoarseness of the voice. He has no neurological symptoms or history of having swallowed any foreign bodies. He has been taking ranitidine which has provided some relief until now. There is no history of taking NSAIDs although he does take paracetamol for an arthritic knee. He has never smoked and rarely takes alcohol. He lives with his wife. He is concerned he may have cancer.

Examiner information

1. Data gathering in the interview

A good candidate would be able to elicit:

- the duration of the symptoms, whether they are getting progressively worse (e.g. cancer) or are intermittent (e.g. motility disorder)
- if there is chest pain between meals or any pain on swallowing
- whether solid food (obstructive) and/or liquids (motility) are equally difficult to swallow (achalasia)
- if the patient can point to where food seems to stick
- any high dysphagia (compression web, pharyngeal pouch, thyroid swelling)
- if swallowing is easier in a different posture
- any history of associated vomiting, haematemesis, regurgitation, heartburn, weight loss, loss of appetite, hoarseness, dyspnoea, cough, choking or spluttering, especially when lying flat (typical in achalasia)
- the past history of reflux oesophagitis with any precipitating and relieving factors
- any neurological symptoms (bulbar palsy)
- any history of a foreign body ingestion
- drug history, e.g. NSAIDs, potassium (which can cause oesophagitis) or aspirin
- any history of scleroderma
- the impact of the symptoms and the concerns of the patient.

2. Identification and use of information gathered

The candidate should be able to interpret the history and create a problem list. The objectives for the candidate are to:

- develop a list of possible differential diagnoses
- explain the possible causes for the dysphagia and the impossibility of totally excluding a cancer without an endoscopy
- describe what an endoscopy entails
- address any concerns with regard to the procedure and diagnosis
- arrange follow-up to discuss these results.

3. Discussion related to the case

- This case tests the ability of the candidate to develop a list of differential diagnoses: benign oesophageal stricture, reflux oesophagitis, oesophageal tumour (e.g. carcinoma, benign such as leiomyoma) or motility disorder (e.g. achalasia, spasm, scleroderma). Other conditions which need to be considered are drug-induced oesophagitis, especially due to NSAIDs, infective oesophagitis (e.g. candida, herpes, cytomegalovirus), neuromuscular disorders (e.g. bulbar palsy), pharyngeal disorder (e.g. pouch or web), globus hystericus (high dysphagia in the throat that is related to anxiety), foreign body obstruction.
- The candidate should give a list of investigations such as routine blood tests, especially looking for malnutrition and anaemia, chest X-ray looking for signs of pulmonary aspiration, barium swallow and an upper GI endoscopy.
- For discussion, the candidate should know what an upper GI endoscopy entails with knowledge of the diagnostic and therapeutic uses of this test, knowledge of motility disorders and their presentation and investigations, diagnosing tumours and their management. The candidate must be able to distinguish certain features of the history that may suggest a neoplasm, for example, unrelenting progressive worsening of symptoms, continuous pain, loss of weight and appetite and aspiration.

Comments on the case

This is a case where the history of dysphagia must be taken carefully, looking especially for symptoms suggestive of cancer. It cannot be certain if this is a neoplasm or not just from the history and, as the concerns will not be alleviated until the results of the endoscopy are known, the candidate must be seen to show a sense of urgency and concern.

Case 17 | Epigastric pain and nausea

Candidate information

You are the doctor in a gastroenterology clinic. Mrs Sarah Thompson is referred to you by her GP.

Please read this letter and then continue with the consultation.

Dear Doctor

Re: Mrs Sarah Thompson, aged 39

Thank you for seeing this lady who has complained of epigastric abdominal pain with nausea on and off for 4 months. I cannot find any abnormalities on abdominal examination. She was prescribed omeprazole for 4 weeks with only intermittent relief of symptoms. Her full blood count, urea and electrolytes and liver function tests were all normal. Her past medical history is unremarkable except that she has had episodes of allergic rhinitis. I wonder if you would consider whether an endoscopy is warranted.

Yours sincerely

Dr G. Practitioner

You have 14 min until the patient leaves the room, followed by 1 min for reflection, before the discussion with the examiners. Be prepared to discuss the solutions to the problems posed by the case and how you might reply to the GP's letter.

Patient information

Mrs Sarah Thompson is a 39-year-old domestic cleaner weighing 82 kg who gives a 4-month history of intermittent epigastric pain and nausea. The symptoms have been progressively increasing in frequency and at present are occurring 4–5 times each week. Each episode is colicky and sharp in nature, lasting 30–60 min and with no obvious radiation to the shoulder or the back. Alcohol may precipitate the pain. The pain is not worse with particular movements or on deep inspiration and is not relieved by food, belching or defaecation. She had some intermittent relief with antacids and omeprazole but admits to poor compliance. The nausea is related to the pain. She has had 2 days off work in the last 4 months. There is no history of heartburn, vomiting, bloating, haematemesis, change in bowel habit, rectal bleeding, jaundice and no loss of weight or appetite. In the past she has had seasonal allergic rhinitis for which she takes a Beconase nasal spray. She also suffers from headaches for which she takes paracetamol. She does not take any non-steroidal anti-inflammatory therapy. She smokes 15 cigarettes a day and occasionally drinks two glasses of wine during the evening. She lives with her husband and has two children. Her mother died from colonic carcinoma and she is worried that she may have a neoplasm as a cause of her symptoms.

Examiner information

1. Data gathering in the interview

A good candidate would be able to elicit:

- a detailed history of her symptoms, particularly the site of the pain, the timing, character, constant or intermittent, radiation (to the back or the shoulder), precipitating factors (e.g. movement, food, inspiration), relieving factors (e.g. food, belching, antacids, defaecation), timing of the nausea
- any other gastrointestinal symptoms such as heartburn, dysphagia, vomiting, haematemesis, change in bowel habit, rectal bleeding, jaundice, pale stools, dark urine, loss of weight and appetite, bloating
- a complete drug history, especially non-steroidal anti-inflammatory drugs, codeine phosphate, coproxamol, aspirin
- her response to omeprazole and possible reasons for the non-compliance – this may be important if further treatment regimens are recommended
- a detailed alcohol and smoking history
- the impact of this pain on her life, e.g. time off work
- her concerns, especially the family history of colon cancer.

2. Identification and use of information gathered

The candidate should be able to interpret the history and create a problem list. The objectives for the candidate are to:

- explain the possible diagnoses
- explain how these may be investigated
- aim to address the worsening nature of the symptoms
- determine any possible precipitating factors, especially NSAID usage
- discuss the possibility of an endoscopy with an explanation of the procedure
- discuss her concerns about cancer
- reassure the patient that cancer is unlikely without any 'alarm symptoms', especially dysphagia, weight loss and GI bleeding.

3. Discussion related to the case

- This case is very common in clinical practice and tests the ability of the candidate to differentiate the diagnosis of non-specific dyspepsia from peptic ulcer disease, gallstones and GI neoplasia. The candidate must be able to elicit any possible 'alarm symptoms' (e.g. GI bleeding, unexplained weight loss, progressive dysphagia/odynophagia, recurrent vomiting, anaemia).
- The candidate should have a plan for investigations. Generally, in young people (<55 years) with dyspepsia and an absence of 'alarm symptoms', GI malignancy is highly unlikely. It would be worthwhile to assess the patient's *Helicobacter pylori* status and treat if positive without the need to do invasive testing.
- Non-invasive tests for *H. pylori* include urease breath test and measuring IgG antibodies in serum. If these are positive then eradication therapy may be instituted. If negative, then a trial of proton pump inhibition may be tried, ensuring that the patient takes the drug regularly.
- The candidate should be able to discuss the pros and cons of an upper GI endoscopy at this stage, as this task has been requested by the GP. Further investigation such as an endoscopy should ideally be reserved for when 'alarm symptoms' develop or when symptoms persist despite a trial of therapy. It is important to review the patient again in clinic to discuss further the need for an endoscopy.
- The candidate should be able to discuss the epidemiology of *H. pylori*, its mechanism of action, clinical features and diagnostic methods (non-invasive versus invasive). The candidate may be asked to discuss the pros and cons of eradication with or without peptic ulcer disease and their side-effects.

Comments on the case

This is a common case in clinic and stresses the importance of taking a detailed history, especially eliciting the symptoms suggestive of neoplasia. This case tests the candidate's ability to explore any concerns the patient may have. The possibility of cancer is always a worry for many of these patients – the referral to a specialist is itself anxiety provoking and so exploration of these worries followed by reassurance is very useful. It is important to address the issue of an endoscopy as requested by the GP.

Case 18 | Facial swelling

Candidate information

You are the doctor in a general medical clinic. Mrs Lorna Smith is referred to you by her GP.

Please read this letter and then continue with the consultation.

Dear Doctor

Re: Lorna Smith, aged 31

Thank you for seeing Mrs Smith who has complained of two episodes of itchy facial swelling in the last 6 weeks. I treated her with chlorpheniramine (Piriton) and prednisolone on both occasions but I am unable to identify the cause. She has no relevant past medical history. Please see and advise.

Yours sincerely

Dr G. Practitioner

You have 14 min until the patient leaves the room, followed by 1 min for reflection, before the discussion with the examiners. Be prepared to discuss the solutions to the problems posed by the case and how you might reply to the GP's letter.

Patient information

Mrs Lorna Smith is a 31-year-old housewife who, over the last 6 weeks, has had two similar episodes, 2 weeks apart, of soft tissue swelling of her face. She is presently asymptomatic. Both episodes developed rapidly over 20 min, with swelling around the eyes, lips and tongue. She had some discrete cutaneous swellings (weals) on both hands that were intensely itchy and erythematous. Her tongue felt numb but there was no laryngeal oedema (no stridor or dyspnoea). On the second occasion her eyes became fully closed, causing her distress. On both occasions, the GP gave oral chlorpheniramine (Piriton) 4 mg 4-hourly and prednisolone (30 mg od) to treat the urticaria. The symptoms improved within 6 h but were not fully resolved for 72 h. Once recovered, there was no lasting rash. There has been no obvious precipitant such as extreme temperatures, local pressure, inhalatory allergens (pollen, moulds, animal dander) or insect bites and she is normally tolerant of foods such as fresh fruits, shellfish, fish, milk products, chocolate, peanuts and medications such as NSAIDs, aspirin or penicillin. There has been no recent unusual contact sensitivity to metal jewellery or dog/cat hair and saliva. She has no other symptoms such as GI symptoms (diarrhoea), respiratory symptoms of dyspnoea, cough or wheeze or other systemic symptoms, e.g. fever, arthralgia, myalgia. She has no other previous history of allergies, asthma, allergic rhinitis, eczema or of recent viral infections. There is no family history of allergy or angio-oedema. She does not take any routine medication and does not smoke or drink alcohol except a glass of beer now and again. She lives with her husband and three young children who are all well. The family is concerned about these swellings and wishes to know what is causing it and how it can be prevented.

Examiner information

1. Data gathering in the interview

A good candidate would be able to elicit:

- the exact description of the weals on the hands and the facial oedema, and the parts that are affected
- how quickly the urticaria appeared and for how long it persisted
- the response of the symptoms to antihistamines and prednisolone
- any associated symptoms, especially those suggestive of laryngeal oedema (stridor, dyspnoea) or gastrointestinal or systemic disorders, e.g. fever, arthralgia, myalgia
- any obvious precipitating cause, e.g. trauma, local pressure, emotional stress, inhalatory allergen (pollen, animal dander, mould), insect bites, extreme cold or heat, solar rays, allergic contact substances such as metallic jewellery or dog/cat hair and saliva
- any previous food allergies, e.g. fruit (strawberries), food colouring, shellfish, chocolate, peanuts
- any past history of atopy, eczema, allergic rhinitis, asthma or recent viral illnesses, SLE, thyrotoxicosis or lymphoma which may present with urticaria
- any family history of angio-oedema
- a full drug history, especially NSAIDs, aspirin, ACE inhibitors, opiates and penicillins
- alcohol and smoking history
- social history
- occupational history
- the concerns of the family.

2. Identification and use of information gathered

The candidate should be able to interpret the history and create a problem list. The objectives for the candidate are to:

- assess fully the past symptoms as she describes them now that she is asymptomatic
- fully assess the possibility of a precipitating allergen
- show empathy and reassure the family that the symptoms are rarely severe and dangerous but explaining what to do if laryngeal swelling should occur

- explain that there is no obvious cause for the urticaria and angio-oedema and it is not uncommon for the cause to remain unknown. So, routine detailed investigations are not justified
- explain that most idiopathic cases may last for a few months before resolving altogether, although occasionally some people go on to have chronic urticaria with recurrent episodes
- have a management plan, including the avoidance of aspirin and opiates and to give regular, non-sedating oral antihistamines for prevention, e.g. cetirizine 10 mg od or loratadine 10 mg od.

3. Discussion related to the case

- This case tests the ability of the candidate to take an accurate history of urticaria (well-circumscribed erythematous weals) and angio-oedema (localized oedema involving subcutaneous or submucosal tissues). It is important to search for an allergic cause although in this case there is no obvious precipitant. If urticaria was due to a physical stimulus such as cold, deep pressure, heat and stress, then avoiding such a known cause is the primary treatment.
- There are two basic pathogenic mechanisms for angio-oedema:
  - *mast cell mediated*: this is usually due to allergens that enhance mast cell release (e.g. food products, insect stings, drugs such as antibiotics or NSAIDs) and is associated with urticaria and pruritus in most cases. In severe episodes, it can lead to bronchospasm or anaphylaxis
  - *bradykinin mediated*: a build-up of bradykinin causes the vasodilation and increased vascular permeability in angio-oedema. A build-up of bradykinin can be due to drugs like ACE inhibitors or to defects in the complement system (e.g. in hereditary angio-oedema due to C1 inhibitor deficiency). Urticaria, pruritus and anaphylaxis are *not* present in this type of angio-oedema.
- Management primarily includes reassurance, avoidance of aspirin and opiates which can degranulate mast cells, and the regular use of oral non-sedating antihistamines which should prevent recurrences. It is important to stress this to the patient, and in the GP letter, that severe angio-oedema with laryngeal

swelling (stridor) will need urgent admission to casualty for emergency treatment and observation.

- The examiner may ask for other possibilities such as contact sensitivity (a vesicular eruption that progresses to chronic thickening of the skin with continued allergenic exposure), atopic dermatitis (a condition that may present as erythema, oedema, papules, vesiculation and oozing), cutaneous mastocytosis (reddish-brown macules, papules and urticaria with pruritus upon trauma), and systemic mastocytosis (episodic systemic flushing with or without urticaria but no angio-oedema).

Comments on the case

This case highlights the importance of taking a good history in the absence of current symptoms, with particular emphasis on precipitating factors.

Case 19 | Funny turns

Candidate information

You are the doctor in a diabetes clinic. Mr Donald Tiverton is referred to you by his GP.

Please read this letter and then continue with the consultation.

Dear Doctor

Re: Mr Donald Tiverton, aged 69

Thank you for seeing this gentleman ahead of his routine appointment. He has been having episodes of altered consciousness occurring mainly during the late mornings. He has type 2 diabetes mellitus on insulin and had a CABG in November last year. He is currently under investigation for leg pain with suspected peripheral vascular disease. His current medications includes Humulin M3 bd, aspirin 75 mg od, furosemide 40 mg od, lisinopril 10 mg od, bezafibrate 200 mg bd, and lansoprazole 15 mg od. I am uncertain if these 'funny turns' are due to hypoglycaemia. Please would you advise.

Yours sincerely

Dr G. Practitioner

You have 14 min until the patient leaves the room, followed by 1 min for reflection, before the discussion with the examiners. Be prepared to discuss the solutions to the problems posed by the case and how you might reply to the GP's letter.

Patient information

Mr Donald Tiverton is a 69-year-old retired market trader who has had type 2 diabetes mellitus for 15 years treated with subcutaneous insulin for the last 7 years. He had been reasonably well until the last 2 months when his wife noticed that he was getting drowsier towards noon (before lunch) on most days. According to the wife, these episodes seem to start around 11.30 am. They come on over about 10 min with a sense of oblivion to what is going on around him and he looks pale, sweaty and he mumbles. He has no limb shaking or tongue biting typical of a fit and no collapses typical of a dysrhythmia. Symptomatically, during these episodes, Mr Tiverton feels light-headed and hungry and sometimes has palpitations. When a blood sugar was done on one occasion, it was found to be unrecordable. He eventually comes round after a 'lucozade drink' from the wife. The wife is adamant that these are hypoglycaemic attacks. Mr Tiverton cannot understand why he may be having frequent hypoglycaemic episodes; his diet has not changed (including the timing) and neither has the insulin dose. Previous to these episodes, his hypoglycaemic attacks would occur approximately once every 3 months, usually after an imbalance between the injected insulin and his diet. His activity has not changed and in fact he rarely does much exercise. His glycaemic control is excellent with home glucose monitoring running mainly between 4 and 8 mmol/L and a recent HbA1c was 6.1%. He takes Humulin M3 using a pen device, 26 units in the morning and 24 units in the evening. His other symptom of note is bilateral leg pains when walking which improve on resting but return when he restarts walking. The pain starts in the left calf followed by the right one. He is awaiting a review by a vascular surgeon for suspected peripheral vascular disease. Two years ago he had persistent, severe, central chest pain and underwent a coronary artery bypass graft (CABG) for coronary artery disease but unfortunately with a suboptimal result due to early graft failure. Presently, his angina is infrequent (treated with sublingual glyceryl trinitrate [GTN] spray) and the cardiothoracic surgeons are not keen to undertake further intervention. His weight is steady. He is under regular follow-up by the ophthalmologist and has not needed retinal laser therapy. His medication includes aspirin 75 mg od, lisinopril 10 mg od, bezafibrate 200 mg bd and lansoprazole 15 mg od and he does not take any extra oral hypoglycaemics. He does not drink alcohol and there is no suggestion of him taking extra doses of insulin surreptitiously. They are concerned about the frequent episodes of possible hypoglycaemia and the wife is worried that she cannot leave him alone at home.

Examiner information

1. Data gathering in the interview
A good candidate would be able to elicit:
- details of the nature of these 'funny turns', i.e. frequency, timing (e.g. before lunch) and any symptoms of hypoglycaemia (e.g. palpitations, aura, hunger, blurred vision, light-headedness, sweating) and any association with posture or movement
- whether any blood glucose testing was done during these episodes
- the possibility of unawareness and any episodes of unconsciousness
- symptoms suggestive of other possible causes of altered consciousness, e.g. epilepsy, dysrhythmia, postural hypotension, vasovagal syncope, transient ischaemic attack (TIA)
- insulin regime and dose, usual level of control (home glucose monitoring or recent HbA1c)
- if a record of home glucose monitoring is kept and if the patient has it with him
- injection technique and 'lumps'
- diet, use of snacks, timing of meals in relation to insulin doses
- patient's usual pattern of activity and any deviations from it related to these episodes
- macrovascular and microvascular complications of diabetes, especially in view of his coronary artery disease and peripheral vascular disease
- drug history, e.g. β-blockers

- smoking and alcohol history
- suggestions of factitious overdosing of insulin and/or usage of oral hypoglycaemics
- symptoms suggestive of other causes of hypoglycaemia, e.g. endocrine (hypopituitarism, Addison's disease), tumours (insulinoma, sarcomas) and hepatic
- fears and concerns of the patient and the wife.

2. Identification and use of information gathered
The candidate should be able to interpret the history and create a problem list. The objectives for the candidate are to:
- consider the differential diagnoses for these episodes
- establish whether the episodes are a fault of the insulin regime or unusual activity or an imbalance with his diet
- appreciate the macrovascular and microvascular complications of diabetes mellitus, giving a differential diagnosis for the leg pain including peripheral vascular disease, neuropathy, nerve entrapment or spinal problems
- provide a management plan (as suggested below) with reassurance.

3. Discussion related to the case
- Hypoglycaemia occurs most commonly as a result of very tight treatment of patients with diabetes melli-

tus. However, a number of other disorders are also associated with hypoglycaemia, including insulinoma (although not in this case), large mesenchymal tumours, end-stage organ failure, alcoholism, endocrine deficiencies, postprandial reactive hypoglycaemic conditions and inherited metabolic disorders. Hypoglycaemia is sometimes defined as a plasma glucose level <2.5 mmol/L. However, the glucose thresholds for hypoglycaemia-induced symptoms and physiological responses vary widely depending on the clinical setting. Therefore, Whipple's triad provides an important framework for making the diagnosis of hypoglycaemia: (1) symptoms consistent with hypoglycaemia, (2) a low plasma glucose concentration and (3) relief of symptoms after the plasma glucose level is raised.

- Hypoglycaemia is a common problem and may result from an imbalance between injected insulin and a patient's normal diet, activity and basal insulin requirements. Before meals are the most hazardous times. Irregular eating habits, e.g. shift work, or exertion and excessive alcohol intake may precipitate an attack. However, changing absorption of insulin (which may be the case here) may also be the cause. It is therefore necessary to take an accurate account of diet including snacks and insulin dose and timing history.

- Worsening renal function (which is not uncommon in a diabetic patient) may also give rise to lower insulin requirements and hypoglycaemic episodes because insulin is excreted via the renal system. Therefore, an assessment of the patient's renal function and possible nephropathy should be in the management plan.

- Hypoglycaemia unawareness refers to loss of the warning symptoms of hypoglycaemia that normally alert individuals to the presence of hypoglycaemia and prompt them to eat in order to abort the episode.

This issue must be addressed during the history taking. Some patients who have previously been treated with animal insulins complain of reduced awareness of hypoglycaemia when changed to human insulin.

- Management of hypoglycaemic attacks includes patient education, frequent self-monitoring of blood glucose, realistic glycaemic goals and ongoing professional support. Appropriate adjustments to medications, diet and lifestyle should be recommended. Non-selective β-blockers may attenuate the recognition of hypoglycaemia and they impair glycogenolysis; a relatively selective β1 antagonist (e.g. metoprolol or atenolol) is preferable if a β-blocker is indicated. Management also includes strict avoidance of hypoglycaemia, possibly a change of insulin regime (e.g. basal bolus insulin regime) or in the case of patients previously on animal insulins (who may have insulin antibodies), converting back to a porcine or bovine insulin. Lifestyle factors and diet may need adjusting.

- If the patient is still driving, this issue should be addressed and he should be advised to stop driving until the hypoglycaemia is resolved (especially if he is at risk of hypoglycaemia unawareness). The DVLA should be informed.

Comments on the case

This patient with diabetes has recently developed episodes of hypoglycaemia before lunch. He has a number of macrovascular complications. Although the 'funny turns' are not difficult to elaborate, the history is very suggestive of hypoglycaemic attacks and importance should be placed on why these episodes have developed.

Case 20 | Haemoptysis

Candidate information

You are the doctor in a respiratory clinic. Mr Gordon Bell is referred to you by his GP.

Please read this letter and then continue with the consultation.

Dear Doctor

Re: Mr Gordon Bell, aged 75

Thank you for seeing this man who has had two episodes of haemoptysis during the last 3 weeks. He has a long history of COPD for which he takes beclomethasone, ipratropium, salmeterol and salbutamol inhalers. He has been a chronic smoker for many years. A chest X-ray done last week is reported as normal but I am concerned that we may be missing a neoplasm.

Yours sincerely

Dr G. Practitioner

You have 14 min until the patient leaves the room, followed by 1 min for reflection, before the discussion with the examiners. Be prepared to discuss the solutions to the problems posed by the case and how you might reply to the GP's letter.

Patient information

Mr Gordon Bell is a 75-year-old man who has had two episodes of haemoptysis in the last 3 weeks. Both occurred whilst at home in the morning about 2 weeks apart. The haemoptysis was fresh blood with mucoid phlegm, and about a spoonful in volume. He has never had any previous episodes of haemoptysis. He has had COPD for many years. This manifests as breathlessness on exertion, especially on an incline, and he has to stop twice when walking up a flight of stairs. He has no chest pains, ankle swelling, palpitations and loss of weight or appetite. There is no previous history of a deep vein thrombosis, pulmonary embolism, bleeding disorders or tuberculosis. Apart from the inhalers, he takes no other medication and no anticoagulants. He has been a chronic 20-a-day smoker since the age of 14 years and has worked as a plumber all his life. He has been exposed to asbestos during his work with pipe insulation. He lives with his wife in a terraced house and she does most of the household chores. The patient is concerned that he may have lung cancer.

Examiner information

1. Data gathering in the interview

A good candidate would be able to elicit:

- when was the haemoptysis first noticed and has he coughed up blood before?
- whether the haemoptysis occurs daily or has he had it only once or twice?

- the volume of haemoptysis, e.g. egg-cup full or spoonful
- whether the haemoptysis is fresh, red blood, discoloured brown or mixed in with sputum (colour of sputum, mucoid versus purulent)
- any other associated symptoms such as pleuritic chest pain, dyspnoea, fever, night sweats, syncope, palpitations, or leg swelling suggestive of a deep vein thrombosis
- full idea of his exercise ability, i.e. stairs, distance on the flat or on an incline
- any past history of cardiac, pulmonary (e.g. COPD, childhood pneumonia, tuberculosis) or bleeding disorders
- drug history including anticoagulants
- smoking history
- occupational history, especially asbestos exposure
- family history of tuberculosis
- daily living abilities
- the concerns of the patient, particularly regarding the possibility of lung cancer.

2. Identification and use of information gathered

The candidate should be able to interpret the history and create a problem list. The objectives for the candidate are to:

- explain the possible differential diagnoses; although the chest X-ray was normal one still has to consider the potential chance of lung cancer
- give a list of investigations
- explain that he needs a bronchoscopy, giving a description of the procedure
- share a sense of concern with some arrangement for a follow-up appointment to discuss the results.

3. Discussion related to the case

- This case tests the ability of the candidate to create a list of differential diagnoses for haemoptysis. Although this patient has a normal chest X-ray, lung cancer is still the main diagnosis to rule out. A chest X-ray does not necessarily exclude a small bronchial neoplasm. Haemoptyses are also common in patients with COPD, especially during exacerbations. A history of increased sputum volume and purulence with dyspnoea may point to this. Other possibilities include bronchiectasis, pulmonary embolism, infec-

tive causes such as tuberculosis and pneumonia and mitral stenosis.
- Investigations should include FBC, U&E, LFT and calcium, ECG, spirometry and oxygen saturation on air. These should help to decide if the patient would be able to tolerate a bronchoscopy. If the bronchoscopy is normal then the next step would be a CT scan of the thorax. Mediastinal nodes are more recently being sampled by endobronchial ultrasound (EBUS) techniques rather than the mediastinoscopy under general anaesthesia (GA) procedure.
- The candidate will be expected to be aware of the bronchoscopy procedure, the use of sedation and the diagnostic and therapeutic scope of this procedure. The examiners will expect the candidate to know the different histological types of lung cancer, the manifestations of lung cancer, i.e. direct/metastatic spread and non-metastatic extrapulmonary manifestations, investigations and treatment, i.e. surgical (including contraindications), radiotherapy, chemotherapy and palliative care. It is recommended that all lung cancer cases are discussed at a multidisciplinary team (MDT) meeting attended by physicians, thoracic surgeons, oncologists, radiologist and pathologists, and that all cases are entered in a national database supported by the RCP in order to assess variations in outcomes across the UK, known as the LUCADA database (LUng CAncer DAta).

Comments on the case

This case tests the ability of the candidate to take a history, paying particular attention to the possibility of cancer. Most patients in these situations want to know if it is cancer or not, so avoiding the matter altogether will do the patient no favours. Although the chest X-ray is normal, the candidate must be able to convey to the patient that this may not rule out the possibility completely and hence it would be wise for the patient to have a bronchoscopy. Most doctors, in the authors' experience, have found that patients are quite keen to undergo such a test for the purposes of reassurance. This case also raises the issue of smoking cessation, though it is usually best to address this at a later date.

Case 21 | Headache

Candidate information

You are the doctor in a neurology clinic. Mrs Sarah Wittington is referred to you by her GP.

Please read this letter and then continue with the consultation.

Dear Doctor

Re: Mrs Sarah Wittington, aged 45

I would appreciate your help with this pleasant housewife who has had migrainous headaches on and off for 3 years. They usually occur around the left side of her head with occasional vomiting. I have tried paracetamol, codeine and sumatriptan without much help. I am now struggling to control her symptoms. She is normally fit and well but does suffer from bouts of depression for which she takes paroxetine 50 mg od. I could not find any obvious neurological deficits on examining her.

Yours sincerely

Dr G. Practitioner

You have 14 min until the patient leaves the room, followed by 1 min for reflection, before the discussion with the examiners. Be prepared to discuss the solutions to the problems posed by the case and how you might reply to the GP's letter.

Patient information

Mrs Sarah Wittington is a 45-year-old housewife who has been complaining of episodes of facial pain for the last 3 years. The pain usually begins around the left eye (always the left side), is excruciating in nature and increases in intensity over about 30 min. It may last for up to 2 h, usually occurring at night and with a strange feeling of heaviness on that side of the face with nasal stuffiness. There is no radiation and there are no obvious precipitating factors. These episodes usually keep her awake and tend to occur around once or twice a day for a fortnight and then there are none for about 6–8 months. There has been little relief from painkillers and sumatriptan. She does get another pain that is different from the facial pain. This is a headache with a feeling of a tight band throughout the whole head, throbbing in nature, lasting for around 2–4 h, with no radiation, usually exacerbated by bouts of depression and normally relieved by paracetamol. She has had these headaches for a number of years but it is the facial pain that causes the most trouble. There are no precipitating factors such as straining, coughing or sneezing, nor do they occur on wakening. There is no history of any previous head trauma or seizures. There are no other symptoms of drowsiness, confusion, weakness, ataxia, photophobia, neck stiffness, visual changes or fever. She has had no problems with the teeth, sinuses and ears or any previous herpetic neuralgia, temporomandibular arthritis or temporal arteritis. She has had depression for 6 years, first presenting as low mood and difficulty in sleeping. She has been on paroxetine 50 mg od during this time. Family rows and worry about the children usually aggravate the depression. She has no other relevant past medical history. Apart from the painkillers and paroxetine, she is on no other medication. She rarely drinks alcohol and smokes five cigarettes a day. She is divorced and has brought up two teenage children single-handedly. Her concerns are that the facial pain is causing the depression to worsen and she is desperate for help.

Examiner information

1. Data gathering in the interview

A good candidate would be able to elicit:

- that two types of pain are present: facial and headache
- confirm how long the pains have been a problem and if they come on suddenly. How long are the longest pain-free periods? When was the last attack?
- ask exactly where each pain is
- whether the headaches radiate anywhere, e.g. back of head and neck
- if the pains are constant or intermittent and whether they are deteriorating
- if they are worse at any particular time of the day, e.g. on wakening. Does the pain wake her up?
- how long the pains last for
- any particular triggers, e.g. coughing, straining, exertion, stress at work, particular food, bright lights
- any associated drowsiness, confusion, nausea, vomiting, weakness, ataxia, photophobia, neck stiffness, visual changes or fever
- when differentiating facial pain – ask about problems with teeth, sinuses, ears, and elicit any history of herpetic neuralgia, temporomandibular arthritis or temporal arteritis
- any suggestions of depression, anxiety and, if so, how they present
- any recent history of head trauma or seizures
- drug and alcohol history – ask in detail the response to painkillers and 5-hydroxytryptamine (5-HT1) agonists
- a past history of hypertension
- a detailed social history with attention to work and family dynamics
- any concerns she may have and what she thinks the headaches are due to.

2. Identification and use of information gathered

The candidate should be able to interpret the history and create a problem list. The objectives for the candidate are to:

- identify and explain the presence of two different pains
- describe the possible causes of these pains
- reassure that it is very unlikely that there is a neoplastic reason for her pains and that there are unlikely to be any serious consequences
- have a management plan, i.e. prevention strategy for the facial pain.

3. Discussion related to the case

- This case tests the ability of the candidate to assemble two lists of differential diagnoses. The facial pain described here is typical of cluster headaches (although more common in males) but other causes of facial pain to be aware of are diseases of the teeth, sinuses, ears and throat, temporal arteritis, postherpetic neuralgia, trigeminal neuralgia, temporomandibular arthritis and glaucoma. The headache she describes sounds like a tension headache exacerbated by depression. Other alternatives include migraine and raised intracranial pressure. If migraine is suspected, the history should also include any prodromal symptoms (classic migraine) with visual symptoms of flashing lights and blind patches together with associated gastrointestinal (nausea and vomiting) and cerebral symptoms and signs such as numbness and weakness of limbs.
- Treatment usually involves reassurance and explanation with particular emphasis on the very remote chance of a neoplasm, particularly in the absence of symptoms and signs such as weakness or paraesthesia.

- The Scottish Intercollegiate Guidelines Network (SIGN; www.sign.ac.uk/guidelines/fulltext/107/index.html) *does not* recommend the need to do further tests such as CT head scans for the investigation of primary headaches unless the following 'red flag' features are present: new onset or change in headaches in patients over 50 years; sudden-onset thunderclap headache; focal neurological symptoms; abnormal neurological examination; headaches that change with posture or wake the patient up from sleep; presence of other comorbidities (e.g. history of cancer, or cerebral venous sinus thrombosis).
- With regard to managing the cluster headaches, prevention is important and in some patients calcium channel blockers (e.g. verapamil) or glucocorticoids have been shown to be useful. The acute attacks can be managed with high-flow oxygen treatment or 5-HT1 receptor agonists (e.g. sumatriptan). The latter has a quicker onset of action and longer pain-free duration if given via the intranasal or subcutaneous routes. Meanwhile, the tension headaches are normally managed adequately with paracetamol (if not, add codeine).

Comments on the case

This case highlights the importance of keeping an open mind after reading the GP's correspondence, i.e. do not assume this is migraine. There are two different types of pain and the candidate must be seen to take a full history of both pains – otherwise it will be impossible to correctly diagnose and manage both symptoms.

Case 22 | Hoarse voice

Candidate information

You are the doctor in a general medical clinic. Mrs Kathy O'Donnell is referred to you by her GP.

Please read this letter and then continue with the consultation.

Dear Doctor

Re: Mrs Kathy O'Donnell, aged 49

Thank you for seeing this lady who has complained of a hoarse voice for 6 months. She smokes 15 cigarettes a day and, after a bout of winter bronchitis 2 years ago, she was started on beclomethasone and salbutamol inhalers. She is also known to have oesophageal reflux for which she takes a maintenance dose of lansoprazole. She has no other past medical history and takes no other medication. Please see and advise.

Yours sincerely

Dr G. Practitioner

You have 14 min until the patient leaves the room, followed by 1 min for reflection, before the discussion with the examiners. Be prepared to discuss the solutions to the problems posed by the case and how you might reply to the GP's letter.

Patient information

Mrs Kathy O'Donnell, aged 49 years, is a Dubliner living in the UK. She works as a barmaid at the local Irish centre. Six months ago she noticed she was becoming a little 'croaky' and 4 weeks later her voice had reached the present degree of hoarseness, remaining unchanged with no particular association with a time of day. She has never had bouts of hoarseness before. She had a lower respiratory tract infection two winters ago manifesting as purulent sputum, wheeze and one episode of haemoptysis (blood mixed in with the sputum) lasting for one day. A chest X-ray at that time was normal. Since then she continues to have a slight cough with mucoid sputum at night and a wheeze in the morning. She was also started on beclomethasone inhaler 200 μg, two inhalations twice a day and salbutamol as needed (usually takes at the same time as the beclomethasone). However, she does admit to having used the inhalers up to four times a day most days of the week for the last 4 weeks. She does not use a volumatic nor gargle after the beclomethasone inhalations. She did not have a hoarse voice when she first started using the inhalers. She still suffers from heartburn particularly at night and she now props herself up with three pillows. She commonly wakes up at night with an acid taste in the mouth. She has had no haemoptysis, chest pain, dyspnoea, dysphagia, loss of weight or noticed any enlarged lymph glands in her neck. She has had no recent coryzal illnesses or sore throat, and no past history of hypothyroidism or exposure to environmental hazards such as coal fires. She lives with her husband who has been insisting that she should have sought advice about the voice earlier. She has been working at the Irish centre for 16 years and admits that she needs a clear booming voice during work; there have been times when she is unable to make herself heard. She has always been a heavy smoker since the age of 12 and currently smokes 15 cigarettes a day. She does tend to have about three measures of gin per day during her work.

Examiner information

1. Data gathering in the interview

A good candidate would be able to elicit:
- how long the patient has noticed the hoarse voice. Has she had a hoarse voice before?
- how the hoarseness started. Was it after a bout of viral laryngitis? Has the hoarseness plateaued or is it still worsening?
- if the hoarse voice coincided with starting the beclomethasone inhaler
- if she uses a volumatic with the beclomethasone and gargles afterwards. Has she been using the inhalers excessively?
- if she has been overusing her voice
- any associated sore throats and upper respiratory tract coryzal illnesses
- any associated dyspnoea, cough, sputum, haemoptysis, chest pain, heartburn – if so, is it worse at night, does she prop herself up at night?
- any associated dysphagia with aspiration
- any associated symptoms suggestive of hypothyroidism
- recent inhalational history, e.g. exposure to fire/smoke
- drug history
- smoking history
- occupational history – whether she needs her voice at work. What does she use her voice for, e.g. announcements, etc?
- her concerns and the impact of the hoarseness on her work and family life
- if she would be receptive to smoking cessation advice.

2. Identification and use of information gathered

The candidate should be able to interpret the history and create a problem list. The objectives for the candidate are to:

- assemble the possible differential diagnoses
- explain the possible causes of the hoarse voice
- explain and describe a plan of investigations
- arrange follow-up soon to discuss any results.

3. Discussion related to the case

- The hoarseness of the voice in this case could be due to a number of possibilities: chronic laryngitis secondary to corticosteroid inhaler or gastro-oesophageal acid reflux disease or even overuse, laryngeal polyp, laryngeal carcinoma, vocal cord paralysis secondary to lung cancer and, rarely, thyroid masses or hypothyroidism.
- Investigations in this case would be firstly a chest X-ray to rule out a bronchial neoplasm with left recurrent nerve palsy (although this does not truly cause a hoarse voice), routine blood tests and most importantly, asking an ear, nose and throat (ENT) surgeon to have a look at the vocal cords with a laryngoscope.
- If there are no vocal cord lesions, e.g. polyps or evidence of *Candida*, but only inflammation, this may suggest acid reflux as the cause and this will need to be addressed appropriately. Evidence of *Candida* suggests that the beclomethasone is the cause. This should be addressed by advising the patient to take the beclomethasone less often, using a volumatic that would prevent the aerosol impacting on the pharynx and larynx, and gargling after inhalation.

Comments on the case

This is a common case and highlights the importance of taking all the details of inhaler usage with particular timing to the onset of hoarseness. The candidate must ascertain the impact of the symptoms on the patient's work.

Case 23 | Hypercalcaemia

Candidate information

You are the doctor in a general medical clinic. Mrs Freda Davidson is referred to you by her GP.

Please read this letter and then continue with the consultation.

Dear Doctor

Re: Mrs Freda Davidson, aged 53

Thank you for seeing Mrs Davidson who, after a routine blood test, was found to have a calcium level of 2.84 mmol/L and an albumin level of 39 g/L. She has a past history of peptic ulcer disease 10 years ago and takes fluoxetine for depression.

Please see and advise.

Yours sincerely

Dr G. Practitioner

You have 14 min until the patient leaves the room, followed by 1 min for reflection, before the discussion with the examiners. Be prepared to discuss the solutions to the problems posed by the case and how you might reply to the GP's letter.

Patient information

Mrs Davidson is a 53-year-old housewife who has been found to have hypercalcaemia on routine testing by the GP. She is normally well although she has bouts of tiredness which she puts down to not being able to sleep at night. She has no obvious GI symptoms apart from a poor appetite and a tendency towards constipation if she is not careful with her diet. She has a history of depression for the last 4 years after the death of her mother. Presently she feels low in mood with some loss of self-esteem. She is on fluoxetine for this. Ten years ago she presented to hospital with dyspepsia and an upper GI endoscopy revealed a duodenal ulcer. This was treated with antacids but she does occasionally have dyspeptic symptoms, particularly after a spicy meal. She has no bony pain, nor any past history of renal stones. She lives with her husband and generally leads a fairly active life running the household, doing the shopping and cleaning. She does not smoke or drink and she takes no other medication. There is no family history of hypercalcaemia. She is on a normal diet with no real excessive intake of dairy products. Mrs Davidson is not quite sure why she has been referred to the specialist.

Examiner information

1. Data gathering in the interview

A good candidate would be able to elicit:

- the history of the symptoms relevant to hypercalcae-mia, e.g. tiredness, malaise, depression, abdominal pain (e.g. from a peptic ulcer), constipation, urinary symptoms and renal colic from stones, bony pain, etc.
- symptoms suggestive of respiratory disorders (e.g. sarcoidosis), gastrointestinal disorders (e.g. peptic ulcer), endocrine disorders (e.g. thyrotoxicosis), malignancy (bony secondaries from breast and lung, lymphoma, myeloma)
- history of the depression
- drug history (i.e. any vitamin D analogues, thiazides, lithium)
- family history (hypocalciuric hypercalcaemia)
- immobility
- concerns of the patient.

2. Identification and use of information gathered

The candidate should be able to interpret the history and create a problem list. The objectives for the candidate are to:

- take a history relevant to hypercalcaemia
- determine any specific cause for the hypercalcaemia
- ascertain the history of the peptic ulcer and the depression and to think about a possible link
- explain to the patient the biochemical findings
- have a plan of further investigations and management.

3. Discussion related to the case

- Hypercalcaemia can be due to:
  - excessive parathyroid hormone secretion (primary, tertiary or ectopic, lithium and hypocalciuric hypercalcaemia)
  - excessive vitamin D (vitamin D intoxication, sarcoidosis and other granulomatous diseases)
  - malignancy (breast, lung, haematological), but unlikely if asymptomatic
  - high bone turnover (immobility)
  - drugs (thiazides, vitamin D analogues)
  - endocrine factors (hyperthyroidism).
- Primary hyperthyroidism is the most common cause of hypercalcaemia discovered by chance.

Hypercalcaemia from any cause can result in fatigue, depression, mental confusion, anorexia, nausea, vomiting, constipation, short QT interval on the electrocardiogram and, in some patients, cardiac arrhythmias. There is a variable relation between the severity of the hypercalcaemia and the symptoms. Generally, symptoms are more common at calcium levels >2.9–3 mmol/L but some patients, even at this level, are asymptomatic. When the calcium level is >3.2 mmol/L calcification in the kidneys, skin, vessels, lungs, heart and stomach can occur and renal insufficiency may develop, particularly if the blood phosphate levels are normal or elevated due to impaired renal function. Severe hypercalcaemia, usually 3.7–4.5 mmol/L, can be a medical emergency as coma and cardiac arrest can occur. Hypercalcaemia in an adult who is apparently asymptomatic is usually due to primary hyperparathyroidism. In malignancy-associated hypercalcaemia it is the malignancy that brings the patient to the physician and the hypercalcaemia is discovered during the routine investigations. Investigations include serum calcium, phosphate and parathyroid hormone levels.

- Parathyroid hormone values are elevated in >90% of parathyroid-related causes of hypercalcaemia; are undetectable or low in malignancy-related hypercalcaemia (which may be due to secretion of an ectopic hormone known as parathyroid hormone-related protein, PTHrP); and undetectable or normal in vitamin D-related and high bone turnover causes of hypercalcaemia.
- Therapy for primary hyperparathyroidism is primarily surgical, particularly in those with stones, bony involvement, calcium levels above 2.9 mmol/L or a previous episode of severe acute hypercalcaemia.
- The candidate will be expected to discuss preoperative localization investigations, especially the role of MRI, radioisotope subtraction scanning and the management of acute hypercalcaemia.

Comments on the case

This case presents with an abnormal biochemical finding and the candidate will be expected to tailor the history towards finding a cause and recognizing that previous medical illnesses may be related.

Case 24 | **Hyperlipidaemia**

Candidate information

You are the doctor in the diabetes clinic and the GP has written a note about this patient whom you are about to see for his annual review.

Please read this letter and then continue with the consultation.

Dear Doctor

Re: Mr David Palmer, aged 54

Please would you advise on the treatment of this gentleman's hyperlipidaemia. He is a known diabetic and his total cholesterol level was 7.0 mmol/L 6 months ago. I started him on a statin and after 3 months his cholesterol fell to 5.4 mmol/L with an HDL cholesterol of 1.5 mmol/L and a raised triglycerides (fasting) level of 4.5 mmol/L. At this recent visit, I also found proteinuria on urine dipstick. He is overweight and dietary advice has been unsuccessful. His medication is currently Novorapid insulin tds, Insulatard insulin noct, metformin, atorvastatin, perindopril and aspirin.

Yours sincerely

Dr G. Practitioner

You have 14 min until the patient leaves the room, followed by 1 min for reflection, before the discussion with the examiners. Be prepared to discuss the solutions to the problems posed by the case and how you might reply to the GP's letter.

Patient information

Mr David Palmer is a 54-year-old ex-taxi driver who was found to have a raised cholesterol (7 mmol/L) 6 months ago after a routine visit to the GP's diabetic surgery. He was started on atorvastatin and a repeat cholesterol 3 months later showed the cholesterol to have dropped to 5.4 mmol/L. He is reasonably well in himself and is self-caring. He has had diabetes mellitus for 8 years for which he takes insulin four times daily by Novopen (Novorapid 12 units before meals tds and Insulatard 18 units at night). He developed diabetic retinopathy for which he has had laser treatment to both eyes 2 years ago; poor vision was the reason for him giving up work. He also has had numbness of both feet and was found to have proteinuria on urine dipstick 3 months ago by the GP. He has a history of hypertension for 8 years for which he initially took bendroflumethiazide. However, 4 years ago he had an episode of gout and the thiazide was changed to an ACE inhibitor (perindopril). He does not have a history of ischaemic heart disease but his father died of an MI when he was young. Despite dietary advice from the practice nurse, he is struggling to keep his weight down (he is presently 92 kg) and he does not want to increase his insulin dose any further as he worries that this may increase his weight. He does not think he eats excessively. He has three meals a day; breakfast includes cereal and buttered toast, followed by lunch which usually consists of salad and buttered sandwiches and in the evening a cooked meal usually pork with potatoes and vegetables. When he increases his insulin, he does notice his appetite increases as well and he has a tendency to have snacks between meals with resulting weight gain. Home monitoring of glucose reveals levels between 8 and 13. Other medications include metformin 500 mg tds and aspirin 75 mg od. He smokes five cigarettes a day and is trying to cut down. He used to smoke 20 a day but, as he does not work, stopping altogether has been difficult. He does not undertake any exercise. He drinks on average 3 pints of beer a day and lives with his wife and three grown-up children. He does not seem too concerned about the hyperlipidaemia as he is not symptomatic from this, but he is slightly concerned about the urine protein finding.

Examiner information

1. Data gathering in the interview

A good candidate would be able to elicit:

- the details of the hyperlipidaemia (some patients will know the exact lipid values)
- cardiovascular history – suggestive of ischaemic heart disease and of peripheral vascular disease
- full diabetic history including micro- and macrovascular complications. Treatment of diabetes
- history of hypertension
- smoking history
- family history of ischaemic heart disease and hyperlipidaemia
- a full dietary, alcohol and exercise history
- concerns of the patient.

2. Identification and use of information gathered

The candidate should be able to interpret the history and create a problem list. The objectives for the candidate are to:

- ascertain the cardiovascular risk factors in this patient
- explain the importance of minimizing these risk factors by improving glycaemic control and hence the need for reducing weight and alcohol intake, increasing insulin, stopping smoking, keeping blood pressure and lipids stringently under control and improving daily life activities, e.g. more exercise, weight control, etc.
- explain that total calorie intake (alcohol and dietary fat) is excessive and this must be reduced. Also explain that increasing the insulin dose increases food intake and hence the weight gain

- explain the possible significance of the proteinuria and the need for doing further tests, i.e. urine albumin/creatinine ratio, 24-h urine protein collection, renal function tests
- address any concerns, particularly the balance between the increase in insulin dose and the possible weight gain.

3. Discussion related to the case

- This patient has numerous cardiovascular risk factors which need to be addressed. He has hyperlipidaemia (although with a relatively good high-density lipoprotein [HDL] level), hypertension, diabetes mellitus, family history and he also smokes and drinks.
- The cardiovascular risk in patients with type 2 diabetes without a history of MI is said to be equivalent to that of a non-diabetic patient who has had an MI. Instead of defining treatment cut-off levels for hypercholesterolaemia, the use of cardiovascular risk profiles ought to be favoured. Previous recommendations have been for the treatment of elevated blood pressure with a cardiovascular risk of >15% over 10 years and treatment of elevated cholesterol with a cardiovascular risk of >30% over 10 years. However, these cut-off levels were believed to be mainly financially driven and recommendations for the treatment of cholesterol with cardiovascular risks of >20% are becoming acceptable. The traditional risk calculations, however, will not apply in this case as the patient has established proteinuria which increases the risk a further 2–3 times. Many physicians would treat as for secondary prevention in these cases. With respect to proteinuria and hypertension, the current debate is whether treatment should be with an ACE

inhibitor, an angiotensin II receptor antagonist or both.

- It has been shown in the Steno-2 study that intensive multifactorial intervention for patients with type 2 diabetes mellitus (i.e. aiming for intensive control of hyperglycaemia, hypertension, hyperlipidaemia and microalbuminuria) reduces the risk of cardiovascular disease and microvascular complications by 50% over an 8-year period.
- As well as improving glycaemic control, general management should include further advice on diet, especially reducing fat intake, alcohol, weight and exercise, considering increasing the dose of atorva-statin, adding a fibrate and considering the use of fast-acting insulins (Humalog and Novonorm) as these possibly help with weight control as there is no need for snacks.

- Discussion with examiners may include the increased risk of side-effects of statin plus fibrate combinations (gemfibrozil and cerivastatin combination led to the withdrawal of the latter) and combined use of thiazides and β-blockers may adversely affect the lipid profile. The candidate will be expected to know the up-to-date guidelines for hyperlipidaemia management.

Comments on the case

This is a complicated case and tests the ability of the candidate to assess the many possible risk factors rather than purely focusing on the hyperlipidaemia.

Case 25 | Jaundice

Candidate information
You are the doctor in a gastroenterology clinic. Mr Brian Jones is referred to you by his GP.

Please read this letter and then continue with the consultation.

Dear Doctor

Re: Mr Brian Jones, aged 56

Thank you for seeing this solicitor who has complained of jaundice with right hypochondrial pain, malaise and nausea for the last 4 days. He has had arthritis of his hip since breaking his femur in a road traffic accident 16 years ago. For this he takes co-codamol. Please see and advise.

Yours sincerely

Dr G. Practitioner

You have 14 min until the patient leaves the room, followed by 1 min for reflection, before the discussion with the examiners. Be prepared to discuss the solutions to the problems posed by the case and how you might reply to the GP's letter.

Patient information
Mr Brian Jones is a 56-year-old solicitor, working in the city centre, who complains of a sudden onset of jaundice 4 days ago with right hypochondrial pain. The jaundice has progressed during these 4 days but there are no pale stools and only slight discolouration of the urine. The pain is a dull, constant ache and is worse on deep inspiration. There is also malaise, nausea with loss of appetite and a loss of weight of 2 kg. He has no abdominal swelling, haematemesis, melaena, vomiting, pruritus, fever, peripheral oedema or altered sleep pattern. Past medical history includes a road traffic accident, as a pedestrian, 16 years ago, when he broke the neck of his femur. Despite repair, he has suffered from subsequent arthritic pain for which he takes co-codamol regularly. This pain is sometimes severe enough to affect his sleep and cause depression. Occasionally, he has taken more than the prescribed dose of co-codamol but has not taken any overdoses. He says he drinks 'socially' but more detailed questioning reveals that he has been a heavy consumer for 12 years, drinking two bottles of wine a day, particularly after work with clients. He does admit to drinking heavily during 'working lunches' as well. He does not drink beer but has some spirits at home in the evening, usually two measures of whisky. He does not drink in the morning nor does he suffer from any early morning withdrawal tremor. He believes he had a blood transfusion at the time of his fractured hip but no recent transfusions. There has been no recent travel abroad nor are there any obvious HIV risk factors. There is no past history of autoimmune illnesses. He was divorced 6 years ago and he lives alone. He has had one conviction for drink-driving 3 years ago.

Examiner information

1. Data gathering in the interview

A good candidate would be able to elicit:

- when the patient first noticed the jaundice, whether it is gradually progressing and if the skin and sclerae are yellow
- any previous episodes of jaundice and any family history of jaundice
- associated pruritus, discoloured stools or urine (implying biliary obstruction)
- any abdominal pain and its nature
- any associated symptoms, including nausea/vomiting, haematemesis, fatigue, malaise, fever, loss of appetite, weight loss, rash, arthritis, peripheral oedema, abdominal swelling, confusion/altered sleeping pattern (encephalopathy)
- any respiratory or cardiac symptoms
- full alcohol history, including drinking at work. CAGE questionnaire, driving offences, psychological and social problems as a consequence
- any relevant past medical history, e.g. liver and gallstone disorders, malignancy, recent anaesthesia (especially halothane), blood transfusions, history of other autoimmune disorders, e.g. coeliac, diabetes, hypothyroidism, etc. important for primary biliary cirrhosis and autoimmune hepatitis
- a full drug history, including antibiotics, paracetamol (any overdoses in an attempt to relieve arthritic pain) and antirheumatic drugs
- any risk factors for viral hepatitis, e.g. A (travel abroad, shell-fish consumption), B and C (intravenous drug abuse, tattoos, sexual)
- other risk factors for hepatitis, such as blood transfusion, contact with environmental sources, e.g. leptospirosis.

2. Identification and use of information gathered

The candidate should be able to interpret the history and create a problem list. The objectives for the candidate are to:

- create a list of differential diagnoses
- ascertain any risk factors for hepatitis
- have a plan for investigations
- be able to approach the patient about the high alcohol consumption with regard to encouraging abstinence and offering help, especially counselling
- address any concerns the patient may have, especially with regard to the possibility of cirrhosis or cancer

- gain an insight into any psychological difficulties which may be associated with the high alcohol consumption, especially depression, and also gain an appreciation of the impact the current illness may have on his work
- arrange a follow-up appointment to discuss the results of investigations.

3. Discussion related to the case

- Causes of painful jaundice include hepatitis (alcoholic, infective, drug induced, Wilson's disease), biliary colic, pancreatitis, cholecystitis, metastatic and Budd–Chiari.
- Causes of painless jaundice are haemolysis (hyperbilirubinaemia, Gilbert's), pancreatic or biliary malignancy and hepatic cirrhosis, e.g. related to alcohol, haemochromatosis (associated with arthritis), primary biliary cirrhosis (itching and malaise).
- This case tests the ability of the candidate to develop a list of differential diagnoses for jaundice (painful versus non-painful) and to ask appropriate questions to decide which particular diagnosis fits the case best. The most likely diagnosis is alcoholic hepatitis. However, questioning should reflect the possibility of other diagnoses such as obstructive jaundice (e.g. gallstones), viral hepatitis and liver metastases.
- The candidate's plan of initial investigations should include FBC, U&E, LFT, GGT, clotting, glucose, viral hepatitis screen, cytomegalovirus antibodies, autoimmune antibodies (antimitochondrial antibodies, anti-liver kidney microsomal antibodies [anti-LKMA], anti-smooth muscle antibodies, immunoglobulins), α-fetoprotein, ferritin and total iron-binding capacity, caeruloplasmin.
- Imaging is extremely important and an abdominal ultrasound would be first line.
- For discussion, the candidate will need to know the causes of jaundice and cirrhosis, the pathological changes of alcoholic liver disease, the consequences of the alcohol dependency syndrome, i.e. physical, psychological and social, management of liver failure and complications of portal hypertension.
- A common discussion topic is management of the alcoholic patient with regard to recognition and counselling. The CAGE questionnaire has been developed to aid the identification of alcohol abuse and a detection rate of up to 70% has been claimed in those who say yes to two or more of the following four questions: (1) have you ever felt you ought to Cut down your drinking? (2) have people Annoyed you

by criticizing your drinking? (3) have you ever felt bad or Guilty about your drinking? (4) have you ever had a drink first thing in the morning to steady your nerves or to get rid of a hangover? (Eye opener).

Comments on the case

This case typifies the common scenario of a patient underestimating the quantity of alcohol he consumes. The candidate must not just assume that 'social drinking' equates to one pint per evening; the candidate's and the patient's definition of a 'social drinker' may have no concordance. The candidate must be prepared to burrow further into the alcohol history with recognition of the possible psychological and social consequences.

Case 26 | Joint pains

Candidate information

You are the doctor in a rheumatology clinic. Mrs Margaret Rees is referred to you by her GP.

Please read this letter and then continue with the consultation.

Dear Doctor

Re: Margaret Rees, aged 35

Thank you for seeing Mrs Rees who has complained of painful, swollen joints in her hands during the past 5 weeks. This is associated with tiredness particularly in the mornings. She is finding that her symptoms are interfering with her work and she has now taken the last 2 weeks off as sick leave. She presently takes co-codamol and she is intolerant of NSAIDs, as they exacerbate her oesophageal reflux. Please see and advise.

Yours sincerely

Dr G. Practitioner

You have 14 min until the patient leaves the room, followed by 1 min for reflection, before the discussion with the examiners. Be prepared to discuss the solutions to the problems posed by the case and how you might reply to the GP's letter.

Patient information

Mrs Margaret Rees is a 35-year-old right-handed lady who works behind the counter at the local LloydsTSB bank. Over the last 5 weeks she has complained of a gradual onset of swollen, painful joints in the proximal interphalangeal (PIP) and metacarpophalangeal (MCP) distribution of both hands (initially the right). This is associated with stiffness particularly in the mornings which improves with usage of the hands, and generalized tiredness that may on occasions persist throughout the day. Her pain, swelling and stiffness are worse in the right hand than the left. The only other joint affected is the right shoulder. There are no obvious precipitating factors but gentle activity may improve the stiffness. There are no associated skin rashes, nodules, nail changes, sensory loss or radiation of the pain in the hands. Other general symptoms of the respiratory, neurological or ophthalmic systems are absent. There have been no acute episodes of swelling. Her symptoms are particularly affecting her ability to write and type, which are essential for work, and because of this and the tiredness she has taken the last 2 weeks off work. This is particularly upsetting as she never takes time off and she is worried that she may be made redundant. Another disability she has noticed is with buttoning up her blouses. She is taking co-codamol without a great deal of relief. She also takes a maintenance does of lansoprazole for oesophageal reflux and because of this she is intolerant to NSAIDs.

There is no other past history of arthritis, autoimmune disorders, recent infections or trauma. Her mother suffered with osteoarthrosis when in her seventies. She does not smoke or drink alcohol. She lives with her husband and two children who are very supportive. She is naturally anxious as to whether this may be rheumatoid arthritis and if so about any potential long-term disability.

Examiner information

1. Data gathering in the interview
A good candidate would be able to elicit:
- which joints in the hands are affected.
- if other joints are affected, e.g. wrists, shoulders, neck, back, hips, knees, feet, etc.
- how long has the swelling been present for, if there are any acute attacks of swelling and if so how often and what precipitates an attack
- whether the swelling affects both hands at the same time (symmetrical arthropathy)
- any associated pain with radiation, morning stiffness, skin rash, nodules, sensory loss
- other general symptoms related to systemic rheumatological disorders, e.g. fatigue, malaise, fever, eye changes, respiratory, neurological
- history of the oesophageal reflux and inability to tolerate NSAIDs
- detailed occupational history with any history of repetitive strain injuries or trauma
- any disability, e.g. dressing, writing, using cutlery, socially and at work, e.g. typing
- any past medical history, e.g. connective tissue disease, vasculitis, autoimmune disorders, infections, GI disorders (cirrhosis, peptic ulcer), skin disorders, e.g. psoriasis
- any family history of rheumatoid arthritis
- a drug history, e.g. thiazides precipitating gout, procainamide or hydralazine causing lupus erythematosus and ask if the patient is intolerant of NSAIDs as this may determine certain pharmacological therapy regimens
- a smoking and alcohol history
- concerns of the patient (social and work).

2. Identification and use of information gathered
The candidate should be able to interpret the history and create a problem list. The objectives for the candidate are to:

- explain the possible diagnoses
- express that the diagnosis may be rheumatoid arthritis but it is impossible to comment at this stage on long-term prognosis
- show full understanding, with empathy, about the restriction on her daily activities
- describe in detail the necessary tests to be performed
- illustrate that you would like to admit her to carry out these tests and to start therapy once the diagnosis is made
- attempt to reassure her that alternative treatments other than NSAIDs are available for rheumatoid arthritis
- endeavour to address any other concerns she may have.

3. Discussion related to the case
- This case tests the candidate's ability to take a detailed joint history and to consider the primary diagnosis of rheumatoid arthritis, with particular relevance to the systemic symptoms. Other possible diagnoses to be considered are other seronegative arthropathies such as psoriasis or Reiter's, both of which may present with asymmetrical distal interphalangeal joint arthropathy. Nodal osteoarthrosis rarely presents under the age of 50.
- The candidate should consider admission with a plan of investigations: full blood count, urea and electrolytes, liver function tests, erythrocyte sedimentation rate (ESR), serology (rheumatoid factor which is present in approximately 70% of cases, anti-cyclic citrullinated peptide [anti-CCP] antibodies), full autoimmune screen (e.g. antinuclear antibodies, antineutrophil cytoplasmic antibody [ANCA], complement levels and other autoantibodies for conditions like SLE, dermatomyositis, etc. if indicated).
- X-rays of the affected joints should be requested and aspiration of a joint performed if an effusion is present with culture for bacteria. Further imaging of the joints, e.g. MRI scan, may be required, especially

if the neck is involved. Physiotherapy input may also be considered.

- The candidate would be expected to have a detailed knowledge of the systemic effects of rheumatoid arthritis, its immunopathology, the role of disease-modifying antirheumatic drugs and their potential side-effects and the development of the new anticytokine therapies such as anti-tumour necrosis factor (TNF)-α monoclonal antibody.

Comments on the case

This case highlights the importance of taking a detailed 'impact of symptoms' history. The history is typical for rheumatoid arthritis but extra marks will be awarded if the candidate can visualize the patient in the social setting with the burden of her illness on work and family life. This case will also test the ability of the candidate to address the anxieties and concerns that the patient may have.

Case 27 | Loin pain

Candidate information

You are the medical doctor in an endocrine clinic and about to see this patient for his annual review. The GP has sent a letter with the patient.

Please read this letter and then continue with the consultation.

Dear Doctor

Re: Mr Ronald Tweedle, aged 76

Thank you for seeing Mr Tweedle whom you see for acromegaly on an annual basis. He has been complaining of recurrent left-sided loin pain which has been getting gradually worse over the last 3 weeks. He was treated for a UTI with trimethoprim but his pain has not resolved.

Please see and advise.

Yours sincerely

Dr G. Practitioner

You have 14 min until the patient leaves the room, followed by 1 min for reflection, before the discussion with the examiners. Be prepared to discuss the solutions to the problems posed by the case and how you might reply to the GP's letter.

Patient information

Mr Ronald Tweedle, a 76-year-old gentleman, presents with a 3-week history of left-sided loin pain. The pain may come on at any time of the day; it is usually severe, sharp and intermittent and may last up to 2 hours. Sometimes the pain radiates anteriorly but there is no dysuria or haematuria. He has had these pains now on two separate occasions. The GP made a home visit each time and gave voltarol, which resulted in some relief, and trimethoprim to cover any infection. He has a previous history of a staghorn calculus in the right kidney which was surgically removed 12 years ago. He has been otherwise well in himself and only suffers symptomatically from prostatism which manifests as postmicturition dribbling with poor stream. He is on finasteride for this. He also has a previous history of acromegaly 20 years ago which was treated surgically and he is under regular yearly follow-up in the endocrine clinic. He has some residual peripheral visual field loss, but the acromegaly is inactive at the moment. A recent CT scan of the head showed no recurrence of the tumour. He has a past history of sick sinus syndrome presenting as dizziness and bradycardia for which a pacemaker was inserted 8 years ago. He takes ramipril for hypertension. He lives alone in a ground-floor flat. He is self-caring and he does not smoke or drink. He is concerned about the possibility of recurring renal stones.

Examiner information

1. Data gathering in the interview

A good candidate would be able to elicit:

- a complete history of the pain, i.e. frequency, position, radiation, nature, relieving/exacerbating factors (e.g. alcohol, drinking large quantities of fluids), associated dysuria, haematuria, history of prostatism
- previous history of renal stones, presence of hypercalcaemia at the time
- history of acromegaly and particularly ascertaining the activity, i.e. worsening visual field defects, sweating, headaches, etc. Other symptoms, e.g. change in appearance, increased size of hands, ring tightening, deep/hollow voice, tiredness, impotence or poor libido
- history of other features resulting from acromegaly, e.g. hypertension, heart failure, arthropathy, carpal tunnel syndrome, diabetes mellitus, galactorrhoea, goitre
- when the pacemaker was inserted and what type – this would be a contraindication for MRI scanning
- other drug history
- social history
- concerns of the patient.

2. Identification and use of information gathered

The candidate should be able to interpret the history and create a problem list. The objectives for the candidate are to:

- ascertain that the history does sound like renal stones and correctly establish the previous history of renal calculi

- link the acromegaly with the renal calculi and the cardiovascular disease
- provide a plan of action for the patient.

3. Discussion related to the case

- Differential diagnoses in this case would be renal stones, pyelonephritis and prostatic obstruction predisposing to hydronephrosis.
- Investigations would include blood tests for calcium and urea/electrolytes, mid-stream urine (MSU), a plain abdominal X-ray and an intravenous urogram.
- Long-term sequelae of acromegaly potentially include the deficiency of other pituitary hormones; visual loss due to compression of the optic nerve; impaired glucose tolerance and diabetes; hypertension; renal stones due to increased urinary excretion of calcium; increased risk of gastric and colonic neoplasms; skeletal problems such as kyphosis, scoliosis and accelerated osteoarthrosis; cardiac problems including accelerated atherosclerosis and cardiomyopathy; overgrowth of soft tissues which may not entirely resolve after treatment, including a goitre and nerve entrapment syndromes such as carpal tunnel syndrome. Skin changes in acromegaly include acral bony overgrowth (frontal bossing), soft tissue swelling, excessive sweating and hypertrichosis.

Comments on the case

This is quite a typical case where the past medical history is 'retrospectively' interlinked and hence it is vitally important not to dismiss past illnesses but to speculate on any possible connection with the present symptoms.

Case 28 | Loss of weight

Candidate information

You are the doctor in a general medical clinic. Mrs Marlene Llewellyn is referred to you by her GP.

Please read this letter and then continue with the consultation.

Dear Doctor

Re: Mrs Marlene Llewellyn, aged 40

Thank you for seeing Mrs Llewellyn who has complained of a 5 kg loss of weight over the last 6 months. Her appetite is good but she has noticed an increasing frequency of bowel actions during the last few weeks. She has a past history of anxiety for which she takes zopiclone. A recent FBC, U&E, LFT and chest X-ray are all normal. Please see and advise.

Yours sincerely

Dr G. Practitioner

You have 14 min until the patient leaves the room, followed by 1 min for reflection, before the discussion with the examiners. Be prepared to discuss the solutions to the problems posed by the case and how you might reply to the GP's letter.

Patient information

Mrs Llewellyn is a 40-year-old housewife who has complained of a 5 kg loss of weight over the last 6 months, from 54 kg to 49 kg. She has always been thin. She first noticed the weight loss when her clothes started to feel looser and the children were saying that she looked much thinner than before. She eats well and there has been no loss of appetite. Her diet is non-vegetarian with fresh fruit and cereals in the morning, followed by a sandwich at lunch and usually a cooked meal with meat and potatoes in the evening. She does no physical exercise apart from her daily living activities. There has been no purposeful dieting and no abuse of laxatives or diuretics. She has no other bowel symptoms apart from occasional loose stools recently but no steatorrhoea. Normally she goes once a day but in the last few weeks it has been up to three times a day. There is no constipation, rectal bleeding, nausea/vomiting, vaginal bleeding, cough, sputum or haemoptysis. Her past medical history includes an anxiety neurosis for which she takes zopiclone. She continues to feel 'on edge' most days with occasional tremors and palpitations during the anxious episodes, which are usually triggered by family rows. Recently she has noticed that she is not sleeping well with early morning wakening. She has smoked 10 cigarettes a day since the age of 16 and does admit to smoking more when she is anxious. She does not drink alcohol but her husband drinks heavily and this exacerbates her worries. She lives in a three-bedroom semi-detached house in a deprived area with her husband and two children. She has always been a housewife. She cannot understand why she is losing weight despite an unchanged diet.

Examiner information

1. Data gathering in the interview

A good candidate would be able to elicit:

- if the patient feels her clothes are looser, whether she is looking thinner and if friends/family have noticed any change
- how much weight she has lost. Take a dietary history with assessment of intake and any change in appetite
- if the weight loss is intentional, e.g. dieting, exercise, laxatives/diuretics
- a previous history of weight loss
- previous body weight
- associated GI symptoms, e.g. dysphagia, abdominal pain, nausea/vomiting, GI bleeding, altered bowel habit, steatorrhoea
- endocrine symptoms, e.g. thyrotoxicosis (tremors, increased appetite, diarrhoea, palpitations, eye symptoms), adrenal insufficiency (weakness, dizziness, excessive sweating)
- other cardiovascular and respiratory symptoms
- drug history, especially diet pills, laxatives, amphetamines
- symptoms suggestive of anxiety and depression
- social history, recent separation or job loss/change
- alcohol and smoking history (smoking reduces appetite)
- other past medical history, e.g. GI disorders, emphysema, neoplasia, diabetes mellitus
- the patient's concerns regarding the weight loss.

2. Identification and use of information gathered

The candidate should be able to interpret the history and create a problem list. The objectives for the candidate are to:

- create a list of differential diagnoses
- plan a list of investigations
- convey these to the patient with explanations
- educate her on the hazards of smoking
- arrange quick follow-up with reweighing and to discuss the results of investigations.

3. Discussion related to the case

- This case tests the ability of the candidate to decide if the loss of weight is non-gastrointestinal, e.g. thyrotoxicosis or anxiety/depression, or gastrointestinal, e.g. primary neoplasm, malabsorption (coeliac disease, Crohn's disease), poor dietary intake as a result of alcoholism or functional dyspepsia/peptic ulcer. Do not forget the possibility of intercurrent disease.
- Investigations including FBC, U&E, thyroid function tests (TFT), LFT, GGT, glucose, chest X-ray and, if these are all normal, one may consider looking specifically for gastrointestinal causes.
- If all investigations are normal, observation of her weight with a daily food diary over a few weeks/months may be necessary.
- The diagnosis here is between an anxiety neurosis and thyrotoxicosis. The anxiety neurosis may well be exacerbated by thyrotoxicosis and it is not uncommon for patients to be labelled 'anxious' only to subsequently find that they are thyrotoxic. The candidate will be expected to describe the systemic effects of thyrotoxicosis, the complications (e.g. crises) and treatment (antithyroid drugs versus radioactive iodine versus thyroidectomy).

Comments on the case

This is a common general medical case of 'weight loss ?cause'. Do not assume the weight loss is psychological or gastrointestinal. The clues are in the history and you must have made a mental note of all the possible causes before the consultation in order to tailor the history along the lines of that list. If you feel the case may be thyrotoxicosis, then you can really concentrate specifically on the long list of possible symptoms to gain extra marks. Again, you must have a plan of investigations on hand and be prepared to reply to the patient's question, 'Have I got cancer?'.

Case 29 | Lower gastrointestinal haemorrhage

Candidate information

You are the doctor in the gastroenterology clinic. Mr John Davies is referred to you by his GP.

Please read this letter and then continue with the consultation.

Dear Doctor

Re: Mr John Davies, aged 53

Thank you for seeing Mr Davies so quickly. He has complained of rectal bleeding for the last 3 weeks without any loss of weight. His past medical history includes osteoarthritis of both knees and haemorrhoids. He takes diclofenac only. I am concerned that he may have a neoplasm. Please see and advise.

Yours sincerely

Dr G. Practitioner

You have 14 min until the patient leaves the room, followed by 1 min for reflection, before the discussion with the examiners. Be prepared to discuss the solutions to the problems posed by the case and how you might reply to the GP's letter.

Patient information

Mr John Davies is a 53-year-old car mechanic who one morning 3 weeks ago noticed dark red blood mixed in with his stools at the bottom of the toilet pan. He thought at first that this was from his haemorrhoids but these normally present intermittently with bright red blood on the toilet paper and not mixed in with the stools. The blood is present every day and he passes stools regularly once a day. There has been no change in his bowel habit, and he has had no haematemesis, loss of weight, abdominal pain, diarrhoea, vomiting, jaundice, hypochondrial tenderness or malaise. He does not suffer from urgency, tenesmus or pain on passing stools. He has not noticed any lumps protruding through his anus. He has had haemorrhoids for many years and the last time he noticed any blood from these was 3 months ago. The new symptom is definitely different. There is no other history of bleeding disorders, other GI history or of food poisoning. He takes diclofenac for his arthritis but does not suffer from NSAID-induced dyspepsia. There is no other relevant drug history, e.g. iron or bismuth. There is no family history of polyps or colonic carcinoma. He does not drink or smoke. He lives with his wife and both lead active lifestyles. Mr Davies is naturally concerned that this may be cancer.

Examiner information

1. Data gathering in the interview

A good candidate would be able to elicit:

- if he had passed blood rectally before and, if so, the nature and frequency of this
- the description of the present blood in the stools, e.g. fresh red blood, dark red or black, mixed with stool, on the surface of the stool or on the toilet paper only. How much blood and mucus is present
- any associated diarrhoea or any nocturnal diarrhoea (sometimes seen in ulcerative colitis)
- how often he passes bloody stools in a day
- any change in bowel habit
- if he has abdominal pain, urgency or tenesmus when passing stools
- any straining, constipation, anal pain (fissure), rectal lumps/masses
- any weight loss and, if so, over how long a period
- any associated symptoms such as loss of appetite, nausea, vomiting, haematemesis, abdominal mass, fatigue and tiredness, and bleeding elsewhere
- other previous GI history, haemorrhoids, bleeding disorders, food poisoning
- drug history especially NSAIDs, anticoagulants, iron and bismuth (black stool not red)
- alcohol history
- family history of GI neoplasia, polyps
- concerns regarding cancer.

2. Identification and use of information gathered

The candidate should be able to interpret the history and create a problem list. The objectives for the candidate are to:

- decide clearly the difference between the previous rectal bleeding and the present symptom
- explain that cancer cannot be totally excluded unless the proper investigations are carried out
- explain what these investigations are and describe what is involved with a sigmoidoscopy, double-contrast barium enema and, if needed for confirmation of doubtful lesions, a colonoscopy, including the description of preoperative sedation, biopsies and retaining of tissue for histology.

3. Discussion related to the case

- The case tests the ability of the candidate to compare the present history with the past symptoms and to judge if these are from the same aetiology or not. The history of the previous haemorrhoids is clearly different from the present symptom. The most worrying differential diagnosis includes a lower GI neoplasm, the history of which can sometimes point to the possible site of the cancer, e.g. altered bowel habit with or without abdominal pain is common in descending colonic lesions, rectal and sigmoid carcinomas tend to present with bleeding commonly mixed in with stools, and caecal lesions may just present with an iron deficiency anaemia and no other obvious bowel symptom. Other possibilities include colonic and/or rectal polyps which may intermittently bleed, particularly the larger ones, colitis such as ulcerative colitis although diarrhoea is more common with bleeding, diverticular bleeding which can occasionally be massive and can be detected on double-contrast barium enema as pouches of mucosa extruding through the muscular wall. Haemorrhoids and anal fissures present with fresh bleeding with pain on defaecation (particularly with the fissures). Angiodysplasia may also be a cause of lower GI bleeding. The candidate should have a plan of investigations including full blood count, routine biochemistry, flexible sigmoidoscopy, double-contrast barium enema (good preparation essential), and colonoscopy to confirm the presence of a suspicious lesion.
- The candidate will be expected to discuss the importance of neoplastic polyps with regard to transformation to carcinoma, genetics of colonic carcinoma, use of faecal occult blood testing, screening and prevention, and treatment (surgical and chemotherapy).

Comments on the case

This case is an important one to stress the importance of collating details of the previous haemorrhoid history and comparing this to the present history. The candidate will get extra marks if he/she makes it obvious to the examiner that the line of questioning is conforming to his/her thought processes whilst searching for the possible site of the lesion.

Case 30 | Macrocytic anaemia

Candidate information

You are the doctor in a general medical clinic. Mr Arthur Evans is referred to you by his GP.

Please read this letter and then continue with the consultation.

Dear Doctor

Re: Mr Arthur Evans, aged 84

Thank you for seeing Mr Evans who was noticed to be pale by his carers. He has been in the residential home for 2 years since the death of his wife. He is normally mobile with a stick. A full blood count shows: Hb 6.3 g/dL, WCC 5.8 × 10⁹/L, platelets 213 × 10⁹/L and MCV 112 fL. He does not normally complain of any symptoms but the carer has noticed a decline in activity levels over the last year. He also has arthritis of the right hip for which he takes paracetamol.

Yours sincerely

Dr G. Practitioner

You have 14 min until the patient leaves the room, followed by 1 min for reflection, before the discussion with the examiners. Be prepared to discuss the solutions to the problems posed by the case and how you might reply to the GP's letter.

Patient information

Mr Evans is an 84-year-old retired machine operator who does not complain of any symptoms but recently has been noticed to be very pale by the residential home carers. He has been in the home for 2 years since the death of his wife. Normally he is mobile with a stick, has no obvious symptoms of dementia, is self-caring and takes an active role in the daily activities at the home. However, over the last year his activity has reduced with increasing tiredness, particularly towards the end of the afternoon, and there has been a tendency to retire to bed early in the evening. Closer questioning reveals that he has lost about 4 kg in weight, his appetite has diminished over the last few months and he has mentioned to the carer that he has a sore mouth. He does not complain of vomiting, dysphagia, abdominal pain, diarrhoea or gastrointestinal bleeding. There are no cardiovascular, respiratory, hypothyroid or neurological symptoms such as limb weakness or numbness. His past medical history includes arthritis of the right hip that does restrict his movement and for which he needs a stick. He has never been referred to an orthopaedic surgeon. He has no past history of liver disorders, alcohol problems, autoimmune disorders such as Graves' disease or Hashimoto's thyroiditis, thyrotoxicosis, idiopathic adrenocortical insufficiency, vitiligo or hypoparathyroidism, or of any GI disorders or previous operations. There is no family history of any of the above mentioned autoimmune conditions either. He eats a normal diet supplied by the home that includes meat, vegetables and fruit. His only medication is paracetamol. He used to smoke five cigarettes a day until 12 years ago and he does not drink alcohol. Although he does not have any concerns about his condition, Mr Evans is aware that the residential home staff have expressed their concern about the pallor.

Examiner information

1. Data gathering in the interview

A good candidate would be able to elicit:
- how the patient has deteriorated with regard to activity at the home
- a description of any tiredness, dyspnoea, weight loss or poor appetite
- his premorbid state, especially mobility, self-caring abilities and dementia
- a full gastrointestinal history, especially loss of weight – how much? Suggestions of small bowel disease, e.g. steatorrhoea (ileal disease, bacterial overgrowth), jaundice, a sore tongue (glossitis) in pernicious anaemia
- a dietary history – ?strict vegetarian
- full systemic history to identify heart failure, vitamin B12 deficiency-related subacute combined degeneration (any paraesthesia?), autoimmune disease
- past medical history, especially of GI surgery (gastrectomy, ileal resection), GI disease (coeliac disease, Crohn's disease, bacterial overgrowth, tropical sprue), malignancy, renal dialysis (folate)
- full drug history, especially antifolate drugs such as phenytoin, methotrexate, trimethoprim
- family history of autoimmune disorders, including pernicious anaemia
- alcohol history (folate deficiency)
- fish tapeworm (very rare)
- the concerns of the patient and his carers.

2. Identification and use of information gathered

The candidate should be able to interpret the history and create a problem list. The objectives for the candidate are to:
- assemble a list of the possible causes of the megaloblastic anaemia
- have a plan of investigations
- explain to the patient that he has an anaemia and that the symptoms of weight loss, poor appetite and tiredness are most likely to be related to this

- address any concerns that he, the carers and the GP may have
- arrange follow-up.

3. Discussion related to the case

- The main problem is the macrocytic anaemia and the consultation needs to address finding a cause for this, i.e. megaloblastic versus non-megaloblastic.
- This case tests the candidate's ability to assimilate a list of differential diagnoses from the information given by the GP and to take an appropriate history. Essentially, this patient describes an insidious illness manifesting with tiredness, loss of weight and appetite and with a sore mouth suggesting a glossitis; these point to a diagnosis of pernicious anaemia.
- Causes of macrocytic anaemia are megaloblastic (bone marrow contains erythroblasts with delayed nuclear maturation) such as B12 or folate deficiency, or non-megaloblastic, e.g. hypothyroidism, alcohol excess, liver disease, reticulocytosis or drug induced. A mean cell volume (MCV) of over 110 fL is more suggestive of megaloblastic than non-megaloblastic anaemia. Pernicious anaemia is common in the elderly and is characterized by atrophy of the gastric mucosa with consequent failure of intrinsic factor production, leading to vitamin B12 malabsorption.
- Investigations should include vitamin B12 and folate levels (values less than 100 ng/L and 4 μg/L are highly suggestive of B12 and folate deficiencies respectively), LFTs looking for a raised bilirubin, parietal cell antibodies (present in 90% of patients) and intrinsic factor antibodies (found in 50% of patients but specific for pernicious anaemia) and, if there are any doubts, a bone marrow examination. A Schilling test may be performed to delineate the cause of B12 deficiency, i.e. pernicious anaemia, or terminal ileal disease or bacterial overgrowth. Further small bowel investigations are only relevant if small bowel disease is suspected.
- Treatment of vitamin B12 deficiency is with hydroxycobalamin 1000 μg intramuscularly every week for 4

weeks and then 1000 µg intramuscularly every 3 months for life. If any GI symptoms persist then endoscopy should be considered as gastric carcinoma has twice the normal incidence in pernicious anaemia as in the normal population.

Comments on the case

This case tests the ability of the candidate to evaluate the results given in the letter. This is a typical case where the candidate must know the causes of a macrocytic anaemia. If not, the history taking will be insufficient to score points.

Case 31 | Neck lump

Candidate information

You are the doctor in a general medical clinic. Mr Abdul Hussein is referred to you by his GP.

Please read this letter and then continue with the consultation.

Dear Doctor

Re: Mr Abdul Hussein, aged 41

Thank you for seeing Mr Hussein who presents with a firm nodule on the right side of his neck of 3 months duration. He seems otherwise well and a recent chest X-ray was reported as normal. There is no tuberculosis in the family and he has no significant past medical history apart from *Plasmodium vivax* malaria 2 years ago. Please see and advise.

Yours sincerely

Dr G. Practitioner

You have 14 min until the patient leaves the room, followed by 1 min for reflection, before the discussion with the examiners. Be prepared to discuss the solutions to the problems posed by the case and how you might reply to the GP's letter.

Patient information

Mr Hussein is a 41-year-old Bangladeshi man who came to the UK 4 years ago. Since then he has worked as a waiter but back in Bangladesh he was a shop assistant. He first noticed a lump in his neck 3 months ago when he was washing. It is situated on the right side of the neck, is firm and has not changed in size. He thinks he has also felt another lump on the right side but towards the back of the neck. The lumps are not tender. There have been no symptoms of cough, sputum, haemoptysis, fever, malaise, pruritus, diarrhoea, weight loss or rash. He feels tired but puts this down to working late nights. There has been no recent history of a sore throat or tonsillitis. There is no family history of tuberculosis, including in the family back in Bangladesh. He smokes up to 10 cigarettes a day, does not drink alcohol and lives with his wife and three children who are all fit and well.

Examiner information

1. Data gathering in the interview

A good candidate would be able to elicit:
- where the glands are and if he has noticed any other glands
- when the gland was first noticed and how

- if the gland is increasing or fluctuating in size
- if the gland is hard, soft, non-tender or tender
- if he has a history of tuberculosis or recurrent sore throat or tonsillitis
- any past history of head and neck cancer
- if there has been any recent family history of sore throats, viral illnesses, tuberculosis

- other associated symptoms of cough, sputum, haemoptysis, fever, fatigue, pruritus, malaise, diarrhoea, weight loss, rash or eye problems (sarcoidosis)
- occupational history and contacts at work
- family history and well-being of present family
- smoking history
- concerns of the patient.

2. Identification and use of information gathered

The candidate should be able to interpret the history and create a problem list. The objectives for the candidate are to:

- develop a list of differential diagnoses (the most likely diagnosis in this case is tuberculous lymphadenitis)
- discuss the possibility of tuberculosis (TB) with the patient
- arrange investigations
- discuss the need for a fine needle aspiration and, if a dry tap, excision biopsy for cytology and microscopy and culture for acid- and alcohol-fast bacilli (surgical referral)
- have an idea about the family members with regard to possible contact tracing if tuberculous lymphadenitis is confirmed
- reassure the patient that in the absence of an abnormal chest X-ray and respiratory symptoms, the patient's chance of being infectious is very low.

3. Discussion related to the case

- This case tests the candidate's ability to determine the probable cause of an enlarged lymph node. The possible diagnoses are (a) TB lymphadenitis (most likely in this case despite a normal chest X-ray), (b) metastatic lymph node from a head and neck neoplasm, (c) non-specific viral (doubtful in the absence of a sore throat and persistence of the nodule for 3 months) or infectious mononucleosis or cytomegalovirus, (d) lymphoproliferative disorder (watch out for weight loss and fever), (e) sarcoidosis (watch out for eye and joint symptoms) and (f) HIV lymphadenopathy (a never-to-be-forgotten contender). TB

lymphadenitis is a common presentation of Mycobacteria, particularly in patients from South Asia and not necessarily associated with an abnormal chest X-ray. The patient may be feeling well but, despite this, full investigation including a fine needle or excision biopsy is imperative to make a firm diagnosis.

- A Heaf test may be considered but is not confirmatory and the investigation of choice is a biopsy looking for Mycobacteria bacilli and caseating granulomas. Commonly the fine needle aspirate is non-yielding and a complete excision biopsy by the surgeon is necessary (tell the surgeon to send part of the node to microbiology in normal saline and not formalin). The histology sample can go in formalin. A raised ACE level in the presence of non-caseating granulomas would support sarcoidosis but the chest X-ray is commonly abnormal. An abnormal chest X-ray such as hilar lymphadenopathy, with fever and loss of weight, may indicate a lymphoproliferative disorder.
- Recently the development of interferon-gamma release assays (known as T spot test) have been able to measure host immune response against mycobacteria, which can reveal the presence of infection with *Mycobacterium tuberculosis* and detecting 'latent' TB. It has the advantage of being quick (results within a day) and less influenced by previous BCG vaccination.
- The candidate may be asked about the other presentations of tuberculosis, treatment of tuberculosis including the side-effects, multidrug resistance, length of treatment, contact tracing and prevention.

Comments on the case

This is a common case and tests the candidate's ability to make decisions. The node has been present for 3 months and hence a biopsy is warranted.

Case 32 | **Painful shins**

Candidate information

You are the doctor in a general medical clinic. Mrs Doreen Fredericks has been referred to you by her GP.

Please read this letter and then continue with the consultation.

> Dear Doctor
>
> **Re: Mrs Doreen Fredericks, age 43**
>
> Thank you for seeing Mrs Fredericks who has been suffering from painful, red, raised lesions on her shins for the last 2 weeks which have been accompanied by malaise. She is otherwise well although I treated her with a course of amoxicillin 1 month ago for a bout of bronchitis. She smokes 15 cigarettes a day.
>
> Your sincerely
>
> Dr G. Practitioner

You have 14 min until the patient leaves the room, followed by 1 min for reflection, before the discussion with the examiners. Be prepared to discuss the solutions to the problems posed by the case and how you might reply to the GP's letter.

Patient information

Mrs Fredericks is a 43-year-old healthcare assistant who works at a residential home. She has had painful, red, raised lesions on both shins for the last 2 weeks. She has felt unwell with malaise and has been off work for the last week. She does not have a fever, arthralgia, loss of weight, any eye complaints, sore throats, bowel symptoms or other skin rashes. One month ago, she had a bout of bronchitis manifesting as cough and purulent sputum for which she had a 7-day course of amoxicillin. She has had a persistent cough with occasional mucoid sputum for the last 6 months but her GP has suggested that this is most likely due to her smoking. She smokes 15 cigarettes a day. She has an unremarkable past medical history and takes no medication apart from the oral contraceptive pill. She lives with her husband and two teenage children who are all well. She has not been abroad for over 15 years.

Examiner information

1. Data gathering in the interview

A good candidate would be able to elicit:
- the features of the skins lesion, i.e. site, shape, size, colour, raised or flat, painful or painless, any deterioration or improvement, relieving or aggravating factors
- other systemic symptoms, e.g. malaise, fever, arthralgia, loss of weight, cough, sputum, haemoptysis, gastrointestinal symptoms
- other symptoms particularly suggestive of sarcoidosis, streptococcal infection, tuberculosis and inflammatory bowel disease
- the details of the recent bout of bronchitis

- any recent history suggestive of infection, e.g. fungal, atypical organisms
- the history of the recent course of antibiotics
- other drug history, especially the oral contraceptive pill
- any travel abroad and any exposure to atypical organisms and tropical infectious agents
- the impact of the painful skin lesions on her life and work
- the concerns of the patient.

2. Identification and use of information gathered

The candidate should be able to interpret the history and create a problem list. The objectives for the candidate are to:
- confirm a history suggestive of erythema nodosum
- explore the possible aetiology from the history
- explain the possible diagnosis to the patient
- detail the investigations to be carried out.

3. Discussion related to the case

- Erythema nodosum presents as painful, tender, dusky blue-red nodules, commonly over the lower limbs or shins, which may fade over a couple of weeks leaving a bruised appearance. It is common in young adults, particularly women, and can be associated with arthralgia, malaise and fever. Inflammation occurs in the dermis and the subcutaneous layer (panniculitis).
- Streptococcal infections and sarcoidosis (accompanied with bilateral hilar lymphadenopathy) are the most common causes in adults. In children, erythema nodosum is most commonly caused by upper respiratory tract infections, especially from streptococci. Less common causes (except in endemic areas) include tuberculosis, mycoplasma, leprosy, coccidioidomycosis, histoplasmosis, psittacosis, lymphogranuloma venereum and ulcerative colitis. The condition can also be a reaction to drugs (sulphonamides, iodides, bromides, oral contraceptives). In some cases, no cause may be found.
- Investigations should include a chest X-ray, ESR, ACE level, throat swab if streptococcal sore throat is suspected and a search for an infective organism, e.g. mycoplasma serology, sputum for *Mycobacterium*.
- Treatment is symptomatic with non-steroidal anti-inflammatory drugs and bedrest. Oral steroids are sometimes necessary and stopping the oral contraceptive pill may need to be considered in this case.

Comments on the case

This case tests the candidate's ability to develop a list of differential diagnoses and to tailor the history towards finding a cause for the patient's symptoms. The history of the cough must be detailed to determine if the patient is describing possible sarcoidosis or tuberculosis. It is possible that no cause will be found.

Case 33 | Painful shoulders

Candidate information

You are the doctor in the general medical clinic. Mr Alfred Swindon has been referred to you by his GP.

Please read this letter and then continue with the consultation.

Dear Doctor

Re: Mr Alfred Swindon, aged 71

Thank you for seeing Mr Swindon who has been suffering for the last 4 weeks with painful shoulders and a stiff neck. I have treated him with diclofenac but with no success. I am worried that he may have cervical myelopathy.

Please see and advise.

Your sincerely

Dr G. Practitioner

You have 14 min until the patient leaves the room, followed by 1 min for reflection, before the discussion with the examiners. Be prepared to discuss the solutions to the problems posed by the case and how you might reply to the GP's letter.

Patient information

Mr Alfred Swindon is a 71-year-old retired shopkeeper who has been suffering from painful, stiff shoulders and neck for the last 4 weeks. These symptoms appeared suddenly and are worse in the mornings, lasting up to 2–3 h. He does not have any stiffness or pain in the lumbar spine or hips. Other associated features include tiredness, fever, weight loss and a feeling of low mood. He does not have any weakness of his limbs and no restriction of head movements once the neck stiffness is relieved. He is otherwise well and has no respiratory, cardiovascular or gastrointestinal symptoms. He does not have any other neurological symptoms such as dizziness, blurred vision, tinnitus, headache, scalp tenderness, claudication of the jaw or tender temporal or occipital arteries. He is on no medication and used to smoke 10 cigarettes a day up to 30 years ago. He has an occasional glass of wine in the evenings and lives with his wife.

Examiner information

1. Data gathering in the interview

A good candidate would be able to elicit:

- the history of the painful stiff shoulders and neck (suggesting polymyalgia rheumatica), including time of onset, the limbs affected, any variation of severity during the day, the duration of symptoms and any proximal muscle weakness (polymyositis if proximal pain is present or myopathy if pain and stiffness are absent)

- any associated systemic features such as tiredness, fever, weight loss or depression

- any suggestion of giant cell arteritis, e.g. painless loss of vision, severe headache, tenderness of the scalp, jaw claudication when eating, tenderness over the temporal and/or occipital arteries
- any other neurological symptoms
- symptoms suggestive of rheumatoid arthritis, e.g. symmetrical arthropathy in both hands, etc.
- any symptoms suggestive of cervical myelopathy, e.g. head movement restriction, pain along the distribution of the dermatomes in the arms, wasting of the small muscles of the hand
- symptoms suggestive of hypothyroidism
- past medical history
- the drug history
- the impact of the illness on the patient.

2. Identification and use of information gathered

The candidate should be able to interpret the history and create a problem list. The objectives for the candidate are to:

- identify the symptoms clearly and to differentiate the three main possibilities: polymyalgia rheumatica, polymyositis and myopathy
- detail a list of investigations
- explain the possible cause for his symptoms and outline a management plan.

3. Discussion related to the case

- Polymyalgia rheumatica (PMR) is an inflammatory rheumatic condition which is part of the same disease spectrum as giant cell arteritis (GCA) – around 15–30% of patients with PMR go on to develop the latter. Both conditions are associated with specific alleles of the HLA-DR4 gene and histological studies show mild synovitis and subclinical arterial inflammation (more prominent in GCA). PMR usually occurs in patients over 50 years old and the female/male ratio is 2/1.
- The onset may be acute or subacute. PMR is characterized by severe pain and stiffness of the neck, pectoral and pelvic girdles, morning stiffness, stiffness after inactivity and systemic complaints such as malaise, fever, depression and weight loss (cachectic PMR may mimic cancer). There is no selective muscle

weakness or evidence of muscle disease on electromyography (EMG) or biopsy. A normochromic normocytic anaemia may be present. In most patients, the ESR is dramatically elevated, often >100 mm/h. C-reactive protein levels are usually elevated and may be a more sensitive marker of disease activity in certain patients.

- Polymyalgia rheumatica is distinguished from rheumatoid arthritis by the usual absence of small joint synovitis (although some joint swelling may be present), erosive or destructive disease, rheumatoid factor or rheumatoid nodules. PMR is differentiated from polymyositis by finding normal muscle enzymes, EMG and muscle biopsy and by the prominence of pain over weakness. Hypothyroidism can present as myalgia with abnormal thyroid function tests and an elevated creatine kinase (CK). PMR is differentiated from myeloma by the absence of a monoclonal gammopathy and from fibromyalgia by the systemic features and the elevated ESR.
- Corticosteroids produce a reduction in the symptoms within 48 h of starting treatment. This should reduce the risk of developing GCA. Non-steroidal anti-inflammatory drugs are less effective and should be avoided. PMR usually responds dramatically to prednisolone initiated at around 15 mg od. If temporal arteritis is suspected, treatment should be started immediately with 60 mg od to prevent blindness. As the symptoms subside, corticosteroids are tapered to the lowest effective dose, regardless of the ESR. Some patients are able to discontinue corticosteroids within 2 years whereas others require small amounts for years. Prevention of corticosteroid-induced bone loss using bisphosphonates should also be considered.

Comments on the case

This case tests the candidate's ability to clearly ascertain the history of painful stiff shoulders and to differentiate the diagnosis of polymyalgia rheumatica from polymyositis and myopathy. The GP wondered if the patient had cervical myelopathy but the history should be able to rule this out.

Case 34 | **Palpitations**

Candidate information

You are the doctor in a cardiology clinic. Mr Colin Jeffreys is referred to you by his GP.

Please read this letter and then continue with the consultation.

Dear Doctor

Re: Mr Colin Jeffreys, aged 78

Thank you for seeing Mr Jeffreys who is normally a fit and healthy man. However, he had an attack of palpitations and dizziness whilst on the golf course 2 weeks ago. I would be grateful if you could rule out any serious cardiac disease. He takes salbutamol for mild, late-onset asthma. He also had a transient ischaemic attack 5 years ago and he takes aspirin for this. He was in sinus rhythm today and his BP was 130/68 mmHg. His recent FBC, U&E and TFT were all normal. Please see and advise.

Yours sincerely

Dr G. Practitioner

You have 14 min until the patient leaves the room, followed by 1 min for reflection, before the discussion with the examiners. Be prepared to discuss the solutions to the problems posed by the case and how you might reply to the GP's letter.

Patient information

Mr Colin Jeffreys is a 78-year-old former city councillor who had one episode of palpitations 2 weeks ago when teeing off at the local golf course. The palpitations came on suddenly, lasted for around 5 min and then abruptly disappeared. He remembers that the palpitations were rapid and regular with no missed beats, and there was a feeling of heaviness in his chest, with dyspnoea and faintness, and he felt extremely ill. Once back home, he felt exhausted for the rest of the day. He visited the GP the next day at which point the referral to the cardiology clinic was made. Currently he feels fine, with no obvious irregular heartbeats. He has had no more chest pain, dyspnoea or any symptoms of hyperthyroidism (such as anxiety, tremor, loss of weight or increased appetite). There were no previous episodes of palpitations or chest pains and he has no symptoms suggestive of an anxiety-depressive neurosis. His asthma is stable with no nocturnal symptoms and he only uses his salbutamol inhaler once a day (he does not have a tremor or any other side-effects from the inhaler). He does not take any other inhalers such as long-acting β2-agonists. He had a transient ischaemic attack 5 years ago which presented as weakness of his right hand but this subsided after 1 h. He had no palpitations then. He was started on aspirin and has had no similar events since. There is no past history of ischaemic heart disease, hypertension, diabetes mellitus or hypercholesterolaemia. He stopped smoking 23 years ago when he used to smoke 10 cigarettes a day. He has a glass of sherry in the evenings but no more. He does not drink tea or coffee and takes no other drugs. He lives alone in a three-bedroom house and has no family. His main concerns are that his GP has told him to stop playing golf until investigations have revealed a cause for his recent illness.

Examiner information

1. Data gathering in the interview

A good candidate would be able to elicit:

- how long ago the palpitations occurred and what the patient was doing at the time
- any previous history of palpitations
- if they started and stopped abruptly (supraventricular tachycardia, SVT) and how long they lasted for
- how fast did the heart race. Ask the patient to tap it out on the desk
- did the patient take his own pulse at the time of the palpitations? If so, how fast was the pulse rate? Was the pulse regular or irregular? If the patient did not take his own pulse, did he feel any thumping in his chest? If so, how fast and how regular was the thumping? Was there a missed beat and if so did the next one feel heavier?
- whether he presently has any palpitations or irregular heartbeats
- any other associated symptoms such as chest pain, dyspnoea, faintness, anxiety, tremor, recent loss of weight and increased appetite (hyperthyroidism)
- a drug history, e.g. sympathomimetics or salbutamol tablets. How often does he use the salbutamol inhaler? Does he also use a long-acting β2-agonist inhaler?
- details of alcohol, caffeine and tobacco consumption. Has he taken illicit drugs or herbal remedies?
- details of the TIA. Did he have a rhythm problem, e.g. atrial fibrillation (AF), at that time?
- any previous history of heart disease, hypertension, thyroid disorders
- any symptoms of anxiety and depressive disorders
- any concerns that the patient may have.

2. Identification and use of information gathered

The candidate should be able to interpret the history and create a problem list. The objectives for the candidate are to:

- explain the possible differential diagnoses
- arrange a set of investigations
- promise the patient that all the tests will be done as soon as possible.

3. Discussion related to the case

- This case tests the ability of the candidate to (a) decide if the palpitations are related to ischaemic heart disease or due to a non-cardiac cause (other causes of palpitations in the clinic situation, particularly in young people, are caffeine/tobacco induced, anxiety disorder and occasionally thyrotoxicosis), (b) aim to decide if the palpitations were regular (SVT, AF, 2:1 block) or irregular (AF, variable block).
- The most likely cause of the palpitations in this case would be related to ischaemic heart disease and sinoatrial disease and investigations would be tailored towards this (GP has said TFT are normal). This would include glucose, cholesterol, resting ECG, chest X-ray, echocardiogram and a 24-h ECG.
- The examiners will expect the candidate to be able to discuss (a) the management of paroxysmal atrial fibrillation including issues of anticoagulation and (b) the acute management of narrow complex and broad complex dysrhythmias.

Comments on the case

This is a typical case where the patient is presently asymptomatic and the emphasis is on taking a detailed history to work out exactly what rhythm the palpitations characterize – a 24-h ECG will probably show 'sinus rhythm with a few ventricular ectopics'. Tapping out the palpitations is a good way of determining rate, rhythm and mode of onset and cessation. Do not expect the patient to have measured his own pulse when he felt ill.

Case 35 | **Personality change**

Candidate information

You are the doctor in a liver clinic. Mr Matthew Hayward is referred to you by his GP. He is accompanied by the wife (whom you will be speaking with during the consultation).

Please read this letter and then continue with the consultation.

Dear Doctor

Re: Mr Matthew Hayward, aged 42

Thank you for seeing Mr Hayward earlier than usual. You see him regularly for Wilson's disease of the liver. Over the last 4 weeks he has been irritable with bouts of anger directed towards his wife for no obvious reason, together with odd sleeping patterns. Compared to the previous investigations, his liver function tests, clotting and albumin have deteriorated.

Please see and advise.

Yours sincerely

Dr G. Practitioner

You have 14 min until the patient leaves the room, followed by 1 min for reflection, before the discussion with the examiners. Be prepared to discuss the solutions to the problems posed by the case and how you might reply to the GP's letter.

Patient information

Mr Hayward, a 42-year-old unemployed man, first presented 7 years ago with a tremor and abnormal liver function tests. Further investigations confirmed Wilson's disease and slit lamp examination of the eyes showed Kayser–Fleischer rings. Since then he has been reasonably well although his tremor has persisted. He was initially started on penicillamine but developed a rash and fever and was switched over to trientine. Over the last 4 weeks his wife has noticed him to be more irritable, with poor concentration, confusion, bursts of temper and sleeping during the day but not at night. These symptoms are variable, with good and bad days. She has not noticed him to be obviously jaundiced but he has been complaining of tiredness and nausea with a poor appetite. There have been no convulsions, loss of weight, constipation or any obvious abdominal swelling suggestive of ascites and no GI bleeding. His diet has not changed although he is probably not eating as much, nor is he on any other medication. There is no history of taking benzodiazepines or any illicit drugs which may cause hepatic damage. He does drink alcohol, usually about 6 pints of beer during the week, but there has been no sudden increase in alcohol consumption. His compliance with trientine has been patchy due to occasional drug-induced nausea.

He does not smoke and has not been abroad recently. There are no other risks factors for concomitant viral hepatic infections. Mrs Hayward is particularly concerned about the personality change as his current behaviour is certainly out of character for him.

Examiner information

1. Data gathering in the interview

A good candidate would be able to elicit:

- the history of the Wilson's disease, i.e. presentation (neurological, hepatic and occular), diagnosis (serum and urinary copper with caeruloplasmin and liver biopsy), treatment, treatment changes, side-effects to treatment
- present history of behavioural and psychiatric changes and the effect of this on the wife, e.g. personality, mood, tempers, sleep pattern, poor concentration, irritability, confusion, disorientation, slurred speech, self-care
- other liver disease symptoms and signs, e.g. jaundice, ascites, ankle swelling, bruising, itching, urine changes, weight loss, convulsions, nausea and vomiting
- factors suggesting reasons for possible precipitation of portosystemic encephalopathy, e.g. high protein diet/poor nutrition, GI haemorrhages, alcohol, constipation, infection (peritonitis), drug induced, e.g. benzodiazepines or illicit drugs, development of hepatocellular carcinoma, or worsening cirrhosis. Other causes include electrolyte imbalance, e.g. hypokalaemia or hyponatraemia (?diuretic usage)
- any suggestions of other hepatic disease on top of Wilson's disease, e.g. viral hepatitis
- poor compliance with medication and if so why
- social and psychological impact on the family.

2. Identification and use of information gathered

The candidate should be able to interpret the history and create a problem list. The objectives for the candidate are to:

- obtain a history of the Wilson's disease
- obtain a history of the present symptoms suggestive of portosystemic encephalopathy
- determine possible triggers for the encephalopathy, especially poor drug compliance
- provide a plan of investigations and management, including admission to hospital
- explain the possible causes for the deterioration.

3. Discussion related to the case

- Hepatic (or portosystemic) encephalopathy refers to a chronic neuropsychiatric syndrome secondary to liver cirrhosis presenting as a fluctuating disorder of personality, intellect, mood and reversal of normal sleep pattern. Other features include nausea, vomiting and weakness. The most important factors in the pathogenesis are severe hepatocellular dysfunction and/or intrahepatic and extrahepatic shunting of portal venous blood into the systemic circulation so that the liver is largely bypassed. As a result of these processes, various toxic substances absorbed from the intestine are not detoxified by the liver and lead to metabolic abnormalities in the central nervous system (CNS).
- Aside from the build-up of metabolic toxins (e.g. ammonia), cerebral function may also be impaired by altered transmission of neurochemicals (such as an increase in γ-amino butyric acid [GABA]-mediated inhibition) and decreased cerebral glucose metabolism.
- Factors precipitating portosystemic encephalopathy include those mentioned above. Signs include a coarse flapping tremor, constructional apraxia and decreased mental function. Investigations include routine biochemistry, clotting and haematology and an EEG which will show triphasic slow waves.
- A number of conditions can mimic the clinical features of hepatic encephalopathy. These include acute alcohol intoxication, sedative overdose, delirium tremens, Wernicke's encephalopathy, Korsakoff's psychosis, subdural haematoma, meningitis and hypoglycaemia. Other metabolic encephalopathies must also be considered, especially in patients with alcoholic cirrhosis.
- Basic management includes identification and removal of the precipitant, protein restriction and intestinal purgation with lactulose (aiming for increased frequency of motions, at least four a day).
- The neurological manifestations of Wilson's disease include both resting and intention tremors, spasticity, rigidity, chorea, drooling, dysphagia and dysarthria. Psychiatric disturbances are present in most patients

with neurological symptoms. Schizophrenia, manic-depressive psychoses and the classic neuroses may occur, but the most common disturbances are bizarre behavioural patterns that defy classification. Improvement in the psychiatric state can occur with pharmacological reduction of the copper excess, but psychotherapy may be required.

- The treatment of Wilson's disease consists of removing and detoxifying the deposits of copper as rapidly as possible, and must be instituted once the diagnosis is secure, whether the patient is ill or asymptomatic. Penicillamine, which functions as a copper chelator and increases urinary excretion of copper, is administered orally in an initial dose of 1 g daily in single or divided doses. Because penicillamine has an anti-pyridoxine effect, 25 mg/day of pyridoxine is also given. In nearly 10% of patients, sensitivity to penicillamine develops early. White blood cell (WBC) and platelet counts should be assessed and urinalysis performed several times during the first month of treatment. Penicillamine should be discontinued and replaced by trientine if rash, fever, leucopenia, thrombocytopenia, lymphadenopathy or proteinuria develops or if neurological worsening accompanies the institution of penicillamine and persists for a week or more. Treatment must be continued for life. Trientine is not recommended as long-term therapy. It is possible to restart penicillamine after a period of cessation. The symptoms may not recur if oral prednisolone is given before restarting penicillamine. Inadequate treatment, or interruption of therapy, can be fatal or cause irreversible relapse.

- Zinc acetate is a useful adjunct for maintenance therapy of Wilson's disease and works by decreasing enteric absorption of copper. It accomplishes this by inducing intestinal cell metallothionein, which binds copper and prevents its transfer into the blood. Because zinc is essentially non-toxic and the other two agents do have toxic side-effects, zinc may be better tolerated. However, the American Association for the Study of Liver Diseases still recommends penicillamine or trientine as first-line treatment and zinc to be used in patients who (a) cannot tolerate the above drugs or (b) are in the presymptomatic or maintenance phase. Zinc must not be given with penicillamine or trientine as both these agents chelate zinc.

- Patients with acute liver failure or decompensated liver cirrhosis due to Wilson's disease should be assessed for liver transplantation.

Comments on the case

This case tests the ability of the candidate to detect a precipitant for the portosystemic encephalopathy and in this case compliance with taking drugs is an important factor.

Case 36 | Pins and needles

Candidate information

You are the doctor in a neurology clinic. Mr Leonard Willis is referred to you by his GP.

Please read this letter and then continue with the consultation.

Dear Doctor

Re: Mr Leonard Willis, aged 64

Thank you for seeing Mr Willis who still works part-time as a gardener. He gives a 2-month history of pins and needles in both hands. He has a past history of hypercholesterolaemia for which he takes simvastatin 20 mg. His last cholesterol level was 4.8 mmol/L. Other previous history includes an inguinal hernia repair 14 years ago. He also takes aspirin 75 mg od. His BM glucose recorded in the surgery today was 5.0 mmol/L.

Yours sincerely

Dr G. Practitioner

You have 14 min until the patient leaves the room, followed by 1 min for reflection, before the discussion with the examiners. Be prepared to discuss the solutions to the problems posed by the case and how you might reply to the GP's letter.

Patient information

Mr Willis is a 64-year-old part-time gardener who has been complaining for the last 2 months of pins and needles with pain, tingling and numbness in both hands. He is right-handed and the pain first appeared in that hand which was soon followed by pain in the left. The symptoms are worse particularly in the thumb, index and middle finger but they do sometimes affect the whole hand. The symptoms are now occurring at night, causing sleep disruption. Shaking the hands sometimes helps but in the mornings his hands feel clumsy and swollen although later in the day the symptoms are better. He does not have similar symptoms in the feet or arms and he does not complain of any burning sensation in the feet. There are no other neurological symptoms such as weakness in the limbs, tremor, headache, blurred vision, muscle wasting, dysphasia or dysphagia. He has no other respiratory, cardiovascular or abdominal symptoms. His past history includes hypercholesterolaemia (cholesterol 8.0 mmol/L), for which he takes simvastatin 20 mg od, and an inguinal hernia repair 14 years ago. The latest cholesterol measurement last year was 4.8 mmol/L. He has no history of ischaemic heart disease, cerebrovascular disease, peripheral vascular disease, diabetes mellitus, trauma or renal disease. He has never smoked and only drinks one bottle of beer a day at home. He has a normal diet and does not take any other medication except for aspirin. He works with another gardener, usually doing weekly contract jobs. He has noticed that during one job last week, where he had to use a stone cutter to take down an old coal shed, his symptoms immediately returned and persisted for much longer during that day and night. He has not suffered from any cuts or injuries to his hands during his work. He lives with his wife and his main concerns are that his job is being affected by the symptoms.

Examiner information

1. Data gathering in the interview

A good candidate would be able to elicit:
- the time-length of the symptoms and whether they are deteriorating
- if the patient is left- or right-handed
- which hand had the symptoms first and which part of the hand is affected, including which fingers. Are the feet affected as well?
- what are the exact symptoms, i.e. pain, burning sensation, numbness, weakness, clumsiness, feeling of heaviness or tingling
- other neurological symptoms, especially weakness, paraesthesia, tremor or muscle wasting
- other cardiovascular, respiratory and abdominal symptoms, looking for the possibility of cancer, vascular disease and diabetes mellitus
- any previous trauma
- a full drug history, including enquiry about drugs which may cause peripheral neuropathy, especially isoniazid, nitrofurantoin
- a full alcohol history
- dietary history (vitamin B1, B6 and B12 deficiencies)
- metabolic history, especially osmotic symptoms suggestive of diabetes mellitus, renal failure, thyrotoxicosis
- positive hereditary history of neuropathies such as hereditary motor and sensory neuropathy
- causes of carpal tunnel syndrome, e.g. obesity, arthritis, previous fractures of wrists, repetitive strain injury, e.g. vibrating tools (stone cutter), hypothyroidism, acromegaly, pregnancy
- any concerns that the patient has.

2. Identification and use of information gathered

The candidate should be able to interpret the history and create a problem list. The objectives for the candidate are to:

- assimilate a list of differential diagnoses
- explain these diagnoses to the patient
- have a plan of investigations
- arrange follow-up to discuss the investigations.

3. Discussion related to the case

- This case tests the ability of the candidate to differentiate carpal tunnel syndrome from one of the many causes of peripheral neuropathy (diabetes mellitus, neoplasia, drugs, alcohol or idiopathic).
- The case presents with the typical features of carpal tunnel syndrome which tend to affect mainly the dominant hand. In this case, the vibrating tool exacerbates the symptoms. For diagnosis and confirmation, nerve conduction studies should be performed which will show a reduced or absent median sensory nerve action potential (SNAP) from the index finger and prolongation of the latency. EMG may show denervation of the abductor pollicis brevis.
- Treatment may include night-time splints, local steroid injections (temporary relief) and, if necessary, surgical decompression.
- The examiners would expect the candidate to be able to discuss the differential diagnoses for a peripheral neuropathy.

> ### Comments on the case
> This case again demonstrates the importance of taking a detailed history in order to provide the probable diagnosis and distinguish this entrapment neuropathy from a peripheral neuropathy.

Case 37 | Polyuria

Candidate information

You are the doctor in a general medical clinic. Mrs Janet Abrahams is referred to you by her GP.

Please read this letter and then continue with the consultation.

Dear Doctor

Re: Mrs Janet Abrahams, aged 42

Mrs Abrahams gives a 2-week history of polyuria, feeling unwell and being generally tired. Four months ago she had a bout of flu followed by acute bronchitis. The cough has persisted despite three courses of antibiotics. Her recent blood glucose test done at the clinic was 5.8 mmol/L. A chest X-ray is reported as showing 'numerous pulmonary infiltrates and bilateral hilar lymphadenopathy. Please refer to a physician'.

Please see and advise.

Yours sincerely

Dr G. Practitioner

You have 14 min until the patient leaves the room, followed by 1 min for reflection, before the discussion with the examiners. Be prepared to discuss the solutions to the problems posed by the case and how you might reply to the GP's letter.

Patient information

Mrs Janet Abrahams is a 42-year-old accountant who presents with a 2-week history of polyuria and thirst. The symptoms came on suddenly over 2 days and she now passes copious amounts of urine daily (volume exceeds 4 L), including during the night. She says she has to pass urine about every 15 min and it is very dilute. In response to this, she has to drink an equivalent amount of liquid (especially cold fluids) during the day. Associated with this is a cough which first presented 4 months ago after a bout of flu. Despite three courses of antibiotics, the cough persists and is non-productive with no wheeze, sputum or haemoptysis. She feels tired with generalized aches in her body. She has no chest pains, feeling of faintness, palpitations, GI, arthritic or eye symptoms. She has not noticed a change in her periods or her weight. The past medical history includes an appendicectomy when she was 6 years old but no recent head trauma or neurosurgery. Presently she takes no medication and she finished her last course of antibiotics 6 weeks ago. She has never taken corticosteroids. She does not smoke or drink alcohol. She has no psychiatric history. There is no family history of note such as diabetes mellitus or asthma. She lives with her husband and two children who are all well. She has now stopped working as it was impossible to do her work whilst having polydipsia and polyuria. She is obviously concerned about her symptoms.

Examiner information

1. Data gathering in the interview

A good candidate would be able to elicit:

- a chronological history of the events
- the onset, volume of urine passed, frequency of micturition (day and night) and volume of fluid intake (type of fluids, e.g. cold drinks), colour of urine
- appetite, weight, cough history (dry or with sputum and haemoptysis, worse in the mornings with wheeze), any associated heartburn and sinusitis. Precipitating factors such as common household pathogens
- other general symptoms which may suggest a cause for the polyuria, e.g. diabetes mellitus (osmotic) or cranial diabetes insipidus, e.g. tumours (primary craniopharyngioma, ependymoma, hypothalamic pituitary glioma, lung and breast metastases), infections (tuberculosis, meningitis, cerebral abscess), infiltrations (sarcoidosis, Langerhans cell histiocytosis), postsurgical (transfrontal or trans-sphenoidal), postradiotherapy, vascular (haemorrhage or thrombosis, aneurysm), and head trauma, or nephrogenic diabetes insipidus, e.g. drug induced (lithium, glibenclamide), metabolic (hypokalaemia, hypercalcaemia), familial, renal tubular acidosis
- symptoms suggestive of pituitary dysfunction, e.g. galactorrhoea, amenorrhoea, hypogonadism, visual field defects, hypothyroidism, hypoadrenalism
- psychiatric history (compulsive water drinking)
- full drug history
- relevant past history, e.g. head trauma, head neurosurgery
- smoking and alcohol history
- impact of symptoms on family and work
- the concerns of the patient.

2. Identification and use of information gathered

The candidate should be able to interpret the history and create a problem list. The objectives for the candidate are to:

- have a complete list of possible differential diagnoses
- explain the chest X-ray findings and to suggest the possibility of sarcoidosis as the cause for the patient's symptoms
- explain what sarcoidosis is
- explain the need to admit for further investigations
- explain the investigations in detail.

3. Discussion related to the case

- This case tests the ability of the candidate to differentiate the possible causes of polyuria and polydipsia. The differentials are stated above. The most likely cause is sarcoidosis with pituitary involvement.
- Initial investigations are biochemistry, including osmolalities of blood and urine, ACE, MRI scan of the head and bronchoscopy with a transbronchial biopsy to confirm a tissue diagnosis of non-caseating granuloma. In this case there is no need to do water-restricting investigations.
- The diagnosis may be made on early-morning paired plasma and urine osmolalities but, if these are normal, a water deprivation test will need to be undertaken. The principle of this test is to withhold fluids while monitoring plasma and urinary osmolalities. If the patient loses more than 3% of the total body weight on hourly measurements during the test and the serum osmolality is >300 mOsm/kg, it should be stopped and a dose of desmopressin given and the patient allowed to drink. Otherwise monitoring is continued by plasma and urinary osmolalities for 8 h, then desmopressin is given and the patient allowed to drink. A normal response is for the plasma osmolality to remain within the normal range (280–295 mOsm/kg) and the urine/plasma (U/P) osmolality ratio to rise to >2.0.
- In pituitary diabetes insipidus the urine osmolality fails to rise appropriately and the urine volume remains inappropriately high in spite of a rising plasma osmolality. Plasma osmolality rises to >300 mOsm/kg and the U/P ratio remains <2.0 with urine concentration increasing normally after administration of desmopressin.
- The treatment should include intranasal synthetic vasopressin analogue desmopressin (DDVAP) 10–20 μg od or bd or orally 100–200 μg tds. The patient should start on high-dose corticosteroids, e.g. prednisolone 40 mg od, for the sarcoidosis and be tailed down slowly. She should be offered bisphosphonates as well because of the long-term steroids.

Comments on the case

This case highlights the importance of the information given by the GP to enable the candidate to direct the history taking.

Case 38 | Pruritus

Candidate information
You are the doctor in a general medical outpatient clinic. Mrs Shirley Baxter is referred to you by her GP.

Please read this letter and then continue with the consultation.

Dear Doctor

Re: Mrs Shirley Baxter, aged 52

Thank you for seeing Mrs Baxter who has been complaining of generalized pruritus and increasing fatigue for the last 6 months. I have tried her with lubricant bath oils initially with some soothing effect but now her itch is worse and keeps her awake at night. She is normally fit and well and I enclose the following routine blood results. She takes no regular medication. Please see and advise.

Hb 11.3 g/dL, WCC 6.8 × 10^9/L , platelets 354 × 10^9/L, Na 139 mmol/L, K 4.1 mmol/L, urea 3.9 mmol/L, creatinine 74 mmol/L, bilirubin 12 μmol/L, alanine aminotransferace 29 U/L, alkaline phosphatase 290 U/L, albumin 39 g/L, glucose 5.1 mmol/L.

Yours sincerely

Dr G. Practitioner

You have 14 min until the patient leaves the room, followed by 1 min for reflection, before the discussion with the examiners. Be prepared to discuss the solutions to the problems posed by the case and how you might reply to the GP's letter.

Patient information
Mrs Baxter is a 52-year-old school secretary who has been normally fit and well without any time off work for ill health. However, over the last 6 months she has been complaining of a persistent generalized pruritus. She has tried various bath oils with some initial soothing effect but the itch has now worsened. She finds that the pruritus keeps her awake at night and she has scratched herself to such an extent that her skin is raw and bleeding. Associated with this is a recent feeling of generalized tiredness and she is finding it hard to concentrate at work. There are no other symptoms of loss of weight or appetite, or of cardiovascular, pulmonary or GI origin, including jaundice, bowel habit alteration, haematemesis or PR bleeding or any thyroid and neurological symptoms. No rashes have been seen and her skin looks quite normal except for the scratch marks. There has been no occupational exposure to fibre-glass or to pruritus-provoking recreational or domestic agents. The past medical history includes a Colles' fracture when she was 8 years old. She does not suffer from anxiety or depression. She takes only paracetamol for occasional head-

aches and no herbal remedies. She lives with her husband and has three grown-up children. Her husband is well with no similar itching. She has not been in close contact with anyone else. She does not smoke and only drinks three glasses of wine per week. Her main concerns are about the possible cause for the pruritus and her poor sleeping.

Examiner information

1. Data gathering in the interview

A good candidate would be able to elicit:
- the timing of the pruritus, and whether this is persistent or intermittent, improving or deteriorating, and the extent and severity of her scratching
- which part of the body has the pruritus and which part of her body started first. Do her eyes itch?
- any relieving factors, e.g. bath oils, or provoking factors, e.g. stress, depression, drugs, certain foods
- whether the pruritus affects sleep and work
- whether there are any associated skin rashes, pruritus ani and/or vulvae
- living conditions and contact history, e.g. anyone with scabies
- occupational exposure, e.g. fibre-glass
- systemic symptoms, e.g. tiredness, jaundice (primary biliary cirrhosis, haemochromatosis), fever, weight loss (malignancy, especially lymphoma), osmotic symptoms (diabetes mellitus), thyroid symptoms (hypo- or hyper-), history of chronic renal failure, history of HIV
- drug history, including herbal remedies
- any recreational and domestic agents, e.g. skin creams, biological washing powders
- psychiatric illness, especially anxiety and depression
- alcohol and smoking history
- impact of the pruritus on her and family.

2. Identification and use of information gathered

The candidate should be able to interpret the history and create a problem list. The objectives for the candidate are to:
- develop a list of differential diagnoses
- explain the possibilities to the patient
- show that one blood test was slightly abnormal (alkaline phosphatase) and to explain that one cause could be related to the liver
- plan and explain the investigations to be arranged, particularly concentrating on primary biliary cirrhosis

- address the problem of the pruritus with general advice such as avoiding soaps but to tell her that follow-up will be arranged soon with results of further tests.

3. Discussion related to the case

- This case tests the ability of the candidate to work out the possible systemic causes of pruritus. The raised alkaline phosphatase possibly suggests primary biliary cirrhosis that can present with pruritus before the appearance of any jaundice. Other possibilities include diabetes mellitus, hypo- or hyperthyroidism, chronic renal failure, haemochromatosis, polycythaemia, HIV infection, and internal malignancy such as a lymphoma. Topical causes, e.g. washing-up liquid/clothes detergents, drug-induced and psychological histories are, however, still very important.
- Other tests not performed as yet can include thyroid function, lipids, iron studies, autoantibody screen (antimitochondrial antibodies). If autoantibodies are positive then the next step would be an ultrasound of the liver and a liver biopsy.
- The candidate would be expected to discuss the management of pruritus (usually difficult) using cholestyramine (4g sachet three times per day), and ursodeoxycholate (10–15mg/kg daily in 2–4 divided doses) in improving liver enzymes and pruritus, prognosis and the role of liver transplantation.

Comments on the case

This case also tests the candidate's ability to read the GP's letter carefully. The finding of an abnormal alkaline phosphatase level should enable the candidate to structure his or her history taking without forgetting the possibilities of other systemic medical causes. The candidate must not forget to ask about other recreational and domestic skin contacts.

Case 39 | Purpuric rash

Candidate information

You are the doctor in a haematology clinic. Mrs Christine Bunch is referred to you by her GP for an urgent assessment.

Please read this letter and then continue with the consultation.

Dear Doctor

Re: Mrs Christine Bunch, aged 36 years

Thank you for seeing urgently this lady who has presented with a 4-day history of a purpuric rash. I cannot detect any obvious bleeding. Her FBC is as follows: Hb 11.1 g/dL, WCC 8.4 × 10^9/L, neutrophils 6.7 × 10^9/L and platelets 20 × 10^9/L. She is normally fit and well and takes no medication. Please see and advise.

Yours sincerely

Dr G. Practitioner

You have 14 min until the patient leaves the room, followed by 1 min for reflection, before the discussion with the examiners. Be prepared to discuss the solutions to the problems posed by the case and how you might reply to the GP's letter.

Patient information

Mrs Christine Bunch is a normally fit and well 36-year-old lady who works in a florist shop and presents with a 4-day history of a gradual onset of a purpuric, non-blanching rash which started in both hands but now covers both arms and legs. The purpuric spots are flat, bright red, well-circumscribed and varying in size with larger lesions seen particularly on the arms. She feels generally quite well though she has always had a tendency towards bruising. There is no associated epistaxis, bleeding gums, haematuria, lymphadenopathy, fever, weight loss, abdominal pain, arthritic pain or vaginal bleeding. Her last menstrual period (LMP) was 2 weeks ago and her periods do tend to be heavy. There is no recent history of a viral illness or any previous history of purpuric rashes, lymphoproliferative disorders or coagulopathies. She has not taken any medication such as anticoagulants, steroids or antibiotics. Her diet is satisfactory with fresh fruit and vegetables and there has been no recent history of trauma or blood transfusions. She has no HIV risk factors and lives with her husband and one son who are both well. She does not smoke or drink. She is obviously concerned about the rash.

Examiner information

1. Data gathering in the interview

A good candidate would be able to elicit:

- how long the purpura has been present for and if it has occurred before
- what distribution the rash covers
- a description, i.e. size, shape, colour, circumscribed, raised, itchy, blanching
- associated symptoms such as epistaxis, bleeding gums, haematuria, fever, weight loss (?evidence of leukaemia or secondary malignancy), abdominal pain, arthritic pain and vaginal bleeding and menstrual blood loss
- if she has noticed any lymphadenopathy
- relevant past medical history of lymphoproliferative disorders, liver disease or recent viral infections (Epstein–Barr virus [EBV], toxoplasmosis, cytomegalovirus [CMV])
- a family history of bleeding and coagulopathies or collagen disorders, e.g. Ehlers–Danlos or connective tissue disorders such as SLE
- a drug history, especially anticoagulants, steroids, sulphonamides, chloramphenicol
- a dietary history, especially vitamin C
- recent trauma, head injury or blood transfusions
- the concerns of the patient.

2. Identification and use of information gathered

The candidate should be able to interpret the history and create a problem list. The objectives for the candidate are to:

- formulate a possible list of differential diagnoses
- explain the possibilities to the patient
- explain that it would be ideal to admit for assessment
- have a plan of investigations and include an explanation of the bone marrow biopsy procedure
- explain that you may have to treat with steroids and explain their side-effects.

3. Discussion related to the case

- This case typically describes idiopathic thrombocytopenic purpura (ITP) in a young woman. She does not have any active bleeding. The other possibilities for consideration are bone marrow failure (e.g. leukaemia, infiltration by secondary malignancy), coagulation deficiency (e.g. thrombotic thrombocytopenic purpura, disseminated intravascular coagulation, haemolytic uraemic syndrome), secondary to other autoimmune conditions (e.g. systemic lupus erythematosus, antiphospholipid syndrome), drug induced (e.g. heparin, quinines, sulphonamides, chloramphenicol, steroids), and infection (e.g. EBV, CMV and toxoplasmosis) and others such as Henoch–Schönlein purpura.
- Most adults with ITP have symptoms that persist for many years and it is then referred to as chronic ITP. Women aged 20–40 are afflicted most commonly and outnumber men by a ratio of 3/1. They may present with an abrupt fall in the platelet count with bleeding similar to that of patients with acute ITP. Usually they have a prior history of easy bruising or menorrhagia. These patients have an autoimmune disorder with antibodies directed against target antigens on the glycoprotein IIb-IIIa or glycoprotein Ib-IX complex.
- The only blood count abnormality is the thrombocytopenia. Bone marrow examination reveals normal or increased numbers of megakaryocytes. Platelet antibodies can be looked for but are not reliably specific. Antinuclear antibody testing is useful in looking for SLE. Patients with splenic enlargement and atypical lymphocytes should have EBV serology and HIV should not be overlooked in high-risk patients. Bone marrow examination may be useful, especially in older patients, to rule out myelodysplasia.
- Treatment is aimed at reducing platelet antibodies with corticosteroids. Haemorrhage can be controlled usually with corticosteroids but, in rare cases, patients may require temporary phagocytic blockade with rituximab or intravenous immunoglobulin (IVIG). Although IVIG is an effective form of therapy, it is quite expensive and should be reserved for patients with severe thrombocytopenia and bleeding and for those who have not responded to other measures. Emergency splenectomy is usually reserved for patients with acute or chronic ITP who are desperately ill and have not responded to any medical measures designed to improve haemostasis.
- The candidate will be expected to discuss the differential diagnoses of purpura, the investigations and the treatment of ITP.

Comments on the case

This case is an important 'describe the rash' history. For all rashes, the candidate should have a set list of questions to ask, i.e. distribution, colour, size, shape, surface, itch, etc.

Case 40 | Pyrexia

Candidate information
You are the doctor in a general medical clinic. Mr Mark Hamilton is referred to you by his GP.

Please read this letter and then continue with the consultation.

Dear Doctor

Re: Mr Mark Hamilton, aged 35

I would be grateful if you could see this man who works for British Petroleum and, after a business trip to Nairobi 4 weeks ago, has developed a fever. A FBC, U&E, LFT, malarial screen and chest X-ray have all been normal. He has no relevant past medical history. Please see and advise.

Yours sincerely

Dr G. Practitioner

You have 14 min until the patient leaves the room, followed by 1 min for reflection, before the discussion with the examiners. Be prepared to discuss the solutions to the problems posed by the case and how you might reply to the GP's letter.

Patient information
Mr Mark Hamilton is a 35-year-old previously fit gentleman who works for British Petroleum overseeing their investment in Africa. He attended a 1-week business meeting in Nairobi 4 weeks ago. Whilst he was there he felt reasonably well and was staying in a four-star hotel. However, 3 days after coming back, he started to feel tired and feverish, particularly at night, although he would not drench the bed sheets. He has not measured his temperature but his wife tells him he feels as if he is 'burning'. The temperature comes and goes for around 12 h. He has had a slight cough but he puts this down to smoking. He has also had one bout of loose stools. He has lost 1 kg of weight as a consequence of a reduced appetite. There are no symptoms of sputum, haemoptysis, shortness of breath, abdominal pain, headaches, weakness of the arms/legs or lymph nodes. His past medical history is unremarkable. Whilst he was out there, he went sightseeing and does admit to being bitten by mosquitoes on one particular day. He took proguanil daily for malaria chemo-prophylaxis throughout his trip but stopped these when he arrived back in the UK. He is intolerant to mefloquine (strange dreams) and chloroquine (sickness). Whilst in Nairobi, he had no bouts of food poisoning nor did he eat uncooked food served at street cafés. There is no family history of tuberculosis or any contact with known cases. Other recent trips include one to Lagos (4 months ago) and one to Cape Town (2 months ago); he was well throughout both these trips. He is heterosexual, never

had contact with prostitutes and has never injected drugs. He smokes 15 cigarettes a day, and drinks about one pint of beer a day. He lives with his wife and has no children. His wife is a teacher who works with young children. She does admit to having felt slightly coryzal recently.

Examiner information

1. Data gathering in the interview

A good candidate would be able to elicit:
- when he came back from Nairobi, how long he was out there for and whether the fever coincided with the trip. Did he have other trips abroad and, if so, was he well during these?
- if he has measured his temperature. If so, how high does it go and is it constant or intermittent? Does the fever ever disappear? How often does it peak?
- other symptoms, e.g. rigors, loss of weight, poor appetite, chills, fatigue, pain, respiratory, cardiovascular, gastrointestinal, neurological (headache, neck stiffness), night-sweats, lymphadenopathy, joint pains and rashes
- if there is any relevant past medical history, e.g. infections, i.e. malaria, pneumonia, tuberculosis, or recent surgery and trauma, neoplasia, connective tissue disorders and liver disorders
- drug history, especially malaria chemoprophylaxis and compliance (ideally 1 week before, during the trip and for 4 weeks after arriving back in the UK), previous immunosuppressives, e.g. corticosteroids, antibiotic therapy
- assess HIV risk, especially contact with prostitutes
- contact history, especially family (viral illness, sore throat)
- alcohol history
- the patient's concerns.

2. Identification and use of information gathered

The candidate should be able to interpret the history and create a problem list. The objectives for the candidate are to:
- assemble a list of differential diagnoses
- explain that the cause of the temperature is uncertain
- explain the possibilities
- highlight a list of investigations to be carried out.

3. Discussion related to the case

- This case describes a pyrexia of unknown origin lasting for 3 weeks or more. The possible diagnoses are extensive and include (a) infective, e.g. malaria, TB, pyogenic abscess, urinary, biliary, joint, subacute bacterial endocarditis (SBE), viral (EBV, CMV), and others (Q fever, toxoplasmosis, brucellosis), (b) cancer, e.g. lymphoproliferative (lymphoma, leukaemia), renal cell carcinoma, hepatocellular carcinoma, (c) immunogenic, e.g. drug induced, connective tissue and autoimmune (e.g. SLE, rheumatoid), sarcoidosis, (d) miscellaneous, e.g. irritable bowel disease (IBD), thyrotoxicosis, (e) factitious and (f) unknown causes.
- The possibilities in this case include malaria (proguanil is inadequate for total chloroquine-resistant *Plasmodium falciparum* and he did not take the full chemoprophylaxis for 4 weeks after returning back to the UK), tuberculosis (cough, loss of weight, tiredness, night-time fever), non-specific viral illness; and always think of HIV infection.
- Investigations include repeating the earlier tests in case something new turns up, especially the malaria screen, blood cultures, repeat chest X-ray, full respiratory pathogen screen including viral, *Chlamydia*, *Coxiella* and *Legionella*, sputum, if any, for alcohol- and acid-fast bacilli and consider giving him a thermometer with a chart and reviewing him again shortly with the chart and blood results. Even if a malarial screen has been normal, it is worth repeating the screen a few more times. Bone marrow aspiration may have to be considered if none of the investigations points to a diagnosis.
- In order to determine tolerance and to establish habit, prophylaxis should be started 1 week before travel and continued at least 4 weeks after leaving. For sub-Saharan Africa where chloroquine resistance is widespread, recommendations include mefloquine 250 mg once weekly or, in the presence of intolerance, chloroquine 300 mg once weekly and proguanil hydrochloride 200 mg once daily.

Comments on the case

This example typifies a case where the diagnosis is not known – and it may never be! Unless a detailed history is taken, the investigator will not be able to focus on his or her pattern of investigations. Do not be afraid to ask about contact with prostitutes, particularly those visiting parts of central and east Africa. Individuals may always conceal such activity and hence one must be vigilant for HIV infection, especially if odd symptoms such as sore throats due to oral thrush (in the absence of antibiotics and corticosteroids) and lymphadenopathy are present.

Case 41 | **Renal colic and haematuria**

Candidate information

You are the doctor in a general medical clinic. Mr Dennis Bingley has been referred to you by his GP.

Please read this letter and then continue with the consultation.

Dear Doctor

Re: Mr Dennis Bingley, age 78

Thank you for seeing Mr Bingley who had an episode of left-sided renal colic accompanied by macroscopic haematuria 3 weeks ago. His past medical history is unremarkable except that he has atrial fibrillation for which he takes digoxin 125 μg od and aspirin 75 mg od.

Your sincerely

Dr G. Practitioner

You have 14 min until the patient leaves the room, followed by 1 min for reflection, before the discussion with the examiners. Be prepared to discuss the solutions to the problems posed by the case and how you might reply to the GP's letter.

Patient information

Mr Dennis Bingley is a 78-year-old former gardener. Three weeks ago he developed a severe, sharp, colicky left-sided pain in the renal area, which lasted for 3 h and was accompanied with macroscopic haematuria. The pain radiated down to his suprapubic area and it was relieved by an intramuscular injection of diclofenac given by his GP. The macroscopic haematuria appeared soon after the onset of the renal colic and was visible throughout the stream. He does not remember passing any stones in his urine. Since this episode he has had no more episodes of renal colic and haematuria. He has suffered with prostatism for many years with symptoms of poor initiation, poor stream and postmicturition dribbling but has no dysuria. He had never noticed any blood in the urine until this recent episode. He was diagnosed as having atrial fibrillation by the GP 5 years ago for which he takes digoxin 125 μg and aspirin 75 mg once daily. He does not take warfarin. He has no respiratory, cardiovascular or abdominal symptoms. He does not complain of any loss of weight or appetite. He does not have diabetes mellitus, any coagulation problems or a previous history of kidney stones. He has not suffered any recent trauma. He lives alone and leads an active life, undertaking his own shopping and house cleaning. He stopped smoking 25 years ago and does not drink alcohol. His GP has told him that he may have kidney stones but he is concerned he may have cancer.

Examiner information

1. Data gathering in the interview

A good candidate would be able to elicit:

- the history of the renal colic, including the site of the pain, the severity, the nature, the time span, radiation, any relieving factors and any aggravating factors
- the history of the haematuria, including if it was frank blood or diluted by urine and whether the haematuria was visible throughout the stream (suggests that the site of the haemorrhage is the bladder or above), at the beginning of micturition with the urine clearing towards the end of the stream (suggestive of bleeding from the urethra) or at the end of micturition (suggestive of bleeding from the bladder base or prostate)
- whether any stones were passed in the urine
- other urinary symptoms such as dysuria, poor stream, postmicturition dribbling
- any past episodes of haematuria and prostatism
- any past history of renal stones or renal disorders
- any history of hypercalcaemia, coagulation disorders or recent trauma to the back
- any medication including anticoagulants
- any family history of renal disorders, e.g. cystic disease
- other respiratory (cough, sputum, fever, haemoptysis), cardiovascular (palpitations, chest pains) and gastrointestinal (change in bowel habit, per rectal bleeding) symptoms
- history of smoking and alcohol
- any known allergies, e.g. contrast
- the impact of the illness on the patient and his concerns.

2. Identification and use of information gathered

The candidate should be able to interpret the history and create a problem list. The objectives for the candidate are to:

- develop a list of differential diagnoses
- explain the possible causes for his symptoms
- arrange relevant investigations
- address his concerns and particularly his worry about a possible cancer.

3. Discussion related to the case

- Haematuria (blood in the urine) can produce red to brown discoloration depending on the amount of blood present and the acidity of the urine. Slight haematuria may cause no discoloration and may be detected only by microscopy or chemical analysis. Haematuria without pain is usually due to renal, vesical or prostatic disease. In the absence of red blood cell (RBC) casts (which usually indicate glomerulonephritis), silent haematuria may be caused by a bladder or kidney malignancy. Such tumours usually bleed intermittently and should not be dismissed if the bleeding stops spontaneously. Intermittent, recurrent haematuria may also occur in IgA nephropathy. Other causes of asymptomatic haematuria include calculi, polycystic disease, renal cysts, sickle cell disease, hydronephrosis and benign prostatic hyperplasia. Haematuria accompanied by excruciating pain (renal colic), as in this case, suggests the passage of a ureteral calculus or a blood clot from renal bleeding. Haematuria with dysuria is also associated with bladder infections or stones.
- The presence of one or more red blood cells per cubic millimetre in an unspun urine sample results in a positive dipstick test for blood and this is abnormal. The test is sometimes too sensitive, giving false-positive results in normal individuals. A positive dipstick test should always be followed up by microscopy of the urine sample to confirm the presence of red cells and so exclude haemoglobinuria or myoglobinuria which may also give false-positive dipstick tests. Microscopy may also demonstrate red cell casts which indicate bleeding from the kidney, particularly in glomerulonephritis.
- Bleeding may come from anywhere within the urinary tract and other investigations include urine cytology, plain abdominal X-ray, ultrasound of the renal tract and intravenous urography. These results will determine any further investigations, e.g. cystoscopy, abdominal CT scan, etc.
- Common causes of bleeding from the kidney include stones, cysts (single or multiple), trauma, carcinoma, glomerulonephritis, tuberculosis, papillary necrosis, infarction, tubulointerstitial nephritis and coagulation defects.

Comments on the case

This case tests the candidate's ability to obtain a thorough history of haematuria and renal colic. The candidate will be expected to discuss a management plan with the patient and to address his concerns about cancer.

Case 42 | Tiredness

Candidate information

You are the doctor in a general medical clinic. Mr Steven Waugh is referred to you by his GP.

Please read this letter and then continue with the consultation.

Dear Doctor

Re: Mr Steven Waugh, aged 48

Thank you for seeing this pleasant man who works for the city council as a personnel manager. He complains of tiredness during the day for the last year. He is regularly found at work by his colleagues asleep at his desk and 5 weeks ago he fell asleep at the wheel of his car, driving off the motorway onto the embankment. Past medical history includes hypertension for which he takes amlodipine 10 mg od and he is overweight at 110 kg. Recent FBC, U&E and thyroid function tests have all been normal.

Yours sincerely

Dr G. Practitioner

You have 14 min until the patient leaves the room, followed by 1 min for reflection, before the discussion with the examiners. Be prepared to discuss the solutions to the problems posed by the case and how you might reply to the GP's letter.

Patient information

Mr Waugh is a 48-year-old man who works for the city council as a personnel manager. He gives a 1-year history of falling asleep at his desk during the day. This may happen up to five times per day and particularly during the afternoon. He has an all-day desk job with very little activity or exercise throughout the day. His colleagues have found him asleep at his desk on so many occasions that presently he is at the receiving end of numerous taunts. He does not sleep well at night and feels tired and exhausted from the time he wakes up in the morning. He has always been a heavy snorer and occasionally his wife has noticed him stopping breathing; this induces his wife to shake him to arouse him and this is then followed by a grunting noise. Unfortunately, the snoring has recently been so bad that his wife now sleeps in a separate room. When he is not at work, e.g. at weekends, falling asleep in front of the television has been a common occurrence but more worrying was the recent car accident. Falling asleep at the wheel of the car and swerving from lane to lane, particularly on the motorway, has been a problem for a number of years, but this is the first time he has had an accident. No alcohol was found when the police breathalysed him. Other symptoms of note are nocturia (three times a night) and occasional morning headaches but there is no obvious dyspnoea, chest pain, cough, sputum or ankle swelling. He has been hypertensive for 10 years and takes amlodipine. He has always been overweight and has a size 18 collar. He does no physical exercise and drinks three cans of lager at home in the evening. He does not smoke. The snoring is obviously causing marital strife (with reduced sexual activity) and problems at work and he is desperate for help.

Examiner information

1. Data gathering in the interview

A good candidate would be able to elicit:

- how long the lethargy has been present and whether it is deteriorating or disabling
- an idea of which daily routine activities are affected by the symptoms compared to before the onset of the illness
- if the fatigue is worse with activity and better during rest (myasthenia)
- symptoms suggestive of obstructive sleep apnoea such as apnoeic episodes during sleep, feeling of poor sleep quality, daytime somnolence (falling asleep at work, in front of the television and whilst driving), loud snoring, nocturia, restlessness at night, morning headaches and reduced libido. Ask for the size of neck collar and weight
- other possible physical symptoms suggestive of endocrine disorder, especially hypothyroidism, cardiac failure, respiratory disease, renal failure and limb weakness
- past medical history of neoplasm, viral illnesses, thyroid disorder or surgery, diabetes mellitus or a psychiatric illness
- psychological symptoms, e.g. stress/anxiety, depression, poor sleep pattern, marital strife
- occupational history
- social history
- smoking and alcohol history, particularly at night which may exacerbate sleep apnoea
- drug history (legal and illegal), especially anxiolytics and benzodiazepines which aggravate sleep apnoea
- the concerns of the patient.

2. Identification and use of information gathered

The candidate should be able to interpret the history and create a problem list. The objectives for the candidate are to:

- decide which diagnosis the story fits with best
- be able to relay the possible differential diagnoses although in this case the likelihood is obstructive sleep apnoea (OSA)

- explain what OSA is (without jargon)
- explain that you would like to arrange a sleep study and what this may entail
- explain that if the findings of the sleep study are suggestive of OSA then continuous positive airway pressure (CPAP) may be considered
- counsel him on the alcohol intake, explaining that drinking at night may exacerbate symptoms and discuss the strategies for losing weight which can improve symptoms.

3. Discussion related to the case

- The case tests the ability of the candidate to take a detailed history and to differentiate the possible causes of tiredness such as OSA (in this case), endocrine disorders, anaemia, postviral illness, heart failure, metabolic or anxiety/depression (with poor sleep quality).
- The candidate should undertake FBC, U&E, LFT, calcium and thyroid function tests if not already done. For sleep apnoea, the Epworth Sleepiness Scale (a questionnaire) is useful to determine the likelihood of OSA. A score of over 15 out of 24 is suggestive (but not totally indicative) of OSA. The scale asks the likelihood of falling asleep when (a) sitting and reading, (b) watching television, (c) sitting in a place of activity (work), (d) passenger in a car for 1 h, (e) lying down to rest in the afternoon, (f) sitting and talking to someone, (g) sitting quietly after lunch (without alcohol), (h) sitting in the car when stopped. A sleep study (polysomnography) is performed and sleep laboratories differ in ways of performing such studies but the majority perform pulse oximetry (looking for hypoxic episodes), heart rate variability monitoring (which reflect arousals during sleep) with videoing, EEG traces and a microphone to detect levels of snoring during the night. Other departments may include recording of thoracoabdominal movements to detect any paradox (excessive movements as a consequence of airway obstruction).
- The candidate should be able to discuss the use of nasal CPAP, the impact of OSA especially with regard to road traffic accidents and discuss other causes of tiredness, especially postviral illnesses, and endocrine causes.

Comments on the case

Tiredness and lethargy are common complaints but the candidate must be aware of not falling into the automatic assumption that there may be no organic explanation. A detailed history must be taken considering all the possibilities, especially as OSA can be treated.

Case 43 | Tremor

Candidate information

You are the doctor in a neurology clinic. Mr Walter Matthews is referred to you by his GP

Please read this letter and then continue with the consultation.

> Dear Doctor
>
> **Re: Mr Walter Matthews, aged 73**
>
> Thank you for seeing Mr Matthews who works as a part-time book-keeper at the local church-run library. He is usually fit and well but recently complains of having developed shaking of his hands and is dropping books at work. He is worried that he may have Parkinson's disease. He takes aspirin for a previous TIA which he had 6 years ago. Please see and advise.
>
> Yours sincerely
>
> Dr G. Practitioner

You have 14 min until the patient leaves the room, followed by 1 min for reflection, before the discussion with the examiners. Be prepared to discuss the solutions to the problems posed by the case and how you might reply to the GP's letter.

Patient information

Mr Walter Matthews is a 73-year-old, generally fit and well gentleman, who continues to work as a part-time book-keeper at the local church-run library. Over the last 8 months he has noticed shaking of his hands. These shakes are worse when he is engaged in an activity rather than when he is resting. His wife has now noticed that when he is making the tea, he cannot steadily pass a cup over without some spillage into the saucer. At work, he is finding that putting books back onto the higher shelves is slightly awkward and that he is often dropping them. His shakes do not seem to be deteriorating and there are no other symptoms such as paraesthesia, tingling, coldness, restlessness, rigidity and immobility, slowness of movements, inability to roll over in bed, dribbling of saliva, loss of memory or attention or any psychological changes. There are no particular exacerbating or relieving factors. He has no other neurological symptoms such as headache or limb weakness and no cardiovascular, respiratory, thyrotoxic or abdominal symptoms. His past medical history includes one episode of a TIA 6 years ago when he presented to his GP with a 1-h history of weakness of the left leg which returned back to full strength. He has taken aspirin 75 mg od since then. He takes no other medication. He is unsure about his family history as both his parents passed away when he was young and he has no siblings. He and his wife are self-caring, generally fit and active, taking part in weekly church activities. He has never smoked and he does not drink alcohol. He lives in a three-bedroom house and the toilet is upstairs. His main concern is the possibility of Parkinson's disease.

Examiner information

1. Data gathering in the interview

A good candidate would be able to elicit:

- the time of onset of the tremor and whether it is slowly or quickly progressive
- whether the tremor is confined to the arms or hands or both; which hand/arm is worse
- whether the patient is left- or right-handed
- whether the tremor is worse at rest (Parkinson's) or on sustained posture (benign essential tremor) or fleeting, purposeless, restless and fidgety (chorea) or intentional (cerebellar)
- examples of difficulty such as bringing a glass of fluid to his mouth, passing a teacup and saucer to his wife, etc.
- any associated tremor of the head (titubation) – in benign essential tremor; or blepharospasm – seen also with Parkinson's
- any symptoms suggestive of Parkinson's disease such as paraesthesia, tingling, coldness, restlessness, rigidity and immobility, slowness of movements, inability to roll over in bed, dribbling of saliva, loss of memory or attention or psychological changes
- other neurological symptoms, especially weakness and numbness of limbs, headaches, blurring of vision, dysphasia, dysphagia, etc.
- other respiratory (e.g. cough from aspiration), abdominal (e.g. constipation in Parkinson's) and cardiovascular symptoms (postural hypotension in Parkinson's)
- history of the TIA
- drug medication (e.g. phenothiazines)
- assessment of any anxiety
- history suggestive of thyrotoxicosis
- alcohol history – does alcohol relieve the tremor?
- the impact of the condition on the family.

2. Identification and use of information gathered

The candidate should be able to interpret the history and create a problem list. The objectives for the candidate are to:

- assemble a list of differential diagnoses for tremor
- reassure the patient that the tremor is a benign essential tremor but that this is persistent and may progress slowly
- reassure the patient that he does not have Parkinson's disease
- explain that treatment is limited but one may try β-blockers
- address any other concerns that the patient may have.

3. Discussion related to the case

- This case allows the candidate to explore the causes of a tremor. This case typically describes a benign essential tremor (about 5–8 Hz) during sustained posture and persisting or worsening during action. This is not a parkinsonian tremor as the other classic features of this disease, i.e. resting tremor, rigidity and bradykinesia, are absent. Other possibilities include a physiological tremor exacerbated by anxiety but this is a small-amplitude tremor and rapid (about 8–12 Hz), best seen in the outstretched hands, absent at rest and attenuated through voluntary movements, cerebellar (on reaching a target), alcohol and drug induced such as those causing parkinsonism (neuroleptics), and β-agonist inhalers such as salbutamol, salmeterol and eformoterol as well as hyperthyroidism particularly thyrotoxicosis.
- Management is purely reassurance and, if symptoms continue to be troublesome, β-blockers may be considered.
- The candidate will be expected to discuss in depth the causes of parkinsonism, the features and the treatment of Parkinson's disease from a multidisciplinary perspective.

Comments on the case

This case demonstrates nicely how, by taking a detailed history and asking when the symptoms are worse (i.e. at rest or during action), one can come to the diagnosis and relieve the patient's anxieties by ruling out Parkinson's disease.

Case 44 | Visual disturbances

Candidate information
You are the doctor in a diabetes clinic. Mr Norman Baron is referred to you by his GP.

Please read this letter and then continue with the consultation.

Dear Doctor

Re: Mr Norman Baron, aged 84

Thank you for seeing this gentleman urgently. He complains of episodes of 'zig-zag' vision lasting for up to an hour. He has previously suffered from migraines but he says these current episodes are different. He takes a twice-daily premixed insulin for his diabetes and his last HbA1c was 8.9%. He is on long-acting nifedipine for hypertension. His past history includes a myocardial infarction (7 years ago) and a CVA (5 years ago) when he was found to have a right carotid artery stenosis. He also takes aspirin and his blood pressure today was 130/72 mmHg.

Please advise on diagnosis and management.

Yours sincerely

Dr G. Practitioner

You have 14 min until the patient leaves the room, followed by 1 min for reflection, before the discussion with the examiners. Be prepared to discuss the solutions to the problems posed by the case and how you might reply to the GP's letter.

Patient information
Mr Baron is an 84-year-old widowed gentleman with diabetes mellitus who has experienced occasional episodes of funny vision over the last 8 weeks – sometimes zig-zag, sometimes blurred with difficulty in reading newspaper print which sometimes becomes shimmery in nature. These may last for up to an hour and they usually resolve spontaneously. There are no triggers and they may come on at any time of the day. There are no associated headaches, loss of consciousness, limb weakness, pain, swelling, redness or any movement problems of the eyes. There is no history of a head injury. His diabetes (first diagnosed 9 years ago) was initially treated with tablets but after an MI 2 years later, coupled with poor glycaemic control, he was changed over to insulin. At present he takes Novomix 30 insulin 16 units am and 12 units pm using a pen device. He has no problems with administering the insulin and his blood sugars are usually stable between 8 and 10. He does not suffer from hypoglycaemic attacks although every few weeks he does have a blood glucose

reading of around 3 and any associated blurred vision recovers after a sugary drink. He has never had any retinal laser therapy. Other past medical history includes a cerebrovascular accident (CVA) 5 years ago presenting as weakness in the left arm, from which he made a full recovery, and hypertension for which he takes long-acting nifedipine. At the time of his CVA, a 50% right carotid artery stenosis was detected but was not operated on. He has had migraine-like headaches but these do not cause any visual problems; only a headache and sickness. He lives alone and is self-caring, mobile and manages to collect his own pension and carry out his own shopping. He stopped smoking 35 years ago and does not presently drink. His only other medication is aspirin od. He is worried about losing his sight and is unsure if these symptoms are related to the diabetes.

Examiner information

1. Data gathering in the interview

A good candidate would be able to elicit:

- if the problem relates to one or both eyes and to which particular area of the visual field
- in detail the exact presentation of the visual symptoms, e.g. clouding (cataracts), painless visual field loss (glaucoma – as opposed to close angle glaucoma presenting with a painful red eye), painless bilateral loss of visual acuity – can he read newspaper print? (macular degeneration), blindness from vitreous haemorrhage and retinal detachment (in diabetes mellitus), progressive night-time blindness (retinitis pigmentosa)
- details of the episodes including frequency, length of symptoms, whether sudden onset and sudden resolution
- establish if the episodes of visual disturbance occur at any particular time of the day or are due to any particular movement or activity
- previous eye problems, retinal screening history and any cataract surgery
- details of the diabetes mellitus and its treatment
- details of the previous stroke, MI and cholesterol levels
- smoking and drinking history
- social history, driving history
- effect of symptoms on daily activities
- the patient's concerns and worries.

2. Identification and use of information gathered

The candidate should be able to interpret the history and create a problem list. The objectives for the candidate are to:

- differentiate the possible causes for the patient's visual problems, i.e. retinal problems (e.g. macular oedema or retinal detachment), migraine, TIAs, postural hypotension or hypoglycaemia, and explain these possibilities
- consider either paroxysmal AF and/or carotid stenosis/emboli as a cause of TIAs. Hypoglycaemia must be excluded as a cause
- recommend that an ophthalmological opinion should be sought unless an alternative diagnosis is obvious.

3. Discussion related to the case

- Further investigation relevant to the differential diagnoses should be considered, i.e. urgent retinal screening/eye hospital referral considered for full retinal examination.
- Postural blood pressure should be measured.
- Further investigations may include CT scan of the head, carotid Doppler, ECG recording (for AF) and a 24-h ECG recording.
- The appearance of neovascularization in response to retinal hypoxia is the hallmark of proliferative diabetic retinopathy. These newly formed vessels may appear at the optic nerve and/or macula and rupture easily, leading to vitreous haemorrhage, fibrosis and ultimately retinal detachment. Not all individuals with non-proliferative retinopathy develop proliferative retinopathy, but the more severe the non-proliferative disease, the greater the chance of evolution to proliferative retinopathy within 5 years. This creates a clear opportunity for early detection and treatment of diabetic retinopathy. In contrast, clinically significant macular oedema may appear when only non-proliferative retinopathy is present. Fluorescein angiography is often useful to detect

macular oedema which is associated with a 25% chance of moderate visual loss over the next 3 years.

- Duration of diabetes mellitus and degree of glycaemic control are the best predictors of the development of retinopathy. Non-proliferative retinopathy is found in almost all individuals who have had diabetes for >20 years (25% incidence with 5 years, 80% incidence with 15 years of type 1 diabetes mellitus).
- Efforts should be made to establish safe control, e.g. diabetes and hypertension, rather than trying to meet targets that may produce sudden effects such as hypoglycaemia or postural hypotension. The choice of the best antihypertensive agent is debatable; calcium channel antagonists and low-dose thiazides have been shown to prevent CVA in this age group but for diabetic patients ACE inhibitors should also be considered.
- New onset of migraine would be unusual at this age whereas the risk of retinal problems from either diabetes or macular degeneration is greater.

Comments on the case

This case demonstrates an elderly gentleman with episodes of disturbed vision possibly due to macular disease or early retinal detachment. The candidate must not forget to ascertain the effect of these symptoms on his daily life. Other causes must be considered and a sense of investigative urgency must be displayed.

Case 45 | Vomiting

Candidate information

You are the doctor in a respiratory clinic. Mr Azhar Khan is referred to you by his TB health visitor.

Please read this letter and then continue with the consultation.

Dear Doctor

Re: Mr Azhar Khan, aged 24

I have asked Mr Khan to come back to clinic today because of his vomiting. He was started on Rifinah '300' 2 od, pyrazinamide 2 g od and ethambutol 800 mg od 2 weeks ago for pulmonary tuberculosis. I have asked him to stop all his tablets until review. Please see and advise.

Yours sincerely

Mrs TB Health Visitor

You have 14 min until the patient leaves the room, followed by 1 min for reflection, before the discussion with the examiners. Be prepared to discuss the solutions to the problems posed by the case and how you might reply to the health visitor's letter.

Patient information

Mr Azhar Khan is a 24-year-old man born in the UK, of Pakistani origin. He works in a fast food chain as a food preparer. He first presented to his GP 6 weeks ago with cough, sputum, loss of weight and feeling generally unwell with a fever. Despite a course of oral amoxicillin, his symptoms persisted and a chest X-ray arranged 3 weeks after the first presentation showed right upper lobe shadowing typical of Mycobacteria tuberculosis. A subsequent sputum sample confirmed the diagnosis on microscopy, making him smear positive. He was started on quadruple therapy 2 weeks ago in the chest clinic: Rifinah '300' two tabs, pyrazinamide 2 g, ethambutol 800 mg, all once a day 30 min before breakfast. He is 54 kg and the doses are correct for this weight. Within 5 days he developed nausea and vomiting after taking the tablets. He would be vomiting up to three times in the morning and the nausea would persist into the afternoon. His appetite has decreased and he has not gained any weight. He has some epigastric tenderness, but no jaundice or right hypochondrial pain. There have been no other symptoms such as diarrhoea, dysphagia, abdominal distension, haematemesis, PR bleeding, skin reactions, peripheral neuropathy or visual disturbances suggestive of retrobulbar neuritis. There are no symptoms suggestive of labyrinthine, endocrine or metabolic disorders. Despite trying to persevere with the medication, his nausea and vomiting continued and the TB health visitor advised him to stop the medication, believing that his symptoms were drug induced. Within 2 days of stopping therapy, his symptoms have improved. LFTs on his first visit to the chest clinic were normal. His cough and sputum persist. Contact tracing has revealed no new cases in his close contacts and, as there were no unusually susceptible individuals such as children or immunocompromised individuals working with Mr Khan at the fast food chain, it was felt that contact tracing should not be carried out here. He has not returned back to work since the microscopic confirmation of the Mycobacteria. He has no past medical history of GI disorders such as oesophageal reflux, dyspepsia, pancreatitis or previous GI surgery. He has no previous or present psychiatric history and he does not take any other medication such as antidepressants, opioids, antibiotics or dextropropoxyphene. He lives with his parents and two younger sisters. He does not drink alcohol or smoke. There is no family history of TB here in the UK or Pakistan. He has only visited Pakistan once when he was 7 years old. He is obviously concerned that his respiratory symptoms have not improved and he has lost confidence in the medication.

Examiner information

1. Data gathering in the interview

A good candidate would be able to elicit:

- chronological events of the symptoms in relation to the medication
- frequency of vomiting and nausea and for how long this persists during the day, i.e. when not vomiting does the nausea persist and if there is any relation to meals
- other GI symptoms, e.g. acid regurgitation, dysphagia, abdominal pain, dyspepsia, bloating, fullness, intestinal obstruction (distension, pain, constipation, borborygmi), diarrhoea, haematemesis and melaena
- any suggestions of hepatitis: jaundice, biliary pain, itching, dark urine
- other side-effects of tuberculosis therapy, especially skin reactions, visual disturbances, peripheral neuropathy (isoniazid). Patient would have spotted orange discoloration of urine due to the Rifinah
- other precipitating factors
- systemic symptoms, e.g. weakness, malaise, weight loss, loss of appetite
- symptoms suggestive of endocrine, metabolic or labyrinth disorders
- past history of GI disorders, e.g. reflux oesophagitis, pancreatitis or endocrine disorders and GI surgery
- psychiatric history (e.g. eating disorders, anxiety), alcohol history and family history of TB
- full drug history, including antituberculous (correct doses related to the weight of the patient), overdosing, antidepressants, opioids, antibiotics, dextropropoxyphene
- information about the contact tracing history and work history, especially contacts there and how long he has been off work
- the impact of the illness on himself and his family, and his concerns.

2. Identification and use of information gathered

The candidate should be able to interpret the history and create a problem list. The objectives for the candidate are to:

- identify quite clearly whether the vomiting and nausea are drug induced or not and to relay this to the patient
- have a list of investigations (e.g. LFTs)
- explain the importance of taking medication for pulmonary TB (6 months) in order to reinforce the importance of compliance
- explain that it is not known which medication is causing the symptoms and that admission to the ward with gradual introduction individually of medication at low doses is needed and this may allow gradual tolerance
- explain that it would be unwise to return to work at this stage until he has had at least 2 weeks of therapy at full doses without any side-effects and with improvement in the respiratory symptoms. He is currently still infectious
- address any other concerns and attempt to reverse any loss of confidence in the treatment
- complete a 'yellow' adverse drug reaction form for the Committee on Safety of Medicines (found at the back of the *British National Formulary*)
- notify this case if this has not already been done.

3. Discussion related to the case

- This case tests the ability of the candidate to make a list of differential diagnoses and to style the history taking appropriately around the symptoms of vomiting and nausea. The history taking should allow the candidate to conclude that the symptoms are related to the antituberculous therapy, particularly as the patient's symptoms eased after cessation of the therapy.
- Other general causes for vomiting include GI causes, e.g. peptic ulcer disease (? with pyloric outlet obstruction), gallstones, pancreatitis, small bowel Crohn's, oesophageal disorders, e.g. stricture, achalasia, functional dyspepsia, alcohol or drug induced and eating disorders and non-GI, e.g. bulimia, alcohol or drug related and psychogenic.
- As the most serious side-effect of antituberculous therapy is hepatitis, urgent LFTs are required to detect any changes in aspartate aminotransferase (AST) and alanine aminotransferase (ALT) levels. Modest elevations of these enzymes are not uncommon and, as a general rule, if levels of ALT and AST rise above five times normal or the bilirubin level is elevated, then the medication must be stopped and smaller doses reintroduced individually once the levels have normalized.
- The British Thoracic Society's guidelines on drug challenges particularly in the case of hepatotoxicity suggest the following: once liver function tests are normal, drugs can be reintroduced sequentially in the order of isoniazid, rifampicin, pyrazinamide with daily monitoring of the patient's clinical condition and liver function. Isoniazid should be reintroduced initially at 50 mg/day, increasing sequentially to 300 mg/day every 2–3 days provided no reaction occurs, and then continued. After a further 2–3 days without reaction, rifampicin at a dose of 75 mg/day can be added to a dose of 300 mg/day every 2–3 days and then to 450 mg (if weight is <50 kg) or 600 mg (if weight is ≥50 kg) as appropriate after a further 2–3 days without reaction. Finally pyrazinamide is added at 250 mg/day increasing to 1.0 g after every 2–3 days and then 1.5 g (for <50 kg body weight) or 2 g (≥50 kg).
- The candidate will be expected to know the side-effects of antituberculous therapy.
- The clinical diagnosis and management of TB, including prevention and control, have been recently updated by NICE (March 2011).
- New recommendations discuss the role of interferon-γ testing for the diagnosis of latent TB.
- Standard 6-month four-drug initial regimen (6 months of isoniazid and rifampicin supplemented in the first 2 months with pyrazinamide and ethambutol) remains the 'standard recommended regimen'.

Comments on the case

The candidate must be able to decide if the vomiting is drug induced or not and he/she has to be able to recognize that the patient may have lost all confidence in the therapy which can possibly endanger future compliance.

Case 46 | Vomiting and forgetfulness

Candidate information

You are the medical doctor on-call. Mr Kenneth French is referred to you by the surgical doctor. The patient is in the toilet so you decide to speak to his wife for more information.

Please read this letter and then continue with the consultation.

Dear Medical Colleague

Re: Mr Kenneth French, aged 75

Mr French was admitted last night with a 1-day history of vomiting. He lives 200 miles away and is currently visiting his son in this neighbourhood. The casualty officer referred him to the surgeons after suspecting small bowel obstruction but the consultant surgeon wonders if in fact the patient is suffering from gastroenteritis, after eating undercooked chicken the day before at a local pub. The reason for referral is for an opinion on the complicated previous medical history of a pituitary adenoma. His electrolytes are as follows: Na 133 mmol/L, K 5.5 mmol/L, urea 9.2 mmol/L and creatinine 123 mmol/L.

Please see and advise.

Yours sincerely

Dr S.H.O. Surgeon

You have 14 min until the relative leaves the room, followed by 1 min for reflection, before the discussion with the examiners. Be prepared to discuss the solutions to the problems posed by the case and how you will respond to your colleague's request.

Patient information

Mr French is a retired 75-year-old librarian. The history is obtained from his wife, Mrs French. Mr French is normally a fit and well, self-caring man who enjoys long walks with the dog. He has a past history of a non-functioning pituitary adenoma for which he first presented 10 years ago to the optician with visual field loss. A CT scan of the head then confirmed the pituitary tumour and this was surgically removed. Since then he has been taking hydrocortisone 20 mg in the morning and 10 mg in the evening, levothyroxine 125 μg per day and testosterone patches. Up until his recent illness there has been no suggestion of lethargy, tiredness or fatigue suggestive of adrenal insufficiency, or weight gain, cold intolerance, constipation and voice changes suggestive of hypothyroidism. He has normal body hair distribution including facial hair. Mr and Mrs French live 200 miles away and 4 days ago they decided to visit their son who lives in the area. On the day before admission, they went out to lunch at the local pub. Mr French did at the time wonder if the roast chicken was undercooked, but decided it was edible. Next day (day of admission), he began to feel unwell followed by continued bouts of vomiting, approximately every hour with nausea in between. There was some non-specific central abdominal pain, but no blood in the vomitus or any diarrhoea. He could not keep any oral fluids down and the son decided that he should come to the casualty department. Mr French wonders if the chicken was the culprit but no other family member had similar symptoms. Interestingly, Mr French forgot to bring his hydrocortisone tablets when visiting his son but felt he might manage without them as he had been feeling so well recently. He does not have a Medic-Alert steroid-dependent card with him either; he cannot remember where he keeps it. The treatment so far has been intravenous fluids and Mrs French says that after he had been given intravenous steroids in casualty, he felt much better and his vomiting has improved. However, Mrs French still wonders if the symptoms are related to the possible gastroenteritis as suggested by the consultant surgeon.

Examiner information

1. Data gathering in the interview

A good candidate would be able to elicit:

- an accurate history of the presenting illness; time of vomiting and its frequency, any blood, presence of nausea between vomiting, associated abdominal pain, swelling, diarrhoea or fever. Any possible food poisoning and, if so, how long before the symptoms was the food consumed?
- a full history of the pituitary problem, e.g. when first presented and with what symptoms, e.g. visual field loss (compression of optic chiasma), any symptoms suggestive of hypothyroidism, e.g. cold intolerance, slowness, weight gain, deepening of voice, skin changes, poor memory, depression, constipation, symptoms suggestive of adrenal insufficiency, e.g. weight loss, malaise, weakness, depression, nausea/ vomiting, abdominal pain, syncope from postural hypotension, or symptoms suggestive of hypogonadism, e.g. poor libido, impotence, loss of secondary hair
- the treatment of the pituitary adenoma and whether he keeps a steroid Medic-Alert card. If not, why and explain the need for this
- the reasons for the steroid non-compliance. Reinforce the importance of compliance
- what treatment has been given so far in hospital
- any concerns.

2. Identification and use of information gathered

The candidate should be able to interpret the history and create a problem list. The objectives for the candidate are to:

- identify the reason for non-compliance
- ascertain the full pituitary history
- decide that the likely cause of the illness is steroid insufficiency and not gastroenteritis (no one else in the family had symptoms suggestive of food poisoning)
- reassure the wife
- reinforce the importance of compliance but accept that the recent lapse was a genuine error due to forgetfulness
- suggest issuing a new steroid Medic-Alert card and counsel for future illnesses, i.e. consider having an ampoule of hydrocortisone at home in case oral therapy is impossible. Say that a referral to an endocrinologist will be made and he/she will be able to advise on this matter.

3. Discussion related to the case

- This patient presents with steroid insufficiency rather than gastroenteritis as the cause of the vomiting and ill health. The omission of his treatment, persistent vomiting, the absence of diarrhoea and the improvement of his condition after intravenous steroids are all suggestive of this diagnosis. The raised potassium would otherwise be unusual if the electrolyte disturbance was due to vomiting alone. It is of note that there was rapid improvement following rehydration and an injection of hydrocortisone. Ongoing management should include intravenous (4 hourly) or intramuscular (6 hourly) hydrocortisone 100 mg or a hydrocortisone infusion together with intravenous rehydration until the vomiting has stopped and the patient is eating. He should then return to his oral hydrocortisone. If there had been a history to suggest an intercurrent illness, then there may be a reason for continuing with a higher dose of an oral steroid for a few days before returning to the patient's standard regime.

• The candidate will need to be able to discuss the management of acute hypoadrenalism, the role of fludrocortisone, investigations for suspected Addison's disease, i.e. synacthen test, and the value of Medic-Alert cards and bracelet.

Comments on the case

This case highlights the importance of thinking laterally for a cause of the illness and not being biased by the surgical colleague's opinion. The history and the urea and electrolytes blood test support the diagnosis of adrenal insufficiency.

Case 47 | **Weakness of the right arm**

Candidate information

You are the doctor on-call in the general medical emergency clinic. Mr Leonard Williams is referred to you by his GP.

Please read this letter and then continue with the consultation.

Dear Doctor

Re: Mr Leonard Williams, aged 74

Thank you for your opinion on this gentleman, whom I have just seen as an emergency, with the complaint that he is unable to use his right arm. He has only recently joined my list so I do not have his full records.

He has been taking aspirin for many years, started by a cardiologist when he had palpitations 10 years ago. Eight years ago he had several episodes of weakness in his left arm and was referred to a vascular surgeon who operated on his neck.

He tells me that this current weakness has improved whilst sitting in the waiting room. On examination, I could detect no weakness or sensory loss in his right arm. Blood pressure is 134/74 mmHg and his pulse is regular.

Please see and advise regarding diagnosis and management.

Yours sincerely

Dr G. Practitioner

You have 14 min until the patient leaves the room followed by 1 min for reflection before the discussion with the examiners. Be prepared to discuss the solutions to the problems posed by the case and how you might reply to the GP's letter.

Patient information

Mr Leonard Williams is a retired 74-year-old right-handed businessman. He has experienced four recent episodes of a sudden inability to use his right arm; the first was 4 days ago, the next two occurred yesterday and the last one was this morning. The first three lasted between 2 and 3 h and the one this morning seemed to persist much longer so he went to his GP for an emergency appointment. His arm was getting better (after about 4 h) as he waited to see the GP. About 8 years ago a similar episode occurred but he is unsure which arm was affected though his daughter remembers it being the left arm. He was admitted to hospital for scans of the head and neck that were then followed by surgery on the right side of his neck to remove a blockage. Ten years ago he saw a cardiologist because of palpitations and was told that his pulse was intermittently irregular during a 24-h ECG recording. He was started on aspirin and digoxin. He has recently become more aware of his palpitations and on one occasion he could feel his heart beating 'very fast'. He has no other relevant history such as hypertension, ischaemic heart disease or diabetes mellitus. His wife has problems with osteoporosis so she cannot do any heavy work. His caring daughter (a senior nurse) lives away and is fully occupied with her three young children. She does not visit very often. He lives in a moderate-sized house that needs a lot of cleaning and maintenance; he thinks that it is all this hard work which has kept him healthy for so long. The neighbours are very helpful but he tends to lead a private life. Mr Williams is worried that there may not be anyone to look after him if he has a stroke or if he needs further surgery.

Examiner information

1. Data gathering in the interview

A good candidate would be expected to elicit:

- a detailed history of the weakness of the right arm, especially the number of recent episodes, which part of the arm first became weak, did this spread to the rest of the limb, any feeling of numbness, etc.
- the disability as a result of the weakness, e.g. lifting cups, doing up buttons, writing; is he left- or right-handed?
- any other associated neurological symptoms, e.g. headache, blurred vision, dysphasia, dysphagia, loss of consciousness, vomiting, seizure, confusion
- a diagnosis of the previous TIA with carotid artery stenosis and a carotid endarterectomy
- the frequency of palpitations, their nature and rate, and to elicit the history of the previous cardiology referral and probable diagnosis
- other general risk factors, e.g. family history, hypertension, ischaemic heart disease, diabetes mellitus, hypercholesterolaemia, smoking history
- that it is probably the daughter who more correctly remembers the side of the weakness. Ask about his daughter's input and ability to provide future care
- a history, including a detailed social history including the details of the house where he lives (including stairs, access to front door, toilet, kitchen facilities) and his activities of daily living
- the concerns of the patient with regard to future care.

2. Identification and use of information gathered

The candidate should be able to interpret the history and create a problem list. The objectives for the candidate are to:

- give a differential diagnosis for the episodes of weakness which includes TIAs and epilepsy

- consider either paroxysmal atrial fibrillation and/or carotid stenosis/emboli as a cause of the TIAs
- pick up the issue of the side of his previous TIAs and how it relates to his previous surgery
- discuss with the patient the possible diagnosis, confirmatory investigations, possible treatment with warfarin and the possibility of further carotid surgery
- appreciate the gentleman's concerns regarding loss of independence and, in particular, his wish not to impose on his daughter.

3. Discussion relating to the case

- This case tests the ability of the candidate to take a detailed history of the current and previous symptoms with an assured and accurate record of the chronological order of events. The patient clearly describes transient ischaemic attacks with a past history of atrial fibrillation (AF).
- Further investigations would include a CT scan of the head, carotid artery Doppler and a 24-h ECG recording. Treatment may include warfarin and/or he may need further carotid surgery. These procedures will need to be explained to him along with the benefits and risks associated with the warfarin treatment. The patient has had invasive carotid surgery in the past so the candidate would need to appreciate that the patient will need to be informed of the changes in surgical approach over the last few years. While it is hopeful that further events, especially cerebrovascular, may be avoided by the anticoagulation, the issue of social care along with the various management options may need to be discussed to reassure the patient that his concerns have been noted.
- Since such patients are always at risk of systemic embolization, particularly in the presence of organic heart disease, life-long anticoagulation must be considered. This is particularly important in the elderly, where the attributable risk of AF for stroke approaches

30%. Several studies have now demonstrated conclusively that the incidence of embolization in patients with AF not associated with valvular heart disease is reduced by life-long anticoagulation with warfarin-like agents. Tools like the CHADS-2 score can help to determine which patients are at high risk of cerebrovascular events due to atrial fibrillation and therefore warrant anticoagulation. Aspirin may also be effective for this purpose in patients who are not at high risk for stroke. Although anticoagulation may be associated with haemorrhagic complications, the risk is largely associated with international normalized ratios (INRs) above the recommended level of 2.1–3.0. Particular risk factors that are relevant here are prior TIAs, systemic embolus or stroke, hypertension, poor left ventricular function, rheumatic mitral valve disease and prosthetic heart valves.

- The candidate will be expected to discuss the issues of anticoagulation, primary prevention of further events, especially controlling blood pressure, and the role of antiplatelet/anticoagulation drugs in cerebrovascular disease.

Comments on the case

While this patient may not be fully abreast of the medical terminology associated with his previous medical history and procedures, he is able to give enough information to allow the candidate to establish his previous diagnoses of intermittent atrial fibrillation, transient ischaemic attacks and carotid stenosis. This gentleman has thought ahead as to what might happen if he were to have a cerebrovascular event and is concerned about the possible loss of independence. These issues need to be discussed.

Case 48 | Weight gain

Candidate information

You are the medical doctor in an endocrine clinic. Mrs Patsy Marlow is referred to you by her GP.

Please read this letter and then continue with the consultation.

Dear Doctor

Re: Mrs Patsy Marlow, aged 44

Thank you for seeing this lady with recent weight gain. She has had type 2 diabetes mellitus for 4 years and until recently has had excellent glycaemic control. In the last 6 months her HbA1c has risen from 7.0% up to 9.8% despite maximal oral hypoglycaemic therapy and the diabetes nurses have arranged for her to change to insulin. Her weight has risen during the last year, from 80 kg up to 91 kg, and she appears to have mainly central obesity. She was found to have raised blood pressure at her recent annual review and I have started her on ramipril. Her free T4 and TSH are both normal. I have explained to her that we need to be sure that she does not have a gland problem for her weight gain.

Please see and advise on management.

Yours sincerely

Dr G. Practitioner

You have 14 min until the patient leaves the room, followed by 1 min for reflection, before the discussion with the examiners. Be prepared to discuss the solutions to the problems posed by the case and how you might reply to the GP's letter.

Patient information

Mrs Patsy Marlow is a 44-year-old housewife who has had type 2 diabetes mellitus for 4 years and is under regular follow-up by the shared primary and secondary care teams. Her main problem is a weight gain of 11 kg, from 80 kg to 91 kg, over the last year. Most of the obesity is around the abdomen and this is accompanied by striae. She has never had striae except during pregnancy. Her diet and appetite have not changed and she is generally quite careful about what she eats. Other symptoms include general tiredness and fatigue during the day when carrying out household work such as washing and shopping, feeling low in mood, poor sleep, thinning of her skin and easy bruising, particularly when knocking herself on the furniture. She has noticed a change in her appearance, with facial acne and hirsutism and her face looks fuller. She has also noticed that her periods are more infrequent with scantier blood loss. Her diabetes has been reasonably well controlled until the last few months and the GP has noticed a rise in the HbA1c over this time. Her blood sugar testing was usually between 4 and 8 but is now more commonly between 8 and 12. The diabetes nurse has suggested the possibility of insulin, about which she has expressed some concern. Recently, the GP has noticed her blood pressure to be raised and she was subsequently started on ramipril. The GP has explained that there may be an 'overactivity of her glands' which may be causing these problems. She was initially quite relieved that there may be a distinct cause for the current problems but further explanations by the GP and warning against the possibility of other co-morbidities such as osteoporosis (if left untreated) have led to considerable anxiety. She is presently on gliclazide 160 mg bd and metformin 850 mg bd. She has never taken steroids, either oral or creams. She does not drink or smoke and is happily married with three children who are in their twenties. Both parents also have diabetes mellitus and her husband works in a petrol station. She is keen to know what investigations will be carried out and whether surgery is needed. Her son is getting married in a few months and she is worried about the changes in her facial appearance.

Examiner information

1. Data gathering in the interview

A good candidate would be able to elicit:
- the details of her weight gain, the distribution, any changes in diet to explain this and length of time of symptoms
- symptoms suggestive of Cushing's syndrome, e.g. change in appearance (?old photos), skin changes, e.g. thinning and bruising, hair growth/acne, striae, weakness especially climbing stairs or standing up from a sitting position (proximal muscle wasting), depression, amenorrhoea/oligomenorrhoea, poor libido, poor sleep
- other secondary clues, e.g. hypertension, worsening diabetes, bony fractures, osteoporosis
- history of the diabetes mellitus, including medication, glycaemic control, family history
- a detailed alcohol history – ?pseudo-Cushing's
- use of steroid medications, including oral, topical and vaginal creams
- her perceptions of the condition, her worries and concerns, particularly about osteoporosis.

2. Identification and use of information gathered

The candidate should be able to interpret the history and create a problem list. The objectives for the candidate are to:
- take a clear history of her symptoms and detect other clues suggestive of Cushing's syndrome

- attempt to gain an idea of a possible aetiology, e.g. alcohol versus an ectopic adrenocorticotrophic hormone (ACTH) cause
- explain the possible diagnoses
- explain the nature of the investigations, e.g. 24-h urine collection for cortisol excretion, dexamethasone suppression tests and blood ACTH levels initially with the possibility of scans (pituitary and adrenal)
- address her concerns regarding facial appearance, osteoporosis, long-term prognosis.

3. Discussion related to the case

- Screening tests include 24-h urinary free cortisol, cortisol circadian rhythm (only on inpatients), overnight and low-dose dexamethasone suppression tests. If cortisol levels fail to be suppressed by low-dose dexamethasone, the diagnosis of pseudo-Cushing's is unlikely but further investigations are directed to the cause of Cushing's syndrome. Suppression of cortisol to <50% on high-dose dexamethasone suppression testing would suggest Cushing's disease (pituitary) and non-suppression would suggest either ectopic ACTH or an adrenal adenoma; in the former, ACTH level will be high and in the latter this should be suppressed. Patients with Cushing's disease show an exaggerated ACTH response to corticotrophin-releasing hormone (CRH).
- Ectopic ACTH syndrome may present with a short history of weight loss with pigmented striae and

pseudo-Cushing's due to alcoholism may also present as obesity.

- The candidate will be expected to discuss the possible causes, including excess alcohol intake and iatrogenic Cushing's due to an excessive use of steroids, and be able to discuss the three main types of Cushing's – pituitary, adrenal and ectopic – and outline the interventions appropriate for these diagnoses.
- Selective trans-sphenoidal resection is the treatment of choice for Cushing's disease. The remission rate for this procedure is about 80% for microadenomas but <50% for macroadenomas. After successful tumour resection, most patients experience a postoperative period of adrenal insufficiency that may last for up to 12 months. This usually requires low-dose cortisol replacement as patients experience steroid withdrawal symptoms as well as having a suppressed hypothalamic-pituitary-adrenal axis. Biochemical recurrence occurs in approximately 5% of patients in whom surgery was initially successful.

Comments on the case

Cushing's syndrome remains a difficult problem to diagnose and manage. The two difficulties, particularly in a case like this, are (a) ascertaining whether patients have a pathological cortisol excess or a physiological disturbance of cortisol production and (b) determining the aetiology of the cortisol excess, which can include iatrogenic administration of glucocorticoids, adrenal adenomas or carcinomas, pituitary adenomas and ectopic sources of ACTH and CRH.

Case 49 | Weight loss and chronic diarrhoea

Candidate information

You are the doctor in a gastroenterology clinic. Mr Paul Jones is referred to you by his GP.

Please read this letter and then continue with the consultation.

Dear Doctor

Re: Mr Paul Jones, aged 23

Thank you for seeing Mr Jones who has returned home from India after 4 months of travelling. He complains of loss of weight and chronic diarrhoea. He has no other significant medical history and takes no medication. Please see and advise.

Yours sincerely

Dr G. Practitioner

You have 14 min until the patient leaves the room, followed by 1 min for reflection, before the discussion with the examiners. Be prepared to discuss the solutions to the problems posed by the case and how you might reply to the GP's letter.

Patient information

Mr Paul Jones is a 23-year-old university graduate who has just spent 4 months travelling around India. He complains of pale, bulky stools which he finds difficult to flush away and this has persisted for around 4 months. He may pass this type of stool up to four times a day and this is associated with a progressive loss of weight from around 75 kg down to 68 kg. Closer questioning reveals that he had had these symptoms on and off for a few weeks before travelling to India. Whilst in India he was generally well apart from these symptoms but he does remember one acute episode of, what he presumed was, 'traveller's' diarrhoea 2 months into his travels. Other symptoms include occasional generalized abdominal discomfort, malaise and tiredness, particularly in the last few weeks. He has no mouth ulcers, jaundice, blood in the stools, vomiting, fever, joint pains or iritis. He has not taken any recent antibiotics, there is no family history of tuberculosis or coeliac disease and he is not aware of being in contact with anyone with tuberculosis in India. There has been no previous bowel surgery or radiotherapy and no other history of autoimmune disorders. He is heterosexual and is living with his girlfriend. He has not been exposed to any HIV risks. He does not smoke or drink alcohol.

Examiner information

1. Data gathering in the interview

A good candidate would be able to elicit:

- the timing of the onset of symptoms in relation to his trip to India
- exactly how long the symptoms have persisted for and whether they are deteriorating
- a full diarrhoea history, particularly frequency, consistency of stools, colour, difficulty in flushing away stools, presence of blood, volume (secretory diarrhoea)
- other abdominal symptoms, including pain and weight loss, and any other systemic symptoms such as mouth ulcers, iritis, joint pains and fever
- possibility of infective episodes of acute traveller's diarrhoea in India
- antibiotic and laxative usage
- tuberculosis history
- previous GI surgery or radiation therapy
- autoimmune disorders, e.g. thyroid disease, type 1 diabetes, idiopathic pulmonary fibrosis, rashes (e.g. dermatitis herpetiformis)
- dietary intake, especially cereals, wheat, rye and barley (coeliac disease)
- the impact of the symptoms on his life.

2. Identification and use of information gathered

The candidate should be able to interpret the history and create a problem list. The objectives for the candidate are to:

- develop a differential diagnosis
- relay these possible diagnoses to the patient
- have a plan of investigations
- address any concerns he may have, e.g. regarding the possibility of a neoplasm.

3. Discussion related to the case

- This case tests the candidate's ability to obtain a detailed history in order to assimilate a list of possible differential diagnoses. The possibilities here are (a) malabsorption, e.g. coeliac disease, bacterial over-growth, tropical sprue, pancreatic disease, (b) infective, e.g. bacterial (*Shigella*, *Yersinia*), protozoan (amoebic dysentery, *Giardia*, *Cryptosporidia*), tuberculosis, parasitic (strongyloides), postinfective irritable bowel, (c) small bowel Crohn's disease causing malabsorption, (d) colonic neoplasm. Irritable bowel syndrome is unlikely with the loss of weight. From the history, the symptoms started before travelling to India which makes postinfective unlikely although *Giardia* can occur in the UK. So, coeliac disease is the probable cause.
- Investigations include FBC, U&E, LFT, serum iron, folate, vitamin B12, calcium and autoantibodies for antireticulin and endomysial antibodies (coeliac) and, if positive, small bowel biopsy. If antibodies are negative, consider small bowel barium follow-through to detect Crohn's disease, diverticulae and fistulae/strictures. Stool samples for infective causes and consideration of ^{14}C-glycocholic acid breath test if bacterial overgrowth is suspected.
- All differential diagnoses cannot be fully explained at this stage and hence it will be important to arrange a follow-up appointment in order to further discuss the results of investigations.

Comments on the case

This case typifies those clinical consultations where the diagnosis can be one of any number of conditions. It is imperative that the candidate does not bombard the patient with technical jargon and keeps the interview simple and reassuring. Explain that you will do all you can to find a cause and then advise on relevant treatment. As in any clinical situation, you must let the patient know which investigations are being performed, and why, and, if possible, when. Patients find it quite distressing to receive requests through the post for tests they are unfamiliar with.

Case 50 | Wheeze

Candidate information

You are the doctor in a respiratory clinic. Mr Jim Barrow is referred to you by his GP.

Please read this letter and then continue with the consultation.

Dear Doctor

Re: Mr Jim Barrow, aged 31

Thank you for seeing Mr Barrow who has been a baker since leaving school. He had asthma as a child and has been perfectly well until last year when he noticed increasing chest tightness and wheeze, despite a trial of salbutamol and beclomethasone inhalers.

Please see and advise.

Yours sincerely

Dr G. Practitioner

You have 14 min until the patient leaves the room, followed by 1 min for reflection, before the discussion with the examiners. Be prepared to discuss the solutions to the problems posed by the case and how you might reply to the GP's letter.

Patient information

Mr Barrow is a 31-year-old baker who works at one of the high street supermarkets. He had asthma as a child but 'grew out of it' at about the age of 9. Until a year ago he managed perfectly well with very few symptoms although a coryzal illness would make him slightly wheezy with a feeling of tightness in the chest. He has not needed any regular inhalers until a year ago when he developed more symptoms, with wheeze and cough particularly during the morning but less so later on in the day. He has minimal sputum and no haemoptysis but has found that he is more tired, with a wheeze, when walking long distances, especially if it is cold. As a baker, his shifts start at 3 am and finish at 11 am. He was started on a beclomethasone MDI inhaler 200 µg two inhalations bd but his symptoms have persisted. His symptoms are definitely worse at work and he finds that he has some relief when he is not at work. When he was away on holiday in Spain 2 months ago, he found he hardly ever needed the inhalers. At work, the most likely allergen to be causing bronchial hypersensitivity is flour. Flour handling, for example when preparing dough, consistently causes him to wheeze and cough whereas the exposure of flour in the actual baking areas is less troublesome. There are no extraction ventilation systems where he works and he does not wear a mask. He has no other allergic triggers apart from viruses and he does have seasonal allergic rhinitis for which he takes loratadine. He does not have a peak flow meter at home. He has no other past medical history of note and he does not smoke. He lives with his partner who also does not smoke. They have no pets at home and their house is not damp. There has been no exposure to TB. His major concerns are the continuing symptoms which are occupationally related. He has never thought of leaving his job as a baker.

Examiner information

1. Data gathering in the interview

A good candidate would be able to elicit:

- a full history of the recent asthma symptoms, especially wheeze, cough, dyspnoea, haemoptysis. What time of the day they are worse. Obtain a chronological order of the events. Ascertain any triggers such as viral illnesses, pollen, house dust mite, animal dander, etc.
- if his symptoms are occupationally related. If so, whether his symptoms improve away from work (e.g. holidays)
- if his symptoms are occupationally related, do they come on straight away or after a time lag during the day?
- what the culprit allergen is. Think about other allergens that may cause occupational asthma, e.g. isocyanates (in varnishes, paints, adhesives) and cleaning solvents at work. Ascertain what exactly he does at work, what his job is (desk job, transportation or is he doing dough preparation/baking most of the time?), how much exposure he gets, etc. Have his symptoms got worse with time?
- past history of allergy and atopy, e.g. asthma, allergic rhinitis, eczema. Any exposure to TB. Any history of oesophageal reflux, sinusitis
- inhaler usage, technique, number of times he has needed the salbutamol as 'rescue inhalations' at work
- other job history since leaving school
- whether he has a peak flow meter at home and, if so, what his readings are
- whether there are any pets at home
- if he is a smoker
- concerns of the patient, e.g. of losing his job due to ill health.

2. Identification and use of information gathered

The candidate should be able to interpret the history and create a problem list. The objectives for the candidate are to:

- identify that the symptoms are occupationally related
- identify a likely allergen, i.e. the flour

- have a list of investigations to prove or disprove occupational asthma
- discuss the consequences of having occupational asthma.

3. Discussion related to the case

- Occupational asthma is caused, in whole or part, by agents encountered at work. Once occupational asthma has developed, the worker's asthma is nearly always provoked, in addition, by other non-specific triggers such as viral infections, cold air and exercise. Individuals with pre-existing asthma are at higher risk of developing an occupational component and the whole pattern of asthma may be transformed, with their livelihoods threatened.
- Looking for trigger factors that precipitate symptoms should be part of the assessment in all patients with asthma. All workers, irrespective of whether they are thought to be exposed or not, should be asked if their symptoms are better on days away from work and on holidays. Workers who have improvement in symptoms away from work may also improve because of avoidance of other allergens such as pets, tree pollen and moulds. Early removal of a sensitized worker from exposure has been shown to improve the prognosis, making early diagnosis particularly important.
- An in-depth occupational history needs to be taken. A chronological account of all jobs, patient exposures to the trigger and the relationship between patient exposure and the onset of symptoms should be documented. The principal points to establish are the materials to which a worker is exposed and the interval between first exposure and the onset of symptoms. If symptoms occur on first exposure, then it is probable that the material is a direct irritant. A period of symptomless exposure would favour occupational sensitization. It is relatively common for bakers to develop symptoms for the first time more than 10 years after first exposure. The problem in this case is chiefly from handling flour.
- Measuring lung function with spirometry in the clinic is relatively unhelpful as the individual is away from work. To obtain satisfactory physiological con-

firmation of occupational asthma, measurements of serial peak flows at work and at home (generally every 2 h), during weekends and during holidays are necessary to see if the peak flows show an occupational influence.

- If occupational asthma is confirmed, issues regarding changing jobs need to be addressed and referral to an occupational physician is recommended. In an ideal world, the material causing sensitization should be substituted but, if this is not possible, relocation within the workplace is recommended.
- In some patients, symptoms may take a long time to reverse and, in a proportion, symptoms with spirometry changes may persist.

Comments on the case

This case stresses the importance of taking an occupational history. It should not be underestimated how common occupational disease is, especially occupational lung disease such as asthma. Physicians should realize that one of the most common causes of occupational asthma in the UK is seen in our own workplace – endoscopy nurses exposed to glutaraldehyde.

Section E
Communication Skills and Ethics

'This included a discussion about living wills, euthanasia, options for pain control and her anger at the "delayed/missed" diagnosis.'*

---

*Section F, Experience 41.

These books exist as they are because of many previous candidates who, over the years, have completed our surveys and given us invaluable insight into the candidate experience. Please give something back by doing the same for the candidates of the future. For all of your sittings, whether they be a triumphant pass or a disastrous fail . . .

Remember to fill in the survey at www.ryder-mrcp.org.uk

THANK YOU

A brief history of the evolution of Station 4

The assessment of communication skills and ethics as a distinct station is now firmly embedded in the MRCP examination. In the early 1990s, the Royal Colleges of Physicians started to test candidates' communication skills by including them in the viva part of the examination. The examiners were asked to engage in role-playing with the candidates. They were expected to ask the candidates to break bad news or to discuss an ethical problem while the examiner played the part of a patient or a relative. An inherent problem with such scenarios was that the examiner often played two or more roles, i.e. they kept changing from being the patient to being the examiner and sometimes they would lapse into being the patient's relative – all without notice and all to the chagrin of the candidate. This was compounded by the fact that the examiners, mostly reluctant at playing these roles, could not play them with any degree of conviction. When the entire examination was being reshaped in 1999, the Colleges took the opportunity of formalizing the assessment of communication and ethics into Station 4. Now you will find a real patient or a professional medical actor who will respond to your skills and behaviour in a way which closely mirrors the reality of human interactions as seen in clinical practice. The examiners watch the interaction for 14 minutes without interfering and then, after you have a minute for reflection as the actor leaves the station, they discuss the issues raised in the remaining 5 minutes.

Although candidates face this station with considerable anxiety, we have heard few complaints about the conduct and fairness of this encounter.

Be prepared for the interview

- You will be given written instructions during the 5-minute interval before you enter Station 4. Read the scenario carefully, identify the principal concerns and work out your approach.
- Once you have entered the room and the examiners have settled you down, greet the actor and verify that they are the person that you are supposed to meet. This is the first step in playing this scenario, as you would do in real clinical practice.
- Address the tasks set in the information given and explain everything clearly in language they will understand. Offer to write things down or draw a diagram if detailed explanations are required.
- Make follow-up arrangements so that the person will have an opportunity to ask you more questions after he has had time to consider what he has been told. If necessary, offer to arrange a second opinion if that becomes an appropriate step to take after your consultation.
- Be prepared to discuss the case, including any ethical dilemmas or legal aspects that have been raised, with the examiners.

In this section of the book, we have covered a diverse range of problems that physicians encounter in their everyday clinical practice. Even if you are faced with a problem not given here, it will be very similar to one of these scenarios and the principles will be the same. Study each scenario and then play it out with a fellow candidate. Communication is sometimes described as a 'soft skill' which is an oxymoron really when we stop to consider how hard it can be! Any doctor who has had to break bad news, contradict strongly held beliefs or diffuse extreme anger will appreciate the impact which their communication skills can have to either positively or negatively influence the outcome of such situations. Self-evaluation of one's own skills can be challenging and, as you prepare for your MRCP PACES, it is prudent to reflect honestly on your strengths and weaknesses. Consider each of the fundamental elements against your current abilities.

This station is about role-playing, both for the actor who plays a patient, relative or healthcare professional and for you – who should, we hope, have little difficulty in playing a sensitive doctor! You must understand that this station is not a test of knowledge of the condition under discussion but a test of your ability to interact and communicate effectively with the patient. Although some knowledge of the ethical and legal issues surrounding such scenarios is important, the essence of the interview is that you should conduct it in a manner that demonstrates that you are in sync with the patient's needs and, when appropriate, can respond with sensitivity and compassion.

The examiners will be scrutinizing how you communicate and will be expecting to see evidence of the core principles that will be present in the capable clinician engaged in using counselling skills or breaking bad news to a patient. The points listed here apply to all professional interviews but are especially important when discussing a sensitive subject. Consider how you communicate as you read through these core principles which will be in the spotlight of the examination room.

Remembering who it's about

'He sailed into my room with his entourage in tow, showing off to the juniors and the nurse and barely acknowledged I was there. I felt like a stuffed exhibit in a museum.'*

You have worked hard to progress in medicine, you are right to be proud of your accomplishments and knowledge but the patient or relative in distress is not there for your benefit or to congratulate you on how clever you may be. What they require from you is that you find out what their problem is, how it is affecting them, have a plan for what to do about it and explain what all of this means to them in a professional and yet compassionate manner.

This principle is especially important when dealing with the angry or frustrated person. Unless you are the specific object of their wrath or displeasure (in which case you need to apologize and sort the situation out as a matter of priority), do not take how they are behaving personally. If you react to 'like with like', then expect the situation to escalate. By maintaining your composure, you give them an opportunity to vent their frustration or anger, which gives you time to hear what is making them so angry. They will soon run out of momentum and then you will be able to let them know that you have understood what they are upset about and acknowledge it and make a plan to help them.

Establishing rapport

'They may forget your name but they will never forget how you made them feel.'†

It is essential that you build a good rapport with the actor/patient in order to develop a dialogue and encourage the person to ask questions. Resist any urge to unburden yourself by giving long strings of information. You need to give them time to pause for thought and formulate questions and voice concerns or anxieties. For example, you should allow space for them to hear what you are saying and leave an adequate pause after which you say, 'I'm afraid I have some bad news to share with you'.

There are numerous resources available which describe body language and behaviours in great depth. If you have difficulty with this then take the time to undertake further reading.‡ Think about what draws you to other people and what alienates you – preoccupation with other things, disinterest, boredom, showing signs of stress or impatience, etc., will all militate against successful rapport; it's exactly the same for patients and relatives!

Pay attention and really listen

'The doctor may also learn more about the illness from the way the patient tells the story than from the story itself.'§

A depressingly recurring criticism in complaints against healthcare professionals is that they have failed to listen to either the patient or their family. Perhaps it would be more accurate to say that we need to *hear what is being said and respond to it.* Our own expectations and experiences can literally block our ears up and make us dangerously presumptuous! For example, looking at the unconscious, frail elderly lady supine in the bed, it may be easy to assume that she is always like that. If her relatives tell you that she is not normally like that and that 2 days ago she was living independently at home and walking to the shops every weekday, you have to hear that and contextualize it with the patient's current status.

Of course, we don't just listen with our ears. A skilled communicator uses their eyes and their brain. Maintaining eye contact throughout the interview is an excellent way of letting the patient know that you are giving them your undivided attention; this does not, by the way, mean fixing the patient with a stare but rather letting their visual focus wander while ensuring that when they next look at you, you are looking at them.

Remember that if the words which are spoken don't match the demeanour or behaviour of the patient or relative, there is incongruence. 'How is the pain at the moment, Mr. Davies?'. 'Oh, it's fine,' replies the patient, grimacing and rubbing his leg vigorously. We ignore incongruence at our own peril and potentially to the detriment of the patient by accepting Mr. Davies' words rather than his actions.

Knowing when to be quiet

'The doctor just kept on talking; I didn't hear what she said after she told me my husband was dying. All I could think about was what we were going to do without him, what about the kids…'*

'Doctor, please be quiet for a minute. All **you** *hear is silence; all* **I** *can hear is noise.'**

Candidates often worry about using silence as they are fearful that they will spend the entire 14 minutes waiting for the patient/actor to say something. Be reassured that this will not happen!

Being quiet is different from really listening. Do not hurry and force the giving of information before the person is ready to receive it. Allow the person to dictate the pace of the interview. The clinician necessarily has objectives which form his/her agenda during a consultation with a patient or a relative. While structure in a consultation is to be commended, it should never degenerate into a tick-box exercise. When it concerns health and life-changing events which may be irrevocable, try to create quiet moments, give the patient time to process what they are hearing and to formulate their own questions which will help you/them to steer the discussion in a direction which is *useful to them*. In clinical practice, the experienced proponent of useful silence soon learns that if they don't fill the gap then the patient will – *when they are ready*.

To touch or not to touch?

'I was so distressed and shocked. As the tears started to come, the doctor just squeezed my hand for a moment and I knew how sorry he felt for us.'*

Some candidates have been told, or they imagine, that using touch in the examinations is a good way to physically demonstrate empathy. Some examiners, we are told, don't like it. So, what to do? We would advise that the individual clinician makes up their own mind about it. Clearly, where cultural standards prohibit the touching of strangers then clinicians will not want to do so and in fact would not be expected to. If you don't like it done to you then don't do it to anyone else.

For those who are naturally more tactile and have touched to comfort before they even realize it, the appropriateness of this and its acceptance by the recipient are instantly recognizable in their reaction. We do not advocate the familiar physical contact which you might demonstrate to a close friend or loved one but, for those in distress who find comfort in a tactile response naturally proffered, we see no harm. Clearly, if the response is one of repugnance then you need to apologize immediately.

Using the right words

'What did the doctor say about that lump in your balls, Fred?' 'Haven't a clue, love, he just kept talking about something to do with orchids . . .'*

You get the drift! Every profession or trade has its own language which is quickly recognized by others and defines the members of that group as belonging together. Unfortunately, it excludes everyone else. Great care needs to be taken to avoid words or phrases which are unfamiliar. The quotation above about Fred illustrates the need to listen to the patient so that you know how they describe their body and *reflect* their own language.

You may find this uncomfortable; however, you have a professional responsibility to ensure that the patient understands that the words you are using relate to the anatomy in question. Ideally, to put the patient at their ease, the skilled communicator will choose to mirror the patient's language.

Euphemisms can cause a lot of misery and misunderstanding. 'Keeping your mum comfortable' may mean to you that the patient is reaching the end of her life and that you are not planning any aggressive medical interventions; however, to the family, it may mean making sure that her pillows are arranged nicely and that she doesn't get cold. Be clear, careful and accurate in what you say.

Breaking bad news

'I could tell that the doctor who told me that I had lung cancer thought I deserved it when he said, 'Well, it should come as no surprise to a man who smokes 60 a day that you have lung cancer.'*

In a case that challenges your own judgement about other people's lifestyles, let's try another one:

'Well, if you had paid more attention to your grandmother than concentrating on your MRCP PACES you would have realized that she had heart failure.'

Both the 60-a-day man and the PACES candidate know that their actions have influenced their outcomes, they don't need to hear it from anyone else or feel as if they are being judged. Give bad news as if you were conveying it to someone who you know and care about. This will help you to draw on your reserves of compassion and sensitivity.

When the situation seems bleak, it can be challenging to find a way to reframe things positively. Using a 'however' can help. The purpose is not to give incorrect information or to make light of the gravity of a serious disease, but rather to find some words of comfort to accompany the bad news. For example, when telling someone that she has multiple sclerosis, you may add, 'I can't disguise the fact that it is an unpleasant thing to have or that it is incurable; *however*, many people with this live a long and active life'. When you have just told someone that he has lymphoma, you may say, 'Yes, it is a form of cancer; *however*, there are many treatment options available'.

Being empathic

*'First you must walk a mile in another man's moccasins.'**

Exhortations to be 'empathic' are commonplace in healthcare today. There are a multitude of definitions available using search engines. For the purpose of this introduction the authors offer the following one. The word 'empathy' (from German *einflügen*, 'feeling into') is described in the *New Collins English Dictionary* as 'the power of understanding and imaginatively entering into another person's feelings'. This graphic, often quoted exemplar of empathy implies that unless you have lived their life, you cannot understand what it is to be them. You cannot say 'I know how you feel'. Clearly, you don't. This isn't happening to you – you are the conveyer of the news and not the recipient! Whilst most patients and relatives will be too inhibited or upset to verbalize this response, they may well think it.

It's probably better to consider how you would want to receive the news that you are about to give. By being genuine and acknowledging the impact of the situation on the patient or relative, you can demonstrate compassion and humanity. 'I can't begin to understand what you are feeling at the moment' or 'I can appreciate why you are angry that I promised to come back to see you and then didn't. I am sorry'.

Being honest

*'I don't know, but I will find out and let you know.'**

Depending on your moral compass, you may need to take a deep breath here.

The pedestal of medicine has crumbled to some degree and patients have risen from their knees. It is clear from coverage in the media that doctors can be fallible and make mistakes, unintentional or otherwise, just like everyone else. Be honest and accept if either you or one of your colleagues has made a mistake. If you do not know something that the person needs to know then say so: 'I'm sorry I do not know this but I will find it out for you'. People who are not doctors are just as skilled at recognizing when health professionals are not behaving honestly. You must explain any legal and ethical issues with honesty and clarity: 'I'm sorry to have to tell you that because of your epilepsy you are barred by law from driving for 1 year. This means that I am obliged to advise you that you need to inform the DVLA and your insurance company. I will have to write it in your notes that I have advised you'.

If the specialty of medicine is seen to be honest then it has integrity and can be trusted. The GMC issues guidance for doctors which explicitly directs clinicians to be honest. Saying you don't know something is perfectly acceptable; it is disrespectful to obfuscate or mislead when you know that you don't know something.

You are not alone

'I am sorry; there is nothing more I can do for you.'*

Your patient or relative may well require expertise or support that extends beyond your profession. It is not enough to do just what is required of you clinically, especially if the patient or relative has other needs. You have an obligation to ensure that those best equipped to meet these needs are involved in the patient's journey. If you need to defer to a senior member of the clinical team, either because your patient asks you to or you know that you have a gap in your knowledge or authority, the patient will appreciate and respect your doing so.

Checking understanding

'I have explained that you have a benign hypertrophy of the prostate and that we are going to proceed to transurethral resection – do you understand?' 'Yes doctor.'*

Find out how much the person knows about the condition in question. This can best be established by asking them what they know about their situation and listening to their response. This enables you to know how to start your conversation with them and provides the base on which you can build your communication. His response can also give you some idea of his level of understanding and conversational ability. For example, you may start by saying, 'Your father was admitted yesterday with pneumonia. May I know what you were told and how much you know about this condition?'. His response, whatever it is, will provide you with an easy beginning to detailing subsequent events. If you are going to tell a patient that he has a lymphoma, you may start with a gentle enquiry such as 'I understand that you were told that you had some glands in your chest which were seen on your X-ray. As you know, we have done some more investigations. Before I talk to you about the results, what thoughts have you had about what we might have been looking for?'. Even if he says he has no idea, you can tell him more about the glands and then build on that.

Most of us don't find it easy to admit that we have not understood something that we think others believe we should have. Misunderstandings create a reduction in co-operation with treatment plans as well as affecting expectations of what can be accomplished for the patient. In the same way that you summarize your diagnosis and treatment plan for the patient, you should ask them to tell you what they have understood. You will avoid potentially frustrating and time-consuming incidents such as repeated reiteration or subsequent formal complaints by adopting this simple tactic.

Ethics

You are very likely to be asked about the ethical dimension in a case for Station 4 so it is worth reviewing your knowledge of the basics of the ethical principles.

Every health professional should have an awareness of the role of ethical practice and thinking in relation to healthcare. The application of an ethical approach to complex situations where conflicting opinions or values may come into play can provide a useful checkpoint in the process of reaching important clinical decisions such as withdrawing or withholding treatment. While you may not be required to be an expert, you should be familiar with the four most commonly cited principles of Beauchamp and Childress (2009) which go some way to inform day-to-day ethical issues.¶

Autonomy

'Personal autonomy encompasses, at a minimum, self-rule that is free from both controlling interference by others and from certain limitations, such as inadequate understanding, that prevents meaningful choice.'¶

In simple terms, this means that if a patient makes *an informed and considered decision* about a proposed treatment or clinical management plan which does not concur with either the clinical team's or the patient's family opinion – *the patient's decision must be respected.*

Beneficence

Most commonly thought of in terms of 'first, do no harm'. The development of biomedical ethics grew out of the revelations about the Tuskegee syphilis scandal, a clinical study that ran in Alabama for 40 years. Patients in Alabama with syphilis were knowingly left untreated after the validation of penicillin as an effective treatment for the condition 6 years after the study commenced. This was wrongly done in order to be able to continue to map their untreated condition and so enable the trial to continue. Clearly, this was a failure to do the right thing.

Non-maleficence

'Non-maleficence – a maleficent act as it may be construed as thwarting, defeating or setting back…' (of her interests).¶

A patient, for example, is not informed about the options available to them because their advising clinician does not favour considering any of the alternatives. Or, a diabetic patient who is directed towards an above-knee amputation in the first instance because their consultant thinks that it will eventually be inevitable.

Justice

'. . . fair, equitable and appropriate treatment in the light of what is due or owed to persons.'¶

In healthcare, resources are not limitless. Difficult decisions are taken every day. On a national level, the work of NICE is focused on the efficacy of drug treatments in the context of national health costs. For the clinician engaged in patient care in the hospital setting, justice is more generally concerned, for example, with weighing up whether or not the overall physiological condition of a patient indicates that they should be admitted to a critical care unit and actively supported where the outcome may not be good against the argument that there is only a limited number of beds available and there may be other patients who may be more likely to have a positive outcome from this level of intervention.

Law

The relationship of law and medicine is important. It informs us of society's expectations about how we conduct ourselves as well as the limits of acceptable practice and behaviour. As healthcare advances are made, they will inevitably be reflected in law. It is your responsibility to keep abreast of the law as it relates to the practice of medicine in the UK. You should in particular be familiar with the Mental Capacity Act and other relevant statutes. It is also important to ensure that you know the requirements expected of you in relation to the Coroner and your professional body's guidance in relation to withholding and withdrawing of treatment, resuscitation and advance directives and that you keep abreast of the developments currently under way regarding physician-assisted suicide and euthanasia.‖

Finally

Being an effective communicator can take time and practice, it can be terrifying when it goes wrong and exhilarating when it goes well. The good news is that you are going to get practice throughout the duration of your life. Spend time with people who are clearly excellent communicators, and ask those you trust to tell you how well you communicate. Learn from those things that you don't do as successfully as you would have liked, as well as from those occasions when you have excelled in your performance. Share your tragedies and your triumphs with your peers and always strive to do your best. Good luck!

*Anonymous quote. Mrs Jane Price, Lead Nurse for Patient Experience, Aneurin Bevan Health Board, kindly enlarged and enhanced this introduction for this edition. The quote was collected by her from conversations with 'real' patients over the course of the years.

†A quote from Maya Angelou. See http://www.goodreads.com/author/quotes/3503.Maya_Angelou [Accessed 2.12.2012]

‡Radcliffe SJ. *Body language for absolute beginners*. Available from http://www.sjradcliffe.com/

Desmond J, Copeland LR. *Communicating with today's patient: essentials to save time, decrase risk and increase patient compliance*. San Francisco: Josey Bass, 2000.

§A quote from James B. Herrick. See http://quotiv.com/quote_12442_The-doctor-may-also-learn-more-about-the-illness-from [Accessed 2.12.2012]

¶Beauchamp T, Childress F. *Principles of biomedical ethics*, 6th edn. Oxford: Oxford University Press, 2009. See in particular pp. 99, 152, 241.

‖Haggert E. *The Human Rights Act 1998 and access to NHS treatment and services: a practical guide*. The Constitution Unit, UCL, 2001. http://www.ucl.ac.uk/spp/publications/unit-publications/78.pdf

Brazier M, Cave E. *Medicine, patients and the law*, 5th edn. London: Penguin, 2011.

Station 4
Communication Skills and Ethics

Case 1 | Consent for a lumbar puncture

Candidate information

You are the medical doctor in the emergency admission unit.

Please read this summary and then continue with the consultation.

Re: Miss Bridget Harvey, aged 31

Miss Harvey has been admitted with blurred vision. On admission, it was noticed that she had bilateral papilloedema and a subsequent enhanced CT scan of the head is found to be normal. The most likely diagnosis is benign intracranial hypertension and the consultant neurologist has asked for a lumbar puncture with measurement of the CSF pressure and, if raised, for therapeutic aspiration.

Your tasks are to: explain in straightforward and succinct terms what benign intracranial hypertension (BIH) is and encourage her to consent to a lumbar puncture.

Subject/patient/relative information

Miss Bridget Harvey is a 31-year-old woman who has had blurred vision for the past 3 weeks. She came to casualty and one of the doctors detected blurring of the optic discs in both eyes (papilloedema). She has just had a computed tomography (CT) scan and is waiting to be told the findings. The medical doctor (the candidate) is about to see her, to explain the most likely cause of her symptoms and to discuss the proposed plan (a lumbar puncture). She is very worried that she may go blind but is very unhappy when she is told that the test will involve having a needle in her back because the idea of a needle going into her spine is frightening.

Thoughts and questions the patient/subject may have

- *What is wrong with me and am I going blind?*
- *I really don't want a needle in my back, what else can you do?*
- *Could I end up paralysed if you make a mistake?*
- *What would happen if I decide not to have the lumbar puncture?*

Examiner information

1. Conduct of interview

- Introduce yourself to Miss Harvey and ask how she is.
- Establish her understanding of her current situation.

- Explain the findings of the CT scan of her head. Reassure her that there is no evidence of a tumour, which is encouraging news.
- Explain that the most likely diagnosis for the blurred vision is a condition called benign intracranial hypertension (BIH). Describe this very briefly, mentioning

that there is increased fluid around the brain and spinal canal and that this is putting pressure on the back of the eyes, hence the blurred vision.

- Ask her if she has ever heard of a lumbar puncture and if she knows how it is done.
- Explain that the best way to diagnose and treat the condition is to have a lumbar puncture which allows the spinal fluid pressure to be measured through a needle in the back. If this is found to be raised, her symptoms can be relieved by taking away some of the spinal fluid.
- Ask her if she has any questions at this stage.
- Address any questions or anxieties which she raises.
- Ask her if she would like you to talk her through exactly what the procedure entails and, if so, explain she has to lie on her left side, keeping very still, and that a needle is inserted into the back after giving local anaesthetic which would numb the skin. The needle is inserted into the space between two vertebral bones (you can indicate this by asking her permission to touch her back or alternatively your own) and into the spinal canal. A certain volume of cerebrospinal fluid (CSF) is removed and the needle is then taken out. Reassure her that the only pain she should experience will be initially when anaesthetizing the area ('a stinging similar to a bee sting').
- Explain that she must then lie on her back for at least 4 h to minimize any risk of headache.
- Ask again if she has any questions at this stage.
- Reassure her that the procedure is carried out under strict hygienic (aseptic) conditions to minimize any risk of introducing infection. Reassure her that she will be conscious throughout with a nurse present to assess any discomfort. Explain that she will need the procedure repeating every few days until the CSF pressure is back to normal and that she may need further CSF pressure assessments in the future. Make sure that she understands this last point by asking her to recap the plan.
- Reassure her that with treatment, the outcome is good but it is important to have regular eye checks and spinal fluid pressure checks to minimize the risk of progressive visual problems.
- If her CSF pressure is found to be raised and she does not want to have serial lumbar punctures to drain it (which is the most effective treatment), explain that there are other options available. This includes weight loss and drugs such as carbonic anhydrase inhibitors (e.g. acetazolamide) which work by lowering CSF production.

- Ask how she feels about going ahead with the lumbar puncture.
- Give her time to allow all the information to be considered.

2. Exploration and problem negotiation

The candidate should be able to:

- reassure the patient that the CT scan of the head is normal
- explain the likely diagnosis and proposed management
- reassure her that treatment for BIH is available
- establish her concerns and respond appropriately
- explain the lumbar puncture procedure
- check her understanding and willingness to consent.

3. Communication, ethics and the law

- Patients have a right to information about their condition and the treatment options available to them. The amount of information you give each patient will vary according to factors such as the nature of the condition, the complexity of the treatment, the risks associated with the treatment or procedure and the patient's own information requirements. For example, patients must have enough information to make an autonomous and informed decision about a procedure which carries a high risk of failure or adverse side-effects, or about an investigation for a condition which, if present, could have serious implications for the patient's employment and social or personal life.
- The information that patients want, or ought, to know before deciding whether to consent to treatment or an investigation may include:
  - details of the diagnosis, prognosis and the likely prognosis if the condition is left untreated
  - uncertainties about the diagnosis, including options for further investigation before treatment
  - options for treatment or management of the condition, including the option of not to treat
  - the purpose of a proposed investigation or treatment; details of the procedures or therapies involved, including subsidiary treatment such as methods of pain relief; how the patient should prepare for the procedure; and details of what the patient might experience during or after the procedure, including the common and the serious side-effects
  - for each option, there should be an explanation of the likely benefits and the probabilities of success,

and discussion of any serious or frequently occurring risks, and of any lifestyle changes which may be caused, or necessitated, by the treatment
- advice about whether a proposed treatment is experimental
- how and when the patient's condition and any side-effects will be monitored or reassessed
- the name of the doctor who will have overall responsibility for the treatment and, where appropriate, names of the senior members of his or her team
- whether doctors in training will be involved, and the extent to which students may be involved in an investigation or treatment
- a reminder that patients can change their minds about a decision at any time
- a reminder that patients have a right to seek a second opinion
- where applicable, details of costs or charges which the patient may have to meet.

> **Comments on the case**
>
> This case highlights the important principles that apply to patients undergoing an investigative procedure. Such principles, as highlighted by the General Medical Council (GMC), can apply to any other procedure, for example endoscopy, bronchoscopy, angiogram, etc. and for treatments, such as radiotherapy or chemotherapy.

Further reading

General Medical Council. *Seeking patients' consent: the ethical considerations. Section 4–5: consenting to investigation and treatment.* London: General Medical Council, 1998.

Case 2 | Consent for oesophagogastroduodenoscopy (OGD)

Candidate information
You are the medical doctor on the gastroenterology ward.
Please read this summary and then continue with the consultation.

Re: Mrs Sandra Okojie, aged 63 years

Mrs Okojie was admitted to hospital yesterday with a 2-week history of melaena. She has had no 'alarm' symptoms such as weight loss or change in bowel habit to report. She has a history of hypertension and rheumatoid arthritis for which she takes amlodipine, co-codamol and meloxicam. She has been haemodynamically stable since admission and aside from a haemoglobin count of 8.5 g/dL and MCV 74 fL, her other blood tests have been unremarkable. She has been transfused with 3 units of blood in the last 24 h and is awaiting an OGD, which is scheduled for this afternoon. She remains on an IV drip and is nil by mouth.

Your tasks are to: explain to Mrs Okojie the likely cause for her symptoms and obtain an informed consent for the oesophagogastroduodenoscopy.

Subject/patient/relative information
Mrs Okojie is a 63-year-old woman who is normally fit and well. She has raised blood pressure and mild rheumatoid arthritis which mainly affects her hands. She takes co-codamol and meloxicam for the arthritis but has needed it more regularly over the last few months as she has also developed back pain. She came in to hospital yesterday after she started passing black, offensive-smelling stools 2 weeks ago. She has no other symptoms, specifically no weight loss, abdominal pains or vomiting of blood. She has been given a blood transfusion and is feeling better now. She lives at home with her husband and is a retired school teacher. She does not smoke and drinks around four glasses of wine a week. She has been told that it is likely that she has had bleeding from her stomach area and will need further investigations for this.

Thoughts and questions the patient/subject may have
- *Can you explain to me why you think I have been bleeding from my stomach?*
- *What can you do to stop the bleeding?*
- *(If the candidate uses abbreviations) What is an OGD?*
- *What is entailed in the procedure you want to do? Is it major surgery?*
- *Will it hurt?*
- *Will I be awake?*
- *Why can't you do an X-ray or a scan?*
- *What would happen if I don't agree to have it done?*

Examiner information

1. Conduct of the interview

- Introduce yourself to Mrs Okojie.
- Ask how she is feeling since the blood transfusion and whether she has had any more episodes of passing black stools or blood from the back passage. Has there been any vomiting (with or without blood)?
- Ask her what she has been told about the possible reason for her symptoms and about what further investigations/treatment has already been proposed – this is important so that you can establish the patient's current understanding of the problem and then set your discussion at the right level.
- Explain in straightforward terms that the symptoms she had when she came in were suggestive of a bleed coming from her stomach or small bowel area. Evidence of blood loss was confirmed by the blood tests carried out. The blood tests did confirm that she was anaemic on admission due to the blood loss which then needed to be corrected first with the blood transfusion.
- The most likely reason for the bleed would be an ulcer or inflammation around the stomach or small bowel and, in her case, the tablets she was taking (specifically meloxicam) would put her at risk of this.
- Ask her if she has heard about a procedure called an oesophagogastroduodenoscopy (abbreviated commonly as OGD) or if she knows of anyone who has undergone this procedure.
- Explain why you want to carry out this test on her, and that it is the best way to be certain about what has caused the blood loss.
- Give a few moments for her to absorb this information before asking if you can explain more about this procedure.
- Tell her in simple terms what the procedure involves – for example 'we help you to swallow a long thin tube – less than the thickness of a pen – which passes into your stomach. The tube has a lens in it which is connected to a video camera that the doctor holds. Images are transmitted to a viewing screen so that the inside of the stomach and small bowel are visualized and any source of bleeding can be treated at the same time, if possible'.
- Use drawings if this would help.
- Give her an opportunity to ask any questions about what you have just told her.
- Explain the proposed benefit of the investigation, including the option to provide treatment – 'if there is any bleeding area seen, then it might be possible to inject it with medications to stop it bleeding further. Alternatively, you may be put on a course of antiulcer medication and/or antibiotics if required'.
- She should be told about whether the procedure will be done whilst she is awake, under sedation or under a full anaesthetic (rarely required for OGDs). If she is going to be awake or lightly sedated, tell her about any pain relief or local anaesthetic she may be given.
- Ask her what she thinks and if she is prepared to have it done.
- If she is prepared to consent, go on to explain how she should prepare herself **before** the procedure (e.g. fasting, omitting any medications), anything she might experience **during** the procedure (discomfort in the back of her throat or choking) and her recovery **after** it (i.e. when she can come back to the ward, any pain she may still experience, etc.).
- You should tell her about the common and rare, but potentially serious, side-effects of the procedure (with the chances of them occurring). In this case, that would include bleeding from any trauma from the endoscope (which may require a blood transfusion), perforation (which may require surgery) and reaction to intravenous sedation (see below for more details). You should also mention that if anything unusual is found during the OGD, the operator may want to take a biopsy of this to be sent to the lab for further analysis.
- You should advise her at this stage about any alternative treatments available, including the option of not to treat, and the likelihood of success for each one.
- Tell her which doctor is overall responsible for the procedure and who else is likely to be present whilst she is having it (including any trainees or students).
- Go through the key points of the discussion and ask her to briefly summarize her understanding as it is important that you know you have explained yourself properly.
- Ask her if she has any questions and if she is willing to sign the consent form or if she would like more time to think about it/discuss with her family. Remind her that she has the right to change her mind at any time.
- Give her any information leaflets or written material you have regarding the procedure.

2. Exploration and problem negotiation

The candidate should be able to:

- explain the likely diagnosis and proposed investigations

- ensure that they have discussed alternative options, benefits and risks which the patient may want to consider
- carry out the process of obtaining informed consent for an OGD (or other similar procedure)
- establish through open questions that the information provided has been understood and that consent is informed.

3. Communication, ethics and the law

- Time is precious and the prudent clinician will always seek to establish a patient's knowledge, experience and understanding of the situation. In the context of exams, why waste time telling someone what they already know? In the context of daily practice, you can make intelligent decisions about the direction and drive of the consultation by establishing the patient's current level of awareness.
- Ensuring the competent adult can make autonomous informed decisions is an ethical cornerstone.
- Providing relevant and accurate information of risks, benefits and outcomes is morally right, as is providing patients with options, including that of doing nothing.
- The basis of informed consent stems from the common law fact that every patient has the right to give or withhold consent to any examination, investigation or treatment that he/she is subject to.
- In order for consent to be valid, three criteria need to be fulfilled.
  - The patient should be **competent**/have the capacity to make the decision.
  - He/she should be **informed** sufficiently about the proposed intervention.
  - He/she should give the consent **voluntarily** (i.e. without coercion from either healthcare professionals or family/friends).
- The overall responsibility for ensuring that informed consent has been given by the patient lies with the doctor (or healthcare professional) who is going to carry out the procedure/examination or provide the treatment (**not** with the doctor who is delegated to obtain the consent).
- In order for the process of obtaining consent to be delegated to another healthcare professional, the consultant in charge should ensure the person to whom the process is delegated:
  - understands the procedure
  - is able to discuss the benefits and risks involved
  - understands about alternatives to the proposed investigation or treatment (as well as what will happen if the investigation or treatment is not done)
  - has received the appropriate training in the process of obtaining consent.
- Written consent is not always required. It should be obtained in the following situations:
  - surgery
  - any invasive procedures or investigations
  - any procedure involving general anaesthesia
  - radiotherapy or chemotherapy
  - use of unlicensed drugs
  - research
  - if there is any reason to believe that provision of consent may be disputed later.
- In the UK, the Consent Forms are standardized across NHS organizations.
  - Consent Form 1: for all patients with capacity who are able to give consent for themselves
  - Consent Form 2: for an adult with parental responsibility who is consenting on behalf of a child
  - Consent Form 3: for a competent adult or a person with parental responsibility consenting on behalf of a child for a procedure that does not involve any impairment of consciousness
  - Consent Form 4: for an adult who does not have the capacity to consent for an investigation or treatment which is clinically judged as being in the patient's best interests (requires two clinicians to sign).

Comments on the case

The ability to take consent is tested in the PACES examination. Therefore, a reasonably good knowledge of what these procedures involve, the intended benefits and how the patient has to prepare for them is required. You should also be aware of the common and serious risks associated with the procedure you are going to talk about with the patient.

Junior doctors may be required to gain consent for certain invasive procedures such as OGD, colonoscopy, bronchoscopy, PEG tube insertion and coronary angiograms. It is your professional responsibility to ensure that you are competent to undertake this. You should only be expected to obtain consent for procedures that you are familiar with and are able to undertake yourself having completed the necessary supervised training and achieved an acceptable level of competency.

In the UK, it is far less common, compared to previous years, that the SHO equivalent would take consent for the consultant undertaking the procedure in advance, and therefore usual practice is now for the consultant or specialist registrar to undertake the consent from the patient. However, the case is a good test of understanding the principles of consent as many trainees in medicine will go on to be trained in specific procedures with strict competency assessments.

Case 3 | Emergency surgery under the principles of 'best interests'

Candidate information

You are the medical doctor on-call. You are about to see Mrs Collins who is the daughter of Mr Watkins.

Please read this summary and then continue with the consultation.

Re: Mr Bill Watkins, aged 75

Mr Watkins is a previously fit 75-year-old man who is brought to casualty unconscious after being involved in a hit-and-run accident. He has been intubated and sedated in casualty by the anaesthetists. A CT scan of the head shows a large extradural haematoma with mid-line shift. He also has a fractured left tibia. After discussing the case with your neurosurgical colleagues, it has been decided to take the patient to theatre directly from casualty to evacuate the haematoma. As he remains intubated and sedated, you decide to speak to the daughter, Mrs Collins, who is waiting in the relatives' room. Mrs Collins, however, is unsure whether her father would ever want to undergo an unpredictable operation, particularly when there is a risk of neurological deficit.

Your tasks are to: explain Mr Watkins's condition to the daughter, explain that an operation is needed and get her opinion in the absence of her father's ability to give his consent.

Subject/patient/relative information

Mrs Collins is the daughter of Mr Watkins, a previously fit 75-year-old, who has just been admitted with a serious head injury after a hit-and-run accident. He also has a broken left lower leg. Mrs Collins is his next of kin and lives two streets away from him. When told by the doctors that her father has to have an operation to remove a blood clot from his head, she is unsure if he would ever want to undergo such a serious operation, particularly with the risk of possible brain damage. He has always been a strongly independent man who has stressed that he would never want to live if he was 'no longer himself', for example, after a stroke. However, he never wrote/made any instructions such as a living will or an advanced directive to support this. He has not given his daughter Lasting Power of Attorney to act for him if he is no longer able to speak for himself. She feels unable to give permission for the operation to go ahead on her father's behalf. She is about to see the medical doctor (the candidate) to discuss his condition. He/she will tell her that her father needs the surgery to try and save his life. She knows that this would be unacceptable to him and will strongly disagree with the doctor giving her this news.

Thoughts and questions the patient/subject may have

- *What are the alternatives?*
- *How much time is there before he would need to have the surgery?*
- *Can I have a second opinion?*
- *What if I say no? Surely it's my right as his daughter to decide this for him when he is unable to?*

Examiner information

1. Conduct of the interview

- Introduce yourself to the daughter, checking that Mrs Collins *is* the daughter of the patient. In a real situation, having a member of the nursing staff present during the consultation would be prudent.
- Explain how sorry you are that her father is in such a critical situation. Say that he has been in a car accident as a pedestrian and describe exactly what has been found on the CT scan without using any medical jargon.
- Give her time to allow all this information to sink in.
- Explain that her father is intubated (explain what this means) and under sedation to keep him free from distress in the emergency room in casualty.
- Explain how critical the situation is, that his life is at risk and that you have spoken to your neurosurgical colleagues who all believe that, without an operation to remove the haematoma, Mr Watkins will die.
- Give her time to absorb this information and ask if she feels able to hear about what the operation will entail.
- Explain the basics of the operation, including the opening of the skull and removal of the clot. Explain that the procedure is relatively straightforward but one cannot wholly guarantee a 100% recovery. Admit that there may be some brain damage and cognitive deficit as a result of neuronal ('brain cells') damage secondary to the haemorrhage or from any other intracranial haemorrhage that cannot be rectified/corrected by the operation.
- The daughter tells you that her father would never agree to such an operation if there was a risk of neurological deficit, even if *not* having an operation could result in death. She asks you to respect this decision.
- Ask Mrs Collins if Mr Watkins has ever made a living will or an advance directive with a solicitor which can be used as a legal document if the need arises. She says no.

- Ask if Mr Watkins has appointed his daughter (or anyone else) as a Lasting Power of Attorney to make healthcare decisions on his behalf, in the event that he is unable to do so. She says no.
- Explain that legally, when the patient is unable to consent, the clinician in charge has to proceed with the treatment that is necessary to save life (as in this situation), when the team feels that this decision is in the best interests of the patient.
- As Mrs Collins is not happy with the decision, you tell her that you will call your consultant to discuss the situation further.

2. Exploration and problem negotiation

The candidate should be able to:

- break the bad news to the daughter clearly but with compassion and empathy
- explain that her father is in a critical condition and give the reasons why
- explain the need for emergency surgery to remove the clot (haematoma) and ask if there has been a living will, advance directive or Lasting Power of Attorney made by Mr Watkins
- appreciate the daughter's feelings with regard to her father's wishes of never wanting to undergo surgery with a risk of brain damage (neurological sequelae)
- explain that although one cannot totally eliminate the risk of neurological sequelae, neurosurgery is necessary to save his life
- gently explain that because of his independence and quality of life before the injury, it is important to give him a chance by carrying out surgery (best interest decision by team) and that you will involve the consultant in this case.

3. Communication, ethics and the law

- In an emergency, where consent cannot be obtained, you may provide medical treatment to anyone who needs it, provided the treatment is limited to what is immediately necessary to save life or to avoid significant deterioration in the patient's health.

- Consent to operate is assumed by the consultant responsible for the patient, unless the patient would have withheld consent. Such evidence may be in the form of a living will or an advance directive.
- The Mental Capacity Act (MCA) 2005 has defined the roles of Lasting Powers of Attorney/Court of Protection in consenting (or refusing) life-saving treatment for persons who do not have capacity to do so (please see Case 38 for details about the MCA 2005).
- It is imperative that doctors should seek such substantial evidence before curtailing treatment.
- When speaking to the daughter, have a senior nurse to accompany you and involve your consultant early and remember to clearly and accurately document all discussions.
- It is important to ask for other members of the family to be involved as different individuals express different views on a situation. However, it is possible that there will be a consensus that their father would not want this surgery. Therefore, a consultation with the medico-legal team at the earliest opportunity would be prudent in such a case.
- A second opinion would also be a wise move in such a situation.

Comments on the case

This is a tricky case with pressure applied by the daughter not to operate. One has to always remember that it is the patient's life at risk and legally, in order to save life, one has to do what is necessary unless there is legal evidence to the contrary. This case tests the candidate's ability to be diplomatic, i.e. appreciating the daughter's views but trying to convey the primary concerns for the patient.

Further reading

General Medical Council. *Seeking patients' consent: the ethical considerations. Section 18: emergencies.* London: General Medical Council, 1998.

Case 4 | A competent patient's refusal of treatment

Candidate information

You are the medical doctor on the cardiology ward.

Please read this summary and then continue with the consultation.

> ### Re: Mr Ronald Higgenbottom, aged 79
>
> Mr Higgenbottom has been admitted to hospital with palpitations and has been found to have atrial fibrillation. An echocardiogram has also revealed moderate left ventricular dysfunction. Your consultant felt that it would be wise to anticoagulate him but, after explaining in depth the pros and cons of anticoagulation, he has made an informed decision not to undertake this and to remain on aspirin. His main reasons are that he does not wish to have his coagulation tested every few weeks for the rest of his life and that he is frightened of having a stroke (cerebral haemorrhage) as he has a tendency to have falls. The daughter, Mrs Anderson, wants to speak to you about this issue. She firmly believes that her father should be anticoagulated as a stroke prevention measure. Mr Higgenbottom, who is capable of making an informed decision, has allowed you to speak to the daughter about his condition.

Your tasks are to: speak to Mrs Anderson about her father's informed decision to decline anticoagulation and discuss the legal and ethical issues surrounding this.

Subject/patient/relative information

Mrs Anderson is the daughter of Mr Ronald Higgenbottom, aged 79. Her father was admitted a few days ago with an irregular heartbeat (i.e. atrial fibrillation). A specific test (an echocardiogram) has shown that the heart was not functioning at its full capacity (moderate left ventricular dysfunction); the implication of this situation is that it increases the risk of stroke. It was felt that anticoagulation therapy with warfarin should be offered as this is the best treatment to reduce the risk of a stroke. Mr Higgenbottom was fully informed of the risks and benefits of anticoagulation by the medical doctor (the candidate). However, after careful consideration, the patient decided to decline anticoagulation and to stay on aspirin. Mrs Anderson is upset that he is not being anticoagulated for stroke prevention.

She wants to talk to the medical doctor (the candidate) about this issue. She is his nominated next of kin and therefore has the view that she has the right to overrule his decision.

Thoughts and questions the patient/subject may have

- *What are the risks of my father not taking the warfarin?*
- *Why aren't you forcing him to take it?*
- *I am his next of kin and know what is best for him so just tell him he must do it!*

Examiner information

1. Conduct of the interview

- Introduce yourself to Mrs Anderson, and establish who she is and her relationship to the patient.
- Ask her what she knows about her father's condition and what her views are on this matter.
- Explain that you do appreciate her feelings but the issue of anticoagulation was fully discussed with her father in terms of the advantages, i.e. reducing the risk of a future stroke, and at the same time he was informed of the possible risks of anticoagulation.
- Explain that following this discussion, he told you that he does not want to be given warfarin.
- Use silence to enable her to absorb this information.
- If she asks why he made this decision then you should explain that you did explore all the reasons why he may not want to be anticoagulated and he remains resolute in his decision.
- Ask her if she has had an opportunity to discuss his decision with him yet and suggest that this would be helpful. Say that you are willing to be present for this discussion if they both agree.
- She may challenge his ability to really know what he is doing, given his age. You should explain that there is no evidence that her father cannot make an informed decision due to incapacity and that her father is legally allowed to decline treatment. As a result of this, physicians are unable to enforce treatment for such patients even if the next of kin is uncomfortable or wants to overrule their decision.
- Try to reassure her that her father is receiving effective treatment and, although admittedly warfarin would have been the treatment of choice, aspirin has been shown to be almost as good in reducing the risk of a stroke.
- Make it clear to the daughter that neither she nor the doctors should put pressure on Mr Higgenbottom to agree to treatment because he has the ability to make an autonomous decision to accept or decline medical intervention.

2. Exploration and problem negotiation

The candidate should be able to:
- ascertain the feelings and wishes of the daughter
- convey the fact that her father has made an informed decision and that they did explore in depth any possible misconceptions about the therapy
- explain that patients who do not demonstrate evidence of being incapable of making an informed decision have the right to accept or decline treatment as they prefer
- explain that despite refusing warfarin, her father will remain on aspirin which will provide some protection against stroke.

3. Communication, ethics and the law

- Health professionals cannot legally examine, or treat, any adult without their valid consent (the management of minors is not addressed here). The principal exception is treatment provided under the Mental Health Act 1983. This authorizes assessment of individuals, their admission to hospital or reception into guardianship and, if necessary, treatment for mental illness. Apart from such compulsory treatment, it is unlawful, would constitute assault and is unethical to treat a person who is capable of understanding and willing to know without first explaining the nature of the procedure/treatment, its purpose and implications and obtaining that person's agreement. Otherwise it would represent a maleficent act.
- People can exercise self-determination by making the autonomous decision to consent to treatment while choosing not to be told the full details of their diagnosis or treatment. If this is their choice, consent remains valid as long as they had the opportunity to receive more information and that they understand that they can ask for information at any stage.
- Competent adults have a clear right to decline medical diagnostic procedures or treatment for reasons which are 'rational, irrational or for no reason'. The person's capacity to refuse treatment is decision specific and time specific. The assessment of capacity is covered in more detail in Cases 38 and 39.
- A patient's capacity cannot be challenged or tested merely because other people don't agree with the choice that they have made. If, however, the patient's present choice appears to contradict previously expressed attitudes then health professionals would be justified in questioning in greater detail that individual's capacity to make a valid refusal in order to eliminate the possibility of a depressive illness or a delusional state.
- In all cases where consent is either uninformed or declined, do remember to clearly and accurately document all discussions.

Comments on the case

This is a common case where the next of kin may blame the physician for not initiating certain therapy for their relative. This response is understandable when a relative cares about a family member and feels helpless in the face of a decision that they consider is wrong. Understanding and acknowledging this response without being drawn into attempts to coerce or cajole the patient is essential. It is important for the physician to be aware of the legal rights of the patient in order to allow them to choose if they want treatment or not.

Physicians who feel pressurized or conflicted can seek advice and support from their professional body, their medical director or their organization's medicolegal team.

Further reading

BMA Ethics Department. *The Mental Capacity Act 2005: guidance for health professionals.* London: BMA, 2007.

Case 5 | **Obesity management**

Candidate information

You are the doctor in the endocrinology clinic.

Please read this summary and then continue with the consultation.

Re: Mr Michael Manos, aged 46 years

Mr Manos has come as a new patient to the clinic for his long-standing weight problem. His height is 1.65 m and his weight 118 kg, giving him a Body Mass Index (BMI) of 43. He has been battling with weight issues for over 20 years without much success. His GP tried him on orlistat briefly but he did not tolerate it well due to gastrointestinal side-effects. He has no other comorbidities such as type 2 diabetes mellitus, hypertension or ischaemic heart disease. He has been reading up on some effective surgical procedures for obesity treatment and has come to clinic to discuss this with you.

Your tasks are to: make an assessment of Mr Manos's weight problem, including any relevant lifestyle factors, and address his questions about management options.

Subject/patient/relative information

Mr Michael Manos is a 46-year-old self-employed businessman. He has always been on the heavier side since adolescence but has steadily gained weight over the last 10–20 years. He has tried a few commercial dietary programmes but cannot stick with them for long because he finds it difficult to regulate his diet due to his unpredictable work hours and, as a consequence, he has very little time to engage in exercise. He is prepared to admit that he indulges in 'fatty foods and sweet treats' every now and again, especially at stressful times, and at the moment the economic downturn is seriously affecting his business. He has seen his GP several times asking for help as he really does want to do something about his weight and eventually she gave him a drug called orlistat. However, he stopped it after a few months because of loss of bowel control when he coughed during an important meeting. He has no other medical problems. He is a non-smoker and drinks about 40 units of alcohol a week. He is married and has three teenage children. One of his friends mentioned that there are new surgical techniques which can make people lose weight dramatically and that he should ask about these. He has come to the clinic today with an expectation that he can ask for, and will be offered, the surgery.

Thoughts and questions the patient/subject may have

- *I have been told about this operation and want to have it.*
- *When he is told that he will have to try and lose weight first, he thinks this is ludicrous because if he had been successful in losing weight the conventional way, why on earth would he be here now?*

Examiner information

1. Conduct of interview

- Introduce yourself to Mr Manos.
- Ask him what he hopes to achieve from today's visit to the clinic. Provide an opportunity for him to explain his needs and expectations without interruption. Listen respectfully and then ask him if you can clarify some information for him.
- Ask him for more information about his weight problem (how long he has suffered with it, what steps he has taken to reduce weight, how it is affecting his life/relationships, etc.).
- Take a brief but targeted social history with regard to his job, smoking and alcohol history, diet and exercise habits.
- Explain that, regrettably, no decision can be made today and outline the process: obesity management is done by a multidisciplinary team including dieticians, physical trainers and doctors (sometimes with psychologists as one's relationship with food can be complex). He will need to try out a dietary and exercise programme first and, although he has had challenges in the past, this team will do their utmost to help him overcome these.
- If he is insistent that dietary advice has not worked for him in the past, then explain the benefits of speaking to a dietician again. This may be particularly relevant because even if he does go on to have bariatric surgery, he will need to follow specific dietary guidance to ensure that desired weight loss is achieved and to prevent side-effects from the surgery (e.g. dumping syndrome).
- Having given him a few moments to consider what he has just heard, ask him what he thinks about what you have said before providing information about what happens after surgery, if he were to be accepted.
- If he is still asking to be referred for weight loss surgery immediately, explain that the surgeons will be very unlikely to operate on him until they know that his diet and lifestyle factors are optimized. Also try explaining that the surgical procedures are not without risks (including the risks of anaesthesia in an obese person, postoperative complications, etc.).
- Reassure him that he will be followed up in the clinic and his progress monitored regularly.
- Ask him if he is prepared to have some basic tests before leaving clinic today and if he asks what they are, explain very briefly what needs to be done: blood pressure, waist–hip measurements and blood tests (including fasting glucose +/− oral glucose tolerance test [OGTT], thyroid function, lipid levels, etc.) to look for coexisting medical problems.
- Before finishing the consultation, explain to him that, in the meantime, you will discuss with your consultant about his request for a referral for surgery and promise him that you will discuss the outcome with him at his next visit to clinic. You may even wish him well with his appointment with the dietician.

2. Exploration and problem negotiation

The candidate should be able to:

- establish the patient's expectations and give a clear and sensitively delivered explanation of the process and the expectations which the clinical team would have of him
- evaluate the patient's weight problem in a sensitive, respectful manner and establish his suboptimal dietary and lifestyle factors
- suggest a management plan for him, including involvement of a multidisciplinary team (including a specialist doctor, dietician, physical trainer and psychologist, if necessary)
- listen to his reaction to what he has heard and address his concerns in an empathetic manner
- be understanding and encouraging throughout the consultation.

3. Communication, ethics and the law

- This is an issue which needs to be dealt with very sensitively and empathically by doctors because patients can have complex insecurities and psychological issues which are either related to their current body image or may be a contributory factor to their weight gain. It is frequently the case that people who have severe weight control problems have often tried countless methods to lose weight. They may have a long history of losing then regaining weight and can be extremely frustrated at the lack of permanent success.
- The possibility of medical causes of weight gain should not be ruled out and all reasonable and relevant investigations should be done. If investigations eliminate a medical cause then the patient needs to be told this, particularly if they are attributing their weight gain to a cause which is not the case. This can of course be done kindly and firmly and aimed at encouraging them to reflect on why they have gained weight.
- The prospect of further dieting and exercising may seem disheartening to a patient who has tried and failed several times in the past. It is important to

consider this requirement from a 'best interest' perspective; it is possible to argue that while the patient may not recognize it as such, weight loss through surgical intervention carries risks as well as benefits. Patients who feel they are not being supported in the NHS may consider private surgery in the UK or abroad. It is worth asking if this is something they have thought about. The clinician has a responsibility to mention to the patient that they must be sure to find out as much as possible about the procedure, risks and benefits and most importantly the aftercare. There have been reports in the UK of incorrectly fitted gastric bands slipping or tightening and causing serious clinical problems.

Comments on the case

Discussing weight-related issues can be tricky. Managing such a consultation tactfully, while at the same time imparting the desired messages to the patient, is the hallmark of a good communicator.

Obesity (in both children and adults) is rising at an alarming rate in the UK and there are now many specialist weight management clinics set up in both primary and secondary care.

The National Institute for Health and Clinical Excellence (NICE) issued guidelines in 2006 with the recommended approach to managing obesity. The candidate is advised to have a working knowledge of these guidelines, particularly with regard to recommended drug treatments and referral criteria for bariatric surgery.

Despite the existence of the NICE guidelines, currently some primary care trusts (PCTs) (to be transformed into Clinical Commissioning Groups) do not strictly adhere to them on commissioning for bariatric surgery and therefore it is not uncommon to see some PCTs only funding bariatric surgery if the BMI is over $50 \, kg/m^2$.

Further reading

National Institute for Health and Clinical Excellence. *Clinical Guideline 43. Obesity: guidance on the prevention, identification, assessment and management of overweight and obesity in adults and children.* London: National Institute for Health and Clinical Excellence, 2006.

Case 6 | Side-effects of cardiac medication

Candidate information

You are the doctor in the cardiology clinic.

Please read this summary and then continue with the consultation.

> **Re: Mr Arthur Palmer, aged 70 years**
>
> Mr Palmer is an elderly gentleman who has had permanent atrial fibrillation (AF) for over 5 years which has been notoriously difficult to treat. He has had failed cardioversions three times before and is now only for medical management by the cardiology team. He was started on amiodarone 15 months ago after his last failed cardioversion and has been reasonably well controlled on this and other rate-controlling medications such as bisoprolol. Other medications include lisinopril, simvastatin, metformin and the anti-coagulant warfarin. Over the last 6 months he has been complaining of a non-productive cough and progressive dyspnoea. A high-resolution CT scan of his chest has shown patchy ground-glass opacities and coexisting reticulonodular fibrotic changes believed to be due to the amiodarone. He has come to the clinic to find out about the results of his CT scan.

Your tasks are to: give Mr Palmer the results of his CT scan and explain to him how the changes may have occurred as a result of his medications.

Subject/patient/relative information

Mr Arthur Palmer is a 70-year-old man, and he used to be reasonably fit and well except for a history of hypertension and tablet-controlled type 2 diabetes mellitus. Around 5 years ago, he started developing recurrent episodes of palpitations and chest pain associated with a feeling of faintness. Doctors told him that he has a 'fast irregular heartbeat' (atrial fibrillation) and, when the tablets were not working, they suggested a method of 'shocking his heart out of it' (cardioversion). They tried this three times without any success. Around 15 months ago the cardiology specialist put him on a medication called amiodarone which he said would control his heart rate and rhythm. Aside from developing sunburn more easily, he hadn't had any problems with this drug. Over the last 6 months, however, he has noticed increasing breathlessness when walking up the small hill to his house and a dry cough but he had put this down to his age. He remembers his GP telling him recently that his oxygen levels were slightly on the low side. He had mentioned this to his cardiology consultant during the last clinic visit and he arranged a CT scan of the chest. He has come back to clinic to find out the result. He is very worried that, if there is something wrong with his lungs, he may end up on lifelong oxygen like his brother who had 'severe emphysema'. He is a lifelong non-smoker and used to work in a clothes warehouse, but was never exposed to any asbestos.

Thoughts and questions the patient/subject may have

- *He may be told that the cause of his breathlessness could be due to his medication and this would understandably make him react!*
- *He may want to ask the doctor (the candidate) if they think that the cardiology doctor should have told him about the risk from the medication.*
- *'I was put on the medication to keep me well, now it's made me sick and you are telling me to stop taking it – does this mean I am going to become even sicker than I am at the moment?'*

Examiner information

1. Conduct of interview

- Introduce yourself to Mr Palmer.
- Enquire about his general health, asking specifically about his respiratory symptoms and how they are affecting his activities of daily living.
- Ask him if he was told anything prior to having the CT of his chest and if he has any thoughts on what might be causing his shortness of breath and cough.
- Explain that the CT scan of his chest was not normal and has shown changes consistent with 'scarring' of the lungs which in the medical field is called fibrosis.
- Ask him briefly about other risk factors that he may have for developing respiratory disease such as smoking and occupational history. As there is nothing remarkable in terms of other risk factors, one has to assume that his interstitial lung disease is a consequence of his amiodarone, especially due to the temporal relationship between starting the drug and the development of his symptoms.
- Explain that there is a possibility that the breathing problem is due to the medication he has been taking.
- Give him a moment to absorb this information.
- Ask him briefly about any other side-effects he may have noticed from the amiodarone (e.g. jaundice, corneal deposits, thyroid abnormalities, peripheral neuropathy).
- He may well respond with annoyance on learning that his chest problems have developed due to the drug started by the cardiology consultant and say 'but no-one told me that this drug could destroy my lungs'. Apologize for the fact that he was not made aware of this side-effect of amiodarone but the cardiologist had felt that this was the best treatment for his atrial fibrillation at the time as it was not responding to other treatment options.
- Inform him that lung complications are a rather uncommon side-effect of amiodarone and it is usually reversible by stopping the drug (however, due to the long half-life of the drug, the improvement may not be apparent for a while). Tell him you will discuss with your consultant the plan from here on but he will most likely need to come off the amiodarone. You will also refer him to the local respiratory consultant urgently and there is a possibility that they may want to start him on a course of steroids 'to reduce the inflammation in the lungs'. Reassure him that you will keep a close eye on the cardiac side of things and start him on different medication if needed to ensure that his atrial fibrillation is optimally controlled.
- You should address any other concerns he might have. If he wants to complain about the cardiology consultant you should acknowledge that and promise to give him the appropriate information to do this later. However, explain that you first want to refocus on the current situation in order to help him now.
- Tell him that amiodarone-induced lung toxicity is reversible in ~75% of people on discontinuing the drug and it is extremely unlikely that he will deteriorate or end up on long-term oxygen.
- End the consultation by giving him your contact details in case he has any other questions and arrange a follow-up appointment.

2. Exploration and problem negotiation

The candidate should be able to:

- explain the CT chest findings to the patient and that they are likely to be due to the drug amiodarone which he was started on for his atrial fibrillation
- give him time to absorb this information and then ask how he is feeling about what you have told him
- deal with the situation in a calm, professional manner. If the patient becomes discontent with your explanations, then stress that giving any drug is a balancing act between benefit and side-effects. Reassure him that the drug was clinically indicated at the time it was started
- make sure that he is provided with information about making a complaint if he wishes to do so later

- ask him if he would like you to explain more about the amiodarone-induced lung toxicity. If he wants to know details, tell him
- impress upon him its potential reversibility if he discontinues the drug
- suggest a plan of action from here on, including referral to a respiratory specialist and that close monitoring by the cardiology team will continue.

3. Communication, ethics and the law

- It is important to understand that when patients are given information that a treatment has had an unwanted adverse effect, the clinician recognizes that this is likely to be upsetting and may even provoke anger. Patients place a considerable amount of trust in health professionals and can feel really let down when things go wrong (whether or not the outcome was a mistake or bad luck). Acknowledging that something has gone wrong is not an admission of liability; neither is saying you are sorry that this has happened.
- We recognize the need to obtain informed consent prior to invasive procedures. However, it is less usual in clinical practice to consider obtaining consent from patients who may be prescribed a drug which is known to have significant adverse side-effects, particularly where there are pre-existing risk factors. Careful discussion with such patients needs to be undertaken before starting a treatment regimen as ethically they should be able to make an autonomous, informed decision to agree or decline this treatment option. In this scenario, the patient could rightfully feel aggrieved and it is arguable that although the clinician prescribed with the best intentions, the patient took a drug which did harm him. Had he been given the information prior to starting then a discussion could have ensued about what to look out for if he took the drug, or whether there were other options to consider.
- Discussing the side-effects of medication requires a fine balance between giving the patient adequate information (especially if being done prior to drug commencement in order to enable him to make an informed decision) but not to put him off the drug. As in the above case, some patients might place the blame on the doctor for 'starting them on such a risky medication' or 'not warning them of the side-effects'. Whilst you need to allow the patient to express his frustration and listen to him, you need to stress that the medication was recommended in his best interests to treat another potentially serious condition.

Comments on the case

Medications which are often brought up in such scenarios include amiodarone, warfarin, statins, digoxin and certain antibiotics.

All drugs may cause adverse effects. The two types of adverse drug reactions that are described are dose-dependent and dose-independent. The former is characterized by an increasing pharmacological effect as the dose is increased. As a rule, such reactions are less serious and rapidly resolve on stopping the drug. Dose-independent reactions are usually more serious with a large variability between individuals in their susceptibility to an adverse effect.

Amiodarone can give rise to several systemic side-effects such as photosensitivity, bluish discolouration of the skin, thyroid abnormalities, deranged liver function tests and corneal deposits.

Pulmonary toxicity is the most feared of the side-effects of amiodarone and can affect 5–10% of patients taking it. Risk factors for this are older age, daily dose >400 mg, treatment duration >2 months and pre-existing lung disease.

Case 7 | Presentation of a first seizure

Candidate information

You are the doctor working on a medical ward.

Please read this summary and then continue with the consultation.

> **Re: Miss Zarina Ahmed, aged 18**
>
> Miss Ahmed is a young girl who is studying for her A-levels in college. She was brought into hospital as an emergency by her parents yesterday evening after a witnessed seizure. This was managed with diazepam given by the ambulance crew and she was subsequently drowsy for a couple of hours in the A&E department. She had a CT head scan which was normal. She feels much better this morning and is keen to go home. Her parents would like to speak to you about the circumstances of the recent admission, but you need to gain the patient's permission in order to do this.

Your tasks are to: explain to the patient, Miss Ahmed, about the seizure she had, how she is going to be managed (including the implications on her lifestyle) and find out to what extent she wants her parents to be informed.

Subject/patient/relative information

Miss Zarina Ahmed is an 18-year-old British Pakistani woman who has been excelling at school. She is hoping to study media studies at university after A-levels this year. Yesterday, she came home from college complaining of a headache. Shortly afterwards she collapsed on the sofa and doesn't remember anything else until she woke up in hospital. She has since been told by her father that after she collapsed, her arms and legs started jerking and this lasted about 5 min. Apparently she was frothing at the corner of her mouth and bit her tongue. She woke up gradually over the next few hours and feels much better this morning. Zarina is usually fit and well and is not on any regular medication. She abstains from cigarettes, alcohol and recreational drugs. She recently passed her driving test – she doesn't have a car yet but hopes to buy one when she goes away to university in the autumn. She has been under quite a bit of stress recently in preparation for her A-level examinations as there are high expectations. She is keen to know if she can be started on medication to prevent such an event from recurring because she is worried it might happen again during her examinations. She realizes that her parents are going to want to talk to the doctors about what has happened but is scared about them finding out too many details, including the risk of recurrence of seizures, because they will worry too much.

Thoughts and questions the patient/subject may have

- *What happened to me? When she is told that she had a seizure, she will ask if this means that she has epilepsy.*
- *Why did it happen?*
- *What can you do to stop it?*
- *Will it happen again?*
- *If she is told that she won't be able to drive for a year she will react as any normal young person would who is about to embark on an independent university life and is looking forward to driving!*

Examiner information

1. Conduct of interview

- Introduce yourself to Miss Ahmed and ask if she prefers to see you in private first before bringing her parents in. Explain that this is an important question to ask as you will need to discuss some sensitive issues, such as drugs and alcohol, which she may not want her parents to know about.
- Ask her how she is feeling this morning and if she remembers anything about what happened last night.
- Explain that the recent event was a seizure. Ask her if she knows what you mean by this – don't assume! Say that the doctors were quite confident of this diagnosis based on the history given by her parents and the paramedic crew.
- Give her a moment to digest this information. She may have already been told what happened but hearing it now could still be difficult.
- Establish if she has had any seizures in the past (including febrile convulsions in childhood), any head trauma or significant medical history, ask about any drugs (prescribed or otherwise) and take an alcohol history. Ask if there are any stress-related issues in her life.
- Reiterate the fact that a single seizure does not equate to a diagnosis of epilepsy (which is regarded as 'a disordered electrical activity in the brain causing recurrent fits').
- Explain that the scan of the head she had was normal but that you would like to arrange another test to look at the electrical activity of the brain ('EEG') as an outpatient. She will be referred to the neurology specialists for follow-up in clinic.
- She may ask about starting on treatment to prevent further seizures. Inform her that it is not usual practice to start patients on treatment following a single fit because the chances of recurrence, especially if she does not have any risk factors, are indeterminate and

variable. If she is keen to know, you can mention briefly about the difficulties with antiepileptic drug regimens, their side-effects, and risk of foetal damage (teratogenicity), etc. However, if she has another fit, or is believed to be at high risk of recurrent seizures as deemed by the specialist, there is a chance she may need to be commenced on treatment.

- Ask if she drives. Inform her that she is not allowed to hold a Group 1 licence for 1 year after a fit (10 years for a Group 2 licence, e.g. heavy goods vehicle [HGV] or people service vehicle [PSV]) and she needs to inform the DVLA and her insurance company about the seizure.
- Deal with any reaction to the news about the driving prohibition with understanding and sensitivity. It may be helpful to be positive, particularly if it is clinically unlikely that she will have a recurrence. A year must seem like a long time at the moment. However, she is likely to be a responsible young adult and will hopefully appreciate that other people could be put at risk if she were to have a seizure while driving.
- Establish her understanding by asking her to recap your discussion.
- Ask if she has any more questions and let her know about the follow-up arrangements before her discharge. Ask her if she is happy for you speak to her parents next to update them on what is happening.

2. Exploration and problem negotiation
The candidate should be able to:
- elicit a brief and targeted history looking for any provoking factors
- explain the diagnosis of a seizure (and the possibility of it constituting epilepsy, if recurrent) with sensitivity and explain the likely impact on the patient and her lifestyle
- explain the DVLA regulations regarding driving after a solitary fit.

3. Communication, ethics and the law

- The DVLA has provided clear guidelines regarding the regulations for driving after a solitary seizure. In summary, they state that persons who have had a single unprovoked seizure (including if this was related to alcohol or drugs) will have their licence revoked for 1 year if they hold a Group 1 licence (or 10 years for a Group 2 licence such as HGV or PSV). Following this, the DVLA may agree to provide a new licence if investigations (such as CT head and EEG) do not suggest a high risk of seizure recurrence. It is the licence holder who is legally bound to inform the DVLA of any medical condition that may affect their driving and they should do this by filling out the 'Declaration of Surrender for Medical Reasons' form. Following the stipulated period, the DVLA can reissue the licence, but will usually ask for a medical report from the patient's medical practitioner first. Note that in some cases, the DVLA may reissue a Group 1 licence after 6 months (5 years for Group 2) if the seizure was a solitary one, provided the individual has been assessed by a neurologist and investigations such as a CT head and EEG have been normal.
- It is your responsibility to inform the patient that she is not allowed to drive for 1 year after an unprovoked fit and it is the patient's responsibility to let the DVLA know about this. You should also let the patient know that her insurance is invalid until the change in her medical status has been reported by her and is on her motor insurance record.
- If you come to know subsequently that the patient is still driving, GMC guidelines state that you should once again remind the patient that she should not be doing so and that she is legally bound to inform the DVLA. This should be clearly documented in the notes. If you find out that the patient is continuing to drive despite repeated warnings, you can inform the medical adviser at the DVLA but should tell the patient first that you are going to do so.

Comments on the case

Scenarios involving seizures, epilepsy and DVLA regulations are a firm favourite in Station 4 of the PACES exam. It is advisable that all candidates read these guidelines thoroughly (link given below). Other popular situations where counselling regarding driving may be required are a diabetic patient on insulin (with or without hypoglycaemic attacks), after myocardial infarction or stroke, after surgery, sleepiness and obstructive sleep apnoea, and collapse with unknown cause.

The above scenario may also be presented in another way whereby you are asked to speak to the patient's mother or father about the event. While it is generally acceptable to give them an overview of what happened and reassure them, you need to be aware whether the patient has disclosed any personal matters to the doctors that she has specifically requested should not be mentioned to her parents. In such situations, patient confidentiality should be maintained.

Further reading

Drivers Medical Group, DVLA. *At a glance guide to the current medical standards of fitness to drive.* 2011. www.dft.gov.uk/dvla/medical/ataglance.aspx

Case 8 | Rheumatoid arthritis

Candidate information

You are the doctor in a rheumatology clinic.

Please read this summary and then continue with the consultation.

Re: Miss Charlotte McInnes, aged 25 years

Miss McInnes is a young woman who was diagnosed with rheumatoid arthritis 3 months ago after presenting with painful, swollen joints in her hands and knees. The diagnosis was confirmed by your consultant during her last appointment and Miss McInnes was not keen on starting treatment at that time, saying 'she would like to go home and think about it'. She only takes paracetamol and ibuprofen for the joint pains as required and is on no other medication. Your consultant feels that she should be given steroids if she has another flare-up of the rheumatoid arthritis. He is also considering disease-modifying agents (such as sulfasalazine or methotrexate) as she already has 8–10 joints affected, albeit not severely. She works as a chef in a top London restaurant and lives at home with her parents.

Your tasks are to: discuss the management options of the rheumatoid arthritis with Miss McInnes and address any other concerns she might have.

Subject/patient/relative information

Miss Charlotte McInnes is a 25-year-old woman who was fit and well until about 9 months ago when she noticed stiffness, pain and swelling of her fingers and wrists, especially in the morning. Her GP referred her to the rheumatologist for this whom she last saw around 3 months ago. After doing a thorough examination of her joints, with X-rays and some blood tests, she was told by the rheumatology consultant that she had early rheumatoid arthritis. He suggested starting her on medication for it but at that time she was not keen on this and wanted to find out more about the treatments first. She has been reading up on these and is clear that she does *not* want to take steroids if she has an acute flare-up, due to the side-effect of weight gain. She is taking paracetamol and ibuprofen for the joint pains when required. She has not noticed involvement of any new joints but feels the inflammation of her finger and wrist joints is becoming more troublesome now. She works as a chef in a Michelin five-star restaurant in London and lives at home with her parents. She has recently started a relationship with James, a 30-year-old lawyer, but has no plans to get married or have children soon. She is concerned what will happen if the arthritis in her hands worsens and how it will affect her job as a chef. She has worked so hard to get to this level and is worried whether her bosses will make her leave the job if her ability to prepare food and organize kitchens suffers as a result of her arthritis. She wants to talk to the doctor today about the side-effects of steroids, what other treatment options are available and whether she needs to inform work about her diagnosis.

Thoughts and questions the patient/subject may have
- *There is no way I am going on steroid tablets – can you give me any other medication for the arthritis?*
- *Do I have to tell my work about this diagnosis?*
- *I am worried what will happen if they find out at work. Can they lay me off if they think the arthritis in my hands will affect my ability to prepare food?*

Examiner information

1. Conduct of interview
- Introduce yourself to Miss McInnes.
- Ask her how she is feeling (specifically about the pain and swelling of her joints) and if there have been any new joints involved. Also ask if the analgesia is working and if she is aware of non-pharmacological interventions (e.g. exercises to increase muscle strength which support the joint, the use of splints for inflamed or deformed joints, relaxation techniques).
- Ask her what the rheumatology consultant discussed with her last time about treatments for her rheumatoid arthritis (RA) and find out her thoughts on this. Explain that you (and your consultant) feel that she needs to be started on treatment for her RA to prevent any spread of the arthritis and destruction of her joints. Check that she is on the same wavelength with you regarding this.
- She will express her concern about the side-effects of steroids and you may need to go into more detail about these with her. Tell her that the use of steroids in her case would hopefully be for a short course whilst she is established on more long-term medication and also to treat any acute flare-ups. Explain that the frequency of side-effects (e.g. weight gain, hyperglycaemia, thinning/bruising of the skin) are relatively low if she is on a low dose of steroids for a short duration and that side-effects are generally reversible.
- Reassure her that she will be monitored closely in the clinic for side-effects of steroids and any other medication she is started on. Also reassure her that she will not be forced to go onto any medication that she is not keen on.
- Briefly tell her that there are other treatments available for RA which can stop its progression and prevent involvement of more joints. If she is agreeable, tell her that you will discuss with your consultant about starting one of these.
- Find out if she is married, in a relationship or planning any pregnancies. Tell her that one of the medications, methotrexate, is absolutely contraindicated in pregnancy so we need to be extra careful in women of child-bearing age.
- Ask how the RA is affecting her life and work. She may express her anxiety about being dismissed from work if her bosses feel that the arthritis will affect her job. She may also ask if she or the doctors will have to tell her employer about the diagnosis.
- Reassure her that she is not required by statutory law to tell her employers about her diagnosis and the doctors will also maintain patient confidentiality. Also, tell her that if her RA is reasonably well controlled (especially if she goes on medication), she should be able to carry out her job without restriction.
- However, if she does face any difficulty in performing her job, she should be encouraged to speak to the occupational health department in her workplace. Agencies such as the National Rheumatoid Arthritis Society (NRAS) can also be a good source of support for patients with RA.
- Close the consultation by telling her that you will discuss with your consultant about starting her on disease-modifying treatment for the RA, if she is agreeable, and you will be in touch soon. Give her the contact details of the rheumatology specialist nurse who may be able to help her further.

2. Exploration and problem negotiation
The candidate should be able to:
- establish the extent of the patient's RA and empathically explore how it is affecting her life and work
- discuss briefly the treatment options available (including side-effects of steroid treatment)
- sensitively deal with her anxieties regarding her diagnosis and employment

- be aware of whom she can turn to for more help and support (in her workplace, community and hospital).

3. Communication, ethics and the law

- It is not possible to do a thorough review of a chronic systemic condition such as rheumatoid arthritis (RA) and go through all the possible treatments and their side-effects within the time allocated for the station (or a single real-life consultation, for that matter).
- In a situation such as the one above, you can assume the patient has an understanding of the diagnosis so you can focus on making a brief assessment of her symptoms (particularly if there have been any new joints affected since her last consultation or any deterioration of her joint function) and go on to discuss the treatment options.
- It is estimated that RA costs the UK economy £3.8–4.8 billion a year in terms of direct costs to the NHS and indirect costs in terms of work-related disability, early mortality, etc. This is in addition to the impact the disease has on a person's personal and family life and overall well-being, including psychological impact. Therefore, this is something you have to bear in mind during every consultation with a patient and address their issues and concerns.
- Be aware of tools like the Disease Activity Score 28 which allows clinicians to make an assessment of how active/symptomatic a patient's RA is by incorporating examination of tender or swollen joints, blood results (such as erythrocyte sedimentation rate [ESR] or C-reactive protein [CRP]) and the patient's global assessment of pain and discomfort on the day.
- The National Institute for Health and Clinical Excellence recommends starting combination disease-modifying antirheumatic drugs (DMARDs) in patients with active RA. This includes methotrexate and one other drug, such as hydroxychloroquine, sulfasalazine or leflunomide. In situations where certain drugs may be contraindicated (e.g. methotrexate in women who are or planning to become pregnant), one single DMARD agent may be started.
- Glucocorticoids should be used in the short term to manage flare-ups as they work well to reduce inflammation quickly. They can be particularly useful in the initiation phase of therapy when waiting for the DMARDs to take effect. Side-effects are rare when steroids at a dose equivalent to 10 mg of prednisolone a day are given for less than a few months at a time and they are reversible on stopping the drug.
- All patients with RA should have access to a multidisciplinary team for specialist advice regarding occupational therapy and physiotherapy, and podiatry review if they have foot involvement.

> **Comments on the case**
> Discussion about any chronic disease, especially one that can cause physical disability such as rheumatoid arthritis, can be difficult particularly if it involves younger people. It is important to address any particular concerns they have, regarding the effect of their disease/symptoms on their job and personal life or questions about management and particular drugs. It is not uncommon for the issue of pregnancy to come up when discussing such diagnoses with young women (or even young men who may be thinking about starting a family) so the candidate should have a rough idea about the genetics of the condition and effects of medications.

Further reading

National Institute for Health and Clinical Excellence. *Clinical Guideline 79. Rheumatoid arthritis: the management of rheumatoid arthritis in adults.* London: National Institute for Health and Clinical Excellence, 2009.

Case 9 | Valvular heart disease in a young woman

Candidate information

You are the doctor in a cardiology clinic.

Please read this summary and then continue with the consultation.

Re: Mrs Karen Thomson, aged 26 years

Mrs Thomson is a 26-year-old Caucasian woman who works as a solicitor in the city. She was admitted to hospital about 3 months ago with an episode of fast atrial fibrillation and an echocardiogram which was done following this showed severe mitral stenosis. She went on to have cardiac catheterization studies which confirmed the diagnosis (valve area 1.4 cm² and pulmonary artery pressure 45 mmHg). Your cardiology consultant has discussed this with the cardiothoracic surgeon who agrees that Mrs Thomson needs to be considered for mitral valve surgery (possibly valve replacement). You are seeing her in clinic to discuss this issue.

Your tasks are to: explain the diagnosis and the proposed management plan to her, and address any concerns she might have.

Subject/patient/relative information

Mrs Karen Thomson is a 26-year-old woman who works as a solicitor for a private company. She has been noticing palpitations and breathlessness whilst running at the gym for a few months and, during one of these episodes, she needed to be admitted to hospital. She was told at this time that she had a 'fast heart rate' and needed further investigations for it. She went on to have a 'scan of the heart' (echocardiogram) and a cardiac catheterization test. The consultant has mentioned to her that she has a tight heart valve known as mitral stenosis. She has been reading about this on the internet and is aware that she may need to have a valve replacement and be on warfarin for life. She got married 6 months ago and is planning a pregnancy within the next year or two. She has also read about the ill effects of warfarin during pregnancy and is keen to postpone the surgery until after she has had a baby because she feels quite well from the heart side of things now.

Thoughts and questions the patient/subject may have

- *Do I really need to have the surgery on my heart – I feel quite well in myself now!*
- *I really don't want to go onto warfarin; can the valve be replaced without me needing to take warfarin after that?*
- *I am really keen on having a baby soon; I don't want to go on any medication which could be harmful for my baby.*

Examiner information

1. Conduct of interview

- Introduce yourself to Mrs Thomson.
- Check her understanding of the diagnosis of mitral stenosis as proven on the echocardiogram and the cardiac catheter studies that she has had recently. Explain this diagnosis to her briefly and in simple terms if you suspect she has not understood this adequately (e.g. 'one of the valves in your heart is narrow and this was confirmed on the heart scan and catheter test'). Explain that this is likely to be a congenital abnormality in her case (as she does not appear to have had rheumatic fever in the past).
- Reiterate the fact that her hospital admission for atrial fibrillation was 'due to strain put on the heart' by her mitral stenosis and this often manifests initially during exercise in young people.
- Ask her if she has spoken to any doctors or heard about any treatment options for this condition. She will tell you that she has read on the internet that she may need surgery for it (which she is not keen on currently).
- Say that your cardiology consultant has discussed her case with the cardiothoracic surgeons and they feel that she will require heart valve surgery, most likely a replacement, as the condition is likely to be progressive and can result in more complications. If she asks whether there are alternatives, explain that there are other treatment options (e.g. percutaneous mitral balloon valvuloplasty/valvotomy, commissurotomy) and the surgeons will be able to advise which procedure is best for her particular circumstances. She may ask how long she will need to stay in hospital and how long she will be off work. Other queries may include life insurance issues.
- Explain that if a metallic valve is inserted she will require warfarin for life following the procedure. If she asks about other types of valves (i.e. tissue bioprosthetic), mention that these would not be recommended in her case due to their lifespan.
- When she brings up the issue of pregnancy, say that warfarin is contraindicated in early pregnancy because of the risk of congenital malformations and placental and maternal bleeding. She will need to be changed to low molecular weight heparin (LMWH) prior to pregnancy until delivery. Inform her that when she becomes pregnant, she will be monitored closely by specialists.
- If she asks about the possibility of postponing the surgery until after she has a baby, discuss the risks of progression of the mitral stenosis and possible cardiac complications brought on by the physiological changes in pregnancy.
- To end the consultation, ask if she has any questions and give her leaflets about valve replacement surgery and anticoagulation in pregnancy. Ensure that an appointment is made with the cardiothoracic surgeon shortly, where she can ask more about the different surgical procedures, etc.

2. Exploration and problem negotiation

The candidate should be able to:

- discuss the diagnosis of the mitral stenosis and the need for surgery with the patient
- sensitively address her concerns regarding pregnancy and explain about the anticoagulation management in pregnancy
- deal with any other questions or concerns she may have.

3. Communication, ethics and the law

- Mitral stenosis is most commonly caused worldwide by rheumatic fever but, in countries with a low prevalence, congenital heart disease needs to be considered. It is often asymptomatic in the early stages but, as the disease progresses, it can present with complications such as atrial fibrillation, pulmonary hypertension and left or right ventricular failure (initially on exertion).
- Intervention is recommended in the following situations: in asymptomatic patients with moderate or severe mitral stenosis (determined by valve area and development of pulmonary hypertension) and in symptomatic patients with mild stenosis, especially if pulmonary hypertension is present. (The normal mitral valve area is $4–6\,cm^2$. Mild, moderate and severe disease are defined as less than 4, 2.5 and $1.5\,cm^2$ respectively).
- There are various surgical modalities available: percutaneous mitral balloon valvotomy (PMBV), open or closed valve commissurotomy and mitral valve replacement. PMBV is usually preferred for rheumatic mitral stenosis if the valve morphology is favourable and there are no other coexisting valve pathologies. It is not often recommended for congenital mitral stenosis due to complex valve morphology and valve replacement is done instead.
- A mechanical valve is usually preferred to a bioprosthetic valve in patients under the age of 65 years, especially if there is coexisting atrial fibrillation and no other contraindications to taking warfarin (the

lifespan of a bioprosthetic valve is around 10–15 years).

- Warfarin is contraindicated in pregnancy because it crosses the placenta and can cause placental and foetal haemorrhage. In the first trimester, it is associated with higher rates of spontaneous abortion and developmental malformations of bone and cartilage. Women on warfarin planning a pregnancy should attend preconceptual counselling with obstetricians and haematologists and they will be converted to LMWH for the duration of their pregnancy.

- Low molecular weight heparin does not cross the placenta and is administered safely via subcutaneous injection, according to body weight, during pregnancy. Women are usually asked to withhold LMWH for 24 h before delivery to reduce the chances of perinatal bleeding. They can be restarted on warfarin after the delivery, with a few days of cross-cover with LMWH. Both warfarin and LMWH are safe in breastfeeding.

Comments on the case

The issue of cardiac problems in a young patient can be very difficult to deal with, especially when it comes to discussing things like surgery and lifelong anticoagulation, etc. Bear in mind that this is a very specialist area and you will not be required to know details of surgical procedures (at least for Station 4). A brief idea of the causative factors and severity of the patient's condition will enable you to outline treatment options and you will then seek senior/specialist help. More often than not, you will need to discuss anticoagulation with the patient and assess the individual's risk versus benefit of being on it. Discussions regarding surgery will be undertaken by a multidisciplinary team consisting of surgeons, cardiologists and cardiac anaesthetists.

The topic of anticoagulation in pregnancy frequently comes up in various formats (in addition to the one in the case), such as:

- preconceptual or pregnant woman with deep vein thrombosis (DVT) or pulmonary embolism (PE)
- preconceptual or pregnant woman with a known thrombophilic condition or family history.

When a person has mental capacity, they are perfectly entitled to make their own informed decisions regarding treatment and intervention options which may be available to them.

Some insight into the history of the woman in terms of attempts to conceive or previous successful pregnancies is essential. If pregnancy has been a long pursued goal, then she may well be inclined to put the needs of her unborn child above her own. Convincing her to do otherwise may be extremely difficult.

Case 10 | Air travel with chronic obstructive pulmonary disease

Candidate information

You are the doctor in a respiratory clinic.

Please read this summary and then continue with the consultation.

Re: Mr Barry Summers, aged 66 years

Mr Summers was diagnosed with COPD 4 years ago. He is normally on salbutamol, seretide and tiotropium inhalers and has a nebulizer machine at home but only uses it very occasionally. He used to be a heavy smoker with a 90 pack-year history but has given up since his COPD was diagnosed. His only other medical history is psoriasis for which he is on topical treatment. His saturation levels on air are 94% and his most recent spirometry shows a forced expiratory volume (FEV)$_1$/forced vital capacity (FVC) ratio of 60% and a FEV$_1$ of 65% predicted. He was admitted to hospital a month ago for 2 days with an infective exacerbation of COPD but this was during a bad winter spell and prior to that he had not had any exacerbations for nearly a year. He is coming to see you in clinic because he has booked a holiday in Florida to visit his son and wants to know if it is safe for him to fly with his lung condition.

Your tasks are to: assess the severity of his COPD and advise him on whether it is safe for him to fly or if any further assessments need to be done.

Subject/patient/relative information

Mr Barry Summers is a 66-year-old man who was diagnosed with 'smoker's lung disease' (chronic obstructive pulmonary disease or COPD) around 4 years ago. This is relatively well controlled with three different inhalers and although he has a nebulizer machine at home, he very rarely uses it. He is not on home oxygen. During the particularly cold winter about a month ago, he came down with a bad chest infection and needed to be admitted to hospital for 2 days as it exacerbated his COPD. Prior to this he had not had any exacerbations for a year. He feels back to his normal self now although still slightly breathless when walking a mile or two on level ground. He last had lung function tests in the chest clinic 6 months ago and was told that 'they were all right'. He has booked a month's holiday to Florida to visit his son and is very keen to go as he has not been abroad for nearly 10 years. He has read about the dangers of flying with COPD and wonders if he will need oxygen on the flight. He used to be a heavy smoker but gave up when his COPD was diagnosed. He used to be a bus driver before he retired.

Thoughts and questions the patient/subject may have
- *Can you arrange for me to have some oxygen on the flight?*
- *Look, I have to go on this holiday. I have been saving for the last few years for this!*

Examiner information

1. Conduct of interview
- Introduce yourself to Mr Summers. Ask about how he is feeling after his discharge from hospital for exacerbation of COPD and try to determine what might have triggered it.
- Establish if he is back to his baseline level of functioning, exercise tolerance, etc.
- Check about compliance with his treatment (e.g. how often he is using his inhalers, does he need his nebulizer machine at home on a regular basis, etc.) and confirm that he has given up smoking.
- When he mentions his planned flight to the USA, say that in view of his lung disease and recent hospital admission with an exacerbation, he will need further assessments before being given the reassurance he is looking for.
- Briefly go through his past medical history to make sure he has no other concomitant respiratory problems that may be an issue while flying (e.g. previous thromboembolism, pneumothorax, fibrotic lung disease, heart failure, coronary heart disease, etc.). Confirm that he is not on long-term oxygen therapy (LTOT).
- Explain that he will need further tests to determine his fitness to fly, such as measurement of oxygen saturations on air, and arterial blood gas testing whilst on air and whilst breathing oxygen that will simulate being on a flight at 30,000 ft.
- Give general advice on flying, such as remembering to carry all his inhalers in his hand luggage, asking for in-flight nebulizers if he may need them and asking for a wheelchair to assist him to and from the aircraft if his exercise tolerance is limited (unlikely in this patient's case). He should be advised to keep mobile during the flight. He is also advised to take out travel insurance especially if he is going to the USA as the health service there is private.
- Advise him that he should inform the airline company as soon as possible about his diagnosis of COPD, whilst further assessments are pending.
- Arrange a follow-up appointment with him in the near future to discuss the results of the respiratory physiology fitness-to-fly tests and close the discussion.

2. Exploration and problem negotiation
The candidate should be able to:
- assess the reasons for, and the severity of, Mr Summers' recent hospital admission and find out about his recovery
- evaluate his current quality of life
- address the issue of flying with respiratory disease
- explain in layman's terms about the respiratory physiology tests necessary in order to determine fitness to fly in a patient with chronic lung disease.

3. Communication, ethics and the law
- With air travel becoming more common these days, it is possible that you will meet patients with various health conditions asking for advice before they travel.
- The specific concern with regard to patients flying with respiratory diseases arises due to hypoxia at high cabin altitudes, prolonged immobility and reduced barometric pressures.
- The British Thoracic Society has provided guidance on identifying patients at risk of developing problems while flying, what assessment needs to be done and advice regarding the need for in-flight oxygen.
- At a cabin altitude of 8000 ft, the partial pressure of oxygen is equivalent to 15.1% at sea level (but remember that the concentration of oxygen in air at 30,000 ft is still the same as at sea level). An individual's PaO_2 can fall to between 7 and 8.5 kPa with associated hypercapnia and tachycardia. Naturally, this can have implications for those with COPD, asthma and pulmonary fibrosis. Those with a recent pneumothorax or venous thromboembolism should not be flying unless seen by a consultant respiratory physician to guarantee safety of flying.
- Patients with COPD should initially have resting oxygen saturation measurements done on room air. If this is <92%, oxygen should be advised on the flight.
- If this is 92–95%, they should have further assessment with a hypoxic challenge, especially if they have an additional risk factor such as FEV_1 <50%, coexist-

ing hypercapnia, coexisting restrictive lung disease and discharge from hospital within the last 6 weeks for exacerbation of chronic lung or heart disease.

- The hypoxic challenge test involves getting the patient to breathe 15% FiO_2 for 20 min and then checking arterial blood gas. If PaO_2 is less than 6.6 kPa, oxygen should be advised.
- Patients with chronic lung disease should inform their airline, in advance, of their condition and their likely requirement for inhalers, nebulizers or oxygen during the flight. A doctor's letter will need to be provided to the airline company.
- Those who require in-flight oxygen should be made aware that it is usually given at a rate of 2 L/min via nasal cannulae and usually commenced when the plane is at cruising altitude (similarly, the flow rate will be increased for patients on supplementary oxygen at ground level).
- Patients with open tuberculosis and current closed pneumothorax are advised not to fly.

Comments on the case

With more and more people undertaking air travel, having a respiratory disease, especially a chronic well-controlled one, should not be seen as a barrier to flying. It is important for all doctors to have some knowledge about what assessments need to be undertaken in order to establish a patient's fitness to fly and what basic advice should be given to them. Organizations such as the British Lung Foundation (BLF) are good sources of information for patients who are on long-term oxygen therapy to find out more about the logistics of travelling abroad with oxygen.

Other groups of patients who may come for advice prior to flying include:

- the diabetic patient on insulin (e.g. how to alter the insulin regime with regard to long-haul flights and time difference abroad)
- patients with previous venous thromboembolism
- patients with muscular dystrophy.

Further reading

British Lung Foundation. *Air travel with a lung condition.* www.blf.org.uk/Page/Air-travel-with-a-lung-condition/

Shrikrishna D, Coker R. Managing patients with stable respiratory disease planning air travel: British Thoracic Society recommendations. *Thorax* 2011;66(9):831–3.

Case 11 | Polypharmacy

Candidate information

You are the doctor in a diabetes clinic.

Please read this summary and then continue with the consultation.

Re: Mr Henry Beaumont, aged 68 years

Mr Beaumont is a 68-year-old man who has a 15-year history of type 2 diabetes mellitus, hypertension and hypercholesterolaemia for which he is on several medications including metformin, gliclazide, pioglitazone, amlodipine, bendrofluazide, furosemide and simvastatin. He was previously on ramipril but this was stopped due to side-effects. The investigations before his clinic visit show an HbA1c of 8.2%, creatinine 146 mmol/L, estimated glomerular filtration rate (eGFR) 53, total cholesterol 6.5 mmol, triglycerides 2.4 mmol and urine albumin creatinine ratio (ACR) 38 mg/mmol. His blood pressure is 158/92 mmHg and weight 88 kg. You are concerned about his cardiovascular risk profile and renal impairment and would like to add further medications to help.

Your tasks are to: explain to Mr Beaumont your concerns about his test results and risk factors and discuss your intention to start further medications to lower his risk.

Subject/patient/relative information

Mr Henry Beaumont is a 68-year-old man who was diagnosed with type 2 diabetes mellitus and hypertension around 15 years ago and was initially started on one tablet for each but over the last few years this has steadily increased to about six different ones. One year ago, his GP mentioned that his cholesterol levels were also high and started him on a tablet called simvastatin which he only takes a few times a week because of the muscle cramps that he had. He was previously given another tablet called ramipril for his blood pressure and kidneys but had to stop it because of an irritable cough and he is now wary about going on other drugs similar to this. He does not understand why the doctors keep putting him on more and more medications because he feels well in himself, and in fact is leaving shortly for a 3-week holiday to the south of Spain.

Thoughts and questions the patient/subject may have

- *I don't know what all you doctors are playing at – I've told everyone I'm feeling perfectly fine but yet you keep putting me on tablet after tablet!*
- *There is no way I am going on another medication for my blood pressure, the last time I had that horrible tablet which gave me such an annoying cough!*
- *Are all these different problems I have really serious? Could they be life-threatening?*

Examiner information

1. Conduct of interview

- Introduce yourself to Mr Beaumont and ask him generally about how he is feeling.
- Establish that the purpose of the consultation with him today is to review his diabetes, blood pressure and other medical problems and to see if anything needs to be changed (ask an open question to ensure that you understand his current level of knowledge).
- First ask him if he understands the different conditions he is being treated for and the reasons.
- Say that you have reviewed his test results and there are a few things of concern (namely his blood pressure and cholesterol levels, kidney function and diabetes control). Explain that the reason you are worried about these various issues is because they work in combination to put him at high risk of heart disease and stroke and this is the reason that we need to control these various health concerns (be careful not to sound too pessimistic or bleak).
- Go through his current medications and determine if he is taking all the ones prescribed and if there are any other barriers to adequate compliance (e.g. forgetfulness, complicated dosing and timing, etc.).
- Check if he has any particular side-effects (he may mention about the simvastatin and myalgia). Reiterate that it is crucial that his cholesterol levels are well controlled and that he needs to take his lipid-lowering treatment regularly. Suggest changing to another statin such as atorvastatin or rosuvastatin which may have a different side-effect profile.
- Express your concern about his deteriorating renal function, which is likely to be due to a combination of his poorly controlled hypertension and diabetes mellitus. If this is an acute deterioration, you may need to consider doing further investigations such as an ultrasound scan of his renal tract. Otherwise, suggest adding in a drug such as an angiotensin receptor blocker which would control his blood pressure as well as protecting his kidneys.
- If Mr Beaumont is reluctant to do this due to the side-effects he had from ramipril previously, reassure him that the drug you are proposing is not likely to have the same effect.
- Give him a written record of the medications he is meant to be on (including any changes you have made) and see if he wants you to speak to his partner/other family member. Offer practical solutions to help with any other barriers identified.
- Tell him you will follow him up closely to monitor the response to treatment or any side-effects and he can always discuss any concern he has with your team, his GP or practice nurse.
- Ask him to see the diabetic nurse in the clinic before he goes.
- Check when he last had his eyes and feet checked for microvascular complications.

2. Exploration and problem negotiation

The candidate should be able to:

- explain to the patient the concerns about his cardiovascular risk profile and his test results in a sensitive manner
- establish, together with the patient, the importance of addressing and controlling these risk factors
- explore the reasons for the patient's non-compliance with the medication and suggest practical solutions and alternatives.

3. Communication, ethics and the law

- Compliance with treatment in general is notoriously poor among patients with chronic diseases. Studies have shown that only around 40–50% of people with chronic diseases take their medication as prescribed and figures of those who attend follow-up appointments or follow dietary advice are also poor (20–70%, depending on the studies quoted). Analysing the prescription ordering rate (by patients) is a commonly used method in studies investigating drug concordance but it has been shown that over 10% of patients do not take the tablets despite picking up the prescription, suggesting that the figures we have for non-compliance may be an underestimate.
- Possible barriers to a patient adhering to treatment can be broadly divided into patient-centred, clinician-centred and medication-centred factors.
- Patient-centred factors include memory problems, depression, poor eyesight, the embarrassment of taking the tablets and/or injections in public places, reluctance to share their diagnoses with family and friends, and variable perceptions about the severity of their illnesses.
- Clinicians need to consider their role in patient non-compliance too. It is essential that clinicians spend time educating patients about the importance of each of their medications and the potential side-effects (depending on the individual patient, you may need to go into more detail about morbidity and mortality figures if they need to understand the seriousness of the condition they are receiving treatment for).

Involvement of family members in the discussion and giving contact details of a member of the medical team should the patient have any queries can also help.

- Medication-related factors that can act as a barrier to compliance include polypharmacy, multiple daily regimes, drug interactions and media reports about potential safety issues of particular drugs.
- It is essential to assess these various factors in turn when assessing a patient who is non-compliant with treatment and consider how the relevant ones can be modified for the benefit of that particular patient. Using aids like written reminders, dosette box reminder alarms and polypills are some ideas which can be helpful.

Comments on the case

Discussing medication regimes and assessing concordance with treatment is an essential skill that all doctors need to have. It needs to be done in a tactful way so as to avoid coming across as authoritative to the patient, which may only encourage them to conceal things from their clinicians.

Case 12 | Blood transfusion

Candidate information

You are the doctor in a haematology clinic.

Please read this summary and then continue with the consultation.

Re: Mr Edgar Madeley, aged 82

Mr Madeley has been referred because of tiredness and a normocytic normochromic anaemia. His haemoglobin count is 7.2 g/dL. Investigations have included a normal upper gastrointestinal (GI) endoscopy and a barium enema which only revealed mild diverticulosis in the large bowel. The consultant wonders whether the anaemia may be due to myelodysplasia in the presence of normal haematinics and no obvious GI pathology. He suggests offering a blood transfusion of 2 units.

Your tasks are to: explain the results of the tests and offer Mr Madeley a blood transfusion.

Subject/patient/relative information

Mr Madeley, an 82-year-old gentleman, was found to be anaemic by the GP 3 weeks ago and he was subsequently referred to the clinic for investigations. He is essentially well apart from tiredness but the consultant physician wanted to rule out a GI malignancy. A barium enema has shown mild diverticulosis only and an upper GI endoscopy was normal. The consultant is keen to give him 2 units of blood. The patient does not have any major objections to the blood transfusion but he wants to be certain that the transfusion is in his best interests and that it is safe. He wants to speak to the medical doctor (the candidate) to discuss this.

Thoughts and questions the patient/subject may have

- *Do you know what the cause of my anaemia is?*
- *Are you sure it is not cancer? My doctor said that was a possibility and that's why he wanted to investigate my bowels.*
- *Will this blood transfusion sort the problem out once and for all?*
- *I've heard of people getting nasty infections from blood transfusions – is that going to happen to me?*

Examiner information

1. Conduct of interview

- Introduce yourself to Mr Madeley and ask how he is.
- Say that, as a result of the anaemia, he has undergone a few tests.
- Explain the results of the barium enema and the endoscopy.
- Say that it is unlikely that the diverticulosis itself would have caused the anaemia and it is possible that the bone marrow is not as active as previously and so fewer blood cells are being produced, contributing to the anaemia.

- Say that the best way to treat this is to give blood through a transfusion. Explain what a normal blood count is and say that, as a result of his anaemia, he has been getting symptoms of tiredness.
- Ask how he feels about having a blood transfusion. He says he is not sure and wants to know the risks.
- Firstly, reassure him that the blood is being offered in the best interests of his health and that the advantage of having blood is that his improved blood count would help improve the tiredness.
- Explain that there is no suitable alternative in terms of tablets to reverse the anaemia.
- Appreciate his concerns but say that in the UK a blood transfusion is safe and that strict regulations are now in place to ensure that wrong blood is not given, i.e. checking that the correct blood type is correctly cross-matched, checking patient identification labels with the labels on the blood bag, etc.
- Reassure him that in the UK all blood donated is checked for viruses such as human immunodeficiency virus (HIV), hepatitis B and C and the risk of contracting an infection is extremely small.
- Other risks with a blood transfusion include allergic reactions to the blood and this presents with an itch and weals within minutes of commencing the transfusion. Reassure that if this happens, treatment is available to counter it.
- Again, reassure him that a blood transfusion is safe and if he decides to have the blood then you can arrange a date for this to be done, with the prospect of going home the same day after a post-transfusion blood test. He will then be seen again in clinic to have the blood count checked again. Say that there is a chance that he will become anaemic again and so he may need blood transfusions several times a year.
- Ask if he has any questions and ask whether he feels he would like to have more time to think about it.

2. Exploration and problem negotiation

The candidate should be able to:
- give the results of the tests
- explain why the patient may have anaemia
- explain that to treat the anaemia, he needs to have a blood transfusion
- discuss the pros and cons of blood transfusion
- give time and space for the patient to decide.

3. Communication, ethics and the law

- Adverse effects of blood transfusion include:
  - non-haemolytic febrile transfusion reactions including allergic reaction and anaphylaxis
  - acute haemolytic transfusion reaction due to incompatible transfused red cells
  - bacterial contamination of the blood product
  - virus infection, although this is rare, e.g. hepatitis B and C, HIV (1 and 2). *Treponema pallidum* is routinely checked as well
  - being given the wrong blood, i.e. due to a mix-up in cross-matching, wrong labelling, human error
  - late complications of repeated transfusions, e.g. iron overload
  - circulatory overload if too much is given.
- Recent pressures on the blood transfusion service have arisen because of:
  - increased demand for blood compared with the increase in donations
  - likely additional demand for blood associated with waiting list initiatives
  - the rise in the cost of blood with leucodepletion and nucleic acid testing
  - recommendations from the Serious Hazards of Transfusion (SHOT) enquiry on how the safety of patients receiving blood could be improved
  - the theoretical risk of new-variant Creutzfeldt–Jakob disease
  - the implications of clinical governance for the blood transfusion service.
- The latest SHOT report, published in 2010, stated that 2010 was the first year in which there was no confirmed case of transfusion-transmitted infection in the UK and that there was a 29% reduction in the number of incorrect blood component transfused reports. This is probably due to better training and competence of clinical staff handling blood transfusion and better reporting systems such as that provided by the National Patient Safety Agency.

Comments on the case

This case demonstrates how such a common procedure in hospital is taken for granted. The doctor must allow an informed decision to be made before getting consent and the patient has every right to refuse.

Further reading

Department of Health. *Better blood transfusion*. London: NHS Executive, 1998.

Serious Hazards of Transfusion (SHOT) *Annual Report 2010*. Summary: www.shotuk.org/wp-content/uploads/2011/07/SHOT-2010-Summary1.pdf.

Case 13 | Hormone replacement therapy

Candidate information

You are the doctor in a medical follow-up clinic.

Please read this summary and then continue with the consultation.

Re: Mrs Jacky Lorimer, aged 55 years

Mrs Lorimer was admitted 6 weeks ago with a community-acquired pneumonia. She was treated with amoxicillin and made a full recovery. The chest X-ray today shows complete resolution of the pneumonia. Her main concern now is about her intermittent hot flushes. She suspects that she is menopausal and wants advice on whether she should try hormone replacement therapy (HRT). She is a little concerned about the risk of thromboembolism in light of the scares she has read about in the press.

Your tasks are to: determine whether Mrs Lorimer would benefit from HRT and discuss the pros and cons of HRT.

Subject/patient/relative information

Mrs Lorimer is a 55-year-old housewife who was admitted 6 weeks ago with a community-acquired pneumonia. She has made an excellent recovery and has had no more respiratory symptoms. While in clinic, she thought she would get some advice from the medical doctor (the candidate) about the use of HRT. She has been getting intermittent hot flushes over the last 5 months. She has noticed some vaginal dryness but no urinary symptoms. There is also reduced libido. She is otherwise well and has no past history of thromboembolism, cardiovascular disease or breast cancer. There is also no significant history of these illnesses in the family. She did, however, have a hysterectomy 14 years ago for uterine fibroids. She feels as if she is coming towards her menopause but she cannot be totally certain because of the lack of menstrual periods. She is quite keen to try HRT but is unsure about the risks of thromboembolism. She has been reading a few women's magazines recently and the articles on HRT have scared her. She does not smoke or drink and she lives with her husband.

Thoughts and questions the patient/subject may have

- *What are the risks of taking HRT?*
- *I've heard HRT can cause dangerous blood clots and breast cancer – is that true?*
- *Is there anything I can do to prevent the harmful effects of HRT? Are there any alternatives?*
- *What do you think I should do, doctor?*

Examiner information

1. Conduct of interview

- Introduce yourself to Mrs Lorimer. Ask how she is. Tell her that her chest X-ray is normal and that the pneumonia has fully resolved.
- She tells you that she may be menopausal and is wondering if she should have HRT.
- Ask her why she thinks she is menopausal. She tells you that she has had a hysterectomy and so she does not have any periods but she tells you about the hot flushes.
- Ask her what other symptoms she has been having, e.g. urogenital atrophy (vaginal dryness, dyspareunia, dysuria, urinary frequency and urgency), mood changes, loss of libido.
- Ask what she knows about HRT.
- Firstly, explain what the menopause is, i.e. declining ovarian function with falling levels of oestrogens. Tell her that you can confirm this by testing her blood oestrogen levels. Then, explain that the reason for giving HRT is to increase the oestrogen levels and so prevent or treat clinical features associated with the menopause.
- Describe the components of HRT, i.e. natural oestrogens with or without progesterones.
- Explain that since she does not have a uterus, progesterone is not needed in addition to oestrogen (in women with a uterus, the former is required to prevent endometrial hyperplasia and carcinoma).
- Describe how HRT can be given, i.e. systemically or topically. Systemically includes tablets by mouth, on the skin (transdermal) or a subcutaneous oestrogen implant. Topically is via vaginal creams, rings or pessaries.
- She asks about the advantages of HRT. Say there will be an improvement of the menopausal symptoms. Tell her that HRT also helps to prevent osteoporosis and hip fractures.
- She asks about the disadvantages of HRT. She is particularly worried about thromboembolism. Explain that there is a suggestion that the risk of developing venous thromboembolism is 2 to 4 times higher in women on HRT (whichever route of administration) but reassure her that, even on HRT, the risk of developing a deep vein thrombosis is very small. Inform her that women on long-term HRT, e.g. over 10 years, have a slightly increased risk of developing breast cancer though this needs to be confirmed by further long-term studies.
- Explain that until recently, the association between HRT and heart disease and stroke was unclear but a recent large study showed that women on HRT were definitely at higher risk of heart attacks and strokes. Therefore, doctors are now more careful about putting menopausal women on HRT.
- Ask if she has a past history of thromboembolism, breast cancer or coronary heart disease and enquire about family history as well. Ask if she smokes.
- Reassure her again that in those women without risk factors, the benefits outweigh the disadvantages.
- Inform her of the side-effects of HRT, i.e. oestrogen-related unwanted effects such as breast swelling and tenderness, nausea, increased appetite with weight gain, and vaginal discharge, but these tend to resolve within 3 months.
- Say that given the above evidence, many doctors now do not recommend the routine use of HRT in post-menopausal women. However, it can be used, at a low dose, for a few months to relieve menopausal symptoms.
- Ask if she has any other queries. Say that you will try to get some leaflets from the gynaecology and bone clinics and that you will send these to her in the post. Tell her you will let the GP know of today's discussion.

2. Exploration and problem negotiation

The candidate should be able to:

- reassure the patient that the pneumonia has fully resolved
- obtain the history of the symptoms the patient has that are suggestive of the menopause
- determine any contraindications to HRT
- discuss the pros and cons of HRT
- be aware that progesterone is not needed in those without a uterus.

3. Communication, ethics and the law

- Specific issues related to misperceptions and fears regarding HRT need to be clarified, and specific, patient-focused educational pamphlets can help to address common concerns about HRT. Doctors should communicate effectively with the patient. Doctors must focus on the emotional and physical aspects of HRT choices and tailor any therapies to the individual patient. It is important to discuss frankly the very serious concerns a woman may have regarding the association with breast cancer and endometrial cancer. Discussing, and preparing, women for possible side-effects helps patients to cope better if and when side-effects occur. Finally, offering a wide variety of HRT therapies provides women with a broader choice if an initial regimen is unsuccessful.

- The findings of the Women's Health Initiative (WHI), a randomized controlled trial of over 16,000 women over 5 years, have provided more evidence on the effects on cardiovascular outcomes. This showed that the risk of coronary heart disease (CHD) was nearly 30% higher in women taking combined HRT compared to placebo although mortality due to that was not increased. Therefore, HRT is no longer recommended for primary prevention of heart disease. This study also showed increased risk of strokes and venous thromboembolism with HRT use.
- With regard to the secondary prevention of heart disease, the Heart and Estrogen/Progestin Replacement Study (HERS) showed no reduced risk of CHD over 5 years in those using HRT but CHD deaths were increased in the first 3 years in the HRT group.
- A woman who has undergone a hysterectomy can take oestrogens without a progesterone. An oestrogen implant is one option, although the individual may wish to use tablets or patches. A woman who still has a uterus must take a progesterone with an oestrogen. This also applies to a woman who has undergone an endometrial ablation procedure because some endometrial tissue may not have been destroyed. The

progesterone can be given cyclically or continuously. During a 28-day cyclical treatment, progesterones are given for 10–14 days, so producing monthly withdrawal bleeding. During 3-monthly cyclical treatment, progesterones are given for 14 days with the aim of producing a quarterly withdrawal bleed. The cyclical progesterone therapy minimizes the development of oestrogen-induced endometrial hyperplasia.

Comments on the case

This case highlights the importance of informing the patient of the pros and cons of a therapy. The patient must be able to make an informed decision. It is not uncommon for patients to exhibit fears originating from the media.

Further reading

Hulley S, Grady D, Bush T, *et al*. Randomized trial of estrogen plus progestin for secondary prevention of coronary heart disease in postmenopausal women. *JAMA* 1998;280(7):605–13.

Writing Group for the Women's Health Initiative Investigators. Estrogen plus progestin in healthy postmenopausal women. *JAMA* 2002;228:321–33.

Case 14 | Lifestyle adjustments after a myocardial infarction

Candidate information

You are the doctor on a postcoronary care ward.

Please read this summary and then continue with the consultation.

Re: Mr Johnny Giles, aged 73

Mr Giles was admitted 5 days ago with chest pain. An ECG and cardiac enzymes confirmed an anterior ST elevation myocardial infarction (STEMI). He was successfully treated with primary percutaneous coronary intervention (PCI) and he is now 5 days post myocardial infarction. He has never been in hospital before and all this has come as a bit of a shock to him. He has been started on aspirin, clopidogrel, bisoprolol, ramipril and simvastatin. He is sitting in the day room waiting for a taxi to take him home. He sees you and summons you over to speak to him. He has a few unanswered questions.

Your tasks are to: answer his queries regarding his MI and give him advice on adjusting his lifestyle relevant to having had an MI.

Subject/patient/relative information

Mr Johnny Giles is a 73-year-old retired painter and decorator who was admitted 5 days ago with an anterior ST elevation myocardial infarction (STEMI). He has never been in hospital before and never previously took any medication. The suddenness of his illness has taken him by surprise. He is about to go home but he doesn't really understand what has been happening. He has got to know the medical doctor (the candidate) quite well over these last few days and sees him walking through the ward. Mr Giles calls him over to ask him a few questions. His first query is whether he really has had a heart attack. No one has actually sat down with him and explained what a heart attack is. His next query is that he cannot understand why he is on so many tablets when he feels so well. Finally, he wants to know what happens next. Will he see the specialist again and should he change his lifestyle and if so in what way? He used to smoke 20 cigarettes a day 5 years ago and he does admit to having an unhealthy diet, especially with fried food, and he never does any exercise. He is not overweight.

Thoughts and questions the patient/subject may have
- *Have I really had a heart attack?*
- *It all happened so fast – and the procedure they did when I came into hospital, has that sorted the problem out completely?*
- *What should I do now to prevent any more problems?*
- *I'm afraid of what to do if the same thing happens again – will anyone from the hospital keep an eye on me?*

Examiner information

1. Conduct of interview

- Say hello to Mr Giles. Ask how he is.
- He asks you if he has had a heart attack.
- Then, tell him that he has had a heart attack and how it was confirmed. Explain in simple language what a heart attack is, i.e. that doctors and nurses call it a 'myocardial infarction' or 'MI', that it is caused by a blockage of a blood vessel that supplies blood to the heart and that this causes damage to part of the heart muscle which presents as chest pain.
- Reassure him that he was given the best possible treatment with immediate intervention to 'open up the clogged-up arteries'. Reassure him that many people do well after a heart attack and that the reason for all the tablets is to offer some secondary prevention.
- He asks you why he is on so many tablets.
- Explain why he is on aspirin, clopidogrel, bisoprolol, ramipril and simvastatin, with individual drug descriptions. Explain the importance of simvastatin in secondary prevention of ischaemic heart disease. Reiterate the need to take these tablets.
- He asks what happens next.
- Say that he will have a scan of his heart (echocardiograph) within the next 6 weeks to look for any complications from the heart attack.
- He will also be enrolled in a cardiac rehabilitation programme and the specialist nurses responsible for this will be in touch with him within the next couple of weeks.
- He asks whether he should change his lifestyle.
- Ask him what his diet consists of, whether he smokes and whether he does any exercise.
- Say that you are pleased that he does not smoke any more and that he is not overweight. However, he ought to cut down on his fat intake. Emphasize that he is on simvastatin for a high blood cholesterol level and having a high-fat diet will contribute to keeping it high. Say that you will ask a dietician to give him advice at an outpatient appointment.
- Point out that regular exercise has benefits for preventing further heart attacks and encourage him to go for regular walks, recommending a 30-min brisk walk at least five times a week, after gradually increasing his activity to this level.
- Determine if there is an element of anxiety or depression. Tell him that the cardiac rehabilitation programme will allow him to meet other people like himself, enabling him to share his experiences with them. Reassure him that the rehabilitation team will be there to support him and to answer any other queries. Reassure him that the rehabilitation programme will consist initially of simple basic exercises which will be slowly increased as he gains more confidence in his exercise ability. Tell him if he has any problems with anxiety and stress, then the programme will give him relaxation therapy.
- Offer him pamphlets from the rehabilitation team of the British Heart Foundation. Say that he should not drive for a month and he can have sex only after increasing his activity level, say, to going briskly up two flights of stairs with no difficulty.
- Ask if he has any other queries. If not, then reassure him again and say you, or your consultant, will see him in clinic again in a few weeks.

2. Exploration and problem negotiation

The candidate should be able to:

- explain what a myocardial infarction is and how it was treated
- explain why he is on the tablet regimen
- reassure him that, with these medications and appropriate lifestyle improvements, his outlook should be promising
- discuss that referrals will be made for an echocardiogram, dietetic advice and for cardiac rehabilitation
- establish if there is an element of anxiety or depression.

3. Communication, ethics and the law

- Secondary prevention includes managing medical comorbidities associated with ischaemic heart disease, e.g. hypercholesterolaemia, hypertension and diabetes mellitus.
- Improving outcome in patients with a myocardial infarction includes not only the acute management but also the aftercare following this major life event. Cardiac rehabilitation pays attention to physical remedies, education and psychological support. It reinforces advice to adopt a healthier lifestyle and so achieve secondary prevention that way.
- Patients should not drive for a month, longer if they feel that their activity and reflexes are not back to their usual level. They must inform the DVLA and their insurance company.
- Patients should be able to cope with the physical demands of sex after 2–4 weeks of the exercise programme.
- Rehabilitation includes strong encouragement to stop smoking, physiotherapy-led exercise programmes with an initial warm-up followed by an individual

exercise prescription consisting of the cycle and/or floor circuits. Patients should be advised to undertake physical activity for 20–30 min a day to the point of slight breathlessness. Close observation of the heart rate is needed, with particular reference to reaching target heart rates and maintaining these rates during exercise.

- Stress management, particularly in a group setting, can be undertaken after the exercise class. High levels of depression and anxiety are common in patients after having an MI.
- Education is also an important component with practical advice on lifestyle changes, help with going back to work and discussion of delicate topics such as sex.
- Studying information leaflets given by the cardiac rehabilitation team should be encouraged.

Comments on the case

This case highlights the importance of post-MI rehabilitation. This case is not a test of the candidate's knowledge about myocardial infarction but of counselling for a patient's fears and worries after such a life event.

Further reading

National Institute for Health and Clinical Excellence. *Clinical Guideline 58. MI: secondary prevention. Secondary prevention in primary and secondary care for patients following a myocardial infarction.* London: National Institute for Health and Clinical Excellence, 2007.

Case 15 | Smoking cessation

Candidate information

You are the doctor in a general medical clinic.

Please read this summary and then continue with the consultation.

Re: Mr Morris Little, aged 58

Mr Little has come to your clinic for investigation of progressive breathlessness. After full lung function testing, a diagnosis of severe COPD is made. Unfortunately, he smokes 40 cigarettes a day. You feel he should be persuaded to stop smoking.

Your tasks are to: explain the hazards of smoking, the beneficial reasons for stopping and suggestions on how to stop.

Subject/patient/relative information

Mr Morris Little is a 58-year-old man who has been referred to the clinic because of increasing breathlessness on exertion. He has a chronic cough with sputum. He has found getting out of the house to visit friends more difficult in the last 2 years. He has smoked 40 cigarettes a day since he was 12. His father smoked until his death from a heart attack at the age of 50. He lives on his own as his wife died 4 years ago and he regards smoking as his only pastime. Every Monday, when he collects his pension, he goes straight to the local tobacconist to buy the week's supply. He has never thought of stopping as he believes his breathing problems are due to his occupational exposure to the coal furnaces rather than to smoking. He always reminds doctors about the 1950s smogs which is another reason for his bad health – and not necessarily smoking. He is about to see the doctor (the candidate) who will try and persuade him to stop smoking. He appreciates the advice and will think about it before he comes back to clinic next time.

Thoughts and questions the patient/subject may have

- *How can you be so sure that all my breathing problems are because of smoking?*
- *But smoking is my only hobby – you can't take that away from me!*
- *Can you offer me any help?*

Examiner information

1. Conduct of interview

- Explain the diagnosis of chronic obstructive pulmonary disease (COPD, which is a chronic lung disease) and the implications of this disease with regard to prognosis.
- Explain that smoking has contributed to him developing COPD and that this condition will worsen rapidly if he continues to smoke.

- Ask him why he smokes and whether he has ever considered stopping. If he has a family, explain the effect of smoking on the family.
- Ask about family history. Are there any smokers in the family and what is their health like?
- Tell him that it is never too late to stop smoking and reiterate that stopping smoking now will help to slow down the rate at which his lung disease will deteriorate.
- Tell him that smoking causes premature death and a number of other cardiovascular and respiratory diseases. If he stops, then his risk of developing lung cancer will also start to fall.
- Tell him he will notice a difference in his breathing soon after stopping and also he will be financially better off.
- Encourage him by saying that many people have successfully stopped smoking.
- Tell him, however, that to have a better chance of succeeding, he must have the desire and willpower to stop.
- Explore any fears of nicotine withdrawal symptoms.
- Tell him that there are ways to prevent nicotine withdrawal. Describe the types of nicotine replacement therapy available, i.e. gum, patches, inhalator.
- Describe other forms of smoking cessation therapy such as varenicline (Champix) and bupropion HCl (Zyban), although the latter is used less frequently now.
- If you are considering the possibility of suggesting a course of varenicline, you must determine whether there is a previous history of severe depression and suicidal thoughts. Patients with psychiatric disease should be monitored very carefully as recommended by the MHRA (Medicines and Healthcare products Regulatory Agency).
- If he sounds interested in bupropion, enquire about possible contraindications such as a current seizure disorder, severe hepatic cirrhosis, bipolar disorder, bulimia/anorexia nervosa, known central nervous system (CNS) tumour, abrupt withdrawal of alcohol or benzodiazepines, concomitant usage of monoamine oxidase inhibitors (MAOIs), antimalarials, tramadol, quinolones, sedating antihistamines.
- Deal with any fears of weight gain.
- Tell him you will provide smoking cessation leaflets and a 'quit smoking' helpline number. He can also get more information from his GP or local pharmacist.
- If he is unsure about quitting, see him in 2 weeks to reinforce the issues discussed just now.
- You may be lucky enough to have a smoking cessation specialist nurse in your trust to whom you can refer him.

2. Exploration and problem negotiation
The candidate should be able to:
- explain the patient's lung condition and how it is related to smoking
- explain clearly the benefits of stopping smoking and the health risks of continuing to smoke
- offer suggestions on how to stop
- make sure that follow-up is arranged to reinforce the issue.

3. Communication, ethics and the law
- About 13 million adults in the UK smoke cigarettes – 28% of men and 26% of women. In 1974, 51% of men and 41% of women smoked cigarettes – nearly half the adult population of the UK. Now just over one-quarter smoke but the decline in recent years has been heavily concentrated in the older age groups, i.e. almost as many young people are taking up smoking but more older established smokers are quitting. Smoking cessation is a major current health drive in the UK and forms part of the CQUIN (Commissioning for Quality and Innovation) framework.
- Advice on stopping smoking (adapted from Action on Smoking and Health [ASH]):
  - provide numbers for professional helplines, e.g. NHS Smoking Helpline and Quit for information and advice
  - explain to the patient that he must prepare mentally
  - dispel smoking myths
  - explain about nicotine withdrawal, i.e. restlessness, irritability, lack of sleep
  - make a list of reasons why the individual might want to stop, e.g. health, setting a good example to others (children), financial, social, e.g. smell, managing without a smoke in public places
  - set a date which will help mental preparation
  - involve family or friends; it is easier to quit if a smoking partner wants to quit as well
  - deal with nicotine withdrawal; nicotine products include Nicorette, NiQuitin CQ and Nicotinell and the strength of gum or patches will depend on how heavily he has smoked
  - hypnosis, acupuncture or other treatments may help some people, but there is little formal evidence supporting their effectiveness. ASH advice is to use them with caution but if they help mental

preparation, then they will have had some value. Herbal cigarettes are pointless – the individual gets all the tar but nothing to help deal with the nicotine withdrawal
- deal with any weight gain worries
- avoid temptation. In the difficult first few days, he can change his routine to avoid situations where he would usually smoke
- stop completely. Although it might seem like a good idea to cut down and then stop, this is actually very difficult to do in practice. If the individual cuts down, the likely response is that he will smoke each cigarette more intensely. The best approach is to go for a complete break and use nicotine replacement products to help take the edge off the withdrawal symptoms
- watch out for a relapse.

Further reading

National Institute for Health and Clinical Excellence. *Public Health Guidance 10. Smoking cessation services.* London: National Institute for Health and Clinical Excellence, 2008.

Comments on the case

All medical practitioners have a duty to offer smoking cessation advice to all patients they see. Unfortunately, the management of smoking cessation can be done badly but the above points should help to provide a basis for advice. Candidates should be able to discuss the types of replacement therapy available as well as the use of bupropion.

Case 16 | Starting insulin therapy

Candidate information

You are the doctor in a diabetes clinic.

Please read this summary and then continue with the consultation.

> **Re: Mrs Kathleen Hayden, aged 45**
>
> Mrs Kathleen Hayden has poorly controlled type 2 diabetes mellitus despite maximum therapy with oral hypoglycaemic agents and apparent compliance with a diet. Home glucose monitoring has revealed continued levels between 10 and 15 mmol/L. She tried but could not tolerate metformin due to the gastrointestinal side-effects and is presently on gliclazide and sitagliptin. The diabetic nurse has informed you that Mrs Hayden has been having more osmotic symptoms during the last 6 months and wonders if it is time to change her to insulin. Her last HbA1c taken 6 weeks ago was 13.4%. Mrs Hayden is not keen to have insulin. Her BMI is 34 kg/m^2 and she has normal renal and liver function.

Your tasks are to: discuss her present glycaemic control, recommend insulin as the means of improving her diabetic control and ascertain her opinion on this matter.

Subject/patient/relative information

Mrs Hayden is a 45-year-old woman who has had diabetes for 5 years. She has been on oral hypoglycaemic therapy and, despite adhering to a diabetic diet, her glucose levels remain around 10–15 mmol/L. She had to stop taking metformin due to intolerable side-effects of nausea and diarrhoea. She is presently on two other tablets known as gliclazide and sitagliptin. She has, over the last 6 months, been developing more osmotic symptoms, particularly polydipsia, with a feeling of tiredness during the day. She is aware that many diabetics eventually need to be transferred to insulin but this idea is totally abhorrent to her. She has a needle phobia and she used to witness her mother, who had diabetes, self-inject with subsequent bruising, pain and skin lumps. Her mother used to have hypoglycaemic episodes and she remembers, when young, that her mother had a bad episode where she could not rouse her from the hypoglycaemic attack and she had to call an ambulance. Her mother later had a cerebrovascular accident (CVA) and Mrs Hayden had to administer the insulin to her. She remembers the needles being long as well as the trouble of storing the needles in disinfectant. She is about to see the medical doctor (the candidate) to discuss the present state of her diabetes and she is aware that the doctor may discuss the possibility of changing to insulin. Mrs Hayden is determined to defer the change-over for as long as she can.

Thoughts and questions the patient/subject may have

- *There must be another solution without having to go on insulin.*
- *I'm terrified of needles – can you give me the insulin in any other form?*
- *The patient has already made her mind up that she is not going to accept insulin treatment – so is a little bit annoyed that the doctor seems to be pushing the issue!*

Examiner information

1. Conduct of interview

- Introduce yourself to Mrs Hayden and ask if she knows why she is here.
- Ask how her diabetes is and whether she is having any osmotic symptoms.
- Tell her that the diabetic team is worried that her diabetic (glycaemic) control is not very good and that her HbA1c is very high. If she wants to know more, explain the risks of poor glycaemic control in terms of micro- and macrovascular complications.
- Say that it is common for such patients to be changed over to insulin. Ask how she feels about this.
- If she is not keen then explore, with empathy, why this may be so.
- Say how much you appreciate her concerns but that you feel that insulin is in her best interests, particularly with the increased risk of complications. Explain that insulin treatment has improved over the last few years to minimize the difficulties that patients face.
- Try to persuade her that some patients do have a needle phobia and that there are ways to overcome this. Persuade her to come to the diabetic centre to have one of the nursing staff demonstrate the new equipment and techniques available. Also explain that even if she feels totally incapable of self-administering insulin, a district nurse can do that for her or even a relative can be taught to do it.
- Appreciate that there are potential risks of insulin treatment such as hypoglycaemic episodes but these can be minimized by regular monitoring of her blood sugars. Say that she will be started on the lowest possible dose of insulin and the diabetes specialist nurses will keep a close eye on her.
- Explain that there are a lot more support staff available these days and she can get advice and help whenever she needs to.
- Emphasize with delicacy that changing to insulin is inevitable but she can defer it for a couple of months while she attends the diabetic centre.

- Suggest that there are newer therapies for diabetes (such as the GLP-1 agonists like exenatide or liraglutide), which are not insulin and may be indicated in some patients. Explain that these are also injectable preparations. However, due to her significantly high HbA1c and symptoms, these drugs are unlikely to improve her control that much and insulin will still be the next recommended step.
- However, if she wants to consider these drugs instead of insulin, say that you will give her more information about them.
- Discuss any other concerns not already addressed.

2. Exploration and problem negotiation

The candidate should be able to:
- discuss the importance of converting to insulin
- explore any fears about insulin therapy
- provide suggestions on how to overcome these fears.

3. Communication, ethics and the law

- Although this patient cannot be forced to take insulin, it is important that in her best interests she is fully informed of the risks of progressive disease. It is important to explore the real reasons for rejecting therapy and to address these in a positive and sensitive way.
- This lady's view of insulin therapy has been influenced by her previous experiences with her mother and so it is important to educate her about the new therapies available.
- Even when patients absolutely refuse insulin therapy the first time, it is important to review them regularly in case they change their mind (which they usually do).

> **Comments on the case**
>
> This case is influenced by previous psychological experiences and it is a test for the candidate to address these in order to convince the patient that the therapy recommended is in her best interest.

Case 17 | Refusal of analgesia

Candidate information

You are the doctor in a medical clinic.

Please read this summary and then continue with the consultation.

Re: Mr Donald Murphy, aged 74

You are about to see Mr Murphy in clinic. He had a right apical bronchial carcinoma (Pancoast's tumour) diagnosed 8 months ago. He had radiotherapy for a bony metastasis in the right clavicle. His pain, however, has been worse over the last 4 weeks and he was started on morphine sulphate tablets (MST) and is presently on 30 mg bd, in addition to the voltarol he was already taking. However, the hospital nurse specialist tells you, before the consultation, that she believes he is refusing to take his analgesia and, as a result, he is suffering greatly from the pain. Mr Murphy is fully aware that he has a terminal illness.

Your tasks are to: analyse the patient's pain control and explore the possible reasons for non-compliance.

Subject/patient/relative information

Mr Murphy is a 74-year-old man who was diagnosed as having a right-sided lung cancer 8 months ago. At that time, a bony metastasis was discovered in the right clavicle (i.e. spread of the cancer to his collarbone) and radiotherapy was given with some relief. However, for the last 4 weeks his pain has recurred in the same area and it keeps him awake at night. The GP, in conjunction with the local Macmillan nurse, started him on morphine sulphate tablets (MST) in addition to the voltarol and this has been slowly increased to 30 mg bd. However, over the last week, Mr Murphy has not taken any of the morphine tablets and only takes his voltarol when he feels like it, which is rarely. He is concerned that he is becoming addicted to them and he has never liked taking tablets; he would rather put up with the pain. Deep down, behind a jolly 'what will happen, will happen' exterior is a fear of dying. Because the morphine tablets make him slightly drowsy, he is worried he may never wake up when he goes to sleep. There is also a problem with constipation. His diet has never been very good and the morphine has not helped his bowels at all. So, due to a combination of these factors, he has decided not to take the morphine tablets. He has no family and lives alone. He is about to see the medical doctor (the candidate).

Thoughts and questions the patient/subject may have

- *I'm really managing all right – why does everyone keep going on about increasing my tablets?*
- *OK, sometimes the pain gets too much, but I don't want these morphine tablets.*
- *If the doctor puts Mr Murphy at ease and demonstrates that he/she is able to understand his concerns, he may admit that his real fear is about dying in his sleep.*

Examiner information

1. Conduct of interview
- Introduce yourself to Mr Murphy and ask how he is (open question).
- If he tells you that all is fine, explain that the specialist cancer nurse is worried about the pain he has.
- Explore the pain more deeply, i.e. where is it, where does it radiate to, is it constant or does it come and go, does it keep him awake, exacerbating features, e.g. movement, do the tablets relieve the pain, etc.
- Ask him about his pain relief medication (open question). Ask him what he is taking.
- Approach the subject gently by saying that the team is worried that he may not be taking the tablets regularly, or at all.
- If he tells you that he is taking tablets and he has no pain then there is not much else you can do apart from believe him. However, you can still remind him of the benefits of treatment, with information on the possible side-effects.
- If he tells you he does not like taking the tablets, explore why. Is it a fear of the drugs, e.g. addiction, side-effects from the morphine, e.g. constipation? What is his mental state like – confusion (as a result of the drugs)? Is there any influence from the other members of the family? Is he in denial about the cancer or is it a fear of the cancer? He may feel that taking morphine equates with dying.
- Find out what is the patient's understanding of the pain.
- What fears does he have about the disease? Has it resulted in depression? Has he any other symptoms of vomiting, poor nutrition, weight loss, etc?
- What is his opinion regarding the other analgesics he has tried?
- Explain the nature of the pain he has, describe the experiences of other patients with morphine, explain the likely side-effects and, if other family members are present, discuss future or alternative treatment plans.
- Explain that you would like to do an X-ray to look for any other bony deposits and, if this is suspicious, that you would like to proceed to an isotope bone scan. Ask whether he would consider further local radiotherapy if another metastatic deposit is detected.
- He may not agree to restart medication straight away but, in conjunction with the specialist nurse, further meetings fairly soon would be useful to discuss the situation – he may change his mind at the next visit.

2. Exploration and problem negotiation
The candidate should be able to:
- take the full history of pain, the drugs being used and their side-effects
- explore the possible non-compliance with morphine tablets and reasons why
- explore any fears the patient may have about his disease
- suggest he speaks to the specialist nurse about this issue in order to produce a positive change in the patient's attitude towards his treatment
- consider investigations looking for further metastatic deposits with the possible consideration of radiotherapy.

3. Communication, ethics and the law
- Fears about the disease, the pain and the medication need to be explored compassionately.
- Refusing treatment raises difficult dilemmas. Firm coaxing by a trusted member of the family or even by the staff may help. Effective communication from the outset between staff, patient and family can allay much of the possible fear and anger. It is unprofessional to suggest to relatives (if present) that they should try concealing the medication in the patient's food and drink, as this would heighten any mistrust if discovered.
- As far as opioids are concerned, psychological dependence, i.e. addiction, does not occur when used for terminal pain and so a fear of addiction is unwarranted.

Comments on the case

This case tests the ability of the candidate to explore deeply into the feelings of terminally ill patients, their fears and their beliefs. The candidate should show compassion and understanding rather than dismissing simple misconstrued beliefs as 'nothing'.

Case 18 | Human immunodeficiency virus testing

Candidate information

You are the medical doctor in an infectious diseases clinic.

Please read this summary and then continue with the consultation.

> **Re: Mr Alex Whittle, aged 35**
>
> Mr Whittle presented to his GP 3 weeks ago with fever, a maculopapular rash, headache and myalgia. On examination, the GP noted pharyngitis and oral mucocutaneous ulceration. The GP knows that Mr Whittle is gay and also that he has a history of intravenous drug use, and therefore wondered about the possibility of a primary HIV infection. He has referred him to the clinic for further advice and testing. The routine blood tests and chest X-ray recently carried out were unremarkable.

Your tasks are to: discuss the possibility of HIV infection as a cause of Mr Whittle's symptoms and counsel him for an HIV test.

Subject/patient/relative information

Alex Whittle is a 35-year-old man who used heroin intravenously for a total of 8 years up until 2 years ago. He used to inject over 100 mg of diamorphine a day and often shared needles. He gave up using heroin completely 2 years ago and was feeling good about it as he got a job, moved into a permanent address and made new friends. However, 2 months ago he lost his job and couldn't afford to stay in his accommodation. He started using drugs again, albeit only two or three times during that period, but thankfully he asked for help and a couple of good friends supported him. They are letting Alex stay with them and he has stopped the drugs again now. Until 3 weeks ago he was well but then started feeling generally poorly with a fever, sore throat, headaches and muscle aches. He noticed a faint red rash over his body and arms and went to see his GP about it; he had some blood tests and a chest X-ray which came back clear. However, his GP has now referred him to an infectious diseases clinic 'as a precaution' just to get him checked out. He has never allowed himself to consciously think about HIV infection because he is afraid to. His friends with whom he has shared needles or had sex with in the past all seem OK, as far as he is aware. As he has been abstinent from regular intravenous use for 2 years, he has convinced himself that the likelihood of acquiring HIV is negligible. He has never had an HIV test. He is gay but has not been in a sexual relationship with another man since he separated from his long-term partner over 5 years ago.

Thoughts and questions the patient/subject may have
- *Everyone will know if I have the test and that could be bad for me.*
- *Are you saying that you think I have AIDS?*
- *If I agree to have the test what will happen?*

Examiner information

1. Conduct of interview

- Pace the consultation so it is unhurried.
- Make it clear that this discussion is confidential.
- Briefly ask Mr Whittle about the symptoms he had 3 weeks ago and ask how he is feeling now.
- Ask him if he has ever thought about his previous lifestyle and the risk of exposure to HIV infection.
- Give him time to think for a few moments before continuing.
- Ask him about his history of heroin use; whether he injected heroin and whether he shared needles. If he did, were any of his associates known to be HIV positive? Has he been abstinent from injecting heroin and, if so, for how long? Does he use heroin by other means, e.g. smoking?
- Give him a bit of space so that he doesn't feel that he is being interrogated (his thoughts are likely to be racing now).
- Explore whether he has other risk factors for HIV infection.
- Tell him you are concerned that his current clinical presentation may be related to HIV infection.
- Give him a few moments before asking how he feels about this. Check that he is OK to continue.
- Now ask him if he has ever had a test for HIV and if he would consider one now.
- He may express concerns about everyone finding out if he has the test. Reassure him that the test is confidential to the staff looking after him and that the result would not be released to anyone without his consent.
- Be honest with him that, if he does undertake a test and it is positive, he will need to tell any sexual partners (essential) and his GP (encouraged), who will be able to provide more appropriate healthcare if he/she is aware of his positive status.
- Explain that the test is not a test for acquired immunodeficiency syndrome (AIDS) but a test for the HIV virus and emphasize the difference.
- Explain that a sample of blood is taken and that the result should be available within a day or two. Go on to explain that sometimes the first test can be negative but that a repeat test is recommended in up to 2 weeks time.
- He may ask if he has AIDS. Explain that if the HIV test is positive, he will need further assessments and tests to determine if he has signs of a severely compromised immune system or other illnesses/infections. Depending on these, it will be determined if he

has AIDS. However, reassure him that many patients with HIV infection will not develop AIDS, especially if he has early diagnosis, regular monitoring and timely treatment.
- Acknowledge that this news must be difficult to take in and ask him if he wants time to decide or whether he is comfortable to have the test straight away.
- Explain to the patient the benefits of getting tested (for example, if the test is positive he can start treatment and monitoring early, can take precautions to avoid transmitting the infection to others and engage in healthier behaviour).
- However, acknowledge that it can raise anxiety levels and possibly cause discrimination at the patient's work place or affect future insurance policies if tested positive (unless done at an anonymous test centre).
- Tell him that there is support available at this hospital's genitourinary medicine clinic, as well as via other groups, and he is free to see a member of staff any time during the day. Give him contact details of these services before he leaves.
- Provide him with leaflets that may answer some of his questions.
- Advise him that if he has sex before the results of the test are known, he should make sure he uses a condom, regardless of whether or not he knows the person he has sex with.
- Ask if he has any concerns that have not been addressed.
- If he does decide to have the HIV test, ask him who he would like to give him the result and who he wants with him at the time. Tell him when and by whom the blood is going to be taken and reiterate what the follow-up arrangements are going to be (regardless of whether the patient consents for the test or not).
- Close the discussion by asking the patient to summarize the key points, to enable you to establish what his understanding of the situation is, and invite questions.

2. Exploration and problem negotiation

The candidate must be able to:
- make an assessment of the patient's recent illness and prepare the patient through thoughtful discussion for the possibility that he may be HIV positive
- maintain a non-judgemental attitude towards the patient in relation to his lifestyle choices and situation
- do a brief risk assessment for HIV infection in this patient

- pace the consultation and provide 'warning shots' before discussing the possibility of HIV
- ensure that they make the patient aware of their responsibilities in relation to other people and risk
- clarify the difference between HIV-positive status and AIDS
- provide information about the HIV test and, if possible, secure his agreement
- if time allows, outline what will happen after the test.

3. Communication, ethics and the law

- Preparing a patient prior to an HIV test is a skill any medical trainee should be able to perform competently because this is a situation that is not necessarily only done in a specialist infectious diseases clinic. Any in- or outpatient with a presentation that is suspicious of an HIV- or AIDS-related illness, or is otherwise considered to have risk factors, should be offered an HIV test with appropriate information given beforehand.
- Obtaining informed consent for an HIV test should generally follow the same principles as obtaining informed consent for any other investigation or procedure.
- The amount of information that a patient will want will vary from person to person. Ask what they want to know and provide as much or as little detail as they need at the time. Remember that consent is always grounded on the principle of informed decision making. If a patient just waives their right to be given sufficient information then you need to explain that there are implications for them and that they should think seriously about having more information. If they are still prepared to proceed from a position of ignorance, you should document this carefully and remind them that they can ask for more information at any time.
- All communication can be enhanced by the use of diagrams and written material where appropriate and available.
- It is ethically important to carry out a risk assessment to enable the individual to identify his personal risk for acquiring the infection and also consider who he might be at risk of transmitting the infection to. Be unequivocal in clearly advising the use of condoms, to stop sharing needles and other risk-taking behaviour until the test result is known to avoid exposing others to the risk of infection.
- The issue of life (or other) insurance policies following an HIV test is often brought up in such a scenario. Generally, if the test is negative, then an individual should not be discriminated against when taking out life insurance. If the test is positive then all insurance policies taken out prior to this will be honoured, although he may find difficulty taking out future policies.

Comments on the case

Obtaining consent from a patient for an HIV test is commonly encountered in Station 4 of the PACES examination. Remember that you should not limit yourself to talking about the actual test alone but also make an assessment of the patient's risk factors and encourage him or her to consider risk-reducing behaviour regardless of the test result.

If talking about HIV testing with a woman of child-bearing age, discuss the implications of having HIV during pregnancy, and transmitting the virus to her child during pregnancy, during delivery or while breastfeeding.

Following this, discuss when and how the results will be communicated to the patient. This will typically be in about 2–3 days, unless you have the facilities to do a rapid antibody test. It is best done face to face together with an HIV specialist nurse or counsellor. You also need to mention what the planned follow-up arrangements will be, including the option of retesting if the patient is still in the 'window period' where they have not mounted the antibody response yet. Also stress that a negative test does *not* mean that the person is immune to or will never get the infection in the future.

Epidemiological studies estimate that up to one-third of all adults in the UK with HIV infection are undiagnosed. There is now a universal 'opt-out' policy to HIV testing which means that individuals coming into contact with healthcare services at specific settings are offered an HIV test as routine but they can refuse it. These settings include sexual health clinics, antenatal or pregnancy termination services, and drug dependency programmes, services caring for people diagnosed with tuberculosis, hepatitis B/C or lymphoma and in areas where the local prevalence exceeds 2 in 1000. This is in addition to offering the test to people who are felt to be at particularly high risk (e.g. partners of HIV-positive individuals, men who have sex with other men and their female partners, intravenous drug users, people from a country with high HIV prevalence or their sexual partners).

The UK national guidelines for HIV testing recommend that first-line testing should now be fourth-generation assays which test for both HIV p24 antigens and IgG antibodies to them simultaneously. Such a combination test can give a positive result within 4 weeks of acquiring the infection and can have a sensitivity and specificity of over 99%. A positive screening test should be repeated with a second sample and also be sent for confirmatory testing. There is also 'point-of-care' testing which can give a result as quickly as 10 min and can be done from fingerprick or mouth swab samples. However, since these methods only test for antibodies, the reported sensitivity is lower, especially if the patient is still within the window period (currently 12 weeks).

Note that the serological tests usually test for HIV-1 infection. Therefore patients with HIV-2 infection (which is more prevalent in West Africa) can have an indeterminate result. Other possible causes for an indeterminate result include early stages of seroconversion and advanced HIV infection (when the antigen levels are too low).

Further reading

British HIV Association, British Association of Sexual Health and HIV and British Infection Society. *UK national guidelines for HIV testing*. London: British HIV Association, 2008. www.bhiva.org/HIVTesting 2008.aspx

Case 19 | Communication of a human immunodeficiency virus-positive result

Candidate information

You are the medical doctor working in a respiratory ward and you are due to speak to Mr Steve Turner.

Please read this summary and then continue with the consultation.

Re: Mr Steve Turner, aged 48

Mr Turner was admitted to hospital 2 weeks ago with breathlessness and a non-productive cough. He was found to be in severe type 1 respiratory failure and was immediately taken to the intensive care unit (ICU), was intubated and placed on ventilatory support. Chest X-ray and bronchoscopy findings were suggestive of *Pneumocystis jirovecii* pneumonia (PJP), which was confirmed on subsequent culture of bronchial washings. The ICU team carried out an HIV test (whilst Mr Turner was intubated), which came back positive and he has been started on antiretroviral treatment in the last few days. He was extubated 4 days ago, and was transferred to the respiratory ward yesterday. He is unaware of the investigations or any of the results from his ICU admission. The ICU team found out from his brother that Mr Turner is married and that he has been known to have contact with prostitutes whilst on business trips out of the country.

Your tasks are to: explain to Mr Turner the events and tests carried out in ICU, tell him about the positive HIV result and address any concerns that he may have.

Subject/patient/relative information

Mr Steve Turner is a 48-year-old-man who is married with two teenage children. He is a businessman who has to travel abroad for work frequently and has had unprotected sexual intercourse with female prostitutes whilst away. He has been open about this to his brother, whom he is close to, but does not want his wife or children to know under any circumstance. He has never used illicit drugs (intravenous or otherwise), nor has he received any blood transfusions. He does not have any tattoos. He has been losing some weight over the last few months but was otherwise reasonably well until the week before his admission when he became progressively short of breath and developed a non-productive cough. He felt very unwell on the day of his admission and cannot remember subsequent events until about 3 days ago when he was no longer requiring ventilation in the ICU. He is feeling better now apart from extreme tiredness. He has noticed that he is on several new medications and cannot understand what they are for. He is aware that the prostitutes he had sexual encounters with when abroad could be carrying sexually transmitted infections but he never seriously considered the possibility that he could have picked one up. When the diagnosis of HIV is mentioned, he is angry that he was tested without his permission and wants to know why it was done. He is adamant that he does not want his wife to know about it under any circumstance because it will 'jeopardize his marriage'. He also has several insurance policies (including life and property insurance) and wants his HIV diagnosis to be kept confidential.

Thoughts and questions the patient/subject may have

- *What gave you the right to test me without my permission?*
- *What made you think that I might have HIV?*
- *Have you told my wife?*
- *Who told you I was at risk?*
- The 'patient' will respond to the attitude of the candidate as appropriate – if they appear to be detached or judgemental then he may be less open to discussion.

Examiner information

1. Conduct of interview

- Introduce yourself to Mr Turner. Ideally this consultation should take place in a quiet room on the ward so as to maintain the patient's confidentiality and if possible with a specialist nurse present.
- Ask him how much he remembers about the events preceding and during the admission (he may tell you about some breathing difficulties and cough before admission but may not recall much else).
- Tell him in simple terms that he was admitted with a severe form of pneumonia which required admission to the ICU, that ventilatory support and other treatments were required and that he has responded well to this.
- Say that due to the specific type of pneumonia that he had, the team looking after him was suspicious about the possibility of HIV infection and, in his best interests, carried out an HIV test whilst he was sedated in the ICU.
- Give him a few minutes to absorb what you have said before continuing.
- Ask him if the possibility of HIV infection has ever crossed his mind before or if he has been tested for this in the past.
- Give him the positive HIV test result in an unambiguous way (and again pause after this to allow him to take it in).
- Ask him if he is all right to continue talking about this now.
- Sensitively broach the subject of whether he knows of any risk factors he has been exposed to for acquiring HIV infection or if he has considered or even had

an HIV test in the past. Tell him you are going to ask him personal questions that may provide an understanding of his exposure to HIV risks. Ask about his sexuality, marriage/regular sexual partners, other sexual partners (casual contacts, male or female), usage or not of protection, particularly condoms, and then ask about illicit drug use, tattoos, and previous blood transfusions, etc.
- Tell him that he has been started on antiretroviral treatment for the HIV and also on medications for the pneumonia. If he wants to know more, say that due to the PJP that was confirmed, he does fall into the more severe end of the HIV spectrum known as AIDS. Reassure him that although he will need to be on the treatment for an extended period of time, many people with HIV illnesses these days have a reasonably good quality of life and a near normal life expectancy.
- Ask him who he wishes to discuss the test result with. Reassure him that aside from the medical and nursing staff looking after him directly, no one else has been informed to ensure patient confidentiality. Ask him whether he will inform his wife (essential) and GP (he should be encouraged to let the GP know).
- Give him details of what is going to happen from here. For example, when he will be seen by the specialist HIV doctor or nurse, how they will monitor his response to treatment, and what the discharge plans are, etc.
- Ensure that you arrange another time to come back and speak to him again. Ideally this should be later the same day or the next day to ensure that he has understood the information given to him and to give him the opportunity to ask any questions.

- Address any other issues he has before ending the consultation.

2. Exploration and problem negotiation

The candidate should be able to:
- briefly explain to the patient the reason for his admission to the ICU and what he was treated for whilst there
- sensitively bring up the topic of HIV infection and its relation to his respiratory illness, and break the news of the positive test result to him
- deal calmly with any challenges which arise about testing without his consent and give cogent reasons for the decision to test
- briefly assess any major risk factors he has for HIV infection (including current and past sexual partners) and talk to him about contact tracing/partner notification.

3. Communication, ethics and the law

- In this case, the patient's lack of capacity was temporary but the HIV test was indicated in his best interests to ascertain the cause of his severe PJP infection/respiratory failure and so that he could be started on the appropriate treatment to aid his recovery and wean him off the ventilator.
- It is important for the clinicians managing this patient to be conscious of their own values and judgements and to ensure that they maintain a professional demeanour which does not prejudice their behaviour or attitude. Encouraging a husband to tell his wife that he is HIV positive and how this has happened will be doomed to failure if you convey disapproval and disgust towards him.
- There is no easy way to communicate a positive HIV test result, especially if the patient was not aware of the test being carried out and so had no adequate preparation beforehand. It requires a lot of sensitivity on the part of the doctor. It is best not to get sidetracked and to come to the point as quickly as possible.
- HIV testing is usually done in a planned setting after an assessment of an individual's risk factors and after obtaining informed consent. However, there are circumstances when it may need to be done in the patient's best interests or without his prior consent which, unless undertaken with justifiable clinical reason, could represent a violation of his autonomy.
- It is likely, when told that an HIV test has been carried out without discussion and consent, that the patient will be angry and shocked, and you may need to

conduct this interview in a 'breaking bad news' style, allowing a lot of time for him to take it in and to deal with any reactions he may have.
- Fear of discovery and rejection is a normal human response in many people and so the consequences of disclosing this information are understandably frightening. Acknowledging this and suggesting that there may be professional colleagues who can help to support the patient while he tackles these challenges should certainly be offered. The sexual and reproductive health multidisciplinary team is an excellent resource which should not be overlooked in encouraging the patient to let his spouse or other sexual partners know. In fact, the patient should be encouraged to contact trace his previous sexual partners (or, if an intravenous [IV] drug user, people who might have shared needles with him) to ask them to get the appropriate counselling to be tested too.
- UK national guidelines for HIV testing recommend that any individual who tests HIV positive should see an HIV clinician, specialist nurse or sexual health counsellor within 2 days and definitely within 2 weeks of being given the result. Therefore, you need to know about the local specialist services in your area, the planned treatment and recommended follow-up for the patient before breaking the news.
- Following the Mental Capacity Act 2005 for England and Wales, there are guidelines available regarding HIV testing in patients who do not have the capacity to consent for the test. In situations where the lack of capacity is deemed to be temporary, the medical team need to consider if the test can be postponed until the patient regains capacity 'unless testing is immediately necessary to save the person's life or prevent a deterioration of his condition'. If the test was carried out, the result should be communicated to the patient as soon as possible after he/she has regained consciousness.
- In situations where the lack of capacity is likely to be permanent (e.g. due to a mental disability), it is essential to note that capacity is 'decision specific' and 'time specific'. Therefore, just because a person lacks the capacity to make more complex decisions (such as in relation to property or finances), it cannot be assumed that he/she cannot make other decisions (for instance, in relation to healthcare or consenting for an HIV test). The capacity to do this needs to be assessed in relation to the specific decision at hand and at the time it needs to be made. The person needs to be given as much information as possible, in a form easily understandable to them, in order to help

them make the decision. If they are still unable to, you should consider if there are any people with Power of Attorney or court-appointed deputies to speak on behalf of the patient or if there is an advance directive in place. If none of the above is available, the test can be done in the patient's best interests if clinically indicated.

- The sharing of a positive HIV result with third parties raises several ethical dilemmas in terms of protecting the patient's confidentiality/autonomy balanced against the responsibility we have towards the general public – i.e. justice (for example, if the patient continues to engage in risk-taking behaviour and is potentially transmitting the infection to others). The ideal situation would be for you to gain the patient's consent to communicate the result to his GP and other healthcare professionals looking after him.
- In situations where the patient refuses to give consent for disclosure, you need to weigh the harm that may arise from non-disclosure, in terms of public interest, against breaching doctor–patient trust by disclosing the information. GMC guidance states that public interest refers to 'protecting individuals or society from serious harm such as a serious communicable disease or serious crime'.
- The GMC document 'Disclosing Information about Serious Communicable Disease' states that 'you may disclose information to a known sexual contact of a patient with a sexually transmitted serious communicable disease if you have reason to think that they are at risk of infection and that the patient has not informed them and cannot be persuaded to do so'. *However, you should let the patient know that you are going to disclose this information.* Also, when undertaking contact tracing or partner notification, you should maintain the anonymity of the patient if possible.
- According to GMC regulations about disclosure of patient information for employment or insurance purposes, you need to ensure that the patient has sufficient information about the consequences of disclosure and obtain their written consent to do so if possible. You need to make it clear to the patient that you cannot withhold any relevant information. You should only reveal factual information relevant to the request and offer to show the patient a written copy of your report. If the patient refuses to consent to disclosure, make it clear to them that you may need to breach confidentiality if it is in the public interest or required by law.

<table>
<tr><td>

Comments on the case

Following a positive HIV serology result, you will need to send more blood off to determine the severity of the patient's immunosuppression by checking viral load and CD4 counts. The viral load levels are typically very high in acute HIV infection (>100,000 copies/mL usually) and are detected by polymerase chain reaction (PCR) testing to components of the HIV virus. Another way of detecting the severity of HIV infection is to check host CD4 cell counts (because the virus attacks the host's T-lymphocytes which express CD4 molecules). The above two indices are used to determine the status of HIV infection, to monitor response to treatment and to provide guidance about when to initiate prophylaxis for opportunistic infections.

This case highlights two important issues in HIV medicine. Firstly, the conduct of an HIV test in a patient who did not have the capacity to consent to the test when it was carried out and, secondly, the communication of a positive result. It is important for candidates to be familiar with the Mental Capacity Act 2005 and the principles regarding consent for investigations and treatment in patients who lack capacity. The GMC website provides excellent guidelines on maintaining doctor–patient confidentiality and situations where it may need to be breached.

</td></tr>
</table>

Further reading

Department for Constitutional Affairs. *Mental Capacity Act 2005: Code of Practice.* London: Department for Constitutional Affairs, 2007.

General Medical Council Supplementary Guidance. *Confidentiality: disclosing information about serious communicable diseases.* London: General Medical Council, 2009.

General Medical Council Supplementary Guidance. *Confidentiality: disclosing information for insurance, employment and similar purposes.* London: General Medical Council, 2009.

Case 20 | New diagnosis of tuberculosis

Candidate information

You are the doctor in a respiratory clinic.

Please read this summary and then continue with the consultation.

Re: Miss Angela Adeyemi, aged 25

Miss Adeyemi is a lady from Nigeria, living in the UK for the last 4 years. She works as a carer in a residential home for elderly patients. She presents with a 6-month history of weight loss, night sweats and a non-productive cough. She was referred to the respiratory clinic and a bronchoscopy was carried out which came back positive for alcohol- and acid-fast bacilli and also *Mycobacterium tuberculosis* was grown on the culture. Miss Adeyemi has come back to the clinic to find out the results of her bronchoscopy.

Your tasks are to: explain to Miss Adeyemi the diagnosis of pulmonary tuberculosis and how she will be managed from here on.

Subject/patient/relative information

Miss Angela Adeyemi is a 25-year-old woman, who was born and brought up in Nigeria. She moved to the UK 4 years ago with her mother and two younger brothers and lives with them at home. She works full time as a carer in a residential home. She is the sole breadwinner of the family and her income is needed to pay the rent for the family's flat as well as her brothers' education. One month ago, she was referred to the respiratory clinic with a 6-month history of weight loss, night sweats and a dry cough. The consultant did not give her much more information except that she needed a bronchoscopy to look for certain types of infection. She went on to have this shortly after and has come back to clinic for the results. She suspects at the back of her mind that tuberculosis is a possibility because of its prevalence in Nigeria and she has seen other people suffer from it in her home town. She is very worried about the possibility of a positive diagnosis as it would have serious implications for her job since her family are completely dependent on her income. She is also concerned about the possibility that other family members might be infected. She is uncertain as to whether it can be completely cured.

Thoughts and questions the patient/subject may have

- *What is the result of the test I had done?*
- *Can you make me better?*
- *How long will it take?*
- *Could my family have it/get it?*
- *What am I going to do if I can't work?*

Examiner information

1. Conduct of interview

- Introduce yourself to Miss Adeyemi and ask about her general health (e.g. if there is any improvement in her symptoms).
- Establish her understanding of the bronchoscopy and the reason for today's appointment. If she says that she was not told anything, ask if she has any thoughts on what might be going on or if she has any particular concerns.
- Explain that today you would like to discuss the results of her bronchoscopy and what needs to be done from here.
- Tell her, in simple terms, that the bronchoscopy results have confirmed that she has tuberculosis (TB) of her lungs.
- Ask if she knows about TB or if she knows of any family or friends who have been diagnosed with it before. Since she is from a country of high prevalence she was probably exposed to it in the past but it can become clinically apparent at any time subsequently.
- Explain that she will need to be started on medications for TB and if she completes the course of antibiotics (which is for 6 months), she can be completely cured of it, although there is a chance of reactivation in the future should she become unwell or immunocompromised for any reason.
- Tell Miss Adeyemi that she will be closely followed up by the local TB services and her response to treatment monitored carefully. She will have a named key worker and should be given the contact details of the key worker before she leaves the clinic.
- Tell her that TB is a notifiable disease in the UK and her details will need to be passed on to the Department of Health.
- She needs to be informed that all her household and other close contacts will be offered screening for TB (i.e. people who share a bedroom, kitchen, bathroom with the index case, their boyfriends/girlfriends and other frequent visitors to their house). Find out who these household/close contacts are and mention that you will inform her GP as well as the local TB service representative regarding the offering of screening to these individuals. Depending on whether these contacts are found to have latent or active TB, they may be offered treatment, further investigation, bacille Calmette–Guerin (BCG) vaccination or advice and follow-up.
- If she asks about her job, say that she needs to contact her occupational health department as soon as possible if she has one, but it is likely that she will be asked to refrain from carrying out any direct patient care until she has been established on treatment for at least 2 weeks or is sputum smear negative.
- Address any other concerns she has and end the consultation.

2. Exploration and problem negotiation

The candidate should be able to:

- establish what the patient was told during her initial consultation and prior to the bronchoscopy (i.e. was the possibility of TB ever mentioned?)
- give her the result of the cultures from the bronchoscopy which confirms pulmonary tuberculosis
- discuss the procedure of initiating antituberculous treatment (ATT), the likely duration of treatment and screening of her household contacts
- sensitively appreciate her concerns about losing her job as a carer.

3. Communication, ethics and the law

- When discussing the diagnosis of TB with patients who are employed in the healthcare sector, it is important that they understand the implications for the infection risk to others. This may mean a change of occupation which is likely to have a significant impact on them and any dependents that they may have. You should ideally put them in contact with someone who can give them advice or at least signpost them – for example, a TB nurse specialist or social worker.
- All patients with confirmed or suspected TB should be referred to the local Health Protection Agency (HPA) so that contact tracing can be carried out.
- Healthcare workers new to the NHS should be assessed for the risk of having TB by means of a questionnaire, examination of BCG scar and the result of a Mantoux test within the last 5 years, if available. If the Mantoux test was positive and they have not been vaccinated previously, they should be offered the BCG injection.
- If a healthcare worker or NHS employee is diagnosed with TB and/or is commenced on ATT, they need to inform their occupational health department immediately. Occupational health is likely to consider the case on an individual basis, taking into account if the patient has latent or active TB and the risk associated with their job. It is possible that the healthcare worker will be asked to refrain from contact with patients (especially children, pregnant women

and immunocompromised people) until they have been on treatment for a few weeks or have three consecutive sputum samples which are smear negative.

Comments on the case

Tuberculosis is a very commonly encountered topic in Station 4 and the focus can vary from diagnosis to treatment concordance to occupational health issues and infection control/public health matters. This case looks at communicating a new diagnosis of pulmonary TB and it is possible that the discussion will centre on contact tracing, occupational risks and management in high-risk groups (e.g. homeless people, coexisting HIV-positive infection). Depending on the exact scenario and availability of time, you may also be expected to consent the person for an HIV test at the same time.

Tuberculosis is on the rise in the UK, with around 7500 new cases diagnosed each year. Pulmonary TB accounts for around 60% of TB cases here.

Tuberculosis infection may be latent or active, and can be predominantly pulmonary or affect other sites (e.g. lymph nodes, meninges, joints, etc.).

For latent, non-active TB, NICE recommends carrying out a Mantoux test and if this is positive or the results unreliable then to consider interferon-γ immunological testing, if available.

A Mantoux test (i.e. tuberculin skin test) should be interpreted in the context of the patient, i.e. if they are likely to be immunosuppressed or at increased risk of TB (e.g. HIV infection, on chemotherapy, on renal dialysis, or have been in close contact with an active TB case). People who have been vaccinated with the BCG can have false-positive reactions to the Mantoux test, especially if they have been vaccinated in the recent past.

Interferon-γ immunological testing is a serological test which measures the interferon-γ released by T-cells in response to stimulation by M. tuberculosis antigens. It has a specificity of more than 95% for a diagnosis of latent TB infection. The results are not affected by prior BCG vaccination.

Suspected active pulmonary TB should be investigated initially with a chest X-ray followed by at least three early-morning sputum samples for TB microscopy and culture. If the patient is not able to produce sputum, the samples should be obtained by bronchoscopy and bronchial lavage.

For suspected active, non-pulmonary TB, tissue should be obtained for TB culture by, for example, lymph node biopsy, pleural biopsy, cerebrospinal fluid or any other aspirate or histology sample.

Laboratories will first detect acid-fast bacilli (AFB) by microscopy in the stained smears. Rapid diagnostic tests for Mycobacterium tuberculosis complex, which use PCR techniques to amplify certain RNA or DNA sequences in M. tuberculosis, can be used to confirm the diagnosis, especially when the smear is also AFB positive. Culture of the organism will then be done for species identification and drug susceptibility testing.

If the clinical signs and risk factors are strongly suggestive of TB, treatment should be commenced before waiting for culture results.

Once a diagnosis of TB is made, the patient should be referred to a specialist in the management of the condition (usually a respiratory physician). The team would normally include specialist nurses, pharmacists and health visitors.

The standard recommended regime for treatment is 6 months of a four-drug regime (isoniazid and rifampicin, together with pyrazinamide and ethambutol for the first 2 months). A thrice-weekly regime of the above-mentioned drugs may be used in cases of directly observed therapy (DOT). However, this is not usually recommended if the infection has affected sites other than the lungs (e.g. meningeal, lymph node, bone/joint, etc.).

For meningeal TB, the initial treatment is the same with four drugs for the first 2 months but, following this, the isoniazid and rifampicin should be continued for a total of 12 months. A glucocorticoid (normally prednisolone 20–40 mg) should be given initially with gradual withdrawal after 2–3 weeks.

Treatment of latent TB should be considered for high-risk patients (e.g. HIV positive or healthcare workers) with positive Mantoux (or interferon-γ) results or with TB scars on chest X-ray. Treatment is with 6 months of isoniazid or 3 months of isoniazid and rifampicin.

Further reading

National Institute for Health and Clinical Excellence. *Clinical Guideline 33. Tuberculosis: clinical diagnosis and management of tuberculosis, and measures for its prevention and control.* London: National Institute for Health and Clinical Excellence, 2006.

Case 21 | Non-compliance with anti-tuberculous treatment

Candidate information

You are the medical doctor in a respiratory clinic.

Please read this summary and then continue with the consultation.

Re: Mr Connor Morley, aged 19

Mr Morley was diagnosed as having pulmonary tuberculosis 2 months ago (smear positive). He is now being reviewed in clinic by yourself. He is not unwell but his cough and sputum persist and he has not gained any weight. His chest X-ray is no better. He works in a nightclub collecting glasses; he drinks about eight pints of strong lager a day and smokes 40 cigarettes a day (including cannabis). He does not have HIV infection. He lives in a hostel for the homeless. He migrated from Ireland when he was 12 and essentially comes from an unhappy family background. His father is in prison and his mother committed suicide 4 years ago. You have spoken to the TB health visitor and she is not convinced that Mr Morley is taking the antituberculous tablets every day. In fact, the TB health visitor has confirmed with the GP that Mr Morley has only picked up one prescription (2 weeks supply) on the first day of treatment, 2 months ago. Presently he should be on Rifinah '300' two tablets a day, pyrazinamide 2g a day, ethambutol 800mg a day and pyridoxine 10mg once a day. You are concerned that he is still symptomatic, that he is poorly complying with the medication and that he is still infectious. Mr Morley has let it be known that he would not want to be admitted to hospital.

Your tasks are to: approach Mr Morley on the issue of non-compliance and negotiate ways of improving his compliance.

Subject/patient/relative information

Mr Morley is a 19-year-old man originally from Ireland who was diagnosed 2 months ago with lung TB (i.e. pulmonary tuberculosis). He had presented with cough, sputum and loss of weight. The chest X-ray showed shadowing and TB was confirmed by a smear-positive sputum sample. Cultures have revealed fully sensitive Mycobacteria tuberculosis. He settled in the UK when he was 12 and comes from an unsettled and unhappy background; his father is in prison and his mother committed suicide 4 years ago. Presently he lives in a hostel for the homeless and works part-time as a glass collector in a nightclub. He drinks excessively and smokes heavily (including cannabis) as well. He has been started on a total of nine tablets a day, which consist of Rifinah '300', pyrazinamide, ethambutol and pyridoxine. His compliance has been poor, in fact non-existent, over the last 2 months. He finds the pyrazinamide difficult to swallow, and feels sick with the others (especially the Rifinah). He is awake most of the night and, because he drinks heavily, he forgets to take his tablets. He has seen the TB health visitor only once because each time she visits the hostel he is either sleeping or out drinking with friends. He has failed to attend clinic four times but thankfully has turned up today. His symptoms of cough and sputum persist and he has not gained any weight. He is in denial of his illness and will not admit to poor compliance. He is due to see the medical doctor (the candidate) in clinic. The candidate will be trying to convince him to agree to participate in a programme of directly observed therapy (DOT).

Thoughts and questions the patient/subject may have

- Mr Morley's life experiences make him feel uncomfortable around authority figures and, having spent years with a dominant father pushing him around, it is hard for him to be told what to do. He recognizes this in himself and tries to work against it.
- He knows that he is unwell and really does want to feel better but he doesn't believe that he deserves to.
- *Why are you accusing me of not taking my tablets? do you have any proof?*
- *Why are all of you suddenly so concerned about me? I have spent most of my life alone and know what is best for me.*

Examiner information

1. Conduct of interview

- Introduce yourself to Mr Morley and thank him for coming into clinic today.
- Ask how he is with regard to his symptoms.
- Ask how he has been getting on with the tablets – you may want to say that you know it can be difficult for people with TB as there are quite a few to take and they aren't very pleasant.
- This approach should give him the opportunity to start to explain why he hasn't been taking the medication. Give him some prompting if needed; for example, ask about side-effects (real or perceived), forgetfulness, inability to get hold of the tablets and poor information about how to take the tablets. Other possibilities may be that the purpose of taking the medicine is not clear, a perceived lack of benefit (feeling better), unpleasant taste/difficult to swallow (pyrazinamide is notorious for this), complicated regimen, etc.
- Listen attentively to what he is telling you with minimal interruption.
- If he denies missing his medication then you will need to be frank with him and explain that the lack of improvement is causing concern and the team have to query whether he is taking the medication. Give him a moment to absorb this and then if necessary explain that his GP has told the TB health visitor that he has not picked up any prescriptions except for

the first one which was 2 months ago (hopefully he will admit to non-compliance).

- If he still denies non-compliance, explain calmly and clearly that he really needs to take the medication as it will make him better and also avoid spreading the TB to other people. Explain that there is a scheme which might be helpful for him, given that he has difficulties with taking the medication at the current time. Give him a minute to think about this and potentially ask questions.
- Emphasize the benefits of the DOT scheme: it is only three times a week – although this will be altered according to how he is doing. He doesn't need to remember to go to the GP and chemist to get the prescription sorted out, etc.
- If you have not made progress then you need to tell him that his current circumstances mean that a decision has to be made with regard to the medication for him. He will be placed on the DOT scheme so that he can be watched taking his medication.
- Ask him how important working in the nightclub is before advising him that he should not work there because of the risk of infecting others.

2. Exploration and problem negotiation
The candidate should be able to:
- establish a rapport with the patient, treating him with dignity and respect
- make an assessment of the patient's current health

- refrain from making judgements about the patient and his lifestyle
- carry out a constructive discussion about his non-compliance
- work with the patient and negotiate a plan that will improve compliance.

3. Communication, ethics and the law

- Non-compliance with medication is very common in TB patients and the factors causing this are stated above. Every consultation should have some assessment of compliance.
- Balancing the individual's autonomy against the need to manage TB for the greater good of the community (i.e. justice) is important. Whilst they may not agree, it is arguable that enforced DOT is in the individual's best interest. They are likely to improve, have regular interaction with a health professional and it reduces the risk to other members of the community.
- Effective communication which takes account of a patient's life experiences, lifestyle and relationships with authority, and avoids confrontation, will pay dividends in discussions about improving compliance. Avoiding making judgements or treating the patient in a paternalistic and authoritarian approach is more likely to earn trust and enable you to establish facts and negotiate solutions.
- It is worth considering the support of the psychology services for some patients where social circumstances and behaviour may indicate poor or low self-esteem. It is arguable that if patients don't value themselves then they have poor motivation to comply with healthcare measures.

Comments on the case

The doctor in the clinic must involve the patient's GP immediately. Ring the GP and inform him of the problems as he may be able to carry out the DOT using a practice health visitor and especially if the practice has had experience of this before.

Directly observed therapy in tuberculosis treatment is where ingestion of every drug is witnessed. Cohort studies with historical controls receiving self-administered therapy have shown improved cure rates from DOT. In the UK, where TB is usually managed by experienced physicians with the help of specialized nurses, DOT is recommended in non-compliers, particularly the homeless, alcoholics, drug abusers, drifters, the seriously mentally ill, patients with multiple drug resistance, and those with a history of non-compliance either in the past or during the present treatment. It should be considered in refugees especially from countries where multidrug resistance is particularly high (e.g. Eastern Europe).

Directly observed therapy can be daily but an intermittent regimen is usually more convenient. The most common is rifampicin, isoniazid, pyrazinamide and ethambutol (or streptomycin) three times weekly for 2 months, then rifampicin and isoniazid three times weekly for 4 months.

Ways to help compliance include better education, explanation of side-effects, alternative regimens, simplified drug regimens, e.g. in antituberculous therapy, rifampicin, isoniazid and pyrazinamide can come as a combination product, e.g. Rifater, which is much easier to swallow.

Use your investigative skills to work out the degree of compliance, e.g. from clinical and radiological improvement. The colour of the urine can sometimes help to check if the patient has taken rifampicin the same day. Do not necessarily go for the easy alternative and admit the patient to hospital. Circumstances will not change when he is discharged.

Case 22 | Multidrug-resistant tuberculosis

Candidate information

You are the medical doctor working for a respiratory team.

Please read this summary and then continue with the consultation.

Re: Mr Bobby Singh, aged 44

Mr Singh is a 44-year-old man who was diagnosed with TB 5 months ago and was started on standard anti-tuberculous treatment. However, he admits to not taking the tablets very frequently because of the side-effects and also because they were not making him feel any better. He has become more unwell over the last 2 months with ongoing weight loss, extreme tiredness and a productive cough. He has been unable to eat or drink and was admitted to hospital a week ago with general malaise and dehydration. Blood tests were unremarkable apart from mild renal impairment (treated with iv rehydration), and an HIV test was done which was negative. Sputum samples obtained on admission are suggestive of multidrug-resistant TB and his treatment is due to be changed in view of this. Your consultant feels that Mr Singh is too unwell to be discharged until he is established on his new treatment and his clinical condition improves. Mr Singh has been in a sideroom in an isolation ward for a week now and Sister has told you that he is unhappy about this and wants to speak to you regarding this and other concerns, including the restrictions on his family visiting.

Your tasks are to: discuss Mr Singh's TB treatment with him and respond to his questions about the infection control policies in place on the ward.

Subject/patient/relative information

Mr Singh is a 44-year-old man who was born in India but has been resident in the UK for over 30 years. Five months ago he was diagnosed with tuberculosis (TB) after returning from a 2-month holiday in India. He was started on antituberculous drugs, but has found it hard to tolerate the side-effects and doesn't feel that there has been any improvement, so he has not been taking them. He has become increasingly unwell over the last 2 months with ongoing weight loss, extreme tiredness and a productive cough. It got to the stage where he was unable to eat and drink and was admitted to hospital a week ago as a result. He was asked to provide sputum samples on admission and has been told by the nurse that he may need to go on further medication. However, he is not aware of the exact details of this. He lives at home with his wife, parents and three young children between the ages of 3 and 10. He does not smoke or drink alcohol. He is quite unhappy at the moment because he feels that he has been left in a sideroom on the ward for the last week without any explanation and wants to know when he can go home. He is really missing his children and he has been told that they are not allowed to visit him on the ward.

Thoughts and questions the patient/subject may have

- *Why do I have to be shut up in this room?*
- *How long will I have to stay in here for?*
- *I am getting really upset about not being able to see my children; it is not fair on my family or me.*
- *I am seriously thinking about packing my bags and going home.*

Examiner information

1. Conduct of interview

- Introduce yourself to Mr Singh and find out how he is feeling.
- Explain that you have come to see him because you understand from the ward sister that he is concerned about a few things and you hope to be able to help.
- Ask him what he knows about his diagnosis of TB and briefly ask how he was getting on with the medication (he may admit to non-compliance and you could briefly explore the reasons for this but remember that this is *not* the main objective of this station).
- If necessary, you should explain to him that the sputum tests that he provided on admission confirm that he still has active pulmonary TB but, unfortunately, it also appears that he has drug-resistant *M. tuberculosis*. Explain that this is the likely reason why he still has the symptoms of weight loss, lethargy, etc. If he wants to know more, mention some of the causes why he might have acquired drug-resistant TB (e.g. poor compliance to treatment or previous treatment failure, acquisition of TB in a country with a high prevalence of drug-resistant TB).
- Give him an uninterrupted moment to absorb this information as this may enable him to ask questions.
- Tell him that your consultant is still waiting for more results to come back from the laboratory but it is possible that he will need to be started on a different regimen of medication that will work for the type of TB he has. If he wants to know more, say that it is possible that this may involve medication straight into the bloodstream via a vein (intravenous) for a period of time but emphasize it is not necessary for him to stay in hospital for the whole duration of the

treatment if he starts showing clinical improvement and he is felt to be non-infectious. However, say that he will need to be monitored very closely while he is on the new medication (including the possibility of directly observed therapy).

- If he mentions that he is unhappy at being left in the side-room for so long without information, apologize and acknowledge that it must be very difficult being cut off from the day-to-day activity of the ward and contact with other people. Explain to him that due to the concern about him having a particularly drug-resistant strain of TB, it is important to make sure that other patients and staff on the ward are protected as much as possible from the risk of picking up the infection.
- Explain to him that an additional benefit of keeping him in a room of his own is that it protects him from picking up other infections from the hospital while his body deals with the TB infection as his immunity is currently lower than usual. It is also for this reason that any visitors are asked to wear a mask when they come in to visit him.
- Give him a moment, then ask if he is OK for you to explain why his children are discouraged from visiting him on the ward. Go on to explain that since young children often have an immature/underdeveloped immune system, they can be at greater risk of being infected, so it is important to make sure that they only have minimum contact with people with TB. Mr Singh will readily understand the above reasoning if explained to him in a clear non-confrontational manner.
- Ask if there have been any other reasons why he is unhappy about his isolation, e.g. if he felt he was being ignored or his needs not attended to by the nursing or medical staff. If so, take note of these and tell him that you will raise the matter further and get back to him.

- Address any other questions he has.
- Reassure him that you are working hard to help him improve and recover enough to go home and then conclude the discussion.

2. Exploration and problem negotiation

The candidate should be able to:

- explain to the patient the possibility that drug-resistant TB is the cause of his ongoing symptoms and that he may need to go onto more medication for it
- acknowledge the personal impact that these restrictions impose on the patient and his family
- concisely discuss the infection control policies the hospital has for patients with TB
- address the patient's concerns in an appropriate and compassionate manner.

3. Communication, ethics and the law

- The clinician's, and indeed the patient's, responsibilities extend in this type of case to the wider community which needs to be protected as much as possible from the risk of contracting TB from a known carrier.
- The individual patient still has a family and it could be argued that depriving him and his children of an opportunity to have contact is contrary to Article 8 of the Human Rights Act which sets out the right to a family life, although it is equally possible to cite the rights of everyone to be healthy.
- Social isolation may contribute to increased levels of anxiety and depression in the person who is isolated. If the patient is likely to be isolated for some time, it would be compassionate and prudent to have discussions with the infection control team about the possibility of strictly controlled short visits.
- It should not be necessary to admit patients with TB into hospital (drug-sensitive or drug-resistant cases) unless there is a definite clinical or social need to do so.

Comments on the case

This case is challenging in that it tests the candidate's knowledge about an uncommon and difficult issue, drug-resistant TB, but also requires you to deal with a frustrated patient on the ward. Even if you do not know much about the subject matter, you need to reassure the patient that the medical team are taking his condition very seriously and that you will come back with your consultant later to talk about the exact treatment plan. Awareness of the infection control policies in your hospital will be worthwhile.

Patients who are smear positive are considered to have open/infectious TB and hence should be contained in a side-room, unless they are in a ward with immunocompromised patients, when they should be nursed in a negative-pressure side-room. They should remain there until they have completed 2 weeks of standard antituberculous therapy or are discharged home earlier. If they are going to be in contact with HIV-positive or other immunosuppressed patients, they should additionally have three negative sputum smears, show tolerance to treatment and their cough should be resolved before being nursed outside a side-room, in accordance with NICE guidelines.

The NICE guidelines do not recommend the routine use of masks, gloves or other forms of barrier nursing when seeing to drug-sensitive TB patients on treatment, unless staff are going to be administering aerosol products or come into direct contact with the patient's sputum or other body fluids.

Drug-resistant TB refers to cases of tuberculosis where the strain of *M. tuberculosis* is resistant to one of the drugs used in the standard treatment regime (i.e. isoniazid, rifampicin, pyrazinamide, ethambutol or streptomycin). Multidrug-resistant TB (MDR-TB) refers to strains that are resistant to at least isoniazid *and* rifampicin and possibly other agents as well. Extensively drug-resistant TB (XDR-TB) is where the isolate is an MDR-TB but additionally is resistant to any fluoroquinolone *and* to at least one of the three injectable second-line drugs (capreomycin, amikacin and kanamycin).

(Continued)

Drug-resistant TB is rare in the UK except for London, where 6–7% of cases of TB may be resistant to one of the first-line drugs and around 1% are multidrug resistant.

Risk factors for MDR-TB should be assessed for every patient on TB treatment and these include history of previous TB drug treatment or treatment failure; birth in a foreign, high-incidence country; HIV infection; age 25–44 years; male gender and resident in London.

Patients with MDR-TB who are admitted to hospital should be in a negative-pressure side-room and, for as long as they remain in hospital, should be nursed there until they are non-infectious, non-resistant and the cultures negative. Staff and visitors should wear an FFP3 facemask when coming into contact with them.

Case 23 | 'Hospital superbug' 1 (*Clostridium difficile*)

Candidate information

You are the doctor on a medical ward.

Please read this summary and then continue with the consultation.

> **Re: Mrs Joan Fisher, aged 83 years**
>
> Mrs Fisher is an elderly lady who was admitted to hospital 10 days ago after a fall and was given a course of antibiotics for a urinary tract infection in accordance with the drug sensitivity profile of the organism on urine microscopy, culture and sensitivities (MC&S). Yesterday, she developed a few episodes of type 7 diarrhoea (according to the Bristol Stool Chart) and stool cultures have been sent off for *Clostridium difficile* toxin (results awaited). She is otherwise well and the plan is to discharge her once her diarrhoea resolves. Her son, her next-of-kin, has come to the ward to see her and finds that she has been moved into a sideroom because of the diarrhoea. The nurse in charge of the shift has already explained the situation to him but he is insistent that he speaks to a doctor. He was already aware from speaking to other patients' relatives on the ward that 'there has been an outbreak of diarrhoea in the hospital recently'.

Your task is to: address the son's concerns about his mother's infection and isolation.

Subject/patient/relative information

Mr Mark Fisher is the son of Mrs Joan Fisher, an 83-year-old lady who was admitted to hospital 10 days ago after a fall. The doctors found that she had a urine infection and put her on antibiotics for 5 days (she was given them intravenously for the first 2 days). She seemed to be doing well and her son was expecting to take her home soon. However, when he came to see her today, he was told by the nurse in charge that she had developed diarrhoea over the last few days and had been moved to a sideroom. He has also been asked to wear an apron and gloves when going in to see her. While waiting to speak to the doctor, Mr Fisher has been chatting to the relatives of another patient on the same ward who mentioned 'an outbreak of diarrhoea in the hospital'. He has read in the newspapers about 'a hospital superbug, known as *C. diff*, which can cause severe diarrhoea and even death' and is very concerned that his mother has contracted this diarrhoea because of poor hygiene in the hospital. He wants to speak to the doctor looking after his mother (the candidate) to find out more about this and is considering making a formal complaint to the hospital if substantive reasons are not given. (He is at no point aggressive towards or blaming the doctor for the events.)

Thoughts and questions the patient/subject may have

- *Why have you moved my mother to a side-room?*
- *Did the antibiotic for the urinary infection cause the* Clostridium difficile?
- *You are telling me that antibiotics may have caused this and yet you are planning to give her more . . .*

Examiner information

1. Conduct of interview

- Introduce yourself to Mr Fisher and establish the nature of his relationship with the patient.
- Explain that the nurse in charge has told you that he is asking for an update on his mother's current medical condition which you understand is causing him some concern. Give him an opportunity to tell you what is troubling him before asking if you can 'fill in the gaps' by explaining the situation.
- Explain that when she was initially admitted, it was found that she had a urinary tract (or 'water') infection which was confirmed on the urine sample and she was treated with appropriate antibiotics for 5 days.
- Acknowledge that, since yesterday, she has developed a few episodes of diarrhoea and a sample has been sent to establish the cause of it, but the results are not back yet.
- Reassure him that regardless of the stool culture result, the hospital takes all cases of diarrhoea seriously in case it is due to an infectious agent, and precautions have to be taken to avoid the spread of infection.
- Give him a few moments to process this and then ask if you can carry on explaining what happens now.
- Clarify the reason why Mrs Fisher has been moved to a side-room and what precautions are required of all staff and visitors: namely to wear an apron and gloves when going into her room to reduce the chances of picking up the bug or transmitting it to others.
- He may ask whether it is true that there has been an outbreak of diarrhoea in the hospital and if his mother's problem has been caused by staff not taking adequate hygiene measures. Give him an honest answer about the outbreak – if you don't respond to the question he may think you are being evasive.
- Listen to his concerns and ask if he has witnessed any specific situations when he felt there was inadequate hygiene practised (e.g. a member of staff not cleaning their hands between patients, use of unclean equipment, incomplete commode cleaning, entry to dirty

patient areas, etc.). If so, note down these specific examples and say you will speak to the ward manager about it and get back to him. Otherwise, explain that there are several patients in the hospital who may have diarrhoea or other infections for a variety of reasons. However, if there is any suspicion of an outbreak, the infection control team will advise on the containment of infectious diseases on the wards. This team is responsible for carrying out a thorough investigation, reporting it to higher authorities and prescribing measures to reduce the risk of spread by closing off certain wards or bays.

- He may mention that he has read about a 'hospital superbug' which can be serious and can even cause death and he is worried that his mother may have contracted this. Acknowledge his anxieties. Be honest with him and say that this is one of the concerns that the team have and that Mrs Fisher's stools have been sent to the lab to be investigated for the bug called *Clostridium difficile* (or *C. diff* for short).
- Reassure him that if Mrs Fisher's diarrhoea is confirmed to be due to *C. diff*, she will be given the right treatment and monitored closely for any complications with daily examinations, X-rays or blood tests if needed, etc. and that he will be kept informed of her progress.
- Ask him what else he wants to know at the moment. Then, if necessary, you can explain that *C. diff* is a type of bacterium that can cause diarrhoea, and it can occur when an individual's normal gut defence mechanisms have been breached by factors such as antibiotic treatment.
- Reassure him that in most people it is completely treatable with specific antibiotics but very rarely can lead to complications such as severe inflammation of the bowel and obstruction.
- Be prepared to explain, if asked, why, when the antibiotics may have contributed to the problem, you now plan to give her more.
- Ask him if he has any other questions or if he needs more detailed information.
- It is prudent to fire an anticipatory warning shot about the possibility of *C. diff* infection when patients are clearly more vulnerable, such as the elderly, hos-

pitalized patients, and especially those with other comorbidities who are particularly susceptible.

- If he asks whether the antibiotic she was given for a urinary tract infection (UTI) may have caused this, say that it is a possibility but when Mrs Fisher was initially admitted, she was unwell with the UTI and treatment was absolutely indicated. Reassure him that she was given the correct antibiotics (according to the drug sensitivity profile) and for the minimum duration required to clear the infection.
- Remember that if Mrs Fisher's son has raised concerns about specific staff members' hygiene practice or the cleanliness of the ward, you need to be seen to take this very seriously and to tell him how exactly you are going to ensure that it is brought to the attention of the ward manager and the infection control team.
- Tell him clearly who you are going to speak to and provide him with their names and job titles. Explain that he should expect to hear from one of them in the next 48 h and that if he does not, he can contact the ward manager to ask for an update.
- If he is not happy with your explanation then give him the contact details of the Patient Advisory Liaison Service (PALS) or complaints department of your hospital.
- Remember, all patients and their relatives have rights to voice their opinion if they feel their medical care has been suboptimal. If you convey an air of defensiveness or annoyance, you are more likely to elicit a mirror response in the person who is unhappy with treatment and care and that has a deleterious effect on therapeutic relationships and trust that can be hard to win back. Only if sufficient concerns are reported and enquiries made can actions be taken to improve the situation.
- Thank Mr Fisher and close the discussion.

2. Exploration and problem negotiation

The candidate should be able to:

- provide Mrs Fisher's son with clear, honest information on her condition, its possible aetiology

and the infection control policies adopted by the hospital

- address his concerns regarding 'diarrhoea outbreaks in the hospital' and antibiotic-associated diarrhoea
- provide him with information about the channels he can go through if he wants to take the matter further.

3. Communication, ethics and the law

- Members of the general public are understandably afraid about the risks of infections such as C.diff. It is certainly the case that the media in general seem to devote their attention to those cases where patients have succumbed to C.diff or it has been a major contributory factor in their death. Headlines such as 'Clostridium Difficile kills ten patients a day', 'Fatal hospital bug inquiry unveiled' and 'Superbug killed my dad but we were not told' will significantly heighten anxiety of patients and their families when C.diff is diagnosed. As a result of this, it is important that clinicians understand the fear that people may hold and therefore should use core communication skills to explain why C.diff occurs, what the implications are and the projected risks for individual patients. This is particularly critical where underlying co-morbidities may put the patient at significant risk of serious complications, such as colitis, toxicity or organ failure.
- Patients and relatives need to understand the importance of infection control measures, what they need to do and the rationale behind ensuring that they follow the guidance. Whilst it may be considered to be a nursing role to communicate this information, the clinician has a responsibility to at least ensure that patients and families are aware that there are special measures to be taken by them as well as by the health professionals.

Comments on the case

With the increased public awareness of *Clostridium difficile* (or *C. diff*)-induced diarrhoea amongst hospital patients, such a case is not an uncommon scenario in the hospital setting that can be simulated in a

PACES examination. Remember that the patient in this case did not actually have confirmed *C. diff* infection yet but the discussion is likely to go down this line. Therefore familiarize yourself with the national document on *C. diff*

(Continued)

infection and also your trust's infection control/antibiotic-prescribing guidelines.

In the UK, *C. diff* infection rose from the 1990s to the mid-2000s, especially in the over-65s, but since 2007 it has been on the decline. However, even as recently as 2007, over half of acute NHS trusts reported rates of two cases per 1000 admissions in the over-65s. Epidemiological studies have also shown that a more virulent strain of the *C. diff* bacterium, known as NAP1, has emerged in the UK since 2003 and is responsible for some of the outbreaks seen. This strain causes more severe disease and resistance to treatment.

The Department of Health and the Health Protection Agency jointly released guidance in 2008 amalgamating previous guidelines and providing a framework for tackling the problem on individual, trust-wide and national levels. Some of the key recommendations in this document include the following: all staff should have a high index of suspicion for potentially infectious diarrhoea; a patient's diarrhoea should be monitored using a tool like the Bristol Stool Chart; staff should wear gloves and aprons during all contact with the patient or patient's environment and wash hands with soap and water before and after any patient contact.

On a trust-wide level, there should be provision to isolate suspected or proven cases of *C. diff* in single isolation rooms, or in cohort bays or wards. Cohort wards are isolation wards which are not composed of individual isolation rooms.

Trusts should have comprehensive antibiotic guidelines to encourage the use of narrow-spectrum, empirical or definitive antibiotics for different infections and this should be reviewed by doctors, nurses and ward pharmacists on a daily basis. There should be an antibacterial management team comprising a microbiology or infectious diseases consultant and an antibiotic pharmacist to support ward staff.

Cleanliness should be a priority in all clinical areas (in accordance with the National Specification of Cleanliness guidelines) and regular auditing and feedback for all staff should be encouraged.

Antibiotic-associated colitis is caused most commonly by the anaerobic, gram-positive *C. diff*. It is transmitted as spores in the intestinal flora and converted to the toxin-producing form. Studies have shown the rate of carriage of *C. diff* bacteria can range from 20% to 50% among people in long-term homes and hospitals.

Antibiotics disrupt normal colonic flora, thereby providing a suitable environment for growth and multiplication of *C. diff* organisms. Among the antibiotics commonly used in medical practice, the following have been particularly implicated in increasing the likelihood of *C.diff*: clindamycin, fluoroquinolones, broad-spectrum penicillins and cephalosporins. However, all classes of antibiotics (including metronidazole and vancomycin, which are used to treat *C. diff*) can predispose an individual to it. Extended courses of antibiotic treatment and the use of multiple agents also put a patient at increased risk.

Aside from antibiotics, other factors which have been reported to have an association with *C. diff* colitis include advanced age, patients with general ill health and those on proton pump inhibitor treatment (which suppresses gastric acid production). *C. diff* infection can range clinically from asymptomatic colonization to diarrhoea and mild abdominal discomfort to pseudomembranous colitis to toxic megacolon in the most severe cases. Management should consist of stopping the responsible antibiotic if possible and providing general supportive measures. Treatment with oral metronidazole or vancomycin for a period of 10–14 days is usually sufficient to clear the diarrhoea but patients can have positive *C. diff* toxin in stool cultures for up to 6 weeks after treatment.

Further reading

Health Protection Agency and Department of Health. *Clostridium difficile infection: how to deal with the problem*. London: Department of Health, 2008.

Case 24 | 'Hospital superbug' 2 (methicillin-resistant *Staphylococcus aureus*)

Candidate information

You are the medical doctor on the ward.
Please read this summary and then continue with the consultation.

Re: Mrs Gladys Winterburn, aged 91

Mrs Winterburn has been a resident on the ward for 4 months. She was initially admitted after a fall at her home. She has heart failure and has had bilateral chronic leg ulcers for a few years. It has become quite clear that she would be unable to look after herself in her own house and so an application for a nursing home place has been made. Presently, she can mobilize slowly with the assistance of one person, needs full attention with regard to mobilizing, feeding and toileting and her leg ulcers need regular dressings. Unfortunately, 2 weeks ago a methicillin-resistant *Staphylococcus aureus* (MRSA) screen isolated MRSA in the left leg ulcer although there is no evidence of any systemic effects or invasive infection of the ulcer. Provisionally, a place may be available at a local nursing home and one of the senior carers, Miss Brenda Raglan, has come to assess Mrs Winterburn. She has been told about the MRSA and as a result is slightly concerned about the possible impact on the nursing home.

Your tasks are to: speak to the senior home carer, Miss Raglan, outlining Mrs Winterburn's condition, explain the MRSA finding in the leg ulcer and allay any fears she may have with regard to infection control.

Subject/patient/relative information

Mrs Gladys Winterburn is a 91-year-old lady who was admitted 4 months ago after a fall. She also has heart failure and bilateral chronic leg ulcers for which she needs regular dressings. It has become quite clear that Mrs Winterburn will be in need of care for her activities of daily living, especially for mobility, feeding, toileting and dressing of the ulcers, and so a request for placement in a nursing home has been put into motion. Miss Brenda Raglan is a senior carer at a local nursing home. She has come to assess Mrs Winterburn for placement there. The financial arrangements have been sorted out, so all it needs now is for Miss Raglan to see Mrs Winterburn in order to make a general assessment of her suitability. However, to her dismay, Miss Raglan hears about the isolation of MRSA from the leg ulcer. She is particularly concerned about the risk this may pose to her staff and the other patients with regard to the possible difficulty in treatment and also the risk of overwhelming infection. She feels that this has jeopardized the placement and wants to speak to the medical doctor (the candidate) for further information about the MRSA.

Thoughts and questions the patient/subject may have

- *How dangerous is this MRSA infection for Mrs Winterburn?*
- *What precautions do we have to take in the nursing home for her?*
- *Is Mrs Winterburn's MRSA infection going to be a problem for the other residents in our nursing home?*
- While Miss Raglan would like to accept Mrs Winterburn in her nursing home and provide her with the care she needs, as a senior carer, she also has responsibility towards all the other residents and staff of the home. She hopes that the candidate will understand that.

Examiner information

1. Conduct of interview

- Introduce yourself to Miss Raglan who is from a local nursing home.
- Tell her about Mrs Winterburn with regard to her needs for daily living, i.e. she needs help with mobilizing, feeding, toileting and for the ulcer dressings.
- Explain that MRSA has been isolated from one of the ulcers although this is not causing any problems either locally or systemically.
- Explain:
  - what MRSA is and how long the bacterium has been known to physicians
  - what problems MRSA can cause
  - why MRSA is so different from some other bacteria with regard to resistance to antibiotics
  - how residents with MRSA should be cared for
  - what special precautions need to be taken, especially regarding basic hygiene
  - whether staff or other patients need screening
  - who else to inform
  - the procedure if a resident with MRSA needs to be admitted to hospital
  - other sources of advice.
- Explain gently to Miss Raglan that there can be no justification for discriminating against people who have MRSA by refusing them admission to a nursing or residential home, or by treating them differently to other residents.

2. Exploration and problem negotiation

The candidate should be able to:
- discuss the needs of Mrs Winterburn
- explain the MRSA findings in the leg ulcer
- explain what MRSA is and the implications for the patient of having MRSA

- reassure Miss Raglan that MRSA in a nursing home setting should pose little threat to the health of staff and other residents.

3. Communication, ethics and the law

The following are recommendations from the Department of Health.

- **What is MRSA?** MRSA stands for methicillin-resistant *Staphylococcus aureus*, a form of *Staphylococcus aureus* (SA). SA is the most common type of bacterium which can infect humans. About a third of the population are colonized with it. 'Colonized' means that the organism lives harmlessly on a person's skin or in the nose and does not cause any infection. In around one-tenth of these carriers (i.e. 3% of the population overall), this SA is MRSA.
- **What problems can it cause?** Usually SA causes no problems. If it does, the resulting infection is usually trivial and affects the skin, resulting in infected cuts or boils. These are easily treated. SA is more of a threat to hospital patients with deep wounds, catheters or drips which allow the bacterium to enter the body. People with severely reduced resistance to infection, for instance due to HIV infection, are also vulnerable. For these groups of patients, the resulting infection can be serious – septicaemia or pneumonia, for example.
- **What is special about MRSA?** MRSA acts in exactly the same way as SA and causes the same range of infections. Most people who have it come to no harm at all. What makes MRSA different is its resistance to antibiotics. Some antibiotics are still effective but they may be more difficult to use and cause side-effects. That is why the spread of MRSA in hospitals is a cause for concern and why hospital patients with MRSA may be isolated in side-rooms or special wards.
- **How long has MRSA been around?** MRSA is not a new problem – the strains which can cause outbreaks

in hospitals first appeared in the early 1960s. In some countries, where antibiotics are available much more freely than here, the spread of MRSA has now been accepted as more or less inevitable. In the UK, there has been and continues to be a focus on prevention and control.

- **How should residents with MRSA be cared for?** If good basic hygiene precautions are followed, then residents with MRSA are not a risk to other residents, staff, visitors or members of their family, including babies, children and pregnant women. Good hygiene is important to prevent the spread of all infections, not just MRSA. Like any other resident, those with MRSA should be helped with hand washing if their mental or physical condition makes it difficult for them to wash their own hands. They should be encouraged to live a normal life without restriction and they need not be isolated. They may share a room so long as neither they nor the person with whom they are sharing have any open sores or wounds, drips or catheters. They may join other residents in communal areas such as the sitting and dining rooms, so long as any sores or wounds are covered with an appropriate dressing which is regularly changed. They may receive visitors and go out of the home, for example, to see their family or friends.

- **Are any special precautions required?** People with MRSA do not normally require special treatment after discharge from hospital. If a course of treatment does need to be completed, then the hospital should provide all the necessary details. The only special precautions required are that staff:
  - with eczema or psoriasis should not perform intimate nursing care on residents with MRSA
  - should complete any procedures on other residents before attending to dressings or carrying out other nursing care for residents with MRSA
  - should carry out any clinical procedures and dressings on a resident with MRSA in the resident's own room
  - should seek and follow expert infection control advice from the consultant in communicable disease control and/or community infection control nurse for any resident with MRSA who has a postoperative wound or a drip or catheter.

In Scotland, seek advice from the consultant in public health medicine (CPHM) and/or community infection control nurse. Affected residents with open wounds should be allocated single rooms if possible.

- **Good basic hygiene precautions to prevent infections, including MRSA infections:**
  - good hand hygiene practice by staff and residents is the single most important infection control measure
  - disposable gloves and aprons should be worn when attending to dressings, performing aseptic techniques or dealing with blood and body fluids
  - cuts, sores and wounds in staff and residents should be covered with impermeable dressings
  - blood and body fluid spills should be dealt with immediately according to the locally agreed policy
  - sharps should be disposed of into proper sharps containers
  - equipment, such as commodes, should be cleaned thoroughly with detergent and hot water after use
  - clothes and bedding should be machine-washed, in accordance with the local policy
  - cutlery, crockery and clinical waste should be dealt with in the normal way.

- **What about screening?** Residents and staff in care homes do not need routine screening for MRSA unless there is a clinical reason, for example a wound getting worse or new sores appearing. In that case, the resident's GP should send wound swabs to the local hospital for general microbiological investigations. Screening of other residents and staff is very rarely necessary and would only be done following discussion between the consultant in communicable disease control (CPHM in Scotland) and the microbiologist.

- **What is the procedure for admitting someone with MRSA?** When a person with MRSA is admitted to a nursing or residential home, the following people should be informed: the manager, matron or designated member of staff with infection control responsibilities and the resident's GP.

- **What if a resident with MRSA needs to go to hospital?** If an affected resident needs to go to hospital, then the hospital should be informed beforehand that they have, or have had, MRSA: the hospital's infection control doctor or infection control nurse should be contacted if the person is to receive inpatient treatment. They are available through the hospital switchboard and are usually based in the Department of Medical Microbiology and the relevant department should be informed if the person is to receive outpatient treatment.

- **What if an MRSA infection is diagnosed?** This is uncommon outside hospitals. However, if a resident does become infected with MRSA, their GP should contact the microbiologist at the local hospital for advice on treatment. Meanwhile, any infected wounds or skin lesions should be covered with appropriate dressings.

- **To find out more, or to get specific advice, you should contact:**
  - your local consultant in communicable disease control (CCDC) – this is the person who is responsible for the control of infectious diseases within the community served by your health authority. In Scotland, contact your local consultant in public health medicine. You can find the CCDC (or CPHM in Scotland) through the Department of Public Health Medicine at your health authority or the Health Protection Agency (www.hpa.org.uk)
  - your community infection control nurse (CICN); in some areas infection control nurses have been appointed to help provide advice on infection control in the community. They are the best people to consult about writing and implementing infection control policies and about any infection control problems posed by individual residents. The CICN can usually be contacted through the CCDC (or CPHM in Scotland).

Comments on the case

The Department of Health has recommended that there can be no justification for discriminating against people who have MRSA by refusing them admission to a nursing or residential home or by treating them differently from other residents. Long-term residency in hospital with chronic infections encourages emergence of MRSA. It is vital that the candidate understands what is meant by MRSA and its implications. The above information from the Department of Health should be helpful.

Further reading

Department of Health. *What nursing and residential homes need to know*. London: Department of Health, 1996.

Department of Health. *A simple guide to MRSA*. London: Department of Health, 2007.

Case 25 | Assessing suicide risk

Candidate information
You are the medical doctor in an emergency admissions unit.
Please read this summary and then continue with the consultation.

Re: Mr William Bremner, aged 49

Mr Bremner was admitted today by the Foundation Year 1 doctor following a paracetamol overdose. He took ten 500 mg tablets 24 h ago with the intention of committing suicide. His paracetamol levels are under the treatment level and he does not have any symptoms suggestive of hepatotoxicity. He is sitting alone in the day room watching television. The ward nurse is worried that this episode was a genuine suicide attempt. She wants you to assess him.

Your tasks are to: explore the reasons behind the suicide attempt and assess Mr Bremner's suicide risk.

Subject/patient/relative information
Mr Bremner is a 49-year-old information technology consultant. He has recently lost his job due to poor business and his wife left him 2 months ago after 27 years of marriage. They had been incompatible for a number of years but one day his wife just decided to leave. As a result, he is convinced that his life is now hopeless and worthless and that the future is very bleak. He had never really thought about killing himself until now. Over the last month, he has been having suicidal thoughts most days, but yesterday was his first real attempt. He took 10 tablets of 500 mg paracetamol in one go with two glasses of vodka. He wrote a damning note to his wife before the attempt. He went to bed but woke up this morning with a slight headache and nausea. He told his neighbour who brought him straight to casualty. He does not have any paranoia or persecutory delusions. He has always been a heavy drinker (especially spirits, usually three bottles a week) but, more recently, his consumption has increased. He does not suffer from any physical illnesses and he has had no recent bereavements. Currently, he is clearly depressed with low mood and poor sleep, appetite and concentration. He feels life is not worth living but is not sure if he really wants to kill himself. What he does realize is that he wants some help. He is about to see the medical doctor (the candidate).

Thoughts and questions the patient/subject may have
- *You wouldn't understand how I'm feeling at the moment – my life is not worth living any more.*
- *How can you help me sort my life out?*

Examiner information

1. Conduct of interview

- Introduce yourself to Mr Bremner.
- Explain how sorry you are that he is in hospital and that he had wanted to kill himself.
- Reassure him that you are there to help him.
- Ask him how he is feeling at the moment. Ask if he has any symptoms of nausea, abdominal pain or headaches (from the paracetamol poisoning).
- Determine the history of the self-harm: what tablets, how many, did he take them all at once, with alcohol, planned self-harm, was he alone, timed so that no one could intervene, suicide note, recent change in his will, did he inform anyone after the act, admission of suicide intent, does he still want to die?
- Determine the reasons for attempted self-harm and the problems faced by Mr Bremner, i.e. job loss, marital problems, financial difficulties, legal problems, alcohol and drugs problem, present psychiatric disorders, bereavement or impending loss and social isolation.
- Assess Mr Bremner's mental state: suicidal thoughts, feeling of hopelessness, worthlessness and despair, lowering of mood with symptoms of poor sleep, poor appetite and poor concentration, persecutory delusions, paranoia and any auditory hallucinations.
- Is there a present or past psychiatric history, including previous suicide attempts?
- Assess family and social support.
- Explain again that he needs help. Ask if he understands why he needs help (insight?). Say that you will look after him medically as he gets over the paracetamol poisoning and you will arrange further liver function tests. Then he will be seen by the psychiatrist who may consider transferring him to the psychiatric unit to start antidepressant therapy and to protect him from any further self-harm. Ask how he feels about seeing a psychiatrist.
- Ask if he has any other questions.

2. Exploration and problem negotiation

The candidate should be able to:

- understand and sympathize with Mr Bremner's present psychological state
- obtain a detailed history of the suicide event without being judgemental
- assess the other factors (e.g. medical, social, psychological) which are important when assessing an attempted suicide patient

- assess the risk of further suicide attempt
- reassure him that help is available.

3. Communication, ethics and the law

- Factors suggesting a genuine suicidal intent:
  - act carried out in isolation
  - act timed so that intervention unlikely
  - precautions taken to avoid discovery
  - preparation made in anticipation of death (e.g. making a will)
  - active preparation made for the attempt (e.g. saving up tablets)
  - extensive premedication
  - leaving a suicide note
  - failing to inform potential helpers after the failed attempt
  - admission of suicidal intent.
- Evaluating a patient following an attempted suicide should include assessment of:
  - the events that preceded the act
  - reasons for the act, including suicide intent
  - the problems faced by the patient
  - any psychiatric disorders and psychiatric history, including previous suicide attempts
  - family and personal history
  - the risk of suicide
  - the availability of coping resources and support
  - whether the patient is willing to accept help.
- Factors associated with the risk of a further attempt include:
  - male
  - under 19 or over 45 years old
  - unemployment
  - separated, widowed, divorced and living alone
  - chronic physical health
  - previous attempt with hospital admission
  - problems with alcohol and drugs
  - psychiatric disorder (especially depression, schizophrenia, alcoholism).
- An important minority of patients attempting suicide are unco-operative with medical treatment and they attempt to self-discharge. These patients are in a particularly high-risk group for self-harm and, although patient autonomy is paramount, doctors must be aware of their duty of care. If the patient is suffering from a mental disorder, there may be grounds for treating them under the Mental Health Act. An urgent psychiatric opinion is necessary. Where there is no evidence that the patient is mentally disordered, the patient's capacity to make decisions needs to be assessed. The doctor must determine if the patient is

able to (1) comprehend and retain information on the proposed treatment, including its indications, main benefits and the consequences of non-treatment, (2) believe the information, and (3) use the information and weigh it up as part of the process of arriving at a decision.

Comments on the case

While the situation of an attempted suicide is complex, it is important to make an initial psychosocial assessment, including the patient's mental state, as soon as possible. All doctors in medicine must be able to do this.

Case 26 | Genetic counselling

Candidate information
You are the doctor in a neurology clinic.
Please read this summary and then continue with the consultation.

> **Re: Miss Jackie Cromwell, aged 23**
>
> Miss Cromwell has come to see you in clinic today with her father who has recently been diagnosed with Huntington's disease. There is no family history although this may well be concealed. The daughter wants to speak to you privately about the possibility of a genetic blood test to determine whether she is at risk of developing this disease in later life and possibly passing this condition to her future children.

Your tasks are to: obtain her reasons for a genetic test and counsel her for this.

Subject/patient/relative information
Miss Jackie Cromwell is a 23-year-old woman attending the neurology clinic with her father who has recently been diagnosed as having Huntington's disease. She has been reading various leaflets which have highlighted the autosomal dominant nature of the condition, with children of an affected parent having a 50% chance of inheritance. She is aware of the symptoms and the progressive nature of the disease leading to dementia. Although she is fit and well, she has been considering long and hard whether or not she should have a test done to determine her chance of developing the disease. She does not have much idea about the procedure for the test and so has asked the doctor (the candidate) for more information. She has one younger brother and she herself is unmarried with no children. She is concerned about the risk of possibly passing this condition on to any future children.

Thoughts and questions the patient/subject may have
- *Are you sure the disease my father has runs in the family? We are not aware of my grandparents, uncles, aunts or cousins being affected.*
- *How can I find out if I will get the disease? What happens during the test?*
- *What is the risk that my brother will have it? And any children I may have in the future?*
- *I'm scared about what will happen if I take the test – do you think I should just leave things to nature?*

Examiner information

1. Conduct of interview
- Ask if she has a partner. Ideally, the partner should be present during the counselling.

- Try to obtain a family tree, i.e. number of sisters, brothers, aunts, uncles, cousins.
- Ask if there is anything about Huntington's disease that she is unsure of. If not, then just explain briefly the nature, treatment and prognosis of the disease

and ask if there is anyone else in the family with Huntington's disease who might already be affected.

- Explain the purpose of the screening and that a genetic make-up is ascertained to see if she has the genetic mutation seen in this illness (mutation of distal short arm of chromosome 4) which would indicate a high risk of developing the condition.
- Check, in a sensitive manner, that no one is forcing her into having the test.
- Explain the nature of the test and the possibility of false-positive and false-negative results.
- Discuss any significant medical, social or financial implications of screening.
- Explain that there are several reproductive options for her if she tests positive and wishes to have children in the future: prenatal testing by chorionic villus sampling or amniocentesis, preimplantation genetic testing and embryo selection, adoption, etc.
- Reassure her that there will be time to decide if she is unsure about proceeding and that at the next appointment you will provide her with addresses of appropriate support services.
- Say that you could refer her to a regional genetic centre if she decides to go ahead with the testing. A good source of information is the Huntington's Disease Association.
- Keep the conversation simple and comprehensible. Encourage questions.

2. Exploration and problem negotiation

The candidate should be able to:

- determine why Miss Cromwell wants the test
- determine her understanding of the disease
- explain the nature of the test, i.e. blood test looking at the genetic make-up.

3. Communication, ethics and the law
General comments on genetic testing

- All individuals who may wish to take a genetic test should be given up-to-date, relevant information so that they can make an informed, voluntary decision.
- The subject must choose freely to be tested and must not be coerced by family, friends, partners or potential partners, physicians, insurance companies, employers, or others.
- The test is available only to subjects who have reached the age of maturity (according to the laws of the respective country).

- Subjects should not be discriminated against in any way as a result of genetic testing for Huntington's disease.
- Extreme care should be exercised when testing would provide information about another person who has not requested the test. This issue will arise when an offspring with 25% risk requests testing with full knowledge that his parent does not want to know his own status.
- Testing for Huntington's disease should not be part of a routine blood investigation without the specific permission of the subject and such specific permission should, in principle, also be required for symptomatic subjects.
- Ownership of the test result remains with the subject who requested the test. Legal ownership of the stored DNA remains with the person from whom the blood was taken.
- The consent form should address this issue. Local legal guidance policies may be helpful.
- All laboratories are expected to meet rigorous standards of accuracy. They must work with genetic counsellors and other professionals providing the test service.
- The lay organizations can provide an inestimable service in enquiring about the standards of the laboratory and can assist subjects who want to be, or have been, tested with their enquiries and concerns.
- The counsellors should be specifically trained in counselling methods and form part of a multidisciplinary team.
- Such multidisciplinary teams should consist of a geneticist, a neurologist, a social worker, a psychiatrist and someone trained in medical ethics.
- The subject should be encouraged to select a companion to accompany them throughout all stages of the testing process: the pretest stage, the taking of the test, the delivery of the results and the post-test stage.
- This companion may be the spouse/partner, a friend, a social worker or any individual who has the confidence of this person. It may not be appropriate for the companion to be another at-risk person.
- The counselling unit should plan, with the subject, a follow-up protocol that provides support during the pre- and post-test stages regardless of whether this person chooses a companion.
- Neither the counselling centre nor the test laboratory should establish direct contact with a relative

whose DNA may be needed for the purpose of the test without the permission of the subject.

- Information should be presented both orally and in written form and be provided by the team responsible for the testing service.

- **General information on the disease**
  - Information on Huntington's disease must be given to the subject, including the wide range of its clinical manifestations, its social and psychological implications, its genetic aspects, issues around having children, availability of treatment and so forth.
  - It must be pointed out that, at this time, neither prevention nor cure is possible.
  - Genetic testing may show that the putative parent is not the biological parent; this should be brought to the attention of the subject and discussed. With the availability of techniques such as *in vitro* fertilization, etc., even cases of non-maternity may occasionally be discovered.
  - Psychosocial support and counselling must be available before the test procedure commences.

- **Information about the test**
  - Explain how the test is done.
  - Explain the possible need for DNA from one other affected family member and the possible problems arising from this.
  - Asking an affected subject who may be unaware of, or unwilling to acknowledge, his symptoms to contribute a blood sample may be considered an invasion of privacy.
  - The limitations of the test (error rate, the possibilities of an uninformative test and so forth).
  - The counsellor must explain that, although the gene defect has been found, at the present time no useful information can be given about age at onset or about the kind of symptoms, their severity or the rate of progression.

- **The consequences**
  - All consequences have to be discussed – those related to the presence or absence of the gene defect as well as those related to not taking the test. Consideration should be given to the subject, the spouse/partner and children, the affected parent and the spouse.
  - Socioeconomic consequences of the test result including potential employment, insurance, social security, data security and other problems.

- **Alternatives the applicant can consider**
  - Not to take the test for the time being.
  - To deposit DNA for research.

- To deposit DNA for possible future use by family and self.

- **Important preliminary investigations**
  - It is important to verify that the diagnosis of Huntington's disease in a family member of the subject is correct.
  - Neurological examination and psychological appraisal are considered important to establish a baseline evaluation of each subject. Any other specialized tests are always non-compulsory; refusal may not affect participation in the test.
  - Refusal to undergo these and other additional examinations will not justify the withholding of the test from subjects.

- **The test and delivery of results**
  - Excluding exceptional circumstances, there should be a minimum interval of 1 month between presentation of the pretest information and the decision whether or not to take the test. The counsellor should ascertain whether the pretest information has been properly understood and should take the initiative to be assured of this. However, contact will only be maintained at the subject's request.
  - The result of the predictive test should be delivered as soon as possible after completion of the test, on a date agreed upon in advance between the centre, the counsellor and the subject.
  - The manner in which the result will be delivered should be discussed by the counselling team and the subject.
  - The subject has the right to decide, prior to the date fixed for the delivery of the result, if he does not want to be told.
  - The result of the test should be revealed in person by the counsellor to the subject and his companion. No result should ever be revealed by telephone or by mail or email. The counsellor must have sufficient time to discuss any questions with the subject.

- **Post-test counselling**
  - The frequency and the form of the post-test counselling should be discussed by the team and the subject prior to the performance of the test, but the subject has the right to modify the planned programme. Although the intensity and frequency will vary from person to person, post-test counselling must be available at all times.
  - The counsellor should have contact with the subject within the first week after delivery of the result, regardless of the nature of the result.

- If there is no further contact within 1 month of the delivery of the test result, then the counsellor should initiate the follow-up.

Comments on the case

Genetic counselling is a massive subject but candidates must have a grasp of the basic principles involved rather than leaving it all to the local genetics department.

Further reading

Huntington's Disease Association. *Predictive testing for Huntington's disease: fact sheet.* Liverpool: Huntington's Disease Association, 2011. http://hda.org.uk/download/fact-sheets/HD-Predictive-Testing.pdf

Huntington's Disease Society of America Genetic Testing Group. *Genetic testing for Huntington's disease: its relevance and implications.* New York: Huntington's Disease Society of America, 2003. www.hdsa.org/living-with-huntingtons/publications/index.html

International Huntington Association. *Guidelines for the molecular genetics predictive test in HD,* 1994.

Case 27 | Fitness for anaesthesia/surgery

Candidate information

You are the medical doctor in a general medical clinic.

Please read this summary and then continue with the consultation.

Re: Mr Tom Watson, aged 82

Mr Watson is an elderly man who is under the care of the urologists for benign prostatic hyperplasia. He is known to have heart failure and COPD. The urology consultant wants to know if this patient is fit for a general anaesthetic and has asked for a medical opinion, hence his referral to the medical outpatients. Mr Watson's current medication includes aspirin, ramipril, Combivent nebuliser 2.5 mL qds and beclomethasone 200 µg bd inhaler.

Your task is to: give a medical opinion to the urologist.

Subject/patient/relative information

Mr Watson is an elderly 82-year-old man who lives in warden-controlled accommodation. He has been under the care of the urologists for benign prostatic hyperplasia and his symptoms of prostatism are now so bad that a transurethral resection of the prostate is recommended. The urologist is worried about his medical condition, particularly with regard to tolerating a general anaesthetic. He is known to have COPD and heart failure. He has not managed to get out of his flat for the last year and a friend helps him with his shopping and cleaning. He gets breathless walking upstairs and has a chronic cough and phlegm. He has no chest pain but does have ankle swelling as a result of his heart failure. For these conditions he takes a nebulizer, a diuretic and an angiotensin-converting enzyme (ACE) inhibitor (the names of which he cannot remember). He used to smoke 30 cigarettes a day and stopped 6 months ago. He had a previous femoral neck fracture 5 years ago after a fall and then he remembers undergoing a spinal procedure (an injection in the back and both his legs went numb and floppy as a result). He is not allergic to any medication and he is unaware of any allergy to anaesthetic gases as he has never had a general anaesthetic before. He understands the need for the operation but he is worried about having the anaesthetic.

Thoughts and questions the patient/relative may have

- *I thought the operation is for my waterworks – so why do you want to know all about my breathing?*
- *I'm quite worried about this anaesthetic, can't they do the operation with me awake?*
- *Am I fit for the anaesthetic, doctor?*

Examiner information

1. Conduct of interview

- Explain why you are seeing the patient; he may think you are the urologist or an anaesthetist.
- Explore his symptoms caused by the heart failure and COPD. Ask about other medical problems, e.g. diabetes, cerebrovascular disease.
- Ask about previous operations. Were they performed under general, local or spinal anaesthesia?
- Are there any allergies to medications or anaesthetics?
- An anaesthetist would, as a rule, ascertain the state of the teeth and any possible indications of difficult intubation, e.g. short immobile neck, malpositioning of teeth, high-arched palate, receding mandible, poor mouth opening.
- Address any concerns the patient may have.
- Explain that you are a physician and your job is to give a medical opinion but not to decide on your own whether he is fit for an anaesthetic. Explain that this is the responsibility of the anaesthetist.

2. Exploration and problem negotiation

The candidate should be able to:

- do a medical assessment
- ascertain a drug history and any previous allergies
- arrange a list of investigations which would be useful for the urologist and the anaesthetist, e.g. full blood count (FBC), urea and electrolytes (U&E), glucose, resting electrocardiogram (ECG), oxygen saturations on air, spirometry, chest X-ray

- discuss the case with the consultant as a courtesy and write back to the urologist about the medical opinion.

3. Communication, ethics and the law

- It is common for physicians to be asked for an anaesthetic opinion from surgeons. Remember you are a physician and not an expert in anaesthesia.
- So it is important that you give a medical opinion and relay the results to the urologists. If investigations are done but the results are not available that day, e.g. spirometry, biochemistry, haematology, etc., you must let the urologist know that the results are to follow.
- Patients will ask, 'Am I fit for an anaesthetic, doctor?'. You must be honest and say that you are not the right person to judge that, but you can give your medical opinion to the patient, i.e. how bad or good the patient's COPD and heart failure are.

Comments on the case

Remember where you stand in cases like these, i.e. giving advice where you have no expertise. You need to emphasize to the patient and colleagues that the decision on fitness for an anaesthetic is ultimately down to the anaesthetist but a medical opinion is useful. As a medical doctor, you can assess the cardiovascular and respiratory system and arrange relevant investigations, all of which will help the anaesthetist to make the final decision.

Case 28 | Screening for prostate cancer

Candidate information

You are the doctor in a general medical clinic.

Please read this summary and then continue with the consultation.

Re: Mr Eric Spicer, aged 67

Mr Spicer attends the clinic for hypertension and his blood pressure today is 158/78 mmHg. He tells you that he has read in a newspaper that a blood test now exists that detects prostate cancer (prostatic surface antigen test, PSA). He asks you if it is worthwhile screening him for prostate cancer using this test.

Your task is to: discuss the pros and cons of screening for prostate cancer with Mr Spicer.

Subject/patient/relative information

Mr Spicer is a 67-year-old retired electrician who comes to clinic for the management of his hypertension; he is on amlodipine, ramipril and doxazosin. Recently, the blood pressure has been reasonably well controlled. He has been reading in the paper about a new 'magical' blood test that can decide instantly whether someone has prostate cancer or not. There have been a few scares about prostate cancer in the media, and so he is keen to know if he has it. He has read that this is the most common cancer in men and that one may be symptom free and still have it. Admittedly, there has also been some pressure from his wife to have the test. Mr Spicer is relatively well with no prostatic symptoms. After discussion with the doctor (the candidate), he stills decides that he wants to go ahead with the PSA blood test.

Thoughts and questions the patient/subject may have

- *If this blood test for the prostate is so good, how come my doctor has not done it for me yet?*
- *What will happen if I have the blood test and it comes back positive? Does that mean I have cancer?*

Examiner information

1. Conduct of interview

- Ask Mr Spicer if he has any prostatic symptoms such as poor flow at the start, poor stream, postmicturition dribbling, nocturia, dysuria or haematuria.
- Ask what he knows about prostate cancer.
- Ask why he wants to be screened for prostate cancer. Is he worried that he may have prostate cancer? Is there a family history? Is he being pressurized by a relative?
- Discover what he has read in the papers with regard to screening for prostate cancer.
- What are his worries? He tells you that he is aware that prostate cancer is very common in men and that one can be asymptomatic and still have the cancer.
- First, explain briefly what the prostate gland is.

- Reassure him that, in the absence of symptoms, it is unlikely that he will have prostate cancer. Agree with him that prostate cancer is the most common cancer in men *but* it does not cause the largest number of cancer deaths (in contrast to lung cancer in men).
- Describe the ways to investigate the possibility of prostate cancer: digital rectal examination, with a PSA test and, if these are abnormal, a prostatic biopsy.
- Explain that for a screening process to be effective, there are a number of important factors that have to be met. Explain that there are a number of reasons other than prostate cancer why a PSA test result may be raised, e.g. prostatic infection, recent urinary tract infection and benign prostatic hyperplasia. Say that it is not uncommon to have false-positive results, which could result in undergoing an unnecessary surgical procedure (prostatic biopsy). Meanwhile, there is a risk of the PSA test being negative when in fact he does have prostate cancer. Therefore, reiterate that such screening tests are not 100% guaranteed to detect or dismiss the presence of prostate cancer.
- However, if he did have a prostatic biopsy after finding an abnormal PSA and/or prostate gland (on palpation), and it did turn out to be a prostate cancer, then it could mean that the cancer is detected early and so curative therapy can be undertaken.
- Ask if he wants to have a digital rectal examination and the PSA blood test. He says 'yes'.
- Make sure that there is a follow-up appointment to discuss the results.

2. Exploration and problem negotiation

The candidate should be able to:
- ascertain the reasoning for the patient's request for a PSA screening test
- explain the pros and cons of the screening test
- ensure follow-up plans are arranged.

3. Communication, ethics and the law

- For a screening programme to work efficiently, there are a number of criteria which should be met (Wilson and Jungner criteria).
  - The condition is an important health problem.
  - Its natural history is well understood.
  - There is a recognizable latent or early symptomatic stage.
  - A suitable test exists.
  - A test that is acceptable to the general population exists.
  - Screening is done at repeated intervals as a 'continuous process' (as opposed to a 'once-and-for-all test').
  - Adequate facilities exist to cope with abnormalities detected.
  - There is an accepted treatment for those with early recognized disease.
  - There is an agreed policy as to whom to treat as patients.
  - The cost is balanced against benefit.
- Screening (which may involve testing) healthy or asymptomatic people to detect genetic predispositions, or early signs of debilitating or life-threatening conditions, can be an important tool in providing effective healthcare. But the uncertainties involved in screening may be great – for example, the risk of false-positive or false-negative results. Some findings may potentially have serious medical, social or financial consequences not only for the individuals but also for their relatives. In some cases, the fact of having been screened may itself have serious implications.
- You must ensure that anyone considering whether to consent to screening or not can make a properly informed decision. As far as possible, you should ensure that screening would not be contrary to the individual's best interests. You must pay particular attention to ensuring that the information the person wants, or ought to have, is identified and provided. You should be careful to explain clearly:
  - the purpose of the screening
  - the likelihood of positive/negative findings and the possibility of false-positive/false-negative results
  - the uncertainties and risks attached to the screening process
  - any significant medical, social or financial implications of screening for the particular condition or predisposition
  - follow-up plans, including availability of counselling and support services.
- Controversy surrounds the effectiveness of screening for prostate cancer. Although early detection can lead to curative therapy, many individuals with incidental findings will undergo treatment when in fact the tumour would have been so slow growing that it would not have influenced the length of life for the individual. Prostate cancer therapy has complications including incontinence and impotence.
- It is reasonable to search for prostate cancer in the male patient who is having difficulty voiding (slow

stream, urgency) or haematuria, or who has signs and symptoms of metastatic cancer (bone spread resulting in an elevated alkaline phosphatase level and progressive back pain, sciatica or lower extremity neurological impairment). Either curative treatment for cancers confined to the prostate (radical prostatectomy or radiotherapy) or palliative treatments for metastatic disease (orchidectomy to eliminate androgen stimulation of the tumour) are likely to decrease symptoms and improve quality of life.

- The decision to offer prostate cancer screening must be made on an individual basis, depending on the patient's age, health status, family history, risk of prostate cancer and personal beliefs.
- Once a patient undergoes screening and is found not to have prostate cancer, should the patient undergo further annual screening? Guidelines for annual screening do exist but are not necessarily evidence based.

Comments on the case

Screening is a topical subject and patients will regularly read in the press of a wonder test to decide whether or not they have disease X. Allowing the patient to make an informed decision, with the guarantee that the screening is not contrary to the patient's interests, is paramount.

Further reading

Burford DC, Kirby M, Austoker J. *Prostate cancer risk management programme information in primary care: PSA testing in asymptomatic men.* London: NHS Cancer Screening Programmes, 2010. www.cancerscreening. nhs.uk/prostate/prostate-booklet-text.pdf

General Medical Council. *Seeking patients' consent: the ethical considerations. Sections 33–34: consent to screening.* London: General Medical Council, 1998.

Wilson JMG, Jungner G. *Principles and Practice of Screening for Disease,* World Health Organization, Geneva, 1968. http://wholibdoc.int/php/WHOPHP34. pdf

Case 29 | Malignancy in a young patient

Candidate information

You are the doctor in a chest clinic.

Please read this summary and then continue with the consultation.

> **Re: Miss Joanne Harrison, aged 25**
>
> Miss Harrison saw your consultant 4 weeks ago in clinic after presenting to the GP feeling unwell with a fever and loss of appetite. A chest X-ray in the clinic showed bilateral hilar lymphadenopathy. The consultant did not discuss the diagnostic possibilities but he arranged for a mediastinal biopsy (mediastinoscopy) which was performed by the thoracic surgeons 10 days ago. Your consultant is away today and Miss Harrison has come back for the biopsy result. Unfortunately, this shows Hodgkin's lymphoma.

Your tasks are to: break the bad news to Miss Harrison and deal with the concerns and questions that she will have.

Subject/patient/relative information

Miss Harrison is a 25-year-old clerical officer who first presented about 6 weeks ago feeling generally unwell with a fever and weight loss. She thought she had a virus so naturally was a bit shaken when, after some blood tests, the GP told her that he was sending her to see a consultant at the local hospital. She was even more concerned at the speed with which she received the clinic appointment 2 weeks later. She had a chest X-ray during the initial visit and, although the consultant did not discuss the possible causes, she could tell by his language and general demeanour that the result of the chest X-ray was worrying him (it showed bilateral hilar lymphadenopathy or 'enlargement of the lymph glands around the lungs'). She was sent to the local thoracic surgery department where she had a mediastinal biopsy. She has come back to obtain the results and, after speaking to a friend who is a nurse, she is concerned that this may be cancer. She is single, still lives at home and is employed as a clerical officer in the Civil Service.

Thoughts and questions the patient/subject may have

- If she is asked what she thinks may be the problem, she may say that she is frightened that it is cancer or alternatively she may wait for the doctor's explanation.
- When she is told that she does have Hodgkin's lymphoma, she will ask directly if this is cancer.
- *How far advanced is it?*
- *Will my younger brother get this as well?*
- *My aunt died of cancer when I was small, and my dad tells me that it was awful, she was in so much pain and the doctors didn't seem to be able to do anything to help her. . .*

Examiner information

1. Conduct of interview

- Introduce yourself to Miss Harrison. Ensure that this is the correct patient.
- Make sure the clinic room is quiet and comfortable and ask if she has any relatives with her, e.g. partner or parent. If so, ask if she wants him/her to be in the clinic room as well. Normally, a member of the nursing staff would be available but probably not in the exam.
- Start with an open question such as 'How are you after the biopsy?'. She'll probably say she is OK but that her symptoms still persist.
- Ask her whether the consultant explained the possible diagnoses at the first visit. She'll probably say no.
- Ask her if she has had any thoughts about what might be causing her symptoms.
- If she says that she thinks it may be cancer, tell her the biopsy result and then pause.
- Ask her if she has heard of Hodgkin's lymphoma, and wait a moment for her response.
- Confirm that it is a type of cancer (be honest with the patient). Then pause to allow this to sink in.
- When the timing is right, acknowledge that this must be a big shock for her. Reassure her that there are doctors who specialize in this disease and there are well-established treatments available.
- Ask if she feels up to having a brief explanation now about what Hodgkin's lymphoma is. If she agrees then do so.
- She may believe that having cancer means dying in agony so it's important to dispel these myths. She may ask if the cancer is inherited. Reassure her on this issue.
- Tell her that you will refer her urgently to the relevant consultant (a haemato-oncologist). Explain that the specialist will arrange a CT scan of the chest and abdomen to establish the extent of the disease and will then make a decision about the most appropriate treatment.
- She may want to know what treatment options are available. Don't pretend to be an expert when you're not. Don't be afraid to say, 'I don't know the finer details but . . .'. If she feels up to it, you should give a brief explanation about chemotherapy and radiotherapy, reminding her that it is only after the full assessment has been done that one can decide exactly what form of treatment will be the best for her.
- At all times allow her to make her own comments. Listen sympathetically to all of her concerns.

- If a nurse is present, ask her/him for any further comments.
- Ask who is at home with her to support her. It is wise to inform the GP straight away for primary care support. Check that she is not driving home on her own; let the nurse know if this is the case.
- Offer any suitable information leaflets that are available and ensure she has a contact number for when she needs further advice.

2. Exploration and problem negotiation

The candidate must be able to:

- establish what the patient has been told at the previous outpatient appointment
- tell her clearly what the biopsy shows, but with compassion, and check her understanding
- give her time to absorb the news and to ask questions
- tell her what will happen next
- give her as much information as she feels able to cope with at this time and back it up with written information, including bullet point handwritten notes if necessary
- provide an opportunity for her to tell you what her current concerns are and address them as clearly and honestly as you can.

3. Communication, ethics and the law

The candidate should be able to:

- understand that when breaking bad news, it is very important to confirm who the individual is. Otherwise, if the wrong person or partner is given the results without the consent of the patient, the clinician will be breaking confidentiality
- know what the individual has been told in the past so that the required depth and detail of the explanation can be judged better
- realize that if you lack personal medical knowledge of the specialty, you must not be afraid to admit this and to refer on to a relevant specialist
- refer the patient to a recognized centre with a full multidisciplinary team approach
- realize that an immediate reaction to bad news of any sort is often numbness and denial. The patient may ask, 'Are you sure? Surely you have got the result wrong'. The candidate should have sufficient emotional and professional maturity not to take this anger personally.

Once the numbness and denial have diminished a little, the patient may become angry, which may be directed towards the bearer of the bad news. Gradually, there is sadness, then acceptance and eventually hope (although all these reactions are not likely to be displayed in the short space of a single consultation).

The common faults in breaking bad news are:

- avoiding the breaking of bad news in the first place and hoping that someone else will do it
- stalling/procrastinating over the breaking of bad news with irrelevant discussion, e.g. 'Nice day today, isn't it?'
- failing to recognize or respond to the patient's verbal cues and clues, e.g. 'I've got a bad feeling about this', and body language, e.g. the patient puts their head in their hands (despair) or if the patient gives no eye contact; both of these may indicate that the patient needs more time
- not recognizing when to be silent. It may help to imagine if you were being told something distressing and life changing. You most certainly would want to ask questions but you need a little time in order to be able to formulate them. This is very hard to do when someone is continuing to talk at you
- bombarding the patient with too much information – always be guided by them.

It is commendable to feel compassion and to want to be reassuring. However, it is essential that you don't mislead the patient or be dishonest, e.g. 'I'm sure the specialist will be able to make things better. Don't worry, it's not too serious. You'll be feeling better soon'.

Be honest, but avoid conveying an aura of impending doom, e.g. 'Oh dear, it really isn't good at all and it is worse than I had expected'.

Useful strategies to aid the breaking of bad news:

- always be honest and never tell the patient anything that may be false
- do not tell the patient more than she wants to know. Ask how much she wants to know at this time
- give the patient time. Allow for silences. Being told the diagnosis may be too much for the patient and she may not be ready to be told any further information, e.g. treatment options. You may find that the acceptance phase takes longer than you expect, so say 'This must be a great shock for you. You will need

time for all this to sink in so I suggest we meet again in a few days so I can answer all your questions'. This next meeting will be a better time to discuss treatment options

- never give specific times, e.g. when asked for prognosis
- always provide some hope. The patient needs you to show support
- always be sensitive. Never be abrupt and inconsiderate
- appreciate the different ways in which patients cope with denial
- words that are used, e.g. tumour, mass, lesion, malignant or cancer, may have a different meaning to the patient, so make sure the language you use is both understandable and interpretable
- when dealing with anger, do not allow it to be left unexplored. Say to the patient, 'You look upset' or 'Tell me what is bothering you'.

Comments on the case

This case typifies a common 'breaking bad news' scenario. The candidate has a duty of care to carry out a consultation with empathy, understanding, and due regard and respect for the concerns, priorities and feelings of the patient. You must recognize the limitations of your own knowledge and the scope of your professional behaviour. If you are not an expert in this field, you need to say so. You can help the patient best by telling them what you do know and then explaining that this is why you are referring them on to a specialist. Give them a point of contact before they leave you. Breaking bad news to a patient or family member is always upsetting for the clinician, but the feelings and sensitivities of the doctor can never justify a failure to convey the information in an honest manner.

Case 30 | A chronic illness

Candidate information

You are the medical doctor in clinic.

Please read this summary and then continue with the consultation.

> **Re: Mrs Paula Reeney, aged 47**
>
> Mrs Reeney presented to the clinic 4 weeks ago because of a 4-day history of
> blurred vision in the left eye which had occurred 2 months previously. During
> that appointment the consultant did suggest the possibility of multiple
> sclerosis as there was also a history of an episode of facial weakness 8
> months before. Mrs Reeney has blocked out the possibility of multiple
> sclerosis by 'reassuring herself' that this was very unlikely as she had
> recovered from her earlier symptoms. An MRI scan performed 2 weeks ago
> has shown multiple demyelinating plaques in the brainstem and
> periventricular regions suggestive of multiple sclerosis. Mrs Reeney is now at
> the clinic awaiting the news of the results.

Your tasks are to: explain the results of the MRI scan and to convey the diagnosis
of multiple sclerosis to her.

Subject/patient/relative information

Mrs Paula Reeney is a 47-year-old secretary who presented to the GP 2 months ago
with blurred vision in the left eye. A few months previously she had had an episode
of facial weakness, which thankfully passed very quickly. Following the episode of
blurred vision 2 months ago, she was referred to the consultant physician who wondered if her optic discs were swollen. The consultant did mention that there was a
possibility of multiple sclerosis but Mrs Reeney tried to reassure herself that this
could not be possible, as her eye symptoms had resolved. An MRI scan was performed which shows multiple plaques of demyelination suggestive of multiple sclerosis. Mrs Reeney is an active woman and news such as this will be quite devastating
for her. She lives with her husband and two teenage children.

Thoughts and questions the patient/subject may have

- *Why have I got this?*
- *How did I get it?*
- *Can you cure it?*
- *Will my children get it?*

Examiner information

1. Conduct of interview

- Introduce yourself to Mrs Reeney and briefly ask how
  she is.

- Ask what she was told at the last appointment. Had
  the consultant mentioned any possible causes for the
  blurred vision?
- Explain clearly and gently that the MRI scan findings
  do suggest multiple sclerosis.

- Pause to allow this to sink in. Ask her how she feels about this news.
- When the time is right, ask what she knows about multiple sclerosis, pay attention to what she says – she may know very little or she may have done some research and tells you that she knows about the more serious manifestations such as the difficulty in walking, incontinence and dementia.
- Aim to reassure her that not all patients go on to develop this type of extreme end-stage disease.
- Point out that there are specialists who look after patients with multiple sclerosis and that they will help her with the best available therapy.
- She will ask questions that will be difficult to answer, such as why she has got it, how she got it, will it go away, her chances of leading a normal life, possibility of a genetic link, etc. Be honest and say that it is not possible to answer these questions but what you do know is that many people with multiple sclerosis live very active lives even many years after the diagnosis.
- Be reassuring and explain that patients with relapses and remission, as in her case, may go on for many years without any major disability.
- Tell her about the Multiple Sclerosis Society that will support her through this difficult time. Tell her you will give her the contact number of this society (Multiple Sclerosis Society, 0808 800 8000, www.mssociety.org.uk).
- Try to avoid bombarding her with too much information at this stage, unless she asks for it.
- Arrange an early follow-up to discuss this further. Say you will also refer her to a specialist and tell her that you will inform her GP. Give her a contact number if she wants to ring for advice.

2. Exploration and problem negotiation

The candidate should be able to:

- explain the findings of the MRI scan and the likely diagnosis
- allow the patient time and space to enable her to come to terms with the bad news
- provide support and encouragement to enable her to have hope.

3. Communication, ethics and the law

- Breaking bad news when it is a diagnosis of a chronic illness such as multiple sclerosis, diabetes mellitus, rheumatoid arthritis or motor neurone disease usually results in the patient believing the worst is inevitable. Despite being asymptomatic, impending doom is a common belief and it is natural for people to be fearful.
- The challenge for the candidate is not to explain all that is known in the literature about the disease but rather to support the patient when giving the bad news, and being aware of the different phases that receivers of bad news will go through in the course of time (i.e. denial, anger, acceptance and hope).
- The impact of having a chronic disease is multiple, i.e. physical, psychological and social. There will be concerns with regard to their family and their work as well as their health. Coming to terms with the illness and coping with these impacts will take a while and the patient will need help to support the coping mechanisms, particularly on how to deal with setbacks, loss of self-esteem and confidence, dealing with changing goals in life, etc.
- Reassurance and hope are what the patient needs; only 15% of patients diagnosed with multiple sclerosis experience the chronic progressive type of disease and so there are many patients who may be able to live reasonably normal lives for a significant period of time.
- Supplying telephone numbers of specialist services such as MS nurses and the MS Society is always helpful.
- Providing early follow-up will allow further queries to be answered.
- Always inform the GP.

Comments on the case

Breaking bad news of a chronic illness is a common case. Unless the first breaking bad news session is done properly, with understanding and empathy, all trust and belief may be squandered. The doctor must take time in allowing the patient to take in what has been said; the patient may remain totally shocked for a while. Avoid besieging the patient with too much detail on the condition, i.e. epidemiology, pathogenesis, diagnosis, therapy options, etc.

Case 31 | A patient with a functional illness

Candidate information

You are the doctor in a gastroenterology clinic.

Please read this summary and then continue with the consultation.

Re: Mrs Malika Patel, aged 43

Mrs Patel is an Asian woman who has been suffering from recurrent abdominal bloating and diarrhoea for the last 18 months. She opens her bowels around three or four times most mornings, and this is associated with crampy abdominal pain which is often relieved by defaecation. She has noticed some mucus in the stools. Her GP checked her bloods (including iron studies, thyroid function and coeliac screen) and organized an ultrasound scan of her abdomen, all of which were normal. The GP mentioned a diagnosis of irritable bowel syndrome and started her on some Buscopan but Mrs Patel did not find any improvement and requested a referral to a specialist. The GP has mentioned in his referral letter that she does not have any alarming symptoms such as weight loss or rectal bleeding. She has no other past medical history of note.

Your tasks are to: reassure Mrs Patel of the diagnosis of irritable bowel syndrome and negotiate a management plan with her.

Subject/patient/relative information

Mrs Malika Patel is a 43-year-old lady who is normally fit and well. For the last 18 months, she has noticed a change in her bowel habit. She now has recurrent episodes of diarrhoea, especially in the morning. Sometimes she opens her bowels 3–4 times a day, usually in the morning, and has noticed some mucus, but never any blood, in her stools. These symptoms are associated with cramping pains in her abdomen which improve after she has opened her bowels. She hasn't lost any weight but is feeling more tired than normal with muscular aches in her shoulders and back. She went to her GP who did some blood tests and an abdominal ultrasound scan. He said these were all normal, and suggested that she has irritable bowel syndrome but the tablets he gave her have not worked. She is very anxious that there is something else going on because one of her aunts, who also had a change in bowel habit, was found to have colon cancer and now has a stoma following surgery. She has requested to see a specialist because she feels she needs to have further tests (e.g. a colonoscopy and CT scan) in case it is cancer. She lives at home with her two teenage children and is finding it difficult to cope with them since her husband left 2 years ago after 20 years of marriage.

Thoughts and questions the patient/subject may have

- *How can you be so sure that I don't have cancer?*
- *Why won't you give me a scan?*
- Depending on how the consultation is progressing, she may ask if the doctor thinks it is all in her mind because they have mentioned stress to her.
- She may ask for a second opinion.

Examiner information

1. Conduct of interview

- Introduce yourself to Mrs Patel. Ask her if anyone has accompanied her to clinic today who she would like to bring into the consultation room with her.
- Ask about her general health and how she is feeling in herself.
- Briefly recap her symptoms in relation to her bowel activity, abdominal cramps, etc. Make sure you ask specifically about 'red flag' symptoms including weight loss, rectal bleeding, haematemesis, etc.
- Ask what she has been told by her GP about what the likely diagnosis is and what she thinks is going on (bear in mind that these may not necessarily be congruent).
- Tell her you have reviewed the reports of the investigations done by her GP (i.e. blood tests, ultrasound scan) and you are pleased to be able to tell her all of the results are normal.
- After listening to the description of her symptoms and reviewing the investigations, tell her that you also think the most likely diagnosis is irritable bowel syndrome. Pause for a few seconds to let her take this in. This may or may not be what she was expecting to hear.
- Ask her what she understands about irritable bowel syndrome (IBS). Offer to tell her more about it if she wants to know.
- Tell her that IBS is a relatively common functional disorder of the bowels, affecting up to one in five adults in the UK. Its cause is not entirely known but is believed to be related to 'overactivity of the nerves or muscles of the gut'. Other possibilities are a viral or bacterial infection of the gut which may act as a trigger to the development of IBS.
- Explain that you want to briefly ask her some questions about her social and employment history and any other stresses in her life and ask her if this is all right. Tell her that stress has been shown to be associated with IBS and many patients can identify a stress-

ful event in their life around the time of onset of the IBS symptoms.

- Ask Mrs Patel if there is anything in particular that concerns her. She may mention her aunt who was diagnosed with colon cancer after presenting with bowel symptoms. She may also ask for further investigations (e.g. CT scan or colonoscopy) to ensure there is nothing serious going on.
- Acknowledge that it is understandable that she would worry about her symptoms given her aunt's cancer and reassure her in a clear, simple way that her symptoms and investigations so far are not suspicious of a more serious problem like cancer. Say that there is nothing to be gained with further investigations and the risks of invasive tests (e.g. colonoscopy or OGD) will outweigh the likely benefits in her case and hence cannot be recommended at this stage.
- If she is unhappy with your explanation or is still insistent on being referred for further investigations, accept this with good grace and tell her that you will get a second opinion from your consultant.
- Explain that you want to offer her the general dietary advice recommended for patients with IBS. This includes having regular meals without leaving too long a gap in between them, drinking at least eight cups of fluid a day, restricting tea and coffee to three cups a day, reducing consumption of alcohol or caffeine-rich drinks and limiting the intake of high-fibre food. Some patients find that taking probiotic drinks is helpful.
- Encourage her to try the above-mentioned dietary changes together with antispasmodic agents when required. Also reiterate that a reduction in her stress and anxiety levels is also likely to help her symptoms. Stress relaxation therapy may also help.
- Make it clear to her that, if she develops any of the 'red flag' symptoms described above, she should see her GP or come back to clinic urgently, when further tests may well be warranted.
- Give her information leaflets about IBS to take home.

- Signpost her to practical support such as the website www.ibsnetwork.org.
- Arrange a further appointment for her to come back to clinic.
- Round off and end the consultation if she has no further questions.

2. Exploration and problem negotiation

The candidate must be able to:
- listen to the patient's anxieties and treat them with respect and understanding
- reassure her that there is unlikely to be a sinister cause for her symptoms (after excluding any alarming symptoms in her history)
- discuss the diagnosis of irritable bowel syndrome and offer some basic advice on how she can manage it
- firmly but sensitively tell the patient that there is little to be gained from further investigations and therefore more tests are not indicated at the present time.

3. Communication, ethics and the law

- Good communication is vital when managing patients with conditions such as IBS where the patient's anxiety may be a predominant feature and they may request investigations or treatment which are not clinically indicated.
- The first step would be to discuss the diagnosis with the patient (and family members if the patient chooses to have them present) in a manner that is easily understood by them, using an interpreter when needed and information leaflets if appropriate. In many instances, reassuring them that it is unlikely to be anything more sinister (e.g. malignancy or inflammatory bowel disease) may be sufficient for the patient to accept the diagnosis.
- Informed patients who trust you are likely to be more accepting of your reasoning about not pursuing further investigations.
- The patient who is exercising self-determination, as an autonomous person, may feel that they are entitled to further investigations. In explaining the clinical findings, it is important to ensure that you include information that sets out your obligation to 'do no harm' in the context of further investigations. In this particular case, you are weighing up the risks of inappropriate or unnecessary procedures against the benefits.

- It may appear easier to go along with insistent patients' requests for further investigations, but this would amount to collusion and would be unethical as it places them at unnecessary exposure to risk and may further magnify their anxiety.
- It is important to remember that patients do not have the right to demand any treatment. According to GMC guidance, if a patient asks for an investigation or treatment that a doctor considers to be of no benefit to them, the doctor should discuss in more detail the reasons for the patient's request. If, after this discussion, the patient still requests the intervention, the doctor can refuse to provide it but needs to explain his decision clearly to the patient, document it clearly and inform the patient about other options, including their right to a second opinion.
- When you have established a good rapport with the patient, it is prudent to go into more detail about other events going on in the patient's life such as psychosocial stresses as these may be important factors contributing to their anxiety and symptoms. A moment's explanation about the importance of having this discussion will help to create the right conditions for a potentially delicate conversation.

Comments on the case

Dealing with a patient with a functional disorder (e.g. IBS, fibromyalgia) can be tricky both in real life and in the PACES examination. A good candidate will be able to empathize with the patient, and take his/her symptoms and concerns seriously. An ability to build a therapeutic relationship built on trust and mutual respect is critical so that, when the time comes to be firmly reassuring, the careful groundwork is more likely to yield acceptance from the patient that there is nothing more serious to worry about.

Further reading

General Medical Council. *Consent: patients and doctors making decisions together.* London: General Medical Council, 2008.

National Institute for Health and Clinical Excellence. *Clinical Guideline 61. Irritable bowel syndrome in adults.* London: National Institute for Health and Clinical Excellence, 2008.

Case 32 | Brainstem death testing and organ transplantation

Candidate information

You are the medical doctor in an intensive care unit.

Please read this summary and then continue with the consultation.

> **Re: Mr Alfred Robinson, age 57**
>
> Mr Robinson was admitted by you 48 h ago with a large intracranial haemorrhage. The next of kin is Miss Robinson, his only daughter. The CT scan has shown extensive haemorrhage with mid-line shift. He was intubated on arrival, started on intravenous propofol and transferred to the ICU. Sedation was discontinued 36 h ago. On admission, the neurosurgeons, intensivists and your consultant felt that the prognosis was extremely poor and that neurosurgical intervention would be inappropriate. Since stopping sedation, Mr Robinson has shown no neurological response and now he has been confirmed brainstem dead by two consultants. Presently, he is in sinus rhythm, is normotensive and the ventilator is supporting his respiration. The daughter has been informed of the poor prognosis and has been told that special 'brain testing' is being performed. She is waiting in the visitors' room for an update. She is unaware of what exactly brainstem death means.

Your tasks are to: explain to Miss Robinson the diagnosis of brainstem death, what this means for his outcome and sensitively approach the idea of organ donation.

Subject/patient/relative information

Mr Alfred Robinson is a 57-year-old man who was admitted 48 h ago with a sudden headache. He had been previously well and working as an electrician. A CT scan of the head showed a large left-sided intracranial haemorrhage with mid-line shift. On admission, he was unconscious and was promptly intubated, sedated and transferred to the ICU. It was felt at the time by the neurosurgeons, intensivists and the medical team that neurosurgery would be inappropriate and that his prognosis was extremely poor. Sedation was stopped 36 h ago and he has made no neurological response to any stimuli. His heart is still functioning and the ventilator is keeping him alive by providing artificial respiration. Without the machine Mr Robinson would not breathe unaided. The next of kin, Miss Robinson (daughter), has been fully informed of his condition and is aware of the poor prognosis. She is unaware of the present development, i.e. that brainstem death has been diagnosed by two consultants. She is about to see the medical doctor (the candidate) who will explain what is meant by this. He/she will explain that her father is technically dead but Miss Robinson cannot understand how this can be when his heart is working and he looks pink, as if 'asleep'. The medical doctor will approach the idea of transplantation but this is all too much for Miss Robinson and she will need more time to think and talk to family and friends.

Thoughts and questions the patient/subject may have
- *Surely he can't be dead – his heart is still beating and he is breathing, right?*
- *How long will he have after you turn off the breathing machine?*
- *If we agree to go ahead with the transplantation, will that delay his funeral? Will his body become disfigured?*
- If the candidate has clearly and empathically explained the situation to Miss Robinson, she will at the end of the discussion accept that her father is indeed dead but will still need more time to consider the transplant issue.

Examiner information

1. Conduct of interview
- Introduce yourself to Miss Robinson (you would have met her before during this admission).
- Explain gently and with empathy that Mr Robinson has shown no signs of improvement and that there have been no indications at all that he will recover consciousness.
- Tell her that, as a result of the brain haemorrhage, Mr Robinson has suffered irreversible brain damage (there's no easy way to say this – allow a pause for the daughter to take all this in). Explain that the brain cells cannot be replaced once damaged and so these cells will not recover. As a result, her father will never wake up.
- Explain that, as a result of the haemorrhage, he is now brainstem dead as confirmed by two experienced specialists. Explain what this means and that he is technically dead.
- She will obviously mention that the heart is still working so 'How can he be dead, doctor?'.
- Point out gently that her father is relying on the machine to do the breathing for him and that this would instantly cease to function if the machine is stopped and that his heart would stop soon after. Thus, her father's heart and lungs are being artificially maintained and that brainstem death equates with the death of an individual.
- Explain, therefore, that the next appropriate step is to stop the artificial ventilation. Explain carefully that this is not to cause her father to die but that he is already technically dead so continuing ventilation is not going to bring him back.
- Explain that it is the medical team who are making this decision and *not* the family, who may feel they are 'actually causing the death' by allowing the ventilator to be stopped.
- Again, allow time for the daughter to come to terms with all this.
- Carefully approach the idea that as her father has died and there has been no damage to the other organs, it is common in such situations for the family to be approached about the concept of organ donation.
- Ask the views of the daughter on this matter. Ask if her father had ever made his views on this known. Had he ever expressed an objection to the idea of organ donation? Do the family members have any strong feelings? Are there any religious obstacles?
- If the family are willing to consider this, tell them that you will speak to the transplant team who would then approach them. Check that there are no contraindications, e.g. malignancy, and say that there would be routine microbiological screening tests, e.g. for hepatitis B and C.
- Explain that if the family agrees to organ transplantation, then the ventilation would be continued until the organs are retrieved.
- Once done, ventilation would be withdrawn and reassure the daughter that, as her father is brainstem dead, he will not suffer any distress or pain.
- Ask if there are any queries. The daughter may need time to think this over and if this is so then make sure you all agree to meet again later in the day.

2. Exploration and problem negotiation
The candidate should be able to:
- explain, with empathy, the diagnosis of brainstem death and explain what this means
- answer any obvious misconceptions that the family may have with regard to brainstem death

- approach the subject of organ transplantation with tact and sensitivity.

3. Communication, ethics and the law

General comments
- In the clinical setting, the diagnosis of brainstem death, pronouncement of death and discussion of organ donation are usually compressed into a matter of hours or a few days. Unlike the persistent vegetative state which may take weeks or even months to evolve and establish irreversibility, the diagnosis of the irreversible loss of brainstem function can be determined with a high degree of certainty within a short time. Because of this, family members should be approached in steps so that they are able to fully comprehend the process.
- The first step should be to inform the family of the poor prognosis for recovery of any neurological function. The second step should be to raise the possibility that the patient may be brainstem dead; at this point families should be told that studies are being performed to determine whether this is the case. The third step should be taken when it seems fairly certain that brainstem death has occurred, and the family should then be told clearly and unequivocally that the usual practice at the hospital is to pronounce a person dead once the neurological criteria have been confirmed. With this approach, a family should be able to fully understand that the pronouncement of death is a medical decision and that the pronouncement of brainstem death as death is a medical assessment just as cardiorespiratory death is a medical diagnosis.
- At the same time, practitioners should be sensitive to the feelings of the families who are suddenly confronted with the death of their loved one, who may still look 'alive' and who may have been a healthy and vibrant human being just a few hours ago. So, it is really important to give the family enough time to understand the process and grasp the concept. But for how long, and under what circumstances, should the time be given? There are no clearcut answers to these questions and there never will be. Under what other circumstances and for how long is it permissible to delay, or hasten, the pronouncement of death and termination of support systems? Should the pronouncement of death be delayed, or not made at all, if the family is in a state of denial and completely unable to accept the concept of brainstem death for religious or other reasons? What should be done in cases where brainstem death has apparently been caused by the actions of the doctors providing treatment, or in cases in which the pronouncement of death will cause charges against an alleged assailant to be changed from attempted murder to murder? Should time be taken to find family members to gain consent for organ donation? Or should the need for a bed in the intensive care unit be considered when there is a shortage?
- An essential component of all formal pronouncements, as stated by the Royal Colleges and the Department of Health on this subject, is that once a patient is declared brainstem dead then he/she is also legally dead. The Department of Health's 1983 Code of Practice specifically states that the time of death is the time at which brain death is established and not some later time when ventilation is withdrawn or the heartbeat ceases. Clinicians should emphasize this when explaining the situation to relatives, and they should make it clear that ventilation is not being withdrawn to let the patient die but because continued ventilation is inappropriate for a patient who is already dead. The only justification for maintaining ventilation for a short time is to preserve the condition of the organs when it has been agreed that they are to be made available for transplantation.

Code of Practice
- It should be remembered that there is no legal definition of death. Hospital doctors are recommended to follow the guidelines produced by the Royal Colleges on diagnosis of death and brain death, incorporated in the 1983 revised edition of the Code of Practice on the removal of cadaveric organs for transplantation (Health Departments of Great Britain and Ireland).
- Death entails the irreversible loss of those essential characteristics which are necessary for the existence of a living person. It is recommended that the definition of death should be regarded as the irreversible loss of the capacity for consciousness, combined with irreversible loss of the capacity to breathe. The irreversible cessation of brainstem function (brainstem death) will produce this clinical state and therefore brainstem death equates with the death of the individual.
- Conditions under which the diagnosis of brainstem death should be considered:
  - there should be no doubt that the patient's condition is due to irremediable brain damage of known aetiology
  - there should be no evidence that this state is due to depressant drugs

- primary hypothermia as the cause of unconsciousness must have been excluded
- potentially reversible circulatory, metabolic and endocrine disturbances must have been excluded as the cause of the continuation of unconsciousness
- the patient is being maintained on the ventilator because spontaneous respiration has been inadequate or ceased altogether (relaxants and other drugs need to be excluded as causing respiratory inadequacy or failure).

- The diagnosis of brainstem death means that all brainstem reflexes are absent. The diagnosis must be made by two medical practitioners (one has to be a consultant) who have been registered for over 5 years, who are competent in this field, must not be members of the transplant team and they must test separately. The legal time of death is when the first test indicates brainstem death. Diagnosing brainstem death includes demonstration of the following:
  - pupils fixed and not responding to light
  - no corneal reflex
  - absent vestibulo-ocular reflexes
  - no cranial nerve motor responses to adequate stimulation
  - no gag reflex or reflex response to bronchial stimulation (suction catheter placed down the trachea)
  - no respiratory movements occur when the patient is disconnected from the mechanical ventilator. It is necessary for the arterial carbon dioxide to exceed the threshold for respiratory stimulation, i.e. $PaCO_2$ should reach 6.6 kPa (as measured by blood gases). Hypoxia during disconnection should be prevented by delivering oxygen at 6 litres per minute through a catheter in the trachea.

Organ donation

- Following brainstem death, the retrieval of solid organs (heart, lungs, kidney, liver, pancreas, small bowel and facial tissue) and other tissues (mainly corneal tissue but also bone, skin and heart valves) may be done for transplant purposes. UK Transplant is the co-ordinating body that manages the Organ Donor Register, the national transplant waiting list, and is also responsible for the matching and allocation of organs and tissue. Each hospital trust should have a transplant co-ordinator (usually a nurse specialist) who will act as the link between the medical teams, the deceased person's family, the Coroner's Office and the UK Transplant authority.

- The medical or nursing staff should ideally contact the transplant co-ordinator before brainstem testing is performed and, once the first brainstem tests confirm brainstem death, a meeting should be arranged with the family to discuss organ donation.
- If a patient carries a signed donor card or has been included in the NHS Organ Donor Register, there is no legal requirement to establish lack of objection on the part of the relatives, although it is good practice to take into account the relatives' views.
- The NHS Organ Donor Registrar can confirm if the potential donor was registered as willing to donate all or some of their organs.
- Removal of organs is authorized only if there is no reason to believe that the deceased has expressed an objection to his body being so dealt with after death and had not withdrawn this objection, that the surviving spouse, partner or any other surviving relative of the deceased does not object to the body being so dealt with, and that there are no religious obstacles.
- Following the family's 'lack of objection' for organ/tissue donation to go ahead, the medical team and transplant co-ordinators should inform the UK Transplant authority as soon as possible and carry out blood tests for microbiological screening, blood grouping and tissue typing. The care of the deceased person should then focus on optimizing transplantable organ function (e.g. cardiovascular and respiratory support, correction of hypovolaemia, treatment of anaemia and deranged coagulation, etc.).
- Before removing the organs, the surgeon must personally examine the body of the potential donor and he must, on the basis of his examination and the brainstem tests carried out, be satisfied that the patient is dead. Organs must not be transplanted until microbiological safety to do so has been established.
- In situations where the death has been referred to the Coroner's office or is a police/legal case, permission must be sought from the coroner or procurator fiscal to harvest suitable organs or tissue for donation.

Comments on the case

Discussing brainstem death is never easy, particularly as organ donation may need to be discussed as well. Candidates must be aware of what brainstem death is as it is very likely that they will come across a real case during their medical practice.

Further reading

Department of Health. *A Code of Practice for the diagnosis of brain stem death: including guidelines for the identification and management of potential organ and tissue donors.* London: Department of Health, 1998.

General Medical Council. *Treatment and care towards the end of life: good practice in decision-making.* London: General Medical Council, 2010.

NHS UK Transplant. *United Kingdom hospital policy for organ and tissue donation.* London: NHS UK Transplant, 2003.

Case 33 | Hospital postmortem

Candidate information
You are the doctor on a medical ward.

Please read this summary and then continue with the consultation.

Re: Mr Stanley Patton, aged 73

Mr Stanley Patton was a 73-year-old man admitted 5 days ago with respiratory failure. He was known to have renal failure, chronic obstructive pulmonary disease and ischaemic heart disease and he used to smoke 40 cigarettes a day. A chest X-ray showed a left basal pneumonia which was treated in the usual and appropriate way. Discussions with the patient, the next of kin (his daughter, Mrs Nolan) and the ICU consultant resulted in a decision not to ventilate the patient. Over the next 5 days he remained reasonably stable (but still poorly). Unfortunately, last night, he collapsed in the toilet and died despite attempts at resuscitation. You were quite upset to hear this from your colleague who was on-call last night. You decide to review his X-rays and, looking at the chest X-ray, you feel that there may in fact have been a bronchial carcinoma behind the heart which was technically missed. You speak to your consultant and he suggests asking for the daughter's permission for a hospital postmortem to decide if (a) Mr Patton died from a pulmonary embolism and (b) whether Mr Patton had a bronchial carcinoma which was missed by the team. If the daughter refuses permission, your consultant is happy for you to write the death certificate anyway.

Your task is to: ask the daughter, Mrs Nolan, for permission to arrange a hospital postmortem.

Subject/patient/relative information
Mr Patton has had a long history of renal failure, COPD and ischaemic heart disease. He was admitted 5 days ago with pneumonia. It was decided, with the ICU consultants, that Mr Patton would not be a candidate for assisted ventilation, although he was for resuscitation. Mrs Nolan is the daughter and the next of kin. She was always aware of her father's poor condition but it came as a real shock to be told that her father collapsed and died last night. She is taking the news bravely and realistically and is very grateful for the care provided. She was told by the doctor on-call last night that the probable cause of death was the pneumonia. She has accepted this and wants no further fuss. She has come to the hospital for the death certificate and she is quite keen to take this to the Registrar of Deaths in town today and start the funeral plans. She is slightly surprised to see the medical doctor (the candidate) who has been looking after her father during this admission. The doctor asks her if she would give permission for a postmortem. She asks for more information about this. She

wants to know when, where and by whom the postmortem would be performed, whether the body will be disfigured, if she can find out the results and whether any organs or tissues will be retained. Despite all the counselling by the doctor, she decides not to go for a postmortem and wants to proceed with the funeral arrangements.

Thoughts and questions the patient/subject may have

- *Everyone has told me my father had a bad pneumonia and died because of it – why are you suddenly thinking of something else now?*
- *What will happen to my father's body if you do the postmortem?*
- *This is already a very difficult time for the family – I just want to get on with the funeral arrangements without any delay.*

Examiner information

1. Conduct of interview

- Tell Mrs Nolan how sorry you are to hear about the sudden death of her father and that all the staff looking after him are saddened by the news. Pause to allow Mrs Nolan to express her emotions.
- Explain that he was very sick when he came in with pneumonia and that despite the appropriate management he continued to remain poorly.
- Tell her, however, that you and your consultant were surprised by the suddenness of his death. Explain that it is possible he may have had a pulmonary embolism (explain this with minimal jargon) and that you are also concerned he may have had lung cancer – although you are not sure on either point. Explain that this does not always show up on the chest X-ray, especially if it is behind the heart shadow.
- Go on to explain that one way of knowing exactly what may have caused the sudden deterioration is a postmortem – ask her how she feels about this. Ask her what she understands about a postmortem.
- Discuss what a postmortem is and what the benefits of one are.
- Ask if she knows if the patient himself had any known objection to a postmortem before this illness.
- If she feels uneasy about a full postmortem then do explain that if she prefers she could perhaps agree to a limited postmortem of the chest only.
- Tell her when it would be done, where and by whom.
- Reassure her that the body would not be disfigured, although there will be a scar in the chest (and possibly abdomen) which will be well covered with clothes.

- Reassure her that funeral arrangements should not necessarily be delayed.
- Explain that if something suspicious is found, e.g. lung cancer, then, unless there is a specific objection, this organ may be retained to confirm the diagnosis and possibly used for educational or research purposes. If she objects, then another option is for the tissue of interest to be fixed and examined and returned to the body before release. Then reassure her again that organs would not be retained.
- Tell her that, if she wishes, she can obtain the results of the postmortem as they are sent to the consultant looking after her father, and she can arrange an appointment with him to have the findings explained.
- Ask her if she has any other concerns and ask how she feels about a postmortem – she may say 'yes' or 'no'.
- If she says 'no', tell her that you will respect this decision wholeheartedly and will issue a death certificate straight away. Explain what you are going to write on the certificate, i.e. 1A respiratory failure 1B pneumonia 1C chronic obstructive pulmonary disease, 2 renal failure, ischaemic heart disease.
- Do not forget to let your consultant know of the outcome.

2. Exploration and problem negotiation

The candidate should be able to:

- transmit their empathy to the daughter
- explain that it is not absolutely certain what caused the death, giving the possibilities
- counsel the daughter for a postmortem with full explanation of the procedure
- support the daughter whatever her decision.

3. Communication, ethics and the law

- Organ and tissue retention at hospital postmortem examinations is currently an issue attracting public attention and is subject to independent enquiries. There are concerns surrounding the standards and practices relating to the retention and disposal of organs and tissue, in particular communication and policies for obtaining 'consent' for the retention of human materials.
- The legislation and guidance for the NHS trust pathology services are covered by the Human Tissue Act (2004). This states the conditions for the removal of body parts and the conduct of postmortem examinations. Consent must be obtained for a hospital postmortem examination to be conducted and for the removal and storage of tissue or organs after the examination. Appropriate consent is defined as any of the following (in order of priority):
  - consent given (or refused) by the deceased before his/her death
  - the consent of a nominated person chosen by the deceased person before his/her death
  - the consent of an individual in a 'qualifying relationship' to the deceased (e.g. spouse/partner, parent or child, sibling, grandparent/grandchild, niece or nephew).
- If the deceased person's relatives object to the postmortem examination or donation of organs when the deceased person had explicitly consented to it, the medical team should discuss the matter sensitively with the relatives and encourage them to accept the deceased person's wishes. However, the clinician should bear in mind that the relatives do not have a legal right to overrule the deceased person's wishes.
- The relatives should be invited to sign a consent form for a hospital postmortem examination and removal/storage of tissue only after they have received clear information about the procedure and have had sufficient time to consider the information and reach a decision. Further support (e.g. bereavement counselling) may be required.
- The Chief Medical Officer's Interim Guidance (2001) makes a number of recommendations for obtaining consent for hospital postmortems through a signed form which includes:
  - clear written information about what the examination entails and why it is required
  - agreement to the postmortem and options to limit the examination
  - information about why and which organ and tissues may be retained including (1) an agreement or not to the retention of tissue samples or body fluids for laboratory investigation to establish a cause of death and to study the effects of treatment and (2) agreement or not to the retention of organs or body parts and options to specify which organs or body parts the relatives would prefer not to be retained
  - how this might impact on the funeral arrangements
  - clear information about where any retained organs and tissues are stored, why, for how long and arrangements for reunion with the body before the burial or how the relatives want organs, tissues or body parts disposed of following the postmortem examination
  - whether retention for longer periods for diagnosis, training, research or legal reason is required or unlimited retention for medical education or research
  - details on who is agreeing to the postmortem, their relationship to the deceased, who obtained and witnessed the agreement, their position within the trust and contact details with the date of the agreement.

What is a postmortem examination?

- This is a careful internal examination of the person who has just died and can give valuable information about an illness and its effects on the body. It may tell us more precisely why the person has died but even the most detailed postmortem investigations will often leave some questions unanswered.
- Postmortem examinations are carried out by a pathologist, who is a doctor specializing in the laboratory study of disease and of diseased tissue, assisted by a technician who is a person who has the specialist training needed to assist pathologists. They are carried out with special facilities provided in the hospital mortuary. Pathologists perform postmortem examinations to standards set by the Royal College of Pathologists in a respectful manner and with regard for the feelings of the bereaved.
- The pathologist will first carry out an external examination of the body. The internal part of the examination begins with an incision made down the front of the body and the internal organs are taken out for a detailed examination. When the brain is examined, an incision is made in the scalp at the base of the head, so there are no obvious scars around the face. Small tissue samples are usually kept for further investigation under a microscope. When detailed

laboratory investigations require body parts or organs to be kept, the relative will be asked to give their written agreement.

The benefits of a postmortem examination

A postmortem examination can give valuable information about an illness and its effects on the body and may explain why the relative died. This information may make it easier for the family members to come to terms with the death. Postmortem examinations may provide valuable information which can help doctors to treat other patients with the same kind of illness and can provide vital information for research.

Full or limited postmortem examination

- If the relative agrees to a hospital postmortem examination, the doctor will issue the medical certificate of death before the postmortem so that they can proceed with the arrangements for the funeral.
- A full postmortem involves detailed examination of all the internal organs including brain, heart, lungs, liver, kidneys, intestines, blood vessels and the small glands which are all removed from the body, examined and returned back to the body.
- If relatives feel uncomfortable with a full examination, an alternative would be a limited examination where only those organs directly related to the illness are examined. This would mean that no information about the other organs, which may have contributed to the death, would be known.

When will the postmortem be carried out and will it delay the funeral?

- Usually as soon as possible and within 2–3 working days. The actual examination may take 3 h. Laboratory investigations which are carried out after the postmortem may take several weeks.
- Funeral arrangements need not be delayed. The relative's body will be released to the undertaker on the day of the postmortem (unless the examination is done late in the afternoon). If relatives wish the organs to be reunited after laboratory analysis, then this may delay the funeral as some laboratory analyses take several weeks.

Will the body be disfigured?

After the postmortem the technician will prepare the body for relatives to see again if they wish. The internal incision in the centre of the body cannot be seen when the body is dressed. The scalp incision, if the brain has been examined, will be concealed by the hair at the back of the head.

Why may an organ be kept?

- When a postmortem examination is first discussed, the relative may be asked if the pathologist can keep a specific organ, such as the heart, to enable medical staff to carry out a further examination. The pathologist, on behalf of the hospital, would become the custodian of the organ which would be kept in a safe place under secure conditions in the hospital. The identity of the organ and the diagnosis would be confidential.
- Often the doctors would keep the organ indefinitely which would allow the opportunity to learn important information about the underlying condition and its treatment both now and in the future. If in the future relatives change their mind, then the hospital must dispose of the organ in the legal and proper manner or return it to the relative for cremation or burial as they wish.
- The reasons why pathologists may wish to keep an organ, tissue or body parts include:
  - to determine the cause of death
  - specific current research projects
  - archiving for future research projects
  - medical museums for the education and training of medical students and doctors
  - discussions between other clinicians and pathologists.
- Relatives may:
  - wish to ask about the implications of agreeing to these uses
  - like to ask whether tissue, parts or organs will be sent to medical museums, or used for genetic research
  - wish to know whether parts will be sent to another laboratory, to tissue or organ banks or abroad.
- If relatives do not wish an organ to be kept indefinitely, they may be asked whether they would allow it to be kept for several weeks, so that the pathologist and other doctors can examine it in detail before issuing the postmortem report. The hospital can respectfully dispose of the organ or return it to the relative for cremation or burial.
- It is important that if relatives do not want an organ to be retained, they inform the doctor when permission is obtained for the postmortem examination. It is important to record on a specifically prepared consent form what relatives do agree to.

Comments on the case

Postmortem examinations and tissue/organ retention is a major ethical subject and all candidates must be comfortable requesting one. The above enables the candidate to develop a script for obtaining consent from a relative.

Further reading

Department of Health, Department for Education and Employment, Home Office. *The removal, retention and use of human organs and tissue from postmortem examination: advice from the Chief Medical Officer.* London: Department of Health, 2001.

Human Tissue Authority. *Code of Practice – post mortem examination.* London: Human Tissue Authority, 2006.

Royal College of Pathologists. *Guidelines for the retention of tissues and organs at postmortem examination.* London: Royal College of Pathologists, 2000.

Case 34 | Coroner's postmortem

Candidate information

You are the medical doctor working in the intensive care unit and you have been asked to speak to Mr Keith Webber whose son has been confirmed as brain-dead earlier in the day.

Please read this summary and then continue with the consultation.

Re: Mr Danny Webber, aged 16 years

Danny Webber was a young man doing his GCSEs in school. Yesterday, after school, he became involved in a fight with some other students and it was believed he received a blow to his head. He collapsed and lost consciousness straight away. He was brought to hospital soon after and was found to have a Glasgow Coma Score (GCS) of 3/15 on arrival. He was intubated and admitted to the ICU. A CT scan of the head confirmed major intracerebral bleeding. There were no signs of neurological recovery 24h later and brainstem testing by two consultants confirmed that he was brainstem dead. His parents were informed of this and they were present when the ventilator was switched off. Since it is not known how or why Danny was assaulted or by whom, it is now a police case and an inquest and a coroner's postmortem need to be carried out.

Your tasks are to: explain to Mr Keith Webber with compassion and tact about the need for a coroner's postmortem and what this will mean for the family.

Subject/patient/relative information

Mr Keith Webber is the father of Danny Webber who has died in the ICU around 2h ago. Danny was his 16-year-old son and he was living with his mother after his parents' divorce. Danny did not confide much in his parents about his friends or any problems he was having. Yesterday on his way back from school, he became involved in a fight with some other students and it appeared that he sustained a blow to his head which knocked him unconsciousness. The other boys involved in the fight ran away but one of them called the ambulance first. He was taken to the ICU and put on a ventilator. A CT head showed major bleeding in the brain. His parents were informed and they have been by his bedside since. Earlier today the ICU consultant told them that the tests have shown that Danny is brain-dead and there is no hope of recovery. They switched off the ventilator 2h ago with his parents by his bedside. Since it is not known who assaulted Danny, the police are involved and are now investigating the case as grievous assault. The doctor in the ICU is about to speak to Mr Keith Webber about taking Danny's body for a coroner's postmortem. Mr Webber is not keen on this initially because he feels the death of his young son is devastating enough for the family and they want to grieve in private and arrange for his funeral without delay.

Thoughts and questions the patient/subject may have
- *Why do you want to carve him up? He has been through enough!*
- *We just want to bury our son and you can't stop us.*
- *We have the right to say 'no'.*
- *I won't let you steal our son's organs.*

Examiner information

1. Conduct of interview
- Introduce yourself to Mr Webber. Express your condolences for the loss of his son. Ask if it is all right for you to call his son by his first name and ask how he, Danny's mother and the other family members are coping with the situation.
- Ask him if there are any questions he would like to ask you first or anything he wants to talk about.
- Be prepared to give him sufficient time to express his grief as the loss of his son in such a tragic way may not necessarily have sunk in. You should be prepared for anything, as no particular reaction can be predicted in such a situation. The important thing here is not to take it personally and to accept that, faced with this awful situation, none of us knows how we would react.
- Explain to Mr Webber that you need to talk to him about what needs to happen before they can have the funeral for their son. Ask him if he has already been spoken to by the police or other hospital staff with regard to the procedure of dealing with his son's death.
- Tell him in an unambiguous but sensitive manner that Danny's case is now being considered as grievous assault and it will be referred to the police and the criminal justice system for further inquiry.
- Give him a moment to process this information.
- Acknowledge the pain of what you are about to say – something along the lines of 'I realize that what I say now is likely to be upsetting but it is important, because it isn't clear at this stage exactly what happened to Danny. Therefore a coroner's postmortem (PM) examination of the body will need to be carried out'.
- Give him a few moments to absorb this news – it is likely to be unwelcome and to cause resistance.
- If needed, reaffirm the reasons for this to be done, again acknowledging how upsetting it must be for him.
- Ask him if he knows, or wants to know, what is involved in a postmortem and, if he is unclear, explain it to him in simple terms.
- Mr Webber might try to refuse for the PM to be carried out. Explain sensitively to him that because there is criminal activity here, the case has to go to the coroner and a coroner's PM will have to be carried out. Therefore, the family have no right to object.
- As difficult as the situation might be for the family members, most of them will eventually consent to further examination of the body to be carried out, especially if it will help the police investigation and enable justice to be sought for their son's death. Tell Mr Webber that you realize that he may want to talk about this with his ex-wife and family and that you can let him have some time to do this.
- He may express strong worries about organs being stolen – remember that the Bristol heart babies and Alder Hey Hospital cases were widely reported and have had a lasting impact in the minds of some people. You should mention at this stage that the pathologist may need to retain some of Danny's organs or tissues for further tests or until the criminal investigation is complete. Once the retained organs or tissues are no longer required, they may be returned to the family, if requested, or disposed of by burial or cremation.
- He may voice a need to arrange the funeral as quickly as possible, so reassure him that the coroner's PM examination usually takes place without delay and the body will normally be returned to the family soon after to allow the funeral arrangements to proceed. Explain that a coroner's officer and a police family liaison officer will keep them informed about the situation and offer advice.
- Do remember that while not every family will take up the offer, you must ask them if they have a personal spiritual adviser whom they wish to contact or if they would like you to contact the hospital on-call chaplain.

- Thank him for his patience (even if you don't think he has been patient) and ask him if there is anything else he would like to talk about or if he has any questions about the matters discussed. Arrange a time to come back and speak to him later on.

2. Exploration and problem negotiation

The candidate should be able to:
- demonstrate empathy and compassion in speaking to a father who has just lost his teenage son
- discuss the need for a coroner's postmortem and briefly explain what this will mean for the family.

3. Communication, ethics and the law

- A coroner is an independent judicial office holder, who has to be a lawyer or doctor by profession (sometimes both). They are appointed by local authorities and work, together with deputies and assistant deputies, in the coroner's office.
- The primary role of the coroner's office is to inquire into deaths occurring in violent, unnatural or suspicious circumstances, sudden deaths of unknown cause and deaths which occur in prison or whilst in police custody. This will often require a PM examination of the deceased person's body to be carried out.
- By law, the family's consent is *not* needed for a coroner's PM examination but it is good practice to inform the family of the reasons for the examination, what it involves, and when and where it will take place.
- After the initial PM examination, the coroner may need to retain some tissues and organs for further examinations (which can take several weeks). The family can decide whether to wait for these organs to be returned to the body before holding the funeral or they can go ahead with the funeral and then the retained tissues and organs can either be returned to the family for their own arrangements or disposed of by the coroner in a sensitive and respectful way.
- A coroner's inquest is a fact-finding inquiry carried out to establish who the deceased person was (if unknown) and how, when and where he died. Note that it is *not* within the coroner's jurisdiction to determine who was responsible for the death as this lies within the remit of the criminal or Crown courts.
- If the case is suspected to be murder or manslaughter and is referred to the court for trial, then the coroner's inquest will be adjourned (but not the postmortem) until the results of the trial are known. Since this will usually establish the facts surrounding the death, it will then usually not require a coroner's inquest to be carried out.
- Aside from the above-mentioned scenarios where a coroner's postmortem and/or inquest have to be carried out, there are other scenarios in which the death should be reported to the coroner's office. The coroner or his deputies will then decide if further examination of the body is required or if the death certificate can be issued. These situations include: no doctor attending to the deceased during his last illness (or there is an attending doctor but he had not seen the deceased within 14 days of the death); death during surgery or before recovery from anaesthetic; death due to industrial disease, accident or poisoning; death was sudden or unexpected.
- On completion of the PM examination and/or the coroner's inquest, the death certificate will be issued and the Registrar of Births and Deaths informed.
- There are other situations in which a PM examination may be requested by the deceased person's family or medical team (known as a 'hospital postmortem'). These may be in the following situations: to identify the cause of death; to confirm the nature or extent of a disease; to identify other undiagnosed conditions; to identify complications or side-effects of drugs or other treatments.
- It is possible that the pathologists may need to retain the deceased person's organs or tissues after the PM for further tests to investigate further the cause of death or, for example, in murder investigations. However, if the pathologist wishes to retain these organs or tissues for research or teaching purposes, then explicit consent must be sought from the deceased's relatives.
- Refer to Case 32 for details and guidance about brainstem death testing.

Comments on the case

There is no easy way to communicate with a parent who has recently lost a teenage child in a most tragic manner. The consultation will very much depend on what state of mind the bereaved father is in and what he wishes to talk about. It is important not to appear to rush the family with indecent haste and remember that a degree of flexibility is required in such situations.

Further reading

Department of Health, Social Services and Public Safety. *Post-mortem examinations: good practice in consent and care of the bereaved.* London: Department of Health, 2004.

Ministry of Justice, Coroners and Burials Division. *A guide to coroners and inquests.* London: Stationery Office, 2010.

www.victimsvoice.co.uk. Provides factual and practical information and support for families affected by sudden death.

Case 35 | Do not attempt resuscitation decisions

Candidate information

You are the doctor working on a care of the elderly ward.

Please read this summary and then continue with the consultation.

Re: Mrs Edith Greasley, aged 82 years

Mrs Greasley is an elderly lady who suffered a stroke 3 years ago and has been predominantly bed-bound since then apart from when her carers hoist her out into a chair during the daytime. She still has some verbal communication but her higher cerebral function is slowly deteriorating and she has been diagnosed with vascular dementia. In addition, she has a history of ischaemic heart disease, diabetes mellitus and previous breast cancer which was treated 20 years ago. She was admitted to hospital 5 days ago with a urinary tract infection and has been on intravenous fluids and antibiotics since. She has not made much recovery and the consultant feels it is appropriate to sign a 'Do Not Attempt Resuscitation' (DNAR) form for her should she deteriorate.

Your tasks are to: discuss with Mrs Greasley's daughter, Mrs Knowles, about the DNAR decision and address any other concerns she may have.

Subject/patient/relative information

Mrs Knowles is the daughter of Mrs Edith Greasley and is her next of kin. Mrs Greasley suffered a clinically significant stroke 3 years ago and has become bed-bound since apart from when her carers hoist her out into a chair during the daytime. She has some verbal communication but becomes confused on and off and her GP has mentioned the possibility of her having vascular dementia. She has been living with her daughter since her stroke and has carers coming in three times a day to do all personal care. She also has a history of ischaemic heart disease, diabetes mellitus and previous breast cancer which was treated 20 years ago. Mrs Greasley was admitted to hospital 5 days ago with a urinary infection and has been on antibiotics and fluids. The doctor is about to speak to her daughter about making her mother 'Not for Resuscitation'. Mrs Knowles is not agreeable to this because she feels this means her mother will just be 'left to die in the corner of the ward'. She also feels her mother is showing signs of recovery because she opened her eyes and smiled today and she does not want the doctors to 'give up' on her yet. Mrs Knowles is also worried about her mother's nutrition as she often refuses her food. She has heard about artificial feeding 'through a tube into the stomach' and wonders if her mother can be considered for this.

Thoughts and questions the patient/subject may have

- *I want you to explain very clearly to me why you want to let my mother die.*
- *I am sure she would get better if only she would eat, can't you put a tube into her and feed her that way?*
- If Mrs Knowles doesn't feel that the candidate is explaining in a convincing way, she may want to ask if there is someone else she can speak to.

Examiner information

1. Conduct of interview

- Introduce yourself to Mrs Knowles.
- Ask what she knows about what has been happening with her mother since her hospital admission and, if necessary, offer to give her an update.
- Explain in a clear, but sensitive, manner that Mrs Greasley is being treated for a urinary tract infection but it does not appear that she has made much of an improvement despite this (you can say that this is based on the observations made by the nurses, doctors and ward staff as well as the blood results, etc.).
- Tell the daughter, showing empathy, 'I'm very sorry, but your mother isn't very well' and then pause; 'As you know, your mother has a lot of health problems and this latest infection is taking a heavy toll on her ability to recover'. Use another pause to let the message sink in.
- Ask her if she has thought about what would happen in a situation where her mother's health deteriorates further or she does not recover from an illness such as this one. Ask her if she has spoken to other family members about this eventuality and what her/the family thoughts are about this. She might say that since her mother suffered the severe stroke 3 years ago, she was aware that the prognosis was not very good.
- Tell her that your consultant reviewed Mrs Greasley this morning on the ward round and felt that there is a possibility that she may deteriorate further and die in the near future. There is no easy way to say this but don't be afraid of using the word 'death' to avoid ambiguity.
- In view of her multiple health problems and poor quality of life, the consultant feels that resuscitating her in the event of a cardiorespiratory arrest would be futile and that the medical team feel that adopting a 'Do Not Attempt Resuscitation' (DNAR) care pathway is appropriate. Then pause.
- Explain that the DNAR decision refers only to withholding resuscitation in the event that her heart or lungs stop working suddenly. In her mother's case there will be a gradual slowing down of her breathing and heartbeat as she slips gradually away. Stress that this decision does not mean that her mother will not receive other medical treatment to keep her as comfortable as possible.
- Ask Mrs Knowles if she has heard of this approach and what her thoughts are about it. She might want to know more about what it means or she may straight away express her reluctance about it.
- Listen carefully to her thoughts and feelings, remembering that this is her mother whom she loves and has cared for the last 3 years.
- Take some time to give her the necessary information and you can go into more details about her reservations regarding the DNAR decision. It may help to explain that this is not about her mother's age but rather her general physical health. For cardiopulmonary resuscitation to have any prospect of success, the major organs need to be in good health and this is not the case with her mother. Explain that this is a form of advanced care planning which allows health professionals to think about how best to care for patients in a way that is respectful and that also ensures that they have a peaceful and dignified death.
- If she says something along the lines of 'Does this mean you're just going to leave my mother to die on her own?', reassure her that this is not the case and a DNAR decision in no way implies that.
- Reaffirm that her mother will continue to receive full medical and nursing care, with due attention to all her needs. If she has any concerns at any time that her mother is not receiving basic care then she should inform the ward nurses/manager /doctors immediately.
- Also reiterate, in order to reassure her, that a DNAR decision is not final and is reviewed by the team on a regular basis and if Mrs Greasley shows significant

improvement with the treatment she receives, then the decision may be revoked if appropriate.

- Let Mrs Knowles know that the DNAR decision is a medical one usually made by the most senior clinician in charge of the patient after careful thought and discussion within the team. However, explain that it is good practice to discuss with the family/next of kin first to find out their thoughts about it and, more importantly, to enquire if they know what the patient would have wanted if they were in a position to express their wishes. Ask if an advance directive has been made. This will be reassuring to some family members who might otherwise experience feelings of guilt, as if they were being asked to make the decision about whether their relatives should be resuscitated or not.
- Acknowledge that you appreciate that this news must be hard to hear so ask her if she has any questions or if she needs more time to think about the issues raised. She may wish to discuss this with other family members.
- Arrange another appointment to speak to her if required and say that you can ask your consultant to be present too if she wishes to speak directly to him/her. Thank her for listening to you.

2. Exploration and problem negotiation

The candidate should be able to:

- discuss the patient's current medical status and likely prognosis and the indications for a DNAR relevant to this patient
- acknowledge and appreciate the concerns raised by the subject and deal with them in a compassionate but factual manner.

3. Communication, ethics and the law

- Advance care planning (i.e. making decisions about the future healthcare of our patients) falls under the umbrella of good clinical practice that we, as healthcare professionals, should aspire to provide at all times. Making decisions about cardiopulmonary resuscitation (CPR) is one of the most important (and possibly most sensitive) aspects of advance care planning.
- The issue about how, when and to whom decisions regarding CPR are communicated can be very difficult even for the most experienced of clinicians. Joint guidelines from the Resuscitation Council (UK), British Medical Association and Royal College of Nursing advise that 'if a decision not to attempt CPR is made because it will not be successful and the patient has not expressed a wish to be informed about such matters, it is not necessary or appropriate to initiate the discussion with him/her'. However, if a decision has been made that it is necessary to discuss with the patient about CPR or to find out his/her views about it, then it goes without saying that this should be done in a manner that can be understood by the patient, giving time for reflection and questions. This accepted position does need further thought in practice.

- The primary focus of the clinician, when a DNAR decision is being considered, must always be the patient. It is questionable as to how many patients are asked directly whether or not they have thought about or have an opinion about what they would expect if their heart was to suddenly stop. Admittedly, initiating such a conversation may seem a daunting proposition. However, it can help to bring clarity for all involved. A highly skilled communicator should be able to tentatively explore this very sensitive subject with minimal distress being caused. A patient may not have thought about making an advance directive or living will, but they may have expressed an opinion about how they want the last moments of their life to be.
- Similarly, close family members are likely to be naturally inclined towards every effort being made by the healthcare team to sustain the life of someone they love and value. Involving family members in the discussions and decisions is therefore of paramount importance. Of course, it may be a potential source of conflict which needs to be dealt with in a mature, clear-headed and sensitive manner. Being very clear that the decision is not arrived at arbitrarily or due to bias (old age is often cited) can be enormously helpful to both patient/family and clinician.
- A clear explanation about the overall physical health of the patient and the likelihood, or otherwise, of a successful resuscitation may be extremely helpful in setting some perspective. Equally, establishing what the patient/family priorities are, given the reality of their condition, should include a sensitive but factual discussion about what resuscitation actually involves. Are medical heroics really preferable to allowing the patient to die in a peaceful and dignified way supported and surrounded by those who love them?
- Since survival rates from cardiopulmonary arrests are low (15–20% for in-hospital arrests and 5–10% for out-of-hospital arrests), healthcare professionals need to carefully consider the risks versus benefits of prolonged CPR attempts for a patient. This includes

whether he/she would have an acceptable quality of life if resuscitated from an arrest (i.e. bearing in mind the possibility of hypoxic brain damage and resulting disability, prolonged artificial ventilation or other organ support in intensive care unit, rib or sternal fractures, etc.).

- It is important to note that DNAR decisions must be made bearing in mind the individual circumstances of the person without blanket assumptions based on their age, comorbidities, disability, perceived quality of life, etc. Therefore, it must be a healthcare professional who makes the decision based on an objective assessment of what is actually in the patient's best interests, always taking into consideration the patient's views whenever possible. This practice should be encouraged as a mark of respect for all individuals' humanity and their right to make their own informed decisions (remember there are also patients who are felt to be suitable candidates for resuscitation who may choose to decline it).

- It is of course a clinician's responsibility to ensure that the most appropriate treatment, and the one that will most likely benefit the patient, is offered.

- Therefore, if the clinician believes that CPR is unlikely to be successful in restarting the person's heart or lungs in that situation then it should not be attempted. Some situations in which this might be the case include when the patient is in the final stages of an incurable illness (e.g. cancer, end-stage cardiac failure, motor neurone disease, etc.) or has had a recent severe illness (e.g. sepsis, multiorgan failure) or a past medical history which has significant impact on impaired organ function (e.g. significant myocardial infarction, chronic lung disease or respiratory failure, etc.). As mentioned above, one should not assume that all patients with the above-mentioned diagnoses will not be suitable for CPR – assessment should always be made with regard to and due respect for the individual in question.

- While there is no legal obligation for the clinician to discuss DNAR decisions with the patient/family, it is always prudent and compassionate to talk to them about their expectations if death is considered to be the likely outcome of their current condition. There can be no textbook position on discussing resuscitation as it needs to be carefully considered on a case-by-case basis. Using the Beauchamp and Childress biomedical ethics model may be extremely useful in thinking through any decisions or discussions with the patient/family unless, of course, the patient or family raise it with you or other members of the team.

- It is important to note that neither patients, nor their family or friends, can insist on medical treatment (including CPR) which the clinicians feel is inappropriate for the patient. If such a situation arises, the clinician should try to explain the issue once again to the concerned parties and, if they are still not in agreement, a second opinion should be sought.

- In patients who lack mental capacity, the same principles outlined in the Mental Capacity Act 2005 apply because CPR, by definition, constitutes life-saving treatment (see Case 40 for a more detailed discussion of the Mental Capacity Act of 2005).

- In summary, when dealing with a patient in whom there is a foreseeable risk of cardiopulmonary arrest, the clinician should first establish if CPR is likely to be successful and, if so, whether the potential benefits outweigh the risks. The clinician should then consider any previously expressed wishes by the patient, including consulting with close family or friends to help determine this (noting that the role of relatives and friends who do not have any legal authority should be to help in communicating the patient's views rather than being the final decision makers themselves).

- Some patients may have made an advance directive refusing CPR when they previously had capacity. This should have been signed, witnessed and have a written statement saying that the decision is to stand even if the patient's life is at risk. If such an advance directive exists then it should be taken as valid. However, it is the clinician's responsibility to ensure, as far as possible, that the current circumstance fits into that envisaged by the patient at the time of signing the document.

- If such an advance directive does not exist, or the patient has subsequently appointed a Lasting Power of Attorney (LPA) to make healthcare decisions on their behalf, then this person should be consulted regarding CPR decisions (so long as the LPA document clearly includes a statement giving the LPA authority to decide about withholding life-prolonging treatment).

- Note that welfare attorneys, such as an LPA, cannot demand treatment (including CPR) if it is not clinically appropriate. When there is disagreement which cannot be resolved with a second opinion, then it may be necessary to involve the Court of Protection (NB: these regulations primarily refer to England and Wales, so do refer to the relevant guidelines for Scotland and Northern Ireland).

Comments on the case

Discussions surrounding end-of-life care and DNAR are probably some of the hardest that a clinician will have to conduct, no matter how junior or senior they are.

Caution should be applied if a clinician finds themselves avoiding such a discussion because it is more comfortable for them not to address it. Naturally, no one likes upsetting a patient or their family. However, it may be more upsetting and have longer-term ramifications for bereaved families if they subsequently 'discover' that a DNAR order is in place and feel that they were intentionally excluded.

Further reading

Beauchamp T, Childress F. *Principles of biomedical ethics*, 6th edn. Oxford: Oxford University Press, 2009.

British Medical Association, Resuscitation Council (UK) and Royal College of Nursing. Decisions relating to cardiopulmonary resuscitation. 2007. www.resus.org.uk/pages/dnar.htm

Case 36 | Withholding information from patients

Candidate information

You are the medical doctor on a general medical ward.

Please read this summary and then continue with the consultation.

> **Re: Mrs Yu Chang, aged 67 years**
>
> Mrs Chang is a woman originally from Hong Kong who speaks very little English. She was admitted to hospital 2 days ago with a cough and haemoptysis. Looking back through her medical notes and clinic letters, you understand that she is being investigated by the respiratory team for a suspected lung malignancy which was picked up on a chest X-ray. She has had a CT chest and a bronchoscopy but the consultant was unable to obtain sufficient tissue for histological diagnosis and he is referring her for a CT-guided lung biopsy. The CT scan showed that the mass is resectable depending on the histology. Her present symptoms are likely to be due to the lung mass. The respiratory consultant has told Mrs Chang's children about the possibility of lung cancer but her children have not yet decided whether to tell her for fear that 'she will just give up hope'. Earlier today on the ward round, Mrs Chang seemed to be asking you (in a mixture of Cantonese and English) what was wrong with her. She has previously been offered an official interpreter, but prefers to use her daughter whom you are about to speak to.

Your tasks are to: talk to Mrs Lee (Mrs Chang's daughter) about the likely cause of her mother's symptoms and about discussing the possible diagnosis with the patient.

Subject/patient/relative information

Mrs Lee is Mrs Chang's daughter and her next of kin. Mrs Chang is a 67-year-old lady, originally from Hong Kong and who speaks very little English. Her daughter and son accompany her to all hospital visits and translate for her. She was admitted to hospital 2 days ago with a worsening cough and she has been coughing up some bright red blood. Following a chest X-ray about 4 weeks ago, a CT scan of her chest and a camera investigation (bronchoscopy), the family have been told that Mrs Chang needs a further procedure, known as a CT-guided biopsy, as the previous tests have been inconclusive. The respiratory consultant has been open with Mrs Chang's family about the likelihood of cancer and has said it may be possible to treat it with surgery and then chemo- or radiotherapy, depending on what is confirmed on biopsy. However, Mrs Chang's children have made the decision not to tell her about the diagnosis yet for fear that 'she will just give up and refuse all treatment'. They feel she is not strong enough at the moment to take in the news because she is still grieving following her husband's death 6 months ago. However, Mrs Lee understands that her mother has a right to know her diagnosis, especially since she seems to be asking more about it since coming into hospital.

Thoughts and questions the patient/subject may have
- *How do you know that my mother wants to know what is going on – she doesn't speak or understand English!*
- *I think you should respect the family's wishes in this matter. We are the ones who care for Mum 24/7 and know best when and how she should find out about the cancer.*

Examiner information

1. Conduct of interview
- Introduce yourself to Mrs Lee and confirm her relationship with Mrs Chang.
- Ask her to tell you what she understands already about her mother's diagnosis (this is important because it will probably be the daughter or another family member who will eventually be conveying the diagnosis to the patient in her native language).
- Explain that the reason for her hospital admission this time is likely to be due to an extension of, and bleeding from, her underlying lung mass and this is the reason you would like to speak to her about this matter now.
- Ask Mrs Lee how much she thinks her mother knows about the probability of her having a lung cancer and what the family have told her so far.
- If she admits that the family have deliberately kept the diagnosis from Mrs Chang, then give her enough time to explain why and talk about her own dilemma or worries with regard to this issue. Remember that she too is likely to be grieving for her father's death and at the same time caring for her sick mother.
- Enquire if her mother has been asking about what is going on and if she has expressed a desire to know (you can say that she seemed to be doing so during your ward round that morning but you could not be sure due to the language barrier).
- Discuss the pros and cons of not telling the patient the suspected diagnosis, i.e. the family's desire to 'protect the patient' versus increasing the anxiety of the patient about her own health.
- The daughter might become defensive during the interview and say something along the lines of 'are you accusing me of lying to my mother?'. Ensure that you are not confrontational at any time during the interview and reiterate to her that, like her family, you only have your patient's best interests at heart and

that your duty of care is, first and foremost, to her mother.
- Also say that because Mrs Chang is due for a CT-guided lung biopsy soon, the issue of informed consent becomes relevant. Explain to her that in the UK, no one can give informed consent on behalf of a competent adult and, in order for Mrs Chang to give her consent, she will need to know the indication for the procedure and its intended benefit.
- Offer support to both the patient and the family during this difficult time. Offer to give Mrs Lee details of the patient advocacy team or link nurses if she might find that helpful.
- If, at the end of the discussion, the daughter still insists that she does not want to inform her mother about the suspected malignancy, say that you will need to speak to your consultant (who may ask to meet with the daughter or other family members) and involve the patient advocacy team (or equivalent) to discuss further about what is in the best interests of the patient.
- Mention that you will request the respiratory team (preferably the same consultant who has already been seeing her) to review her on the ward and offer their specialist opinion. Tell her you will also let the palliative care nurses and the lung cancer team know that she is in hospital.
- Thank Mrs Lee for her time and give her your contact details.

2. Explanation and problem negotiation
The candidate should be able to:
- establish with Mrs Chang's daughter her understanding of her mother's likely diagnosis and its relevance to the current symptoms
- discuss the reasons for and against telling her mother the suspected diagnosis, including the implications that this has for patient autonomy and providing informed consent

- formulate a plan with the daughter about how the situation can be dealt with.

3. Communication, ethics and the law

- Decisions about how much information to disclose to patients about their diagnosis, prognosis and treatment options, and when to do this, can be difficult, especially when there are coexisting obstacles such as language and cultural barriers. Traditional Chinese family units are quite different from those in the UK. Following the death of a husband, his wife defers to and comes under the guidance of the head of the household – normally this is the eldest son.
- An honest relationship based on mutual trust is the cornerstone to a successful doctor–patient partnership. Therefore, in a situation such as this where the patient appears to be asking the doctor for information regarding her health, it would be unethical for the doctor to withhold that information from the patient.
- With regard to the autonomous adult who has capacity, there is a moral obligation to give them the opportunity to exercise self-determination in order to make informed decisions. Underpinning this is the precept of confidentiality and, in this particular case, these 'rights' have been effectively negated by the patient's own choice to defer to her family and use them for translation. Thus far, all disclosures have been made to the family and not to her. Now that she is giving indications that she wants more information, it would be prudent, after discussing your intention with the family first, to bring in an independent interpreter. This should be done without the presence of the family (to avoid undue discomfort to the patient or potential pressure from the family). If the patient indicates that she does suspect cancer or wants to know in detail what is going on, then that should be discussed with the help of the interpreter. The next of kin should be informed about the outcome of this discussion and the content of these conversations clearly documented in the notes.
- The guidance set out by the General Medical Council (GMC) for doctors has highlighted the importance of good communication with patients and the need to share information with them about their 'diagnosis, prognosis, treatment and care'. Such communication of information becomes especially important when the patient is required to give informed consent

for a procedure or treatment (for example, in this case, the patient will need to consent for the CT-guided lung biopsy).
- However, according to the GMC document on consent, the information shared with patients can vary from patient to patient and it is important to be aware that individual patients may want 'more or less information or involvement in making decisions depending on their circumstances and wishes'.
- However, doctors should *not* make assumptions about how information is disclosed to the patient based on their age, level of education, command of the English language, disability or other factors. In situations where communication may be difficult, the clinician should take all practicable steps to ensure that information is communicated to the patient in a way that is easily understood by them.
- Remember that no one can make a healthcare-related decision (especially with regard to consent for an investigation or treatment) for a patient who has capacity, even if the patient requests the medical team, partner, relative, carer or another person to do so on their behalf. If, despite discussion with the patient, they do not want to be given information about their health, the clinician should respect this as far as possible but this may have implications for the validity of informed consent if it is required in the process.
- The minimum level of information a patient needs to know in order to give valid informed consent for a procedure or treatment includes the following: the aims of that procedure or intervention relevant to the patient, whether it is invasive or not, the amount of pain or discomfort the patient is likely to experience, if the patient needs to undergo any preparation prior to it and the serious risks involved.
- General Medical Council guidance also states that you should not withhold information necessary for making decisions for any other reason, including when a relative, partner, friend or carer asks you to, unless you believe it would cause the patient serious harm. In this context, 'serious harm' means that the person might become upset and refuse treatment.
- If the doctor still feels that it is appropriate to withhold information from a patient, they should document the reasons for doing so clearly in the notes and be prepared to justify their decision later if required.

Comments on the case

Part of a doctor's duty of care to patients lies in being honest with them about their diagnosis (or uncertainties in the diagnosis), treatment and care. It is sometimes easy to overlook the fact that our priority of care should be the patient, especially when he/she does not speak English as a first language, has cognitive impairment or other disability. In these situations, we need to use available resources to ensure that we still communicate directly with the patient in a manner that can be understood by them.

Further reading

Department of Constitutional Affairs, Department of Health, Public Guardianship Office and Welsh Assembly Government. *Mental Capacity Act 2005 – summary*. London: Stationery Office, 2007.

General Medical Council. *Consent: patients and doctors making decisions together*. London: General Medical Council, 2008.

Case 37 | Maintaining patient confidentiality

Candidate information

You are the medical doctor in a medical assessment unit.

Please read this summary and then continue with the consultation.

Re: Mr Andreas Nikolas, aged 22 years

Mr Nikolas is a 22-year-old man who was brought into hospital yesterday evening with a head injury that he sustained when out in the town. He had a Glasgow Coma Score of 9/15 on arrival in A&E and he had three episodes of vomiting, all of which improved after about 3h. He had a CT head which was normal and he was kept in overnight for neurological observations. He is back to his usual self now and is awaiting a review before discharge. When you come to assess him prior to discharge, he brings up another matter with you. He admits that he was involved in a fight with some other men last night during which he fell and injured himself, but before this he tells you that he threatened one of the men with a knife. He is worried that this will have been seen on closed-circuit television (CCTV) and asks that you do not disclose his identity or tell the police about his hospital admission if they make enquiries after his discharge.

Your tasks are to: respond to this additional news appropriately and assess Mr Nikolas's suitability for discharge (including giving post-head injury advice).

Subject/patient/relative information

Mr Nikolas is a 22-year-old man who was brought into hospital yesterday evening with a head injury he sustained when out in the town. He was out celebrating a friend's birthday and, after having quite a few drinks, became involved in a brawl with a group of young men. The argument escalated and became physical. He has been told by the nurse that he received a blow to his head which caused him to fall and this knocked him out. He does not remember any of the events which followed until he woke up in hospital a couple of hours later. He has not told anyone at the hospital but he remembers that last night, in the heat of the moment, he threatened one of the men with a knife after he was punched in the face. Mr Nikolas does not know the identity of the man he threatened with the knife, how badly he was hurt or if he was taken to hospital. He is worried because he dropped the knife and there is CCTV in that part of town. He is now scared that the police may come looking for him in the hospital or demand to know his identity if they are investigating the knife crime. He is particularly worried because he was prosecuted a year ago by the police for domestic violence against his ex-girlfriend and received a suspended sentence. He wants to ask the candidate not to disclose his identity or to tell the police about his hospital admission if they make enquiries after his discharge. As far as his head injury is concerned, he does not have any symptoms now aside from a mild headache and is anxious to be discharged. He will be going back home and his mother will be able to look after him.

Thoughts and questions the patient/subject may have
- *Was anyone else brought in after the fight?*
- *Has the hospital already told the police?*
- *The doctor's aren't allowed to tell the police because of patient confidentiality, are they?*

Examiner information

1. Conduct of interview
- Introduce yourself to Mr Nikolas.
- Ask him how he is feeling, particularly about any ongoing symptoms of headache, vomiting and confusion.
- If none of these are present, tell him that the medical team, whose care he is under, feel that he had concussion and that you are now happy to discharge him.
- If he wants to know, tell him briefly what happened since his admission to hospital the previous night, i.e. that he was brought in with a reduced conscious level believed to be from a head injury. The CT scan of his head did not show any serious injury such as a bleed in or around his brain and he was kept in hospital overnight for observation.
- Ask him who will be at home and if that person is able to monitor him over the next 24–48 h for any delayed complications.
- Ensure that he has been given written advice about the features to look out for in terms of delayed complications of head injury and who to contact for help. Inform him that he needs to be followed up by his GP in 1 week.
- Mr Nikolas will go on to tell you about the incident which occurred the previous night, when he threatened another man with a knife after he had been punched in the face. He is now panicky because he doesn't have the knife and knows that there is CCTV in that part of town. He will ask you not to disclose any information about him to the police who may be investigating the knife crime.
- Tell him calmly that while you are not making any judgements about him, his request places you in a difficult situation. Give him a few moments to let that information sink in.
- He may ask what you mean. Tell him in a straightforward manner that as a medical professional, you have

a legal duty to assist the police in the investigation of crime (including knife crime and gunshot wounds).
- Explain that if you have no reason to believe that he poses a threat to the public, then you do not need to report him to the police. However, if the police approach you as part of their investigation into this crime, you will have to assist in the investigation.
- He may become angry or threaten you but you need to stay calm and be firm. You need to explain that you understand that he is frightened but that the hospital has a strict 'zero tolerance policy' towards threats to staff.
- Alternatively, he may come across as regretful, perhaps asking you not to say anything to the police. Once again, you must remain non-committal and reiterate that you have a legal obligation to provide the information to the police if required to do so.
- Tell him that in such situations you are allowed to breach patient confidentiality without their consent. However, you would not make such decisions on your own and would check with your consultant and seek medicolegal advice if required.
- Ask him what he plans to do with regard to this issue after discharge. If he is amenable to it, you can suggest that he speaks to the police himself and co-operates with their investigation.
- Ensure that you document all the above clearly in the patient's notes.

2. Exploration and problem negotiation
The candidate should be able to:
- assess a patient's suitability for discharge after a head injury and provide appropriate discharge information
- listen to the patient's anxieties regarding the crime he committed the previous day in a non-judgemental way

- make it clear in a sensitive, but firm, manner that you cannot withhold information from the police who are investigating a potential knife crime.

3. Communication, ethics and the law

- Communicating with someone who is frightened and realizes that they have acted outside the law is probably going to be challenging. As in this case, they may have an expectation that you are obliged to maintain their confidence. You have to tell them the facts in these circumstances. However, you should ensure that you do so in a way that minimizes the risk of antagonizing them.
- If you think that your personal safety may be at risk, you should inform a senior colleague and seek advice/support from the hospital security team in order to minimize any potential danger.
- Maintaining patient confidentiality is the cornerstone of the duties of a doctor. Patients often reveal intensely private details about their health and other personal problems so it is essential that trust is maintained by keeping these in the strictest confidence. A breach of this trust may lead to a patient concealing vital information which may be necessary to provide good clinical care and which could potentially risk professional or even legal sanctions.
- However, patient confidentiality does not mean that information about the patient remains strictly between the doctor and patient. Other members of the healthcare, and sometimes social care, team directly involved in providing care to the patient are bound by the same contractual, professional and legal responsibilities as doctors. Naturally, they will, and should, have access to their patient's/client's records on a need-to-know basis (e.g. nurses, allied health professionals, medical secretaries, etc.).
- The General Medical Council document on confidentiality has identified certain scenarios where patient confidentiality can be breached. In situations where it is a statutory requirement to disclose patient information, it is not necessary to obtain the patient's consent but the patient should be informed about the required disclosure.
- Some of the situations in which patient confidentiality may be breached, and pointers on what to do in such situations, are as follows:
  - notification of certain infectious diseases, births and deaths registration (statutory requirement)
  - in legal cases if patient information is requested by a judge or presiding officer of a court (statutory requirement)

- however, only information about the patient which is *directly relevant* to the case needs to be disclosed. The court should not ask about the patient's relatives or other contacts if not relevant
  - it is not necessary for doctors to disclose patient information to police officers or solicitors unless it is required by law or for purposes of greater public interest
  - in situations where another individual, or a community, is at risk of serious harm due to the patient's condition or behaviour (e.g. at risk of serious communicable diseases or crime), then the doctor may breach confidentiality. The patient's express consent should be obtained if possible before such a disclosure and the patient's identity should be anonymized if possible
  - the police are required to further investigate a case whereby a member of the public is armed with, and has used, a gun or knife in a serious attack. The reason for doing this is to ensure that the said person does not pose another threat to his previous victim, to staff /other patients/relatives in the hospital and to other members of the public.
- In a situation such as the above, it is possible that the another man in the altercation involving Mr Nikolas would have been taken to a hospital for injuries sustained and, if these injuries were due to knife crime, then the police will be informed about it. Thereafter, they will conduct an investigation and Mr Nikolas may be questioned as one of the suspects.
- It is possible that the police will come to the hospital, either before or after Mr Nikolas is discharged, to verify his identity and find out information about the reason for his admission, the injuries he sustained during the fight, etc.
- Legally, it is permissible for doctors to disclose information about a patient, without their consent, if the disclosure 'would be likely to assist in the prevention, detection or prosecution of serious crime'. Such a disclosure is especially justified if you believe that other people are still at risk from the patient and if he/she possesses a weapon, etc. However, you should make efforts to inform the patient about this if it is practicable and safe to do so.
- Additionally, if the healthcare professional has reason to believe that the patient presents a threat to the same victim, another member of the public or staff at the hospital, this should be reported to the police (regardless of whether or not you know the identity of the victim of the previous crime, the details of the attack, etc.).

Comments on the case

This is a challenging scenario for all doctors to deal with and will be particularly common to those who work in A&E. It is likely that such professionals will have had the necessary training to deal with injuries as a result of crime and how to liaise with the police.

The key thing to remember is that you must be truthful and so the patient must be informed that a breach of confidentiality will need to be made if the police approach the hospital for information when a suspected criminal act has occurred. It may be considered good practice to tell a patient when a breach occurs in some circumstances, although the wisdom of such an action in this specific case is debatable if it could place the clinician at physical risk.

There are additional circumstances in which patient confidentiality may be overridden in addition to the ones mentioned above.

- Local clinical audit is part of the duty of all healthcare professionals to ensure that consistently high standards of healthcare provision are maintained within the department, hospital or NHS trust. Patient information must therefore be available for audit purposes unless the patient expressly objects.

- Regulatory bodies who are investigating matters such as a healthcare professional's fitness to practise.
- Research, epidemiological surveys, education and training – provide anonymized or coded information if possible. If it is necessary to use identifiable information, then the patient's express consent should be obtained.
- Patient's insurance companies, employers or government agencies evaluating welfare claims – the patient's written consent should be obtained first and a copy of the report should be offered to the patient before it is sent off.

With regard to discharging the patient after a head injury, ensure that the GCS is back to 15 and sustained. The clinician should also make sure that the patient has sufficient support and care at home, especially in the first few days after sustaining the head injury (in case they develop delayed complications).

All patients should receive verbal and written advice about post-head injury care, including the symptoms and signs of delayed complications that they need to look out for and whom they should contact if any of these occur. Patients who sustained the head injury after alcohol or drug intoxication should be given advice about drug/alcohol misuse.

Further reading

General Medical Council. *Confidentiality*. London: General Medical Council, 2009.

General Medical Council. *Supplementary guidance. Confidentiality: reporting gunshot and knife crimes*. London: General Medical Council, 2009.

National Institute for Health and Clinical Excellence. *Clinical Guideline 56. Head injury*. London: National Institute for Health and Clinical Excellence, 2007.

Case 38 | Advance care decisions

Candidate information
You are the medical doctor in a neurology clinic.
Please read this summary and then continue with the consultation.

Re: Mr Maurice Bennett, aged 71 years

Mr Bennett was diagnosed with Parkinson's disease 10 years ago and this is now progressively deteriorating. He is currently on three different anti-parkinsonian medications which he must take at regular intervals to prevent any end-of-dose effects. However, they are also giving him intolerable side-effects. He lives on his own but is planning on moving in with his son as he is finding it increasingly difficult to manage. During his last appointment with the neurology consultant, Mr Bennett mentioned that his memory was fluctuating and he was having trouble planning and managing his daily activities. The consultant arranged a CT head, some blood tests and also referred him for psychology tests. The results of these are back and your consultant thinks that Mr Bennett is suffering from early Parkinson's disease-related dementia.

Your tasks are to: explain to Mr Bennett about his probable diagnosis of early dementia and address any concerns he may have (you can assume Mr Bennett has insight into his condition and full capacity to make decisions at present).

Subject/patient/relative information
Mr Maurice Bennett is a 71-year-old man who was diagnosed with Parkinson's disease 10 years ago. He was started on medication early on which seemed to work well for the first few years. However, he has recently started to be troubled by the side-effects and the medications are not working as well despite taking them every few hours. He lives alone but is in the process of selling his house and moving in with his son as he is finding it difficult to cope on his own. Over the last 6 months he has noticed his memory deteriorating, especially in relation to managing everyday tasks like shopping, finding his way home and so on. His son has also had to help him manage his financial affairs. Mr Bennett mentioned this to his consultant the last time, who suggested that he may have a form of dementia but wanted to arrange a CT head scan, some blood investigations and psychology tests first. He has had these now and is back in the clinic for the results. He is concerned about what might happen should his mental state deteriorate in the future and he loses all ability to make his own decisions. He has always been a fiercely independent man and does not want unnecessary life-prolonging treatment if taken ill. He has been reading up about the possibility of appointing his son as a Lasting Power of Attorney (LPA) who can make healthcare and financial decisions on his behalf. He would like to discuss

these issues with the doctor (the candidate) in clinic today and find out more about what provisions there are in the healthcare system to ensure his best interests are safeguarded in the future.

Thoughts and questions the patient/subject may have
- *How quickly am I going to deteriorate?*
- *I want to make sure that my interests are protected in the future when I may be unable to do so – can you help me to do that now?*

Examiner information

1. Conduct of interview
- Introduce yourself to Mr Bennett.
- Ask him first if there is anything specific he would like to talk about – he will probably say that he wants to know the results of the CT scan and the other tests he has had recently.
- Tell him in a simple but straightforward way that the test results show that he has an early form of dementia, known as Parkinson's disease-related dementia.
- Explain to Mr Bennett what the signs of dementia associated with Parkinson's disease (PD) are, e.g. executive dysfunction and visual-spatial awareness. This means that he may have progressive difficulty with things like managing finances, tasks involving organization or planning, driving, etc.
- Give him a few moments to take in what you have said.
- Tell him in an empathetic way that there is unfortunately no treatment which can reverse his PD and that management is essentially symptomatic – give him some time to take this in, in case this was not what he was expecting to hear.
- However, explain that there are several avenues of support and he will be put in touch with the PD nurse specialist (if he is not already) as well as the old age psychiatry team.
- He will probably then ask about what provisions there are within the healthcare system for safeguarding his best interests in the future as and when his mental health deteriorates.
- Explore the reasons for him wanting to do this, e.g. 'Is there anything in particular you are afraid will happen to you in the future? What types of treatment will you want, or not want, to be given to you?'.
- Talk to him briefly about the options available, i.e. nominating an LPA who can make decisions on his behalf or signing an advance directive (this is generally thought to be more restrictive than the former).
- Give him the necessary information about the provisions of the Mental Capacity Act 2005 for nominating an LPA and what types of decisions his LPA can make on his behalf (e.g. health, personal welfare, finances and property).
- Ask him if he has anyone in mind to be his LPA.
- Explain that he can nominate his LPA (or several attorneys if he wants more than one) to decide about some, or all, of the above domains for him and that is his decision.
- However, if he wants his LPA(s) to consent to, or refuse, life-saving treatment on his behalf, that needs to be explicitly stated on the form, signed and witnessed.
- Let him know where he can go to find out more information about it. A good starting point would be the government website (www.direct.gov.uk), Age UK/Age Cymru (formerly Age Concern), or to get advice and direction from his solicitor.
- Tell him that if he decides to go ahead with it, he and his nominee (i.e. his son) will need to sign a Lasting Power of Attorney for Health and Welfare document (and a separate document if he wants to nominate an LPA to manage his property and finances). These signatures need to be witnessed and certified by a professional (e.g. patient's GP or solicitor) and then registered with the Office of the Public Guardian.
- Ask him if he has any other questions and then arrange a follow-up appointment for him to come back to your clinic soon. Ensure he has the contact details of the Parkinson's disease specialist nurse before he leaves.
- Close the consultation.

2. Exploration and problem negotiation
The candidate should be able to:
- explain briefly the diagnosis of dementia to the patient in a simple manner, how it links to his

Parkinson's disease and how it is likely to affect his day-to-day life
- address the patient's questions about how the Mental Capacity Act can be used to safeguard his health and welfare in the future. Basic information about the role of a Lasting Power of Attorney and where he can get further information should be discussed.

3. Communication, ethics and the law

- The Mental Capacity Act (MCA) 2005 was adopted with effect from 2007 and it is likely that discussion surrounding a case such as this will focus on a working knowledge of this document. Please note that the MCA 2005 is only applicable in England and Wales. Scotland uses the Adults with Incapacity (Scotland) Act 2000 and in Northern Ireland there is no equivalent legislation, with situations being resolved by common law.
- The key principles highlighted in the MCA are:
  - a person must be **assumed to have capacity** unless it can be established that he does not
  - before concluding that a person lacks capacity to make a decision, **all practicable steps** must be taken to help him/her make that decision (including communicating information in a way that is understandable to him)
  - a person cannot be judged as being unable to make a decision just because he makes an **unwise or eccentric decision**
  - if a person is deemed to lack capacity, any decision made on his behalf must be in his or her **best interests**
  - if a decision is to be made on behalf of someone who lacks capacity, the method which is the **least restrictive** to the person's rights and freedom should be used to achieve the desired purpose.
- In order to establish whether a person has capacity to make a decision, he/she needs to fulfil all the following criteria:
  - **understand** the information relevant to the decision (and **believe** it applies to them)
  - **retain** the information
  - **weigh** up the information and other possibilities before coming to a conclusion
  - be able to **communicate** the decision back (this can be verbally, in writing or by any other means appropriate for the person and the decision to be made).
- Note that a person's capacity is **decision specific** and **time specific**. The patient should not be deemed to

lack capacity just because he suffers from a certain medical condition or diagnosis.
- An LPA is a provision set out by the MCA 2005. This refers to a patient conferring authority to one or more individuals who are able to make decisions on healthcare and personal welfare in the best interests of the person when he does not have the capacity to do so himself. This includes refusing life-saving treatment (although this section needs to be explicitly signed and witnessed on the form).
- An advance directive is another means by which a person can make his wishes about healthcare decisions known in the eventuality that he loses capacity. This is a document that only allows the person to refuse specific treatment or to set out specific circumstances where he would not want treatment to be offered. These decisions need to be clearly set out in writing, signed by the person and witnessed.
- Further advice should be sought from either the employing health organization's medicolegal team or one of the medical professional bodies if the clinician is unclear or uncertain about a patient's advance directive.
- Generally, advance directives are felt to be more restrictive than LPA decisions because the latter give the attorneys authority to make decisions on all aspects of the patient's health and personal welfare, including giving consent to or refusing any life-saving treatment. The former only allows refusal of treatment, and the specific circumstances where treatment is to be refused need to be anticipated by the patient, which can sometimes be difficult. If a person has both an advance directive and an LPA, the one that was signed most recently will generally be considered, provided all the criteria for its validity are met.
- The following is a summary of the other provisions and terms detailed in the MCA 2005.
  - *Court-appointed deputy*: a person who is appointed by the Court of Protection to make decisions on healthcare, personal welfare and finances on behalf of a patient. Essentially it is a similar authority to an LPA except that they do not have the power to refuse life-sustaining treatment.
  - *Court of Protection*: this court has jurisdiction with regard to the whole MCA. It can make decisions on behalf of persons who do not have the capacity or it can appoint deputies to do so. This will also be involved in complex cases where a decision cannot be made regarding a patient's capacity or which course of action is in his best interests. If there is disagreement between an LPA's views and

those of the healthcare professionals or other family members/friends, the case may be referred to this court.

- *Office of the Public Guardian*: this department is responsible for registering and monitoring the operations of LPAs and court-appointed deputies.
- *Independent mental capacity advocate (IMCA)*: this is someone who is appointed to support a person who lacks capacity and who does not have any family or friends to speak for them. IMCAs can express opinions on the person's wishes, beliefs and values which can help the decision-making process. Note that this only applies to decisions concerning serious medical treatment or housing where it is provided by the NHS or local authority.

> **Comments on the case**
>
> The Mental Capacity Act 2005 has provided some very useful guidance for managing patients with possible impairment of their mental capacity and all doctors should have a working knowledge of the principles highlighted in it. Aspects of this subject are popular topics of discussion in Station 4 of the PACES exam.

Further reading

Department of Constitutional Affairs, Department of Health, Public Guardianship Office and Welsh Assembly Government. *Mental Capacity Act 2005 – summary*. London: Stationery Office, 2007.

Office of the Public Guardian. *Making decisions: a guide for people who work in health and social care*. London: Office of the Public Guardian, 2009.

Case 39 | Healthcare decisions for a patient who lacks mental capacity

Candidate information

You are the medical doctor on an elderly care ward.

Please read this summary and then continue with the consultation.

Re: Mr George Andrews, aged 64 years

Mr George Andrews has secondary progressive multiple sclerosis (MS) with severe spasticity, ataxia and little use of his limbs. He also has associated cognitive impairment with virtually incomprehensible speech although he can sometimes understand what is being said to him. He lives in a nursing home, can transfer out of bed with two helpers and needs assistance with feeding, washing and dressing. He was admitted to hospital 5 days ago with a right basal pneumonia, which is being treated with antibiotics. This was diagnosed as aspiration pneumonia because his carers mentioned that he often chokes on his food during feeding. His routine blood tests show an albumin of 28 g/L suggestive of poor nutrition. A speech therapy assessment has shown poor co-ordination of his swallowing with aspiration of fluids. A nasogastric tube was tried three times but Mr Andrews was not able to tolerate them and kept pulling them out. During the ward round this morning, your consultant felt that a more permanent method of feeding should be established and has asked you to put the patient on the list for a percutaneous endoscopic gastrostomy (PEG) tube. You are about to speak to Mrs Jean Andrews, his wife and next of kin, to talk about the procedure as it is felt that Mr Andrews does not have the capacity to consent to the procedure himself.

Your tasks are to: discuss with Mrs Andrews why a PEG tube is being considered and to find out her (and the patient's) views about it.

Subject/patient/relative information

Mrs Andrews is the wife of Mr George Andrews, a 64-year-old man who was diagnosed with multiple sclerosis (MS) around 20 years ago. He had infrequent relapses initially which he recovered from well but he has steadily deteriorated over the last 5 years and 2 years ago he had to be placed in a nursing home. He now has no use of his limbs and is unable to walk or even stand up unsupported. His mental abilities are also deteriorating and his speech is virtually incomprehensible although he does sometimes understand what is being said to him and he nods or shakes his head in response. His neurology specialists have told Mrs Andrews that they would not consider any specific treatment for his MS due to his rapid decline. He can still transfer out of bed with two helpers, but needs help with feeding, washing and dressing. He was admitted to hospital 5 days ago with a chest infection which is being treated with intravenous antibiotics. Although Mrs Andrews understands that her husband's swallowing is affected by his multiple sclerosis, she doesn't think that inserting a feeding tube into his stomach (known as a PEG tube) would be in his best interests. She feels that her husband 'has never been a big eater' and food is not normally a concern for him. He also mentioned to her a few years ago that he wished to be 'free from medical interventions or hospitals as far as possible and die peacefully' when his time came (although he did not actually make an advance directive or sign any other legal documents).

Thoughts and questions the patient/subject may have

- *Has it occurred to the doctors that the reason why George has been pulling the tube out of his nose may be because he doesn't want to be fed any more?*
- *What is there to stop him from trying to pull out the PEG tube and wouldn't this be even worse for him?*
- *Is there no other option available?*
- *Can I stop this procedure being done?*

Examiner information

1. Conduct of interview

- Introduce yourself to Mrs Andrews and confirm that she is Mr Andrews' wife and nominated next of kin.
- Ask her what she knows so far to get an idea of where to start your explanation – only if she seems unsure should you go on to explain that the chest infection is likely to be due to his poor swallowing caused by his severe multiple sclerosis (you may draw a diagram to illustrate how incoordination of swallowing can cause spillage of food into the trachea). Mention that his inability to swallow safely has been confirmed on testing by the speech and language therapist.
- If she tells you that she is not aware of the nasogastric tube attempts, talk to her about this.
- Explain that the team are also concerned about Mr Andrews' overall nutritional status and that there is evidence on his blood tests that he is not getting adequate nutrition orally, which is further exacerbated by his swallowing difficulties.
- Tell her that because of this, the team has discussed another option which is to supplement feeding by means of a PEG tube. Explain (with the help of a diagram) what this is in terms of the purpose, who carries out the procedure, and where, how long it takes, the invasiveness of the procedure, that the feeding will be done through a tube into the stomach through the abdominal wall rather than orally, etc. Let her know the possible complications, e.g. dis-

placement of the PEG tube and cellulitis around the wound. However, explain that the medical team feels that this would be the best solution to his swallowing problems.

- Ask her what she thinks about this and what her husband would want to do if he had the capacity to make his own decision. You should *always* check whether the patient has the capacity to understand or consent to any procedure being carried out, including using all means possible to make the information understandable to him. Stress to Mrs Andrews that you will be doing this with her husband before going ahead with a PEG insertion.
- Also ask whether Mr Andrews has made any advance directives or appointed any LPA who could make healthcare decisions on his behalf.
- She may agree to, or contest, the proposal of PEG feeding and if she disagrees, ask for her reasons and appreciate her concerns. You may need to clarify the legal situation with her at this stage, if appropriate (i.e. if an adult in the UK does not have the capacity to consent to, or refuse, a treatment, the responsibility lies with the consultant in charge to make a decision based on the patient's best interest. Family members can voice their opinion on what the patient may or may not have wanted but cannot sign the consent form or decline treatment on their relative's behalf).
- She should be encouraged to discuss the matter with other members of the family or the consultant in charge.

- Check her understanding of the issues discussed and answer any other questions she has.

2. Exploration and problem negotiation

The candidate should be able to:
- ensure that the patient's wife understands why he is having difficulty swallowing and his poor nutritional status
- discuss how this might be addressed with a PEG tube and explain what that involves, including the main risks and benefits
- elicit the wife's views on the procedure and, more importantly, what she feels the patient would have wanted
- answer any questions she raises accurately and with sensitivity.

3. Communication, ethics and the law

- In order for doctors to make healthcare decisions in partnership with the patient, the GMC advises the following principles which doctors should follow:
  - listen to the patient's **views** about their health and respect them
  - discuss with the patient details about their **medical condition**, including the diagnosis, treatment options and prognosis
  - provide them with necessary **information** for them to make decisions about their healthcare
  - **maximize** their abilities to make decisions for themselves
  - **respect** their decision(s).
- For patients who have the capacity to make their own decisions, the process is more straightforward:
  - the doctor makes an assessment of the patient's medical condition and decides on the management options available
  - using his specialist knowledge and an awareness of the patient's views, the doctor identifies investigations or treatment which will overall benefit the patient
  - the doctor puts these options forward to the patient, including details of the proposed benefits, possible risks and side-effects of the intervention. The option of no treatment should also be discussed
  - the patient then weighs up the above information and decides whether to accept any of the options. Remember that a patient who has capacity can accept or refuse any medical intervention even if the reasons for doing so may seem irrational to other people

- if asked, the doctor may recommend a particular option which they feel would be beneficial to the patient but should not put pressure on the patient to accept it.
- In the UK, **no one else can make a healthcare decision** on behalf of a patient who has capacity.
- It is good practice to ensure that, for a patient who seemingly lacks capacity, all practicable steps are taken to convey the necessary information to him and enable him to contribute to the decision-making process. This would involve using alternative tools to help the patient understand and retain the information (e.g. videos, recordings, written documentation) and, if appropriate, help from colleagues such as psychiatrists and speech and language therapists, etc.
- It is also important to bear in mind that, in some of these patients, their lack of capacity will be temporary or fluctuating. Therefore, the physician should not make a judgement based on a single assessment only.
- For a patient who has been assessed to lack capacity to make their own decisions regarding healthcare, the consultant in charge (or the most senior doctor available) has to make a decision based on the best interests of the patient and to decide on a course of action which will provide overall clinical benefit for the patient.
- Factors which the doctor needs to consider before arriving at a decision on behalf of the patient are:
  - which decision would be least restrictive to the patient's future choices
  - what the patient's values, beliefs and wishes are, as interpreted by the healthcare team
  - the opinion of the patient's family members or others close to them with regard to what they understand of the patient's values/beliefs/wishes as well as what they themselves feel would be in the patient's best interests. The doctor should bear in mind that family members **do not** have the overall final say in what decision should be made but their views should be considered seriously
  - if the patient has previously expressed any preferences such as in the form of an advance directive
  - if the patient has previously nominated someone else to make a decision on their behalf such as an LPA. Once again, the doctor should take the LPA's view very seriously but does not have to abide by it if he does not believe it to be in the patient's best interests. In situations of dispute, a second opinion from another senior doctor or the Court of Protection should be sought (see Case 38 for

more detailed discussion about the Mental Capacity Act 2005 and LPAs).

Comments on the case

This is not an uncommon case where there is a discrepancy between the medical team and family members with regard to the treatment of a patient in his/her best interests. It is important to listen to and then take relatives' views very seriously (remember that they know the patient far better than you ever will). However, while we should be respectful of family views, our obligation and moral responsibility remain to the patient if treatment (or non-treatment) is thought to be in their best interest from a medical point of view.

Further reading

General Medical Council. *Consent: patients and doctors making decisions together*. London: General Medical Council, 2008.

Stroud M, Duncan H, Nightingale J. Guidelines for enteral feeding in adult hospital patients. *Gut* 2003;52(Suppl VII);vii1–vii12.

Case 40 | Care of the vulnerable adult

Candidate information

You are the doctor in a medical admissions unit.
Please read this summary and then continue with the consultation.

Re: Stacey Anderson, 21 years old

Stacey Anderson is a 21-year-old woman who has cerebral palsy and severe learning difficulties as a result of this. She also suffers from epilepsy due to neurological damage in childhood. She has a severe scoliosis which contributes to poor respiratory function, and to her feeding difficulties (she is currently PEG fed). She has no verbal communication but is sometimes able to respond to her father. She lives at home with her father who has been providing all care for her since her mother left the family 3 years ago, but he has been struggling to manage recently. She has been admitted to hospital today with a 3-day history of vomiting and diarrhoea. She is haemodynamically stable and her blood tests show mild dehydration which needs to be treated with intravenous fluids. However, Stacey seems to be resisting all attempts by medical and nursing staff to insert an intravenous cannula to give her the supplemental fluids.

Your tasks are to: speak to Mr Tony Anderson (Stacey's father) about the reason for Stacey's admission, the need to treat her with IV fluids and to address any other concerns he might have.

Subject/patient/relative information

Mr Tony Anderson is the father of Stacey Anderson, a 21-year-old woman who has suffered from severe cerebral palsy and learning difficulties since birth. She also has epilepsy due to brain damage and is on tablets for this. She cannot talk but is sometimes able to respond to her family. Feeding and nutrition have always been difficult as she cannot co-ordinate her swallow properly. She has a bad curvature of her spine (known as scoliosis) which makes her breathless and causes difficulty in swallowing. For the last 2 years she has been fed 'through a tube in her stomach' (known as a PEG tube). She was brought to hospital today as she had several episodes of vomiting and diarrhoea and her part-time carer was concerned that Stacey was becoming dehydrated. Stacey has always been unsettled when admitted to hospitals, and is intolerant to needles and procedures (her PEG tube insertion 2 years ago had to be done under general anaesthesia) and her father is not keen on seeing her suffering with pain whilst the staff try to insert a needle (cannula) to give her intravenous fluids. He thinks he can manage her fluids and feed via the PEG tube and is keen to take her home as soon as her blood results are back and do not show dehydration. During the consultation, he reveals that he has been single-handedly caring for

Stacey since his ex-wife left 3 years ago but he realizes that he is not coping very well with it. Stacey is fully dependent on all care, and is only able to transfer from bed to chair when he carries her out. Mr Anderson still has his part-time job as a gas engineer and works for about 4 hours a day. During this time, Stacey is looked after at home by a private carer who only comes in for an hour or so and he has not asked for extra help. Mr Anderson does not want Stacey to go into care. A successful outcome will be the securing of his agreement for Stacey to be kept in for treatment and also to be referred to the learning disability co-ordinator and social workers.

Thoughts and questions the patient/subject may have

- *Can't you see that Stacey is in so much pain every time you try and insert the drip into her? Can you not just leave her alone?*
- *I have been looking after Stacey all these years – I think I am the best person to judge whether she needs to stay in hospital or not!*
- Ultimately, he appreciates that the doctors are trying to help him and his daughter but he will be adamant that he will not let Stacey go into care at any cost.

Examiner information

1. Conduct of interview

- Introduce yourself to Mr Anderson and establish his relationship to the patient (i.e. father, next of kin and guardian?).
- Ask him what he understands about the reason for Stacey's admission to hospital. Signpost by saying that you would like to go through this with him and discuss the management options.
- Explain in straightforward terms that Stacey's vomiting and diarrhoea are likely to be due to a 'stomach bug she may have picked up' (gastroenteritis) and that, as Mr Anderson will appreciate, her other health conditions make her more susceptible to this.
- There may be other causes for the vomiting or regurgitation of her feeds such as increasing swallowing difficulty. Although Stacey is meant to be fed only through her PEG tube (which would reduce the chances of dysphagia or regurgitation), it is important to check with her father whether there is any possibility that Stacey has been having any oral intake. You should also ask about posture as her position could equally affect her ability to swallow secretions. This needs to be done diplomatically and without confrontation and may be helped by saying something like 'I have a checklist of questions I need to ask as a matter of routine, is that OK?'. If he is offended, you can gently explain that the intention is to try to establish the most likely reason for Stacey's current problem in order for the most appropriate treatment to be offered.

- Explain to Mr Anderson that Stacey's blood tests show that she is dehydrated (presumably due to the diarrhoea and vomiting) which requires treatment with intravenous (IV) fluids. As he will understand, the diarrhoea and vomiting could affect her ability to keep down her antiepilepsy tablets.
- Check that Mr Anderson is familiar with IV medications and fluids; ask him if he needs you to explain anything or refresh his memory. Remember that it is highly unlikely that this is Stacey's first encounter with the health service.
- He will tell you that it is virtually impossible to get needles into Stacey as she always reacts violently so, although he appreciates what you are trying to do, it really isn't feasible. If he is refusing for this to be done, then try and find out his reasons for it. If his main concern is the pain that Stacey may suffer, suggest that the doctors could use a topical analgesic (e.g. Amitope cream) which can help.
- Remember that Mr Anderson does not have the right to decline treatment on behalf of his daughter when it is clinically judged to be in her best interest. However, his opinions about what his daughter may or may not want (if she had the capacity to make her own decisions) should be listened to and his concerns addressed as far as possible.
- Most family members will agree to a relatively minimal invasive intervention such as IV fluids/

medications if the reasons are explained carefully. However, if there is still a disagreement, a second opinion should be sought. If a patient is already known to the learning disability team or home care services it can often be useful to recruit their support as they will understand a parent's anxieties – this can avoid animosity.

- If Mr Anderson feels confident to bring up his difficulties with regard to caring for Stacey on his own, especially feeding issues, then allow him time to talk and listen in a non-judgemental manner. Remember that carers of people with physical and learning disabilities need plenty of support themselves and they may regard their struggles as a shortcoming.
- The candidate should realize that there are issues regarding the care of a vulnerable adult here and should not overlook this. Some of the areas causing concern may be the ability, or lack of ability, of Stacey's father to give the full care that Stacey requires, e.g. caring for her on his own without appropriate equipment or manual handling advice. His reluctance to keep her in hospital when medical treatment is required is going to be of concern to the staff.
- Tell him that the priority of the staff in the hospital is to ensure Stacey's safety and welfare, as well as to support him as the carer.
- Ask him if he has given any thought to having outside help and provide him with an opportunity to think about this for a few moments.
- If he needs your help then prompt him by asking what type of, and how much, extra help he would need, and if he knows which agencies could best help him with that.
- Explain how the hospital can help him with regard to finding this out and in making contact with the learning disability co-ordinator, social worker, and the occupational therapist before Stacey's discharge. You should make it clear that before her discharge there will be multidisciplinary meetings, which will involve him, to explore the current situation and the care that Stacey requires. This will allow the staff to plan properly for a suitable package of care when she is ready to go home again.
- Ask him if he has any questions and then arrange another appointment to come back and speak with him along with your colleagues as mentioned above.
- At the end of the consultation, remember that if you have any serious concerns regarding the safety or care of a vulnerable adult such as Stacey you should bring this up immediately with your consultant, ward manager, duty social worker and other colleagues as

appropriate. Document your concerns and all details of your meeting with the family clearly in the patient's notes.

2. Exploration and problem negotiation

The candidate should be able to:
- explain the diagnosis of gastroenteritis and the reasons for treating Stacey with intravenous antibiotics, medications and fluids
- establish, evaluate and attempt to understand Mr Anderson's views about keeping (or not keeping) his daughter in hospital for treatment
- be mindful that there may be issues with regard to the safeguarding of a vulnerable adult here and address them appropriately.

3. Communication, ethics and the law

- Discussion around the ethical aspects of this case is likely to be centred around treatment of a patient who is considered to be a vulnerable adult. Being vulnerable does not automatically mean that they are at risk – rather that there is a potential for them to be harmed either inadvertently (such as in this case) or intentionally.
- The Mental Capacity Act 2005 has useful guidance on factors to be considered when a physician has to make a decision in the best interest of a patient. Some of these principles include:
  - not making assumptions about what is best for a person based on their age or appearance
  - is there any likelihood that the patient may regain capacity in the future to be able to make a decision regarding the proposed investigation or management plan? If so, can the decision wait till then?
  - the doctor must, as far as possible, encourage the patient to participate in any decision-making process, and make provisions to enhance his/her ability to participate
  - where the decision to be made concerns life-sustaining treatment, the doctor should not be motivated by a desire to hasten the patient's death
  - when considering if a decision is in the patient's best interest, the doctor should consider the patient's wishes and feelings (including any written statements made when the patient had capacity) as well as any beliefs or values which may influence the patient's decision
  - the doctor should also consult with any family members and other persons who care for the patient or who are interested in their welfare. This includes finding out if there is anyone who has a

Lasting Power of Attorney or court-appointed deputy who is able to aid in the decision-making process.

- A vulnerable adult is someone over the age of 18 who is at risk of harm or exploitation due to their older age, a mental health problem (including dementia), a physical or learning disability or any other long-term condition.
- The harm to, or exploitation of, these individuals may come in the form of physical, sexual or psychological abuse, financial exploitation (e.g. theft, fraud, misappropriation of property, benefits, etc.), neglect or discrimination/harassment. This includes subjecting the individuals to unnecessary investigations or treatment which would not have much perceived benefit.
- Healthcare professionals have a duty to ensure that vulnerable adults are safeguarded. The Department of Health released a document in 2010 with some principles that should underpin the safeguarding of vulnerable adults:
  - *empowerment*: the vulnerable adult should be presumed to have capacity to make his own decisions until proven otherwise (earlier mentioned principles to assess a person's capacity should apply here)
  - *protection*: if the person is considered to be a vulnerable adult, one needs to consider what support or representation the individual will need in order to ensure his/her protection
  - *prevention*: preventing harm or abuse to the vulnerable adult (including neglect or other types of abuse which may occur within health services) should be the primary aim
  - *proportionality*: the response to harm and abuse should be proportional to the perceived risk of harm and be least restrictive of the person's rights and wishes
  - *partnership*: any action taken should be in partnership with the patient, those close to or caring for them and with multiagencies in the community

- *accountability*: all persons or agencies should be accountable and transparent in their role in caring for these patients.

Comments on the case

Dealing with this scenario requires tact from the candidate in being able to elicit from the father what has been happening at home with Stacey, and yet not to appear to be accusing him of caring for her incorrectly or neglecting her. The latter almost inevitably will result in him disengaging from services and a deterioration of the doctor–patient/relative relationship and loss of trust. However, one must be able to identify that there are issues with the safeguarding of vulnerable adults here and deal with them appropriately. A sense of balance is required when vulnerable patients may potentially be at risk and this can be difficult to achieve without considerable experience. To this end, all UK NHS hospital trusts will provide training in assessing and managing vulnerable adults and children and such training is regarded as compulsory in many hospital trusts. Many healthcare organizations also employ a Protection of Vulnerable Adults (POVA) nurse or equivalent.

Further reading

Department of Constitutional Affairs, Department of Health, Public Guardianship Office and Welsh Assembly Government. *Mental Capacity Act 2005 – summary*. London: Stationery Office, 2007.

Department of Health. *Safeguarding adults: the role of health service practitioners*. London: Department of Health, 2011.

Case 41 | Blood transfusion for a Jehovah's Witness

Candidate information

You are the medical doctor on-call.

Please read this summary and then continue with the consultation.

Re: Mr Ronald Harrington, aged 61

Mr Harrington is a patient with known chronic liver disease and portal hypertension due to haemochromatosis and he has been admitted from clinic because of feeling generally unwell with numerous episodes of melaena over the last 10 days. A clinic blood sample revealed a haemoglobin of 5.0 g/dL. Your consultant has asked you to cross-match him for 5 units and to put him on the endoscopy list. However, the patient tells you that he is a Jehovah's Witness and he has strong views against blood transfusions.

Your tasks are to: explain clearly the nature of the patient's present illness, explain why a blood transfusion is medically in his best interests whilst taking into account his religious views and discuss any possible alternatives to blood transfusion.

Subject/patient/relative information

Mr Ronald Harrington is a 61-year-old man who follows the Jehovah's Witness faith. He was diagnosed as having haemochromatosis 10 years ago and since then has progressed to cirrhosis with portal hypertension. During the last 10 days he has had numerous episodes of melaena although he did not call the GP or come to casualty as he knew what the outcome would be – a blood transfusion. However, he did keep the outpatient appointment today. The consultant has decided to admit him for an endoscopy for suspected oesophageal variceal bleeding. The result of his haemoglobin has come back as 5 g/dL and the biggest concern for the consultant is a possible life-threatening haemorrhage in the presence of the anaemia. Mr Harrington, however, does not wish to have a blood transfusion because of his faith and he acknowledges that death may result if he does have a massive haemorrhage. He is due to see the doctor (the candidate) with regard to his admission and he/she will be explaining the seriousness of his condition to him.

Thoughts and questions the patient/subject may have

- *I knew you would ask me about a blood transfusion – that is why I did not want to come into hospital!*
- *Why can't you respect my wish not to have a blood transfusion? It is my religious belief and I feel strongly about it!*
- *Is there any point in me having the endoscopy if I am not going to have the blood transfusion?*
- *Can I die because of this?*

Examiner information

1. Conduct of interview

- You should interview the patient with a witness and, if the patient wishes, a relative or religious adviser (Jehovah's Witnesses can provide counsellors at short notice if you apply to a local congregation).
- Explain to Mr Harrington the full nature of his present illness and that the reason for feeling unwell is because of a low blood count due to the continuous loss of blood.
- Tell the patient that the best and most efficient way to replete the haemoglobin count is through a blood transfusion.
- Ask him how he feels about a blood transfusion.
- You should tell the patient the benefits of the blood transfusion and the possible hazards if he does not agree to the course of action you recommend, i.e. that he is at risk of dying if he has a large haemorrhage. You should attempt to help the patient understand the reasons for your recommendation.
- If the patient is adamant, you should draw his attention to the clause on the consent form giving him the right to list the procedures that he does not consent to.
- You should also make a note of the precise nature of the restriction placed upon you by the patient.
- Tell him that although he is declining to accept a specific aspect of treatment, it does not take away his right to reasonable and proper care, including access to any alternative treatment, which would not normally be available to other patients.
- Whilst patients cannot 'demand' treatments (see R (Burke) v GMC and Others [2004] EWHC 1879 (Admin)) if alternatives are available, they should be considered and offered where clinically appropriate. You should discuss this with the haematology team in the first instance for advice. The Jehovah Witnesses have a great deal of knowledge about alternative therapies and many areas have Hospital Liaison Committees who work well with clinicians who are receptive to different ways of thinking and working.
- The patient may refuse treatment when he needs it, either in person or through an advance directive, e.g. the card carried by a Jehovah's Witness. This is the individuals right (see Human Rights Act [1998] 1998 c. 42 and Mental Capacity Act [2005] 2005 c. 9)

- Questions occasionally arise about whether the patient's refusal to accept treatment is free of duress from another relative. (see Re T (adult: Refusal of Treatment) [1992] 4 All ER 649). In these circumstances, consent or refusal could not be said to be voluntary.
- Document all that has been discussed and discuss the case with your consultant. You may want to speak to your defence union for medico-legal advice.

2. Exploration and problem negotiation

The candidate should be able to:

- express the reasons for the patient's present illness and explain that a further large GI haemorrhage, in the presence of such a low haemoglobin count, may be life-threatening
- explore the patient's religious beliefs with respect
- explain where the patient stands legally if he declines a blood transfusion.

3. Communication, ethics and the law

- The courts have ruled that a mentally competent adult has an absolute right to refuse to consent to medical treatment for any reason, rational or irrational, or for no reason at all, even where the decision may lead to his own death. A competent adult has this right even if others, including doctors, believe that the refusal is neither reasonable nor in his best interests.
- Despite the difficulties caused by such restrictions, a doctor's legal and ethical responsibilities towards a patient do not change. Such restrictions do not relieve a doctor of the duty to provide other essential treatment. A refusal to treat the patient would only be acceptable if this posed no additional risk to the patient and a colleague was available to take over the patient's care.
- However, Jehovah's Witnesses' religious understanding does not absolutely prohibit the use of components such as albumin, immunoglobulins and haemophilia preparations, and each Witness may decide individually if he wishes to accept these.
- Witnesses believe that blood removed from the body should be disposed of, so they do not accept autotransfusion of predeposited blood. Techniques for intraoperative collection or haemodilution that involve blood storage are objectionable to them. However, some Witnesses permit the use of dialysis and heart-lung equipment (non-blood prime) as well

as intraoperative salvage where the extracorporeal circulation is uninterrupted; the physician should consult with the individual patient as to what his conscience dictates. Under ideal protection of medical confidentiality, decisions on blood transfusion made by a patient who is a Jehovah's Witness would be known only to the patient and the medical team and not to the congregation. This means that the patient would have almost full control over whether his dissociation from the religion due to his treatment decision is ever revealed to the congregation. If the patient personally believes that the decision to receive blood components, of which the church disapproves, does not violate God's commandment, as some dissident Witnesses do, then he could remain silent about the decision and continue his membership provided medical confidentiality is fully protected. Under the previous policy, any suspicion of receiving blood would prompt a judicial committee which could elicit an involuntary confession from the patient and result in his expulsion from the fellowship.

Comments on the case

A Jehovah's Witness declining a blood transfusion can cause a real ethical dilemma and awareness of the patient's rights in the absence of incapacity must be realized. Support from the consultant and one's defence union is vital. The candidate will be expected to discuss the other possible treatment options such as recombinant erythropoietin, intravenous iron infusion and nutritional support, e.g. folate and vitamin B12.

Case 42 | Eligibility for major surgery

Candidate information
You are the cardiology doctor.
Please read this summary and then continue with the consultation.

Re: Mr Lawrence Boon, aged 74

Mr Boon had a non-ST elevation MI 6 months ago and a subsequent coronary angiogram revealed three-vessel disease, particularly at the distal ends of the arteries. The cardiologist decided that there was no distinct artery amenable to grafting or stenting and so a decision for optimum medical therapy was made at the recent cardiology/cardiac surgery combined meeting. Mr Boon is relatively fit apart from the angina. He smokes 20 cigarettes a day and does not intend to give up. The smoking habit was also an issue raised at the meeting. You are about to see Mr Boon in clinic to discuss the decisions made. He is keen to undergo bypass surgery to relieve his symptoms of persistent angina. His recent medication includes aspirin 75 mg od, simvastatin 20 mg, atenolol 50 mg and Imdur (isosorbide mononitrate) 60 mg od.

Your tasks are to: explain the decisions made regarding the bypass surgery and address the disappointment that he will have.

Subject/patient/relative information
Mr Boon is a 74-year-old retired salesman who had a non-ST elevation MI 6 months ago. Since then, he has continued to have angina which may come on after walking 100 yards on the flat. He does not have any rest pain. An angiogram done at the time of his MI confirmed three-vessel disease particularly in the distal areas but no vessel was amenable for grafting or stenting. At a recent joint cardiology/cardiac surgery meeting, it was felt that optimum medical therapy should be the main management for him. Mr Boon is relatively fit apart from the angina and has been told that a decision will be made regarding the possibility of an operation. He is keen to have the operation as he feels a graft will cure all his cardiac ailments. He has been a heavy smoker for many years and does not intend to give up. He feels very strongly about the prejudice medical staff have against smokers and if he is told he is unsuitable for a bypass graft, he has no doubt that the main reason would be his smoking.

Thoughts and questions the patient/subject may have
- *The consultant told me previously that an operation would be the only way to sort my heart out – why have you changed your mind now?*
- *Are you denying me the treatment because I am a smoker? That is downright prejudice!*
- *Surely you have to do something to help me – I can barely walk 100 yards now!*

Examiner information

1. Conduct of interview

- Introduce yourself to Mr Boon.
- Ask what has been discussed with him so far.
- Explain the main reason for the consultation.
- Convey to him that the surgical team feels that bypass grafting would not be technically possible.
- Explain the reasons, i.e. none of the vessels were amenable for bypass grafting or stenting.
- Listen to Mr Boon and appreciate how he feels about it. He may challenge you by asking if it was the smoking that influenced the decision.
- Explain that the decision is made by numerous experts in the meeting based on technical grounds. Any decision made by the team is in the best interests of the patient.
- Address Mr Boon's challenge by saying that although smoking does affect post-bypass prognosis, this did not influence the decision on the bypass grafting.
- Tell him the plan of management for his angina, explaining that optimizing the medical treatment is the main treatment objective.
- Ask how his angina is at present and go through the list of medications he is on with a view to increasing the doses.
- Address the issue of smoking cessation.
- Address any persisting grievances.

2. Exploration and problem negotiation

The candidate should be able to:

- ascertain what has been explained to him before
- discuss the decision made by the cardiac teams with an explanation of their reasons

- address any concerns and grievances expressed by the patient
- convey a plan of management for the patient with the aim of optimizing his medical therapy.

3. Communication, ethics and the law

- The patient is concerned that he has been denied surgery because of lifestyle issues and that he has been discriminated against because of his smoking habit.
- While it should be explained that discrimination on such issues is unacceptable, it is still important to make the patient aware of the deleterious effect of continued smoking when he already has significant coronary heart disease.
- If surgery was possible, bypass grafting cannot be denied because of lifestyle, age, gender, income and religion ('*The NHS – our commitment to you*': the new NHS charter).

Comments on the case

It is not uncommon for physicians to be faced with a situation where a patient is being denied treatment for some reason, e.g. unsuitability (e.g. cancer resection), poor outcome of surgery (e.g. unfit for surgery), lack of funds (e.g. certain chemotherapy regimens) or lack of expertise (specific specialized surgical procedures, e.g. multiorgan transplantation). The skill of addressing the patient's disappointment and anger will be thoroughly tested here.

Case 43 | Postponement of an investigation

Candidate information

You are the medical doctor in a respiratory team.

Please read this summary and then continue with the consultation.

Re: Mr Malcolm Hatton, aged 69

Mr Hatton has a solitary, left-sided peripheral lung shadow of unknown cause. He has smoked in the past and the consultant is keen to rule out a neoplastic lesion. He has come to the day unit today to have a fine needle percutaneous lung biopsy performed by the consultant radiologist. He is, however, on warfarin for a deep vein thrombosis (DVT) diagnosed 6 weeks ago and, at the last clinic appointment, he was told by the consultant to stop his warfarin for 48 h, have the clotting checked on the day of the biopsy and only proceed if the international normalized ratio (INR) was less than 1.5. Normally he takes 4 mg of warfarin a day and his INR has been steady at 2.8. Unfortunately, he has not stopped his warfarin (because the instructions by the consultant were not clear) and the radiologist has refused to proceed with the biopsy.

Your tasks are to: explain that it would be unsafe for him to have his biopsy carried out today and to come to some compromise.

Subject/patient/relative information

Mr Malcolm Hatton is a 69-year-old man with a solitary left-sided peripheral lung shadow of unknown cause. As he has smoked in the past, the consultant physician is keen to rule out a neoplastic lesion by having him undergo a fine needle percutaneous lung biopsy. Mr Hatton was diagnosed as having a DVT 6 weeks ago and was started on warfarin. At the last outpatient clinic, the consultant asked him to stop his warfarin for 48 h before the biopsy, come to the day unit and have his INR checked and, if this was less than 1.5, then he would be able to have the biopsy. Unfortunately, Mr Hatton has not stopped his warfarin and the radiologist has refused to carry out the biopsy. Mr Hatton is unhappy that the biopsy has now been postponed. He is unsure why it was necessary to stop the warfarin, and he is worried that the lung shadow might be a cancer. He is, therefore, concerned that he may have to wait too long for another biopsy appointment. He is about to see the medical doctor (the candidate) for an explanation. After the consultation, Mr Hatton decides to accept the reasons for the postponement.

Thoughts and questions the patient/subject may have

* *Why did the consultant not tell me properly what I had to do with regard to stopping the warfarin?*

- *If it was that important he should have given me some written instructions or rung me a couple of days ago to remind me.*
- *How long is my procedure going to be postponed for now?*
- *What if this shadow is something nasty? I want to know what is going on sooner rather than later.*

Examiner information

1. Conduct of interview

- Introduce yourself and say that you are sorry that the radiologist has declined to carry out the biopsy.
- Allow him to express his reasons for his unhappiness.
- Ask why he did not stop the warfarin (instructions not clear, fear of developing another DVT, forgetfulness).
- Explain the reasons for the postponement, with emphasis on the risk of bleeding if the biopsy is carried out whilst on warfarin.
- Explain that the warfarin must be stopped for at least 48 h before the procedure to allow its effect to wear off. Say that there is only a minimal risk of developing DVT if the warfarin is stopped for 48 h. Say that usually an INR would be checked before the biopsy to ensure that the blood is not too thin.
- He tells you that he is aware that he might have cancer and he does not want to wait too long for the next biopsy appointment.
- Say that the consultant is unsure if the lung shadow is a cancer or not, hence the reason for the biopsy. Appreciate his concerns and say that you will speak to the consultant radiologist straight away to book another appointment at the earliest possible time. Say to Mr Hatton that you will give him the date before he leaves.
- Again apologize for the inconvenience and ask if he has any other queries or grievances about the postponement of the biopsy.
- Ask how he got here; if he came by ambulance, say you will let the ambulance desk know that he will be going home soon.

- Let your consultant and the histology department know of the postponement and rearrange the next outpatient appointment to fit around the rearranged biopsy.

2. Exploration and problem negotiation

The candidate should be able to:

- understand the frustration felt by the patient, i.e. that the procedure is being delayed when he might have cancer
- tell the patient that there is a safety issue regarding having a lung biopsy with concomitant warfarin therapy
- reassure the patient and arrange another biopsy appointment soon.

3. Communication, ethics and the law

The physician should not undertake a procedure if there is a safety issue. Although the patient may show his frustration towards the doctor, the physician is advised to inform him clearly of the reasons for the postponement and to go ahead with delaying the biopsy.

Comments on the case

This case tests the negotiating ability of the candidate. Many scenarios occur where decisions, such as postponement of procedures, must be made in the best interest of the patient, despite the resulting wrath. It is important to explain clearly and fully the reasons for the postponement.

Case 44 | Clinical error in drug administration

Candidate information

You are the medical doctor on-call.

Please read this summary and then continue with the consultation.

Re: Mrs Irene Singleton, aged 79

Mrs Singleton was admitted from a nursing home earlier today with a history of reduced activity and a cough. A chest X-ray revealed a left lower lobe pneumonia. One of the carers relayed a message to the casualty triage nurse that Mrs Singleton is allergic to penicillin. Unfortunately, due to various breakdowns in the communication pathway, this message was not passed on to you. The GP letter had no mention of the allergy and inadvertently intravenous amoxicillin 1 g (first dose) was prescribed and given by yourself. As a result, Mrs Singleton developed a rash and vomiting which was then treated with intravenous chlorpheniramine, hydrocortisone and metoclopramide. Mrs Singleton remains rather delicate but the vomiting has settled. Mrs Singleton's daughter, Mrs Edwards, is upset about this incident and wants to make a complaint. You decide to speak to her first.

Your tasks are to: speak to Mrs Edwards acknowledging the mistake, listen to her grievances and explain what you will do about the incident.

Subject/patient/relative information

Mrs Irene Singleton is a 79-year-old lady who lives in a nursing home. She has dementia and over the last 3 days she has had a cough and reduced general activity. The GP came to visit and suspected pneumonia. This was confirmed on the chest X-ray in the casualty department. She was accompanied by a carer and was immediately seen by one of the triage nurses. The carer passed over the nursing details, including the known allergy to penicillin. If given penicillin, Mrs Singleton develops a rash and becomes nauseated with vomiting. The A&E department is, as ever, extremely stretched and the triage notes stating the allergy were not received by the medical doctor on-call (the candidate). As the patient was unable to give a proper history, all the doctor had was a GP's letter which did not state the allergy. The doctor, in managing the pneumonia, gave the first dose of intravenous amoxicillin 1 g (prescribed by him/her) but within 20 min Mrs Singleton came out in a rash and started vomiting. The doctor promptly realized what had happened and reacted appropriately by giving intravenous hydrocortisone, chlorpheniramine and metoclopramide and arranged observations every 15 min, checking for any deterioration. The doctor crossed off the IV amoxicillin from the chart and wrote in big capital letters in the notes and on the cover 'ALLERGIC TO PENICILLIN'. The daughter, Mrs Edwards, who arrived after the treatment was started, is angry that, although the carer had relayed the message with regard to the allergy, no one took notice and that this has led to further suffering for her mother. She wants an explanation and is prepared to make an official complaint. She is about to see the doctor (the candidate) to make her feelings known.

Thoughts and questions the patient/subject may have

- *How can such a serious mistake be made by you and your colleagues? My mother is already unwell and did not need to be put through any more suffering.*
- *What systems does the hospital have to make sure such an error does not happen to my mother or other patients in future?*
- If the candidate seems genuinely apologetic and gives an acceptable explanation/plan of action, Mrs Edwards may accept it and let the issue pass. If not, she will ask for details about how to make an official complaint.

Examiner information

1. Conduct of interview

- Provide the daughter with space and do not make her feel threatened. Ideally, in the real situation, you would have a member of the nursing staff with you.
- Introduce yourself and make sure you know who you are speaking to.
- Allow her to say what she wants without interrupting her. Do not take any criticism personally. Find out the exact nature of her complaint.
- Acknowledge her feelings with empathy. Look her in the eye as you are listening.
- Offer an apology, saying how sorry you are that this incident has occurred. The daughter will want to know how and why the penicillin was given. Explain that there was a breakdown in communication which should not have happened, that you sincerely did not know that Mrs Singleton was allergic to penicillin, and that the antibiotic had been given in good faith in the best interests of her mother (i.e. it was the best treatment and was given when you did not know she was allergic).
- Explain that you spotted the mistake as soon as symptoms appeared and that the situation was managed correctly by administering the appropriate drugs.
- Tell her what you are going to do about it. Tell her that you will bring the issue up with the consultant, that you will report this mishap as a 'critical incident' to the risk management team, who will let one of the hospital managerial staff know, and that endeavours will be made for this not to happen again, by for

example better staff awareness and reporting of drug allergies. Filling in a standard critical incident form and letting the relative know that you are going to do it will boost their confidence in the system.
- Also stress to Mrs Edwards that her mother's notes will have 'Penicillin Allergy' written on the outside in large print to minimize the chances of any similar mistakes happening in the future.
- Document everything in the notes and draw up an incident report.
- Again apologize for the error.
- Hopefully she will be a little happier and she may accept your apologies or may take this further by making a written complaint. If she does want to do this, then give her the name and address of the appropriate person she should write to.

2. Exploration and problem negotiation

The candidate should be able to:
- acknowledge that a mistake has been made
- apologize for the incident
- explain how the incident has been managed and what is going to be done about it.

3. Communication, ethics and the law

General comments

- In 1985 the Health and Safety Executive defined untoward incidents (or adverse incidents) as events that give rise to, or have the potential to produce, unexpected or unwanted effects involving the safety of patients. The definition therefore includes near misses.

- It should be made clear that an untoward incident is a serious event in which a patient, or patients, were harmed or could have been harmed; the event was unexpected; and the event would be likely to give rise to serious public concern or criticism of the service involved.
- Adverse incidents can have devastating consequences for individual patients and their families, can cause distress to the healthcare staff involved, and can undermine public confidence in the services that the NHS provides.

Content of a typical adverse incident report form (as recommended by a defence body)

There are now standardized incident reporting forms in most hospital trusts. They generally contain the following information:
- date and time of the report
- date and time of the event
- location of the event
- type of incident (e.g. clinical incident, drug error, accident, violence, faulty equipment, etc.)
- identification of the person affected
- condition of the person affected, including any actual harm or 'near miss' injury sustained
- identity of person(s) witnessing the event
- identity of person preparing report
- identity of person to whom the incident is being reported and what action has been taken
- the factual details of the adverse incident
- details of any equipment/drug/blood product/vaccine involved including the manufacturer, model and batch number where applicable.

A non-punitive reporting system

To encourage staff to report untoward incidents, they need assurances that the system will not be used for disciplinary purposes. On the contrary, it should be made clear that the system is about prevention, education and improving quality of care. The material reported is needed not for apportioning blame but to inform staff at meetings for educational purposes, to improve systems and avoid future problems. Involving practice staff in this way will lead to a more open and blame-free culture.

Legal aspects of the report form

In the context of litigation, an untoward incident report is a disclosable document. This means that, if a clinical negligence claim were to arise from the incident, the report would have to be disclosed as evidence. Concerns about this possible use of reports should not, however, be allowed to dissuade people from instituting an active and effective reporting system. It is always wise, though, to ensure that the details of an incident are confined to purely factual events and do not stray into giving opinion.

Comments on the case

Unfortunately the above case is all too common and, unless handled in the proper way, will lead to unnecessary distress for all parties involved.

Further reading

National Patient Safety Agency. *Seven steps to patient safety. An overview guide for NHS staff.* London: National Patient Safety Agency, 2004.

Case 45 | Fitness to drive

Candidate information

You are the doctor in a general medical clinic.

Please read this summary and then continue with the consultation.

> **Re: Mr Robert Wills, aged 39**
>
> Mr Wills is in clinic today after being discharged from hospital 4 weeks ago. He was admitted with a solitary fit. There were no precipitating factors and an electroencephalogram (EEG) and CT scan of the head were normal. Legally, he is barred from driving for 1 year with a medical review required before restarting driving.

Your tasks are to: determine if Mr Wills has had any more fits and discuss the issue of driving.

Subject/patient/relative information

Mr Robert Wills is a single, 39-year-old man who was admitted from casualty 4 weeks ago with a solitary fit. A CT scan and EEG were both normal. There was no particular precipitant for the fit and he does not drink alcohol. He has had no more fits since discharge and he feels well. He does not take any medication. He works for British Telecom (BT) as a maintenance technician which involves a lot of driving to visit residents who have reported a fault. When he left hospital, he was told that he must not drive for a year, but as he was feeling so well, and with the risk of losing his job, he has decided to go back to full-time work. He has not considered placement elsewhere within BT. He is about to see the medical doctor (the candidate) in the clinic who will approach him regarding the subject of driving. At the end of the consultation Mr Wills will agree to talk to the BT personnel department to discuss placement elsewhere within BT.

Thoughts and questions the patient/subject may have

- *I can't believe you doctors were serious about me not driving for a year! It seemed like the consultant just mentioned it in passing last time.*
- *But I'm feeling completely well in myself and it was only one small fit I had last time.*
- *How can I get around without driving? My livelihood depends on it!*
- *Would you be able to write a letter to my company to ask if I can work in another department? I'm afraid they will ask me to leave my job!*

Examiner information

1. Conduct of interview

- Ask how he has been since discharge. Ask if he understands why he was admitted and reassure him that the EEG and CT scan of the head were both normal. Remind him, however, that there is no doubt that he did have a fit. Find out if he has had any more fits.
- Discuss what his occupation is and whether this involves driving.

- Ask him if he is back at work and check that he is not driving (Mr Wills says he is).
- Inform him that after a solitary fit, patients are legally banned from driving for 1 year and then there has to be a medical review to determine if driving can recommence, as recommended by the Drivers Medical Unit, DVLA, Swansea (in some circumstances, the DVLA may reissue the licence 6 months after a solitary unprovoked seizure, provided the patient has had a satisfactory assessment by a neurology specialist and the CT head and EEG have come back as normal).
- Mr Wills tells you that he cannot stop driving as this is essential for his work.
- You reply by saying that it is those patients who drive for a living who are at greatest risk both to themselves and to the public at large.
- Tell him he must notify the DVLA and that he cannot drive until he fulfils the DVLA guidelines.
- He may tell you that his fit was alcohol related but say that the DVLA does not accept alcohol as an excuse for a solitary fit.
- Point out that whether he notifies the DVLA or not, his insurance policy is now invalid (this may persuade him).
- Mr Wills has a short think and tells you that he still intends to drive.
- Tell him that if he does not inform the DVLA then you are required to inform them yourself. Furthermore, you will record this advice in the notes.
- Ask him if he would be able to see his managers and ask if there is any opportunity for placement elsewhere within BT during this time of no driving. Mr Wills says he will speak to the BT management.
- Make sure you arrange to see Mr Wills again soon to reinforce the advice.

2. Exploration and problem negotiation

The candidate should be able to:
- determine if the patient has had further fits
- check whether Mr Wills is back at work and not driving
- explain to Mr Wills that legally he is banned from driving for 1 year
- inform Mr Wills of the risks and that he is required to inform the DVLA
- know the doctor's responsibilities if Mr Wills refuses to consider stopping driving.

3. Communication, ethics and the law

- The legal basis of fitness to drive lies in the Road Traffic Act 1988 and subsequent regulations including, in particular, the Motor Vehicles (Driving Licences) Regulations 1996. A **prescribed disability** is one that is a legal bar to the holding of a licence unless certain conditions are met. An example would be epilepsy.
- A **relevant disability** is any medical condition that is likely to render the person a source of danger while driving. An example would be a visual field defect. A **prospective disability** is any medical condition which, because of its progressive or intermittent nature, may cause the driver to have a prospective prescribed or relevant disability in the course of time. An example would be insulin-treated diabetes mellitus. A driver with a prospective disability may only hold a driving licence subject to a medical review every 1, 2 or 3 years, depending upon the circumstances.
- It is the duty of the licence holder or applicant to notify the DVLA of any medical condition which may affect safe driving. There are some circumstances in which the licence holder cannot, or will not, do this. Under these circumstances the GMC has issued clear guidelines. These are:
- The DVLA is legally responsible for deciding if a person is medically unfit to drive. It needs to know when holders of a driving licence have a condition which may, now or in the future, affect their safety as a driver. Therefore, where patients have such conditions, you should:
  - make sure that the patient understands that the condition may impair their ability to drive. If a patient is incapable of understanding this advice, e.g. because of dementia, you should inform the DVLA immediately
  - explain to patients that they themselves have a legal duty to inform the DVLA about the condition
  - if the patient refuses to accept the diagnosis or the effect that this condition has, or may have, on their ability to drive, you can suggest that the patient seeks a second opinion, and make appropriate arrangements for the patient to do so. You should advise the patient not to drive until the second opinion has been obtained (in this case there is no doubt about the diagnosis, i.e. a solitary fit)
  - if patients continue to drive when they are not fit to do so, you should make every reasonable effort to persuade them to stop. This may include telling their next of kin

– if you are unable to persuade a patient to stop driving or you are given, or find, evidence that the patient is continuing to drive contrary to advice then you should disclose the relevant medical information immediately, in confidence, to the medical adviser at the DVLA

– before giving information to the DVLA you should inform the patient of your decision to do so. Once the DVLA has been informed, you should also write to the patient to confirm that a disclosure has been made. Inform the GP as well (copy letter) and document all discussions accurately in the notes.

Comments on the case

This is another case where the majority of patients would react sensibly and advise the DVLA themselves and seek a possible change of placement at work. However, there will be occasions where you will be put in a tricky situation such as this and so it is vital that you should know the rules and regulations. The DVLA is very helpful by providing further information.

Other common scenarios with regard to medical conditions and driving regulations are:

the diabetic patient who has poor eyesight, is about to start insulin treatment, suffers from recurrent hypoglycaemia or hypoglycaemic unawareness; a patient with an unexplained collapse, a patient with recurrent transient ischaemic attacks, etc. The candidate is advised to have a sound working knowledge of the DVLA guidelines with regard to these.

Further reading

Drivers Medical Group, DVLA. *At a glance guide to the current medical standards of fitness to drive.* 2011. www.dft.gov.uk/dvla/medical/ataglance.aspx

www.gmc-uk.org/static/documents/content/Confidentiality_reporting_concerns_DVLA_2009.pdf

Case 46 | Limits of treatment in end-stage disease

Candidate information

You are the medical doctor on-call.

Please read this summary and then continue with the consultation.

Re: Mr Roger Barnes, aged 74

Mr Barnes has just been admitted to casualty complaining of breathlessness
and confusion. He has a long history of COPD although his past notes are not
available for any further information (including any previous arterial blood
gases). The GP's letter states that Mr Barnes is on nebulizer treatment and
smokes 30 cigarettes a day. He has been treated by the GP for a 'chest
infection' using oral erythromycin over the last 6 days. However, he has
progressively worsened and now he is drowsy and pyrexial. The chest X-ray
reveals a left lower lobe pneumonia. Arterial gases are PO_2 7.6 kPa and PCO_2
12.5 kPa. He is clearly in need of urgent intervention. You call the intensivist
who, on reading the GP's letter, feels that intubation and ventilation is
inappropriate because of his established COPD. You tell the senior nurse
looking after him that you are going to obtain more information from the
eldest son (Mr Geoff Barnes) who is waiting to see you in the visitor's room.

Your tasks are to: tell the son (Mr Geoff Barnes) how poorly his father is, get an
idea of the father's general premorbid condition and discuss whether ventilation
should be offered.

Subject/patient/relative information

Mr Roger Barnes is a 74-year-old retired welder who has a long history of COPD.
Nowadays, he rarely gets out of the house but does manage to get to the bottom of
his garden most days. He has to stop twice when going up stairs. He has a chronic
cough with sputum and still smokes over 30 cigarettes a day. He has a nebulizer
which he uses in the morning only. He also has an oxygen cylinder which he uses
on a prn basis. He is aware that he must not smoke at the same time as using the
oxygen. In addition, he takes ipratropium and salbutamol inhalers. Apart from
regular visits to the chest clinic in the centre of town, he has never been in hospital
for an exacerbation of his COPD. He has no other comorbidities such as ischaemic
heart disease. Over the last 2 weeks his symptoms have worsened; his sputum is
purulent with some haemoptysis. He was given a course of erythromycin but this
caused a gastrointestinal upset so he did not finish the course. He has deteriorated
and is now breathless at rest, drowsy and pyrexial. A chest X-ray reveals a pneumonia
but his condition is now so critical that a decision about whether to support him
with a ventilator must be taken as soon as possible. The anaesthetist has reviewed

him and feels that Mr Barnes would not be an appropriate candidate for invasive ventilation due to the high morbidity and mortality risk plus a high chance of difficulty in coming off a ventilator. The son, Mr Geoff Barnes, is the next of kin. He is due to see the medical doctor (the candidate) with regard to the issue of ventilation. The medical doctor is keen to obtain details of Mr Barnes' the previous quality of life and whether he has ever said that he does not wish to be considered for intubation and ventilation. As far as the son knows, his father seems to enjoy life very much despite his limitations and is sure he would never object to having a go at ventilation. This is a view echoed by the rest of the family.

Thoughts and questions the patient/subject may have

- *How does it matter what my father can or cannot do at home? What has that got to do with the chest infection he has now?*
- *Surely you have to give him all the treatment he needs for his chest infection . . .*
- *Will my father die if he does not get put onto this ventilator?*
- At the end of the discussion, Mr Geoff Barnes remains adamant that his father (and the rest of the family) would want all active treatment but realizes that senior doctors will need to be consulted before the decision is made.

Examiner information

1. Conduct of interview

- Introduce yourself to the son, Mr Geoff Barnes.
- Explain how poorly his father is from the pneumonia and that his previous history of COPD is contributing to his present ill health.
- Explain that his father is in a casualty bay being looked after by a senior nurse but that a decision will have to be made very quickly with regard to his management.
- Tell him that, in his present state, he may not survive and the only other option is to artificially ventilate his lungs to give them a rest and that would mean being treated in the intensive care unit (ICU).
- Get an idea of his father's normal state, i.e. exercise ability, social life, general quality of life, treatment regimens, e.g. nebulizers, home oxygen (cylinder or long-term oxygen therapy machine), previous illnesses, previous response to treatment, previous admissions to ICU and, if so, length of ventilation, difficulty in weaning off and the need for a tracheostomy.
- Explain what ventilation in the ICU involves, i.e. a tube passed into the windpipe connected to a machine which will help to rest his lungs whilst treatment is given for his pneumonia. There will be tubes in the arm and neck to give antibiotics and fluids, and sedation to overcome the discomfort of the tube.

- Tell him the risks of ventilation and ICU, i.e. further infection and sepsis, difficulty in weaning off the ventilator, delirium and sometimes death.
- Ask if his father has shown any previous objections to ICU admission and ventilation.
- How does the rest of the family feel about this?
- Ask if there are any other queries.

2. Exploration and problem negotiation

The candidate should be able to:
- obtain an idea of the extent of the patient's everyday activities
- decide on the severity of the COPD
- decide if the patient would be a candidate for ventilation or not
- discuss with the son if there are any advance views on ventilation given by the patient and family.

3. Communication, ethics and the law

- If you feel that invasive ventilation should be offered you need to speak to your next senior colleague and then the consultant. If the intensivist disagrees with the decision, get your consultant to speak to the intensivists to come to an agreed plan of action. Conflicting opinions should not be expressed in front of relatives.
- If you feel that invasive ventilation should not be offered then think to yourself, 'Have I made the right

decision or not?'. Never make such a life/death decision on your own – always speak to your seniors.

- There are guidelines that may help to decide if ventilation (invasive or non-invasive) is appropriate but remember that these are only guidelines and each patient should be assessed on an individual basis, considering his/her, and possibly the family's, opinions as well.
- The NICE Clinical Guideline 12 gives the following advice about ventilation.
  - Assess the need for ventilation using the following: age, functional status, Body Mass Index (BMI), comorbidities, previous admissions to intensive care, forced expiratory volume in 1 sec (FEV_1) value (if known).
  - Consider non-invasive ventilation (NIV) in patients who are, or will be, slow to wean from invasive ventilation.
  - Consider NIV for patients with persistent type 2 respiratory failure despite optimal medical treatment.
  - Plan what to do in the event of failure of treatment and decide on the ceiling of care (if appropriate).
- Each case must be assessed carefully. Do not be put off by the patient using home oxygen and home nebulizers. Get an idea of exactly what this means, e.g. long-term oxygen therapy versus prn cylinder or prn nebulizer versus 6× a day nebulizer.
- Obtain an idea of what 'housebound' means exactly. The patient may consider that the inability to get to the local shops equates to being housebound, when in fact he may manage to get to the bottom of the garden. If he does go to the shops, how does he do it – by car or by foot?
- Do not let misconceptions about the difficulty in weaning off a ventilator or poor outcome deny a patient ventilation unless that patient is in end-stage failure with a high premorbid arterial PCO_2.

Comments on the case

Not an easy case but very common in everyday medical practice. Most candidates have probably never appreciated the immense complexities that come with deciding whether to ventilate or not. Never allow a single person to make a 'not for ventilation' decision. There will always be a case for 'yes' and 'no'.

Further reading

National Institute for Health and Clinical Excellence. *Clinical Guideline 12. Chronic obstructive pulmonary disease. Management of chronic obstructive pulmonary disease in adults in primary or secondary care*. London: National Institute for Health and Clinical Excellence, 2010.

Case 47 | Withdrawing treatment

Candidate information

You are the medical doctor in an intensive care unit.

Please read this summary and then continue with the consultation.

Re: Mr Alfred Swallow, aged 80

Mr Swallow has been in the intensive care unit (ICU) for the last 2 weeks being treated for cardiorespiratory and renal failure after an emergency aortic aneurysm repair. Despite all active treatment, he has not improved and the surgical and ICU teams have decided to withdraw treatment. This has been agreed with the ICU sister as well. The consultant feels this should begin by tailing down the inotropes first. This, in the opinion of the consultant, will probably lead to death within an hour as Mr Swallow has been dependent on high doses of inotropes for a while. Mr Swallow is well sedated with opioids and benzodiazepines and shows no signs of distress, pain or discomfort. The ICU sister has just told you that the daughter (Mrs Wild) is waiting in the relatives' room to be briefed on the decision.

Your tasks are to: break the bad news regarding Mr Swallow's condition, explain that the ICU team feel that withdrawing treatment is in the best interests of the patient and explain how this will be done.

Subject/patient/relative information

Mrs Wild is the only daughter of Mr Swallow. Mr Swallow has been in the ICU for the last 2 weeks, since an emergency operation for a leaking aortic aneurysm. He is being treated for heart, lung and kidney failure and is on a breathing machine. However, the doctors have said over the last few days that he is not responding to the treatment. Mrs Swallow, his wife, has severe Alzheimer's disease and has been in a nursing home for over 3 years. She is not aware of Mr Swallow's present condition and Mrs Wild does not feel it would be appropriate to bring her over to the unit. Mrs Wild has been aware of her father's poor prognosis particularly with the past comorbid history (previous heart attack and emphysema) and she has noticed how her father has been deteriorating over the last 4 days. Her personal opinion is that her father will not survive this event but she is unsure about how the withdrawal of treatment would be carried out. She has no objections in principle but wants reassurance that her father will be comfortable and in no distress.

Thoughts and questions the patient/subject may have

- *Is this really the end of the road for my father?*
- *What will happen when you switch off the ventilator? Will he be in pain?*
- *Do you think I should bring my mother here before you switch off the ventilator? I'm not sure how much she will understand and seeing him like this might upset her.*

Examiner information

1. Conduct of interview

- Introduce yourself to the daughter (make sure she is the daughter). In a real situation you would have a member of the nursing staff who knows Mr Swallow with you.
- Ask her what she knows about her father's condition and what she has already been told (she will hopefully say that she knows her father remains very ill).
- Say how sorry you are that Mr Swallow remains very poorly and that, despite all efforts, he has not improved. Allow a pause for the daughter to take all this in.
- Explain that you want to share with her some thoughts about the next step. Say that despite being on active treatment, the ICU team looking after him feels his outlook is poor as he is not responding at all and that he is going to die. Then pause.
- Explain that your team feels that continuing active treatment will not achieve the desired result (i.e. restoring her father back to how he was previously) and bring in the concept of withdrawing treatment.
- Obtain an idea of who makes up the family and ask if she, or any other member of the family, has already expressed a view on this matter.
- Ask if she knows of any opinions expressed by her father when he was well as to how he would like this situation managed. Does he have any advance directives?
- Ask if there is any member of the family who is unaware of the situation who might need to be informed.
- Explain that her father is well sedated, not in pain and that he is not aware of what is happening.
- Explain that if the family are in agreement with the withdrawal of treatment, he may deteriorate quickly and die soon after. Again, reinforce the fact that he will be comfortable, in no pain and unaware of what is happening.
- Point out politely that the final decision to withdraw treatment does not lie with her or the family but with the intensive care staff, so they must not feel as if they are actively causing his death.
- Describe how the withdrawal will be undertaken, i.e. tailing down the inotropes, and give an estimate of how long Mr Swallow may survive after this (explain this is only a guess). This will at least give her an idea of how long the process will last, particularly if she has to inform family who live far away.
- Reassure the daughter that her father will be comfortable and free from pain and distress; her father's heart will probably slow down and stop and explain that the ventilator will eventually be switched off. The haemodialysis machine will also be disconnected when the inotropes are being tailed down.
- Explain that a decision is not needed right away and that she should speak to the other members of the family and that you should meet again later in the day to answer any questions she or other family members may have.
- Ask if she has any other queries now.
- Once again empathize with her and ask the ward sister if she has anything else to add to the discussion (if she is present during the consultation).

2. Exploration and problem negotiation

The candidate should be able to:

- explain in detail the patient's condition
- explain, with understanding and empathy, the reasons why the team feels that withdrawing treatment is in the best interests of the patient
- appreciate that withdrawing treatment is probably not a subject the daughter may be familiar with
- share her grief and say that withdrawing treatment is a hard and emotive decision for the staff as well
- describe how withdrawal will take place and what the process will be, with an estimate of time before death occurs.

3. Communication, ethics and the law

General considerations

- The primary goal of medicine is to benefit the patient's health with minimal harm and this should be explained to those close to them so that they can understand why treatment is given, and why a decision to withhold or withdraw further life-prolonging treatment needs to be considered.
- The approach of the doctor in these difficult and sometimes highly charged circumstances must always accord with the ethical principles of medical practice, with the interests of the patient first and foremost.

Benefits

- Benefits to the patient can result either from treatment or non-treatment, depending on the clinical context. Clearly, if there is a possibility of the patient receiving benefit from treatment then it should be continued, unless the competent patient has refused treatment at the time, or in advance of becoming incompetent. Wherever there is any doubt about this, the balance must be in the direction of treatment. Effective palliation, as distinct from life-prolonging treatment, should never be withdrawn. On the other hand, there are clinical situations where treatment is not beneficial and only prolongs suffering. There may be concern that a course of treatment, once started, may be hard to stop if found to be ineffective. This difficulty can be avoided by the construction of a management plan specifying time-limited goals, drawn up in discussion with the patient (if possible), the relatives and with the clinical team.

- Whatever decisions are taken, it is important to stress that the autonomy of the patient must be respected. In this context an advance statement, if available, would be helpful, particularly if the patient subsequently becomes incapable of consenting to a proposed course of action. However, there is no absolute right to a treatment that a responsible professional opinion considers as inappropriate.

Harm

A further ethical consideration relates to the need to do no harm (part of the Hippocratic oath). It is in this area that there is particular controversy. The bulk of opinion holds to the view that painful, invasive procedures or drugs that have unpleasant side-effects should be avoided in situations where they will confer no material benefit. However, questions remain regarding the withdrawal of measures such as tube feeding from those who are either unconscious or suffering from a persistent vegetative state with no chance of recovery, where such measures may do no more than prolong life. It has been argued that thirst distresses patients and witnessing the patient 'starving to death' when nutrition is withdrawn may certainly add to the distress of the attendants. The rule to be applied, as ever, is that the welfare of the patient comes first, so nothing should be done that could add to their discomfort without benefit.

Equity

There is a further ethical matter which, in these days of healthcare rationing, needs to be acknowledged. With regard to the allocation of treatment, whether or not it is definitive or life-prolonging, it is unethical to deny a patient access to treatment or withdraw treatment (for example in ICU) in order to make treatment available to another individual. The instance where this especially features is in regard to the elderly.

Advance statements

In relation to life-prolonging treatment, there are advantages in people recording their wishes in a formal manner while they are competent to do so. There is no requirement for doctors to obey a request for any particular treatment, but they are under an obligation to withhold or withdraw treatment if that is the competent patient's expressed desire given at the time of treatment or, if incompetent, given as a valid advance refusal, even though the doctor may disagree.

Legal aspects

There are circumstances where the issues are unclear or the decisions of the doctors are challenged. In such cases there may be recourse to the courts. A situation where this has been specifically recommended by the law is when there is a move to withdraw artificial nutrition and hydration from a patient deemed to be suffering from a persistent vegetative state. Despite all the power of the courts, the law itself still looks to authoritative medical opinion for guidance.

Comments on the case

As more and more patients are treated in the ICU, circumstances such as the above are becoming common. The candidate must have the ability to discuss these ethical issues as part of a team and this case illustrates how all angles have to be carefully covered. Never make a decision to withdraw or withhold treatment on your own; someone will challenge you!

Further reading

General Medical Council. *Treatment and care towards the end of life: good practice in decision-making*. London: General Medical Council, 2010.

Case 48 | Enrolling a patient in a clinical trial

Candidate information
You are the doctor in a cardiology clinic.
Please read this summary and then continue with the consultation.

Re: Mr Ronald Stevens, aged 65

You see Mr Stevens in your clinic. He has heart failure and you decide that he would be suitable to enter a double-blind randomized controlled trial looking at the effect of treatment 'X' against placebo. This is being carried out by your department as part of a multicentre trial. Treatment 'X' is a new anti-heart failure drug and is given in a dose of 10 mg once a day for 1 year. Previous phase I and phase II trials have only revealed rare side-effects such as a rash, ankle swelling and headaches. The endpoint is left ventricular ejection fraction as measured on the echo. Your consultant is the main supervisor for the project in your department. At present, the patient is taking furosemide and an ACE inhibitor and he should remain on these throughout the trial.

Your tasks are to: consider if Mr Stevens would like to enter the trial and counsel him for this.

Subject/patient/relative information
Mr Stevens is a 65-year-old man who has moderate left ventricular dysfunction as a consequence of ischaemic heart disease and an anterior myocardial infarction 4 years ago. At present he is reasonably well controlled on furosemide 40 mg od and an ACE inhibitor. He manages to do his usual activities of daily living quite well although he becomes more tired by the end of the day. He has never entered a clinical trial before but is willing to give it a go in the hope that it might improve his condition. His main queries are the side-effects of the new tablet, why there must be a placebo arm to the trial, what happens if he changes his mind halfway through the trial, and whether he can remain on the present medication. He is about to see the doctor (the candidate) who is to consider recruiting him into the trial on behalf of the consultant.

Thoughts and questions the patient/subject may have
- *Does joining the trial mean I will be a guinea pig for this new medication?*
- *Is there a chance this new tablet can make me feel worse? Will I get bad side-effects?*
- If the candidate has given satisfactory information about the clinical trial, Mr Stevens may tell him/her at the end of the consultation that he is keen on joining the trial but will need more time to read the information sheet carefully and speak to his family/GP.

Examiner information

1. Conduct of interview

- Introduce yourself and ask him what he understands about his condition.
- Tell him you would like to invite him to take part in a research study, explaining the aims and purpose of the study.
- Explain that he would be given either the tablet being tested or a dummy (placebo) once a day for 12 months. Which tablet he'll receive is decided at random (like tossing a coin). Explain the need for having a placebo arm, i.e. to test whether there is a benefit from the new treatment, and taking a placebo would allow a double-blinded controlled comparison which would eliminate bias in the handling and assessment of patients. Explain that neither he nor you will know what medication he has received (double-blinded). However, the information would be immediately available if required for medical reasons.
- Explain what would be measured and tell him that the advantage of taking part in the study is that his condition would be monitored by the same doctors more closely than usual. It is also possible that his condition may improve (although there is no guarantee) and it may be helpful in developing a new therapy for others with similar conditions.
- Explain the possible side-effects and reassure him that he will be regularly reviewed for this. Explain that the drug has been tested before and the side-effects are rare. He would remain on all his present medication as well.
- Explain that participation is totally voluntary and he does not have to decide now. If he decides not to take part then his regular management by the team would not be altered in any way. If he does decide to take part, he can still withdraw at any time and this would not affect the future conduct of his treatment.
- His identity in the study would be treated as strictly confidential. Records identifying him would not be made publicly available. If the results of the trial are published, his identity would remain confidential. If reference to him is made, this would only be done by using code numbers. However, in order to meet legal obligations, records identifying him may be inspected by representatives of the sponsor and could be reviewed by the registration authorities or hospital ethics committee. His general practitioner would be informed about his participation in this study.
- Explain that monitoring would include echocardiograms and blood samples.
- Explain there are other patients in other centres taking part in the study.
- Should any illness arise during or from the trial then he would be treated in the usual appropriate way.
- Tell him that he can ring you with any queries or worries that he may have and that you will provide an information sheet. If he decides to take part, he would sign a consent form which is attached to the information sheet.
- Invite him to ask any questions he has now and also after he has studied the information sheet.

2. Exploration and problem negotiation

The candidate should be able to discuss clearly and openly:

- what the study is about
- what the patient has to do
- what are the benefits of the study
- what are the discomforts of the investigations and risks (side-effects of therapy)
- the options if he does not want to take part, e.g. would the patient be treated in the usual way if he refuses to enter?
- what happens to the information obtained and the issue of confidentiality
- who else is taking part?
- what if something goes wrong, would he be treated in the appropriate way?
- who to contact for further information (usually the chief investigator or member of the local ethics committee).

3. Communication, ethics and the law

General guidelines adapted from the General Medical Council

- Research involving clinical trials of drugs or treatments and research into the causes of, or possible treatment for, a particular condition are important in increasing doctors' ability to provide effective care for present and future patients. The benefits of the research may, however, be uncertain and may not be experienced by the person participating in the research. In addition, the risk involved for participants may be difficult to identify or to assess in advance. If you carry out research involving patients or volunteers, it is particularly important that you ensure, as far as you can, that the research is not contrary to the individual's interests and that individuals understand that it is research and that the results are not predictable.

- You must ensure that anyone you ask to consider taking part in research is given the fullest possible information, presented in terms and a format that they can understand. This must include any information about possible benefits and risks, evidence that a research ethics committee has given approval and advice that they can withdraw at any time. You should ensure that individuals have the opportunity to read and consider the research information leaflet. You must allow them sufficient time to reflect on the implications of participating in the study. You must not put pressure on anyone to take part in research. You must obtain the person's consent in writing. Before starting any research, you must always obtain approval from a properly constituted research ethics committee.
- There are separate guidelines available when conducting research studies on children under the age of 18 and adults who do not have capacity to make decisions for themselves (including vulnerable adults and those in emergency situations). Such studies would usually have gone through rigorous review by a research ethics committee before being approved, so you should be aware of the recommendations from such a committee before you begin recruitment.
- According to the National Institute for Health Research (NIHR), everyone involved in the conduct of clinical research must have training to ensure they are best prepared to carry out their duties. This is laid down in the Research Governance Framework for Health and Social Care 2005, covering all research in the NHS in England, and in law for those people working on clinical trials. The principles of Good Clinical Practice (GCP) state that, 'Each individual involved in conducting a trial should be qualified by education, training and experience to perform his or her respective task(s)'.

Comments on the case

Never put pressure on a patient when enrolling into a clinical trial and be informative without using jargon. Candidates must realize that consenting to research is not just the patient 'signing on the dotted line'. Any recruiting to research done in a wayward manner can and will lead to serious consequences. You are relying on the patient's goodwill and so they deserve honesty and openness from you.

Further reading

General Medical Council. *Consent: patients and doctors making decisions together*. London: General Medical Council, 2008.

General Medical Council. *Good practice in research: consent to research*. London: General Medical Council, 2010.

http://www.crncc.nihr.ac.uk/workforce_development/ learning_and_development/gcp

Case 49 | Industrial Injuries Disablement Benefit

Candidate information

You are the medical doctor in a respiratory clinic.

Please read this summary and then continue with the consultation.

> **Re: Mr Alan Clarke, aged 74**
>
> Mr Clarke has been seeing you in clinic because of breathlessness. A chest X-ray has suggested pulmonary fibrosis with pleural thickening and plaques over both lungs. Lung function testing has confirmed reduced lung volumes and impaired diffusion. A CT scan of the thorax has confirmed interstitial lung disease with pleural thickening and plaques. All this is suggestive of asbestos lung disease. Mr Clarke, however, is unaware that he can claim Industrial Injuries Disablement Benefit.

Your tasks are to: explain the findings of the lung function tests and the CT scan, explain the diagnosis of asbestos lung disease and to explain to him how to claim Industrial Injuries Disablement Benefit.

Subject/patient/relative information

Mr Alan Clarke is a 74-year-old retired plumber who is a life-long non-smoker. He has worked for a number of firms including some work at the local hospital. He has been a plumber all his life and has been exposed to asbestos from pipe lagging/insulating material during most of his working life. He has been coming to the clinic with a 6-month history of increasing breathlessness. Investigations (chest X-ray, lung function tests and a CT scan of the thorax) have confirmed the diagnosis of asbestosis with pleural thickening due to the previous asbestos exposure. He is about to see the medical doctor (the candidate) for the results. He is unaware that compensation is available in the form of Industrial Injuries Disablement Benefit from the Department for Work and Pensions.

Thoughts and questions the patient/subject may have

- *How can all my breathing problems be due to my job? I was a plumber for over 40 years but have only been feeling unwell for the last few months.*
- *How bad are my lungs now? Can you give me any medication to make them better?*
- *How do I go about putting in the application for this Industrial Injuries Disablement Benefit? Are you sure I will get the money?*

Examiner information

1. Conduct of interview

- Introduce yourself to Mr Clarke and ask how he is.
- Start off by explaining the results of the tests. Explain that the tests suggest scarring of the lung tissue with thickening of the lining around the lung (pleural

thickening) and hardened patches (calcified plaques). Say that all this is a result of asbestos exposure.
- Ask what his occupation was and whether he has been exposed to asbestos. Take details of the length and degree of the exposure.
- Explain that unfortunately treatment is limited and that the asbestosis does tend to progress slowly.

- Reassure him that there is no evidence of lung cancer or cancer of the lining of the lungs which can occur in asbestos lung disease (mesothelioma).
- Ask if he is aware that, as he has an occupational lung disease, he is able to claim for Industrial Injuries Disablement Benefit.
- Say he should obtain a copy of, and complete, the B1 100PD form, which will enable him to claim for pre-scribed industrial disease (including pneumoconio-sis, asbestos lung disease, diffuse mesothelioma and primary lung cancer related to asbestosis). He can download this form from the Department for Work and Pensions website or contact his regional Industrial Injuries Disablement Benefit centre for a claim form.
- Once he has completed the form, he should send it back to the Industrial Injuries Disablement Benefit office who will assign a decision maker to look at his claim. The decision maker may need to contact certain people like his previous employers and doctors for more information and may ask him to have a medical examination. Following this, a deci-sion will be made about whether he is entitled to a claim or not and, if so, how much he will be paid.
- He is allowed to have this back-dated (by 3 months).
- If he disagrees with the disability verdict (i.e. feels he should receive more benefit), the patient can appeal, although only within a month of the date of the letter confirming the decision.
- Ask if he has any other questions.

2. Exploration and problem negotiation

The candidate should be able to:
- explain the findings of the results
- explain the diagnosis of asbestos lung disease
- inform the patient that he is allowed to claim benefit
- inform the patient how to go about claiming this benefit.

3. Communication, ethics and the law

- Many industrial countries have arrangements for compensation for affected workers paid by the state. In the UK, the conditions for which compensation might be awarded are mesothelioma, asbestosis, bilat-eral diffuse pleural thickening (to a thickness of 5 mm or more at any point within the area affected as meas-ured by a plain chest X-ray) and primary carcinoma of the lung where there is accompanying evidence of asbestosis and/or diffuse pleural thickening. The amount of benefit one can get depends on how badly the individual is disabled. It can be paid 15 weeks from the first day the individual was disabled by the disease, unless it is for a mesothelioma when it can be paid from the first day of disability from this disease. Other industrial diseases for which claims can be made include silicosis, byssinosis and coal-workers' pneumoconiosis.
- The patient must download the B1 100PD form from the Department for Work and Pensions website or contact his regional Industrial Injuries Disablement Benefit centre who will send a copy to him. This should be sent back to the Industrial Injuries Disable-ment Benefit office as soon as possible because any delay could mean a loss of money. Benefits cannot be paid for a period of more than 3 months before the date of the claim (except for mesothelioma).
- A medical officer will meet the patient and estimate the degree of disability which will then determine the amount of weekly benefit that can be claimed. In cases of diffuse mesothelioma due to asbestos exposure, the claimant will get a one-off lump sum payment depend-ing on his/her age when the disease was diagnosed.
- Other allowances available include the Constant Attendance Allowance for a patient who is 95% or more disabled, where the effects of the disease mean that virtually constant care and attention is needed, and Reduced Earnings Allowance which is awarded to those who first suffered from the disease 10 years ago, or cannot go back to their normal job, or cannot do another job of the same standard with similar pay. These industrial benefits do not affect other National Insurance benefits such as Incapacity Benefit or the retirement state pension.
- Patients can appeal to a tribunal within 1 month of the date of the benefit decision.
- Patients who wish to sue an employer may do so with the help of legal representation. However, as many patients will have worked for different employers, establishing responsibility for the disease by a specific employer is difficult. In many cases the previous employers no longer exist, and finally many patients are unable to meet the legal expenses.

Comments on the case

This case highlights the importance of being aware of industrial diseases and the availability of compensation. All too often, patients miss out on benefits because the doctors themselves are unaware that they exist.

Further reading

www.gov.uk/browse/benefits
www.gov.uk/industrial-injuries-disablement-benefit/ overview

Case 50 | Internet therapy

Candidate information

You are the medical doctor in clinic.

Please read this summary and then continue with the consultation.

Re: Mr Harry Webberley, aged 62

Mr Webberley regularly attends clinic for his severe asthma. He has been on high-dose corticosteroids, long-acting β-agonist inhalers and antileucotriene medication for many years. He is well-known to have multiple allergies to common allergens such as house dust mite, cat dander and pollen. He is regularly on steroids and as a result of long-term usage, he has become cushingoid. He is desperate to try anything. He is seeing you in clinic today and he tells you that he saw an advertisement on the internet regarding a new portable breathing device, which claims to cure asthma and which he has ordered from California for $65. He seems convinced that this device will cure all his asthma problems.

Your tasks are to: discuss the pros and cons of internet information technology, discuss the likelihood or not of a possible cure from this new device and remind him of the essential treatment principles of asthma.

Subject/patient/relative information

Mr Harry Webberley is a 62-year-old man who has had asthma for many years and is on maximum inhaler and antileucotriene therapy. He has been taking oral steroids on and off for many years and has now become cushingoid. He is desperate for a cure and recently saw an advertisement on the internet for a breathing device which claims to cure asthma. He has ordered one for $65 from California and is eagerly awaiting its arrival. Currently, his asthma remains troublesome with interrupted sleep and wheeze in the mornings. His peak flow rate is never above 150 L/min. He has no pets at home. He is about to see the medical doctor (the candidate) and wants an honest opinion about this device.

Thoughts and questions the patient/subject may have

- *How are you so sure this breathing machine is not going to work? There are some fantastic reviews on it that I've read!*
- *Have you got any other suggestions that might help my asthma, then?*

Examiner information

1. Conduct of interview

- Introduce yourself to Mr Webberley and ask how his asthma is at present.
- He tells you about the device he has ordered over the internet and asks your opinion.
- Tell him that the purpose of the internet should be to provide general medical information and to allow communication with societies such as the asthma

societies. However, many websites are not peer reviewed and any advertisement for a device has to be looked upon with suspicion, particularly if there has been no assessment by reputable academic groups. Also tell him that there is no control over the legitimacy of material put on websites.

- Tell him, therefore, that you doubt whether the device he has bought will be successful although there is no harm in trying (in an attempt not to disappoint him too much). Also tell him that you have not seen any randomized controlled trials using this device in asthma, explaining to him what this means.
- Remind him of the importance of allergen avoidance and anti-inflammatory therapy in the management of asthma.
- Emphasize that the basic principles of asthma control remain the same.

2. Exploration and problem negotiation

The candidate should be able to:
- listen to the patient's view on the new device he found on the internet
- tell him the pros and cons of the internet
- tell him your views on the possible success of the device
- remind him of the important principles of asthma management.

3. Communication, ethics and the law

- The internet can be a useful source of medical information but many sites are not peer reviewed. It is not unusual for patients to ask their physician about an article on the internet which claims to be genuine. Unless the website is from a reputable source, physicians must remain sceptical and they must convey this to their patients.
- Further ethical issues have arisen from the internet, particularly physicians being asked for medical advice over the internet, i.e. email, the trading of pharmaceutical drugs over the internet, and medical advertising on the internet. Below are the views held by the Medical Defence Union regarding the use of the internet.
  - *Referral between physicians.* When a physician sends an ECG, pathology slide or X-ray to a specialist, does the specialist have duty of care? If he does, the specialist must share liability if something goes wrong but generally the physician taking the advice from the specialist would assume most of the liability.
  - *Who makes a record of the consultation?* As in any doctor-to-doctor interaction, it makes sense for each doctor to make his own record. The record might take the form of a video recording of the telemedical consultation kept on disc or tape.
  - *Who is responsible for confidentiality and security of the system?* Doctors have a duty to ensure that information they obtain from patients is kept secure and is not available to those not entitled to see it. As with equipment, if doctors have doubts about the medium then they should not be using it. A patient's personal identity details should not be divulged on the internet. Any email exchange with or about the patient should only take place with the patient's full agreement and understanding that emails are potentially not a secure form of communication.
  - *An email exchange* between a doctor and one of his patients is essentially an exchange of letters electronically. If the doctor begins the exchange, he should make sure that the patient is happy to continue using the medium.
  - *Medical websites.* The purpose of a website might be to provide general medical information, to advertise a practice or to offer medical advice. The intention of the site should be clear to the reader. If the site is simply for information or education, it should clearly say so. If the site is advertising a practice, it should conform to the law and the guidance issued by the Advertising Standards Authority and the General Medical Council (in *Good Medical Practice*, May 2001).
  - *If the site offers advice,* the site might need an appropriate disclaimer. It might say, for example, that it is *not* the intention to establish a doctor–patient relationship. If this is so, it raises the question as to why the advice is being given in the first place. The usual answer is that the site is a commercial enterprise. Nevertheless, if a doctor gives personal medical advice, he establishes a duty of care and thus potential liability. The site should be as secure and confidential as possible.
  - *Selling/prescribing drugs on the internet.* Doctors who prescribe drugs on the internet may have to justify to their registration body why they are prescribing to someone they do not know, have not seen, have not examined and cannot effectively follow up. Such doctors need to ask themselves if they are serving the unknown patient's interests by prescribing and they must be prepared to justify their actions.

Comments on the case

This case demonstrates the potential ethical dilemmas faced by physicians from the internet and, as more and more patients gain access to the web, more and more will be asking for and questioning new therapies and topics that physicians may not have kept up to date with.

Case 51 | Unrelated live donor transplant

Candidate information

You are the doctor in a diabetes clinic.

Please read this summary and then continue with the consultation.

Re: Mr S. Bowman

Mr Bowman is a 42-year-old man who has type 1 diabetes mellitus and diabetic nephropathy and is now on the renal transplant list. His wife, who is genetically unrelated, has been wondering whether or not to donate one of her kidneys. She has come to see you for more advice.

Your task is to: discuss the pro and cons of live organ donation with Mrs Bowman.

Subject/patient/relative information

Mr Bowman is a 42-year-old man with a long history of type 1 diabetes mellitus. He has diabetic nephropathy and has been on the waiting list for a renal transplant for 4 years. He has not had any calls for a kidney and, despite being fairly stable on dialysis, his concerns are increasing that he may never find a donor. Mrs Bowman, for the sake of her husband, has been considering whether or not she should donate one of her kidneys as she has been reading that unrelated donations are often successful nowadays. Her concerns are about the risks to her and her husband and so she has come to see one of the specialists (the candidate) for further information.

Thoughts and questions the patient/subject may have

- *How come we haven't heard from the transplant authorities despite my husband being on the waiting list for 4 years?*
- *I'm starting to lose hope that he'll ever be given a new kidney from that waiting list.*
- *Will there be any risks to me or my husband if I give him one of my kidneys?*

Examiner information

1. Conduct of interview

- Ideally the husband and wife should both be present at the consultation.
- Ask what the husband and wife know about organ donation so that you have some idea as to what level of knowledge the counselling should be directed at.
- Explain that live organ donation has a better outcome than cadaveric donation and that matching will be assessed. Matching may not need to be perfect and it is not vital that the donor should be a close relative of the receiver.
- Explain that while the patient is on the organ waiting list, it is difficult to know when a suitable organ will be available. A non-related organ donation will take him off the list and will remove the need for continuing dialysis and will minimize his deteriorating health.
- Kidneys from living donors do not need to be transported from one site to another so the kidney is in a better condition when it is transplanted.

- Mrs Bowman will gain psychological satisfaction from helping her husband in this way.
- Although small, there are peri- and postoperative risks to organ donation and the long-term risks of living with only one kidney. There is also a small risk of developing hypertension.
- Kidney donation is a major surgical operation and requires about a week in hospital and a few weeks postoperatively to fully recover.
- The psychological impact of donating a kidney, and having only one kidney left, must be highlighted although one can live perfectly normally with one kidney.
- Explain to Mrs Bowman that she will have to undertake several preoperative assessments, including the compatibility tests which may reveal an illness that may have psychological and medical implications (such as hepatitis B).
- Explain that recuperation will mean time off work and possibly lost earnings.
- Mrs Bowman should check the implications of an organ donation with her insurance agency.
- Make sure there are no third-party interests involved.
- Relay the possible risk of the transplantation not being successful due to rejection.
- The recipient will have to be on life-long medication to prevent rejection which may increase the risk of serious infections.
- Tell them that if they decide to go ahead, both of them will be assessed formally by a transplant team.

2. Exploration and problem negotiation
The candidate should be able to:
- ascertain what the couple know already about live organ transplantation
- discuss the pros and cons of live organ transplantation
- fully inform the couple of the risks involved.

3. Communication, ethics and the law
- A donation may be obtained from a non-genetically related person provided no payment has been made or is to be made. Historically, live non-related donors of kidneys were rarely considered because of the medical difficulties involved – that is, that the kidney thus obtained has no better chance of survival as a graft than an equally tissue-matched cadaveric organ.

Advances in immunosuppression now mean that grafts which are less well tissue-matched may survive. Thus, non-genetically related individuals are now increasingly acceptable as donors.
- The Human Tissue Act 2004 is the primary legislation which governs transplantation in England, Wales and Northern Ireland and the Human Tissue Authority (HTA) is responsible for ensuring that the Act is appropriately implemented. The HTA will need to approve all transplants involving live donors after an independent assessment process. The Human Tissue Act allows for the following types of live kidney donations: directed donation (e.g. from a genetically related or non-genetic but emotionally related donor), and altruistic non-directed donation.
- Living donor kidney transplantation should only be undertaken once the following criteria have been met:
  – the risk to the donor must be low
  – the donor must be fully informed
  – the consent must be fully and freely given
  – the donor must understand that he/she is entitled to withdraw consent at any time before the operation
  – the offer of the organ must be totally voluntary and not made through inducements or rewards
  – the transplant procedure must have a good chance of a successful outcome for the recipient
  – an independent assessor must have conducted separate interviews with the donor and recipient and submitted a satisfactory report to the HTA.

Comments on the case
The candidate must understand the basic concepts of organ transplantation, particularly the advantages of live over cadaveric donation.

Further reading
Joint Working Party of the British Transplantation Society and the Renal Association. *United Kingdom guidelines for living donor kidney transplantation.* Macclesfield: British Transplantation Society, 2011. www.bts.org.uk/transplantation/standards-and-guidelines/

Case 52 | A patient desperate for a diagnosis

Candidate information

You are the doctor in a general medical clinic.

Please read this summary and then continue with the consultation.

Re: Stephanie Collins, aged 37 years

Miss Collins is a Caucasian woman who has a 4-year history of extreme lethargy, persistent muscle and joint pains and headaches, and has become prone to recurrent infections. She used to suffer with chronic abdominal pains and dysmenorrhoea. She was eventually diagnosed with endometriosis for which she has had three laparoscopic surgeries. She feels that her current symptoms have worsened since the time of her last surgery 4 years ago which was complicated by a postoperative infection and a pulmonary embolism. This all resulted in a hospital stay of nearly a month. She has been seen by a rheumatologist, a neurologist and a psychiatrist for her current symptoms, all of whom have been unable to provide her with a diagnosis or any appropriate treatment despite having had many investigations. Her GP has now referred her to you, querying the diagnosis of chronic fatigue syndrome.

Your tasks are to: explain to Miss Collins the likely diagnosis of chronic fatigue syndrome and address any other concerns she may have.

Subject/patient/relative information

Miss Stephanie Collins is a 37-year-old woman who is attending clinic today to discuss her symptoms of extreme tiredness, poor concentration and constant pains and weakness in her shoulders and legs. In fact, her symptoms are so severe that she is unable to get out of bed on some days and at other times even doing a small amount of housework leaves her 'shattered for days'. She is a single mother and lives with her 10-year-old daughter Lily (whom she is unable to fetch to and from school). Fortunately her parents live nearby because she doesn't know how she would cope without them. She feels more vulnerable to picking up infections than she used to and often has painful swollen lymph nodes in her neck. She has previously had recurrent stomach pains and painful, heavy periods since her early 20s. She was told that she has endometriosis by the gynaecologists and has had three laparoscopic surgeries for this. She feels that the most recent surgery around 4 years ago caused a flare-up of her current symptoms as it was complicated by a postoperative infection and a 'blood clot on her lung'. She had to remain in hospital for nearly a month at that time and has never really recovered properly since then. She has seen a rheumatologist and a neurologist for her symptoms and has had extensive investigations including multiple blood tests, X-rays, MRI scans and a lumbar puncture but the doctors still haven't managed to find a diagnosis. Out of desperation, she agreed to speak to a psychiatrist who also could not explain her medical symptoms but started her on antidepressants, which she reluctantly agreed to try. However, these have not improved her problems. She has come to the clinic today as she is at the end of her tether and she feels that she has been messed around enough by the doctors. She is really desperate to find out what is wrong, to start a treatment plan and begin to get better. She is aware that some of the healthcare professionals she has had contact with think that she is making it all up and is attention-seeking and this is extremely upsetting because she really doesn't want, or like, to be feeling this way. She is hoping for answers and a solution today.

Thoughts and questions the patient/subject may have

- *So what do you think is actually wrong with me?*
- *I need my life back, can you help me?*
- If the doctor (the candidate) suggests that there may not be any cause for her symptoms, she is likely to react with annoyance.

Examiner information

1. Conduct of interview

- Introduce yourself to Miss Collins and ask if anyone has accompanied her to clinic today who she might like to be present during the consultation.
- Say that her GP's letter states that she has been referred for an evaluation of her symptoms of extreme tiredness, body aches and poor concentration, etc. Check that this is also her understanding of the reason for the referral.
- Explain that you need her to talk about her symptoms and their impact on her life. Let her speak without interrupting. She may express her frustration at not having had a diagnosis so far or that other doctors are seemingly dismissive of her – listen patiently.
- Show genuine concern and empathy for her symptoms and the impact it has on her life. Use phrases like, 'I can appreciate how this has really affected your life' and 'It must be very upsetting for you especially if you're having difficulty getting out of the house or having a normal life with your daughter'. (Avoid sounding too patronizing, though.)
- Acknowledge how frustrating it must be not to have been given a satisfactory diagnosis so far and reassure her that you will do your best to try and help.
- Explain that you have been asked to go through her previous investigation results. Explain that it is necessary to be sure that there is no reversible cause for her symptoms which requires treatment. Explain that both her GP and you are leaning towards a diagnosis of chronic fatigue syndrome (also known as CFS or myalgic encephalomyelitis or ME).
- Pause for a few seconds to let her take this in.
- Ask her if she has heard of this before and what her understanding of it is. She may get upset and say that she is aware that this is a condition 'which doctors think is all in the patient's mind'.
- Reassure her that the symptoms are clearly real and briefly tell her that CFS is a syndrome which causes long-term significant tiredness and other symptoms such as muscle and joint pains, poor sleep patterns, poor memory/concentration, all of which may exist to variable degrees. Explain that the precise cause is not known but some possibilities include a viral illness or other infective trigger, a genetic susceptibility, depression or a recent traumatic life event.
- Ask her if she would be prepared to complete a CFS questionnaire and explain that this will give you more information about how severe her symptoms are and how they affect her life.
- Ask her if there is anything in particular that she is finding debilitating about her symptoms and what her priorities are at the moment.

- Explain to her that whilst there is no easy treatment to 'cure' CFS completely, there are various interventions which are proven to improve a patient's quality of life and give relief of symptoms (these include a range of approaches such as graded exercise therapy, clinical psychology management with cognitive behavioural therapy [CBT], adapting daily activities with help from occupational therapy, etc.).
- Offer to provide her with more information about these different modalities of treatment and, if she is agreeable, she will be referred on to appropriate colleagues.
- Give her some information leaflets to take away about CFS/ME and also details of websites or self-help groups she can access.
- Provide an opportunity for her to ask any other questions or discuss particular worries or concerns she may have at the moment.
- Conclude by arranging a follow-up appointment before she leaves.

2. Exploration and problem negotiation

The candidate should be able to:
- acknowledge the patient's symptoms and their impact
- explain the diagnosis of CFS/ME to her in a clear and sensitive manner
- elicit her specific concerns and address them appropriately
- convey a positive message by offering practical advice about support and medical management which will aim to help her deal with her CFS/ME and what sources of help there are for her.

3. Communication, ethics and the law

- The very nature of an illness such as CFS/ME, and the uncertainty surrounding the diagnosis, can create frustration on the part of the clinician as well as the patient. However, the patient is the person who is living with these symptoms and the impact which they have, and not being able to pinpoint a cause does not make the patient's situation any less real or valid than a patient for whom you can provide a definitive cause for their symptoms.
- Even after a diagnosis of CFS is made, there are few treatment options which have a sound evidence base. However, patients often feel relieved to receive a clear 'label' for their symptoms and, providing it is not delivered in a manner which stigmatizes, it can be a constructive development.

- The clinician can, during a consultation with a patient with CFS/ME (and other similar conditions), create a positive outcome if they demonstrate the following:
  - a genuine interest and empathy for the patient's symptoms and the impact on their life
  - an honest approach about the diagnostic or management uncertainty – there is nothing worse than giving the patient false hope in this situation
  - an up-to-date knowledge of the latest research findings or management guidelines relevant to the diagnosis, and be prepared to discuss this with the patient. This will reassure them that you are taking their problem seriously and trying to help
  - an awareness of simple, but practical, coping strategies for the patient that will help them deal with their symptoms. This empowers the patient to take responsibility for their illness and can produce very positive outcomes
  - details of self-help books or websites are handy to give to the patient. It would help if you have been through these materials yourself and are able to discuss them with the patient
  - information about self-help and support groups that are available.
- Additionally, the candidate should be able to:
  - offer information and advice about returning to employment or education (tailored to the individual's situation)
  - encourage the patient to involve their partner, family or carers in managing their condition.

Comments on the case

Managing a consultation with a patient with chronic problems such as CFS/ME, fibromyalgia, irritable bowel syndrome and so on can be difficult for some clinicians as there are no categorical diagnoses. Medically unexplained symptoms are very common presenting complaints in a general medical outpatient clinic.

It is important not to let one's own impressions, or prejudices, of the condition affect the consultation or the relationship with the patient. It is best to stick to the facts and give objective advice.

Further reading

National Institute for Health and Clinical Excellence. *Clinical Guideline 53.Chronic fatigue syndrome/myalgic encephalomyelitis (or encephalomyelopathy)*. London: National Institute for Health and Clinical Excellence, 2007.

White PD, Goldsmith KA, Johnson AL, *et al.* Comparison of adaptive pacing therapy, cognitive behaviour therapy, graded exercise therapy, and specialist medical care for chronic fatigue syndrome (PACE): a randomised trial. *Lancet* 2011; 377(9768): 823–36.

Case 53 | **A missed tumour**

Candidate information

You are the medical doctor in a neurology clinic.

Please read this summary and then continue with the consultation.

Re: Tia Giuliani, aged 45 years

Mrs Giuliani has come for her 6-month follow-up appointment after resection of her low-grade benign meningioma. She initially presented 2 years ago to her GP with headaches and he diagnosed her as having migraines. It was only after recurrent visits to her GP that, around 9 months ago, he requested a CT scan which showed a suspicious lesion at the surface of her frontal cortex. This was subsequently confirmed to be a meningioma and was completely resected by the neurosurgeons. She would like advice from the doctor today in clinic about the possibility of taking legal action against her GP, whom she feels should have picked up the diagnosis earlier.

Your tasks are to: assess Mrs Giuliani's recovery after resection of her meningioma and address her questions with regard to the delayed diagnosis by her GP.

Subject/patient/relative information

Mrs Tia Giuliani is a 45-year-old woman who lives with her husband and two teenage children. She works in the City as a chartered accountant. Two years ago she developed symptoms of recurrent headaches (initially occurring a couple of times a week) associated with nausea. These headaches did not wake her from sleep and she had no other symptoms such as weight loss, visual problems or any facial/arm/leg weakness. She made several visits to her GP (Dr R) with regard to this and was repeatedly told that it was a migraine and given some mild painkillers. These seemed to work for a few weeks but the headaches recurred not long after and became more severe and frequent. She made a number of visits to Dr R asking for further investigations which he ignored. Then, around 9 months ago, in an act of desperation, she took her legally trained sister with her. With her support and assertiveness, she convinced Dr R to carry out further investigations. A CT scan of the head was arranged soon after. This showed a suspicious mass in her brain and then an MRI of her head confirmed an early-stage brain tumour, called a meningioma. She was then referred to the neurologists and neurosurgeons urgently. An operation followed quickly and fortunately the biopsies and a repeat MRI scan 2 months later showed that the whole tumour had been removed.

Since then she has felt much better and no longer has any headaches. She has come to the neurology clinic today for her 6-month follow-up and wants to discuss with the doctor (the candidate) her intention to seek legal advice with regard to the possibility of suing her GP for negligence in his duty of care. She believes that the brain tumour would have been picked up earlier if the doctor had taken what she said seriously. She is convinced that he would not have arranged the CT scan had it not been for her persistence and the final intervention of taking her sister along with her. The surgical and nursing team at the time told her that she was lucky and that it might have been too late if her symptoms had been ignored any longer. She hopes that the doctor in clinic today (the candidate) will be prepared to provide a written statement of support to help her launch her complaint against her GP.

Thoughts and questions the patient/subject may have
- *Why didn't my GP send me for investigations 2 years ago?*
- *How long had the tumour been growing for?*
- *What would have happened if it hadn't been found when it was?*
- *Clearly he messed up – the neurology doctors and nurses said as much – what do you think?*

Examiner information

1. Conduct of interview
- Introduce yourself to Mrs Giuliani.
- Ask how she has been recovering after her surgery.
- Ask specifically about any symptoms suggestive of recurrence or incomplete resection of the tumour – e.g. persistent headaches, seizures, visual symptoms, and weakness of the face/upper or lower limbs.
- Reassure her that the neurosurgical team were confident that the tumour was removed completely and the biopsy results and MRI scan 2 months after the operation also suggested this. Therefore, it is unlikely that she will need any further treatment (e.g. radiotherapy) but she will be kept under close surveillance, i.e. having an annual MRI scan for the first 5 years.
- Give her a few moments to absorb this information and then ask her how she feels about this news.
- She will mention that she is unhappy that her GP did not pick up the diagnosis earlier and that she wants the candidate's opinion about this as she feels he failed in his duty of care and she is considering taking the matter further.
- Invite her to elaborate on the sequence of events from when she first presented to her GP with symptoms and what was done at the time.
- Remember that whether or not there may have been a delay by the GP in referring her for a scan or picking up the diagnosis, it is unprofessional to apportion blame to a colleague unless fully conversant with all the facts and the documentation. You can explain that if she chooses to seek legal advice then an expert opinion will be sought that will be able to establish if the GP failed in his duty of care.

- Explain tactfully that while you (the candidate) cannot become involved in the complaint personally, your consultant and the neurosurgeon can certainly be contacted either by the patient, or by a legal representative with a request to send information/clinic letters about her assessment in the hospital and the diagnosis if requested by those investigating the complaint.
- Take the opportunity to suggest to her that she may find it beneficial in the long run to consider going through the formal complaints process as a first step – as solicitors most often will do this before assessing the case for liability and explain that taking this route will not affect her right to pursue legal action at a later date.
- Advise her that the first step in this process would be to write a formal letter of complaint addressed to the practice manager at her GP surgery with details of what had happened previously. There are systems in place to deal with the complaint internally within the surgery first and then at the level of the primary care trust or higher authorities if required.
- Give her the contact details of the Patient Advisory Liaison Service (PALS) who can give her more information about the NHS complaints procedure – they will probably have an office in the hospital so she may wish to go there after this consultation to make an appointment.
- Reassure her that her complaint will be taken very seriously by the relevant authorities and she would expect to receive a formal response from them usually within 28 working days.
- If she is still not satisfied with that and wishes to take legal action, tell her that she will need to consult with

a solicitor and, once again, the PALS team can give her better advice on that. In the absence of a PALS team, the local Community Health Council can advise.

- Ask if she has any further questions and, if not, close the consultation. Ensure that she has a follow-up appointment in the clinic.

2. Exploration and problem negotiation

The candidate should be able to:

- assess the patient's recovery post resection of an intracranial tumour, looking out particularly for symptoms and signs of any recurrence
- carefully listen to her concerns regarding the delay in diagnosis and try to tease out the facts from the opinions
- give the patient factual and objective advice about how she can take her complaint further if she wishes to whilst demonstrating professionalism towards other medical colleagues.

3. Communication, ethics and the law

- Increasingly, patients who are dissatisfied with the medical care they have received are prepared to speak up about their concerns and complain either informally or formally.
- Some patients may complain to one doctor about substandard care they received from another healthcare professional and expect the doctor to deal with it on their behalf. Such a situation needs to be handled carefully as the doctor should not apportion blame to colleagues without establishing all the facts first and should maintain professionalism at all times. However, the NHS complaints procedures have an expectation that the doctor will provide information to the patient about the process of submitting a complaint and explain where they can go for further advice. The most common reason why patients complain is to do with poor communication. So it is wise for the doctor to try and resolve the issues and concerns of the patient in a face-to-face meeting before any escalation is considered.
- People who are upset, distressed or angry need to be heard responsibly – this means carefully, with minimal interruption and without burdening the patient with the excuses or opinions of the doctor. In this way, the doctor will significantly reduce the likelihood of further escalating the annoyed person's magnified feelings and thoughts.
- Apart from being able to deal with a complaint against oneself or one's service, doctors may find themselves in a predicament where a patient wants their support in complaining against other medical or paramedical colleagues. Unfortunately, health professionals are not immune from commenting on the medical management of patients by their colleagues – sometimes in good faith when genuine cause for concern is highlighted by the patient's pathway through the system. The practice of criticizing a colleague's professionalism directly with a patient may be considered appropriate when it is clear that there is an obvious oversight or error. Supposition without establishing the facts should be approached with caution. In most cases, it is advisable to contact the colleague whose judgement is under scrutiny and discuss the case before advising the patient that an oversight or error has occurred.

- In 2009, the government introduced changes to the NHS complaints procedure. What was previously under the umbrella of the Healthcare Commission was revamped into a two-tier system:
  - local resolution, by the NHS trust or primary care trust
  - Parliamentary and Health Service Ombudsman (PHSO) – this is an independent body.
- Although most complaints will be resolved at local level, the complainant needs to be told that he has a right to a review by the PHSO if he is still not satisfied with the outcome of his complaint.
- At the local level, the complaint may be delivered either verbally or in writing. If it is given verbally, the NHS trust should put the complainant's points down in writing and a record should be provided to the complainant.
- The receipt of a complaint should be provided to the complainant in the form of an acknowledgement letter within 3 days.
- The complaints manager within the trust will then go through the case in more detail, obtain statements from the staff members involved and provide a clear and complete response to the complainant within a reasonable number of days as per trust policy (usually 28 working days).
- There are two further services that patients can access to assist them through a complaints process.
  - Patient Advice and Liaison Service (PALS): this is an independent service available in most PCTs and NHS hospital trusts. It is an independent body that can assist patients and relatives by addressing immediate concerns, arranging meetings with staff and advising them on access to other services (e.g. formal complaints procedure).

- Independent Complaints Advocacy Service (ICAS): this is also an independent body which can help patients/relatives in making their complaint or can provide ongoing support whilst it is being resolved.
- In primary care, the process of managing a complaint may be slightly different at the local level. If the patient hands his complaint in to his GP surgery, local resolution may first be attempted by the practice manager and/or the GP(s) involved.
- If this does not lead to a satisfactory outcome, the complaint may then be escalated to the PCT complaints manager.
- The other regulatory bodies are the same whether the complaint is made at primary or secondary care level.

Comments on the case

Remember that managing complaints is an important part of the service we provide and we should use it constructively to review and improve our service.

Further reading

Department of Health. *Reform of health and social care complaints: proposed changes to the legislative framework*. London: Department of Health, 2008.

Department of Health. *Listening, responding, improving: a guide to better customer care*. London: Department of Health, 2009.

Case 54 | An unhappy inpatient

Candidate information

You are the medical doctor on-call during a weekend shift.

Please read this summary and then continue with the consultation.

Re: Tanya Smithers, aged 24 years

Miss Smithers was admitted to hospital on Friday afternoon with a suspected pulmonary embolism. She was started on therapeutic Enoxaparin and was told she would have a CT scan of her chest. It is now Sunday evening and Miss Smithers feels that 'nothing has been done' since she came into hospital. Furthermore, she has been moved a total of four times since she was admitted to A&E and is presently a medical outlier on a general surgical ward. She is extremely upset about the lack of progress and lack of communication since her admission and demands to speak to the doctor on-call (the candidate) about this. Her vital observations are stable and her symptoms have almost completely resolved.

Your tasks are to: find out the reasons for Miss Smithers' concerns and address them in a suitable manner.

Subject/patient/relative information

Miss Tanya Smithers is a 24-year-old woman who is normally fit and well and not on any regular medications except for the oral contraceptive pill. She lives at home with her partner and 3-year-old son, Ryan. Her partner works shifts so Ryan's care is being shared out between him and a cousin, which is unsettling for Ryan. She came into hospital 2 days ago (Friday afternoon) with a 3-day history of shortness of breath, right-sided chest pain and a cough, productive of some yellowish sputum but with a few streaks of blood on one occasion. Following some blood tests, ECG and chest X-ray done in the casualty department, she was told that she probably had a chest infection but that a CT scan of the chest would be done to rule out a blood clot in her lung (pulmonary embolism, PE). She was started on intravenous antibiotics and an injection of 'a blood-thinning medication'. She feels better but is concerned that nothing seems to have been done since she came in. She is worried about the possibility of having a PE as she was told that her grandfather died from one a few years ago. She wants to know why she is still waiting for the CT scan to confirm or exclude this. She feels that she has been forgotten because no doctors have been to see her since she came in on Friday afternoon. She is also upset that she has been moved four times since she arrived (from A&E to a clinical assessment unit to the medical admissions unit and finally to a general surgical ward). The most recent move was at midnight today which disturbed her sleep and she is now tired. She is very angry about the above events and expects an explanation from the doctor (the candidate).

Thoughts and questions the patient/subject may have

- *I am told I might have a clot which could kill me and then nobody bothers to send me for a scan to find out!*
- *No wonder I haven't had it done yet, I have been moved so many times they probably can't find me! In fact, that could explain a lot of things . . .*

Examiner information

1. Conduct of interview

- Ideally conduct the consultation in a private room on the ward and with a nurse present, especially if it is possible the patient is going to be angry and potentially aggressive.
- Introduce yourself to Miss Smithers.
- Explain that the nurse has asked you (the candidate) to come and listen to her concerns about her care since admission and that you are going to try your best to address these now.
- Ask her for her understanding of the reason for her admission and what has been happening since. Allow her to talk and express her version of the events and her frustrations – remember that it is not an easy experience for any patient to be admitted to hospital (more so if they have never been unwell before or have young children at home).
- Remember not to come across as confrontational or defensive if she starts to raise her voice. Listen patiently first, acknowledging her fears and frustrations.
- Address each of her concerns in turn.
- Apologize for the fact that she has not been reviewed by the doctor for the last 2 days. Explain that the system is slightly different on a weekend and there are only a small number of doctors on duty who will attend to the new admissions and critically ill patients first.
- Reassure her that all patients who require frequent reviews for clinical reasons will still be seen without delay regardless of the day of the week or time of the day. There are systems in place to ensure that handovers are done between the day teams and weekend on-call doctors to highlight these patients. Moreover, the nurses who check all patients' observations every 6 h (or more often) have warning systems to identify the sick ones who require urgent review by a doctor.

- Explain that at the present time her situation is stable. However, acknowledge that she is bound to be worried especially if there is a family history of death associated with PE.
- Ask her if she would like you to go through again the suspected diagnoses given her symptoms and the plan made for her on admission. Reiterate that the most likely diagnosis was a chest infection for which she is receiving full treatment with intravenous antibiotics.
- Explain that the decision to carry out a scan of her chest was made because the senior clinician who saw her on admission felt that a blood clot on the lungs could not be clinically ruled out. However, emphasize, to reassure her, that she is already on the blood-thinning injections (low molecular weight heparin) to treat for this whilst awaiting the scan.
- Once again, explain that because of the reduced radiology service over the weekend, the earliest the scan would happen would be Monday unless it was clinically indicated to be done as an emergency.
- Apologize for the fact that this was possibly not mentioned to her on Friday as she should have been forewarned about the reduced staffing levels and services over the weekend. Promise to highlight this issue with the day team on Monday morning and also ensure that her CT scan will be requested for the next day, if possible. Reassure her that one of her team doctors will let her know as soon as possible when her scan is scheduled for.
- Also, apologize for the fact that she has had to move wards so many times since admission. It is certainly not acceptable to move a patient in the middle of the night unless there is a clinical need to do so and tell her that this will be raised immediately with the ward sister and bed manager to ensure it does not happen to her again.
- Encourage her to stay in hospital until the CT scan is done and the intravenous antibiotics are com-

pleted. Ask her if she has any concerns about her son's care.

- Ask her if she has any other concerns she wishes to talk about and then close the consultation.
- Record your discussion with her in the patient's notes and explain that you will fill in an adverse incident form with regard to the inappropriate transfer of a patient between wards out of hours.

2. Exploration and problem negotiation

The candidate should be able to:

- listen patiently to the patient's complaints and address each of them in turn to a satisfactory level
- acknowledge her distress and apologize for those elements which have compounded it
- provide an adequate explanation for the delay in the patient's review and investigation whilst reassuring her that she is still continuing to receive appropriate treatment
- handle the situation with professionalism and patience despite any anger or aggression displayed by the subject.

3. Communication, ethics and the law

- A breakdown in the doctor–patient relationship is fundamentally attributed to lack of communication and that was the reason for this patient's annoyance as well.
- In terms of inpatient care, it is not surprising that a lot of these problems arise out of hours during the night and at weekends.
- There are several reasons for this: reduced staffing levels, interruption in continuity of care, less frequent review of management plans/discharges, reduced availability of investigations, lack of good handovers, etc.
- Anticipating potential delays and difficulties and 'warning' the patient in advance can often ameliorate a significant degree of unhappiness. Regular team doctors should keep their patients (and family members) informed about their care and draw up clear management plans that incorporate what will happen over the weekends and bank holidays.
- A significant number of these conflicts or complaints can be avoided by ensuring good communication with patients.
- If a proposed investigation, procedure or consultation is likely to be delayed for whatever reason, this should be explained to the patient in advance and documented in the notes.
- Providing bullet point written information for patients can be very helpful as it ensures that they have a reminder and other colleagues can use this to check that the patient is receiving consistent messages and information.
- However, in the eventuality that the patient is still dissatisfied, some strategies you can use during the consultation are:
  - maintain eye contact. Do not adopt a defensive posture or attitude
  - make the patient feel that you have time to listen and are taking them seriously
  - apologize for any inadequacies in the care provided or lapses in communication
  - do not promise to do anything or make any arrangements that you cannot see through
  - explain their options, including the right to a second opinion, putting in a formal complaint, etc.

Comments on the case

This is not an uncommon scenario in which a patient wants to express dissatisfaction with the care received from the medical team. Being able to deal with angry or unhappy patients is an essential skill that every doctor needs to have for everyday practice (and the PACES examination).

Case 55 | Delay in investigation

Candidate information

You are the medical doctor in an outpatient clinic.

Please read this summary and then continue with the consultation.

Re: Mr Terry Palmer, aged 65

Mr Palmer presented with haemoptysis 5 weeks ago. A chest X-ray showed a right hilar mass and bronchoscopy a week later confirmed a squamous cell carcinoma in the right upper lobe bronchus. Mr Palmer is a fit man who would be able to tolerate resection. It has been 4 weeks since a staging CT scan of the thorax and upper abdomen was requested. He has not yet had any information about a date for this scan. He is naturally angry and wants to show his displeasure to you in clinic.

Your tasks are to: acknowledge the unacceptable delay and propose a plan to rectify this.

Subject/patient/relative information

Mr Terry Palmer is a fit 65-year-old smoker who was told 5 weeks ago that he had lung cancer. He was told that he needed an urgent CT scan of his chest and abdomen to enable the doctors to decide if his cancer can be removed surgically. He feels fit and ready for surgery but, 4 weeks on, he is still waiting for the CT scan. He is unimpressed and, as each day goes by, is becoming more frightened that the cancer is spreading. He feels like he is a walking time-bomb. His biggest fear is finding out that, by the time he has the scan done, it will be too late to have surgery. He has been following the recent media coverage regarding cancer patients waiting for treatment and feels extremely let down by the system. He is seeing the medical doctor (the candidate) in clinic today to express his distress and disappointment.

Thoughts and questions the patient/subject may have

- *Why is this taking so long?*
- *What are you going to do about it?*
- *At this rate it's going to be too late for me to have the operation . . .*
- *Help me – I'm frightened.*

Examiner information

1. Conduct of interview

- Introduce yourself to Mr Palmer.
- Allow him to voice his anger. Acknowledge the delay and the effect it is having on him.

- Express concern and disappointment about the delay and acknowledge that the scan is essential in planning the treatment of his cancer.
- Ask whether or not he has been offered a key contact person with whom to discuss any concerns or worries during this time. If not, ensure that this is

done in line with local practice before he leaves clinic today.

- Check his address (sometimes the wrong address is put on the request card).
- Promise to raise the situation urgently with the consultant, and speak to a radiologist whilst the patient is still in the clinic with the aim that a date can be obtained before he leaves.
- Check that his telephone number is recorded in the notes so that he can be contacted later the same day if there is a delay in speaking to a radiologist before he leaves clinic.
- If he is still unhappy with the situation, make arrangements for him to speak to your consultant. Ensuring he has a date for a very urgent scan should resolve the situation.
- However, if he is still dissatisfied and wants to take further action about the delay in having the CT scan, explain that there is a complaints process within the NHS and ask if he wants further information to be provided at this stage or after he has seen the consultant.

2. Exploration and problem negotiation

The candidate should be able to:
- listen patiently to the patient's concerns
- agree with the patient that the delay is unacceptable
- formulate a plan of action to rectify the situation
- ensure that he has a support system in place
- offer information about the complaints system.

3. Communication, ethics and the law

- This patient is frightened. He is depending on you for help. Any criticisms are not personal and must not be taken personally.
- Health professional's codes of practice enshrine the professional values of not harming patients either actively or through omission. This patient is clearly being psychologically harmed by the delay in the CT staging process.
- You must be seen to care and to take an active role in rectifying the problem; otherwise he will lose all confidence in you.

- If his cancer has progressed during the delay he would have the right to formal complaint and to consider legal redress.
- Ensure that all the facts regarding the patient's concerns are well recorded in the medical notes in case of further complaint.

Comments on the case

Unfortunately, delay in investigations is a very common scenario. All doctors must be able to sit and listen, with objectivity and compassion, to a patient's negative experience within the health system. The clinician who becomes irritated or dispassionate in this type of situation may find it helpful to stop and consider for a moment what they would think and feel if it were them or someone whom they care about in a similar situation.

Clinicians must be able to show that they care and so one must acknowledge the complaint with empathy. Listening will go a long way in allowing the patient to feel that doctors are humane and that they care about their patients as people. The doctor dealing with the complaint must provide a plan to deal with the problem/complaint. In this case, there may be a reason for the delay, e.g. request card not filled in, wrong address, patient did not receive the scan date, CT scanner broken down, no staff available to do the CT session, scan not reported, etc. Unless the doctor makes an effort to sort it out there and then, nothing will get done. You must let your consultant know, and you must speak personally face to face with the radiologist (avoid phone messages), and then ring the patient back immediately to let him know of the outcome if you are unable to sort it out in the clinic.

Case 56 | A patient wanting to self-discharge

Candidate information

You are the doctor on a general medical ward.

Please read this summary and then continue with the consultation.

Re: Miss Stella Newman, aged 19

Miss Newman was admitted 7 days ago with a stiff neck and a reduced level of consciousness. Meningitis was diagnosed and *Listeria monocytogenes* was isolated though the exact source was unknown. She has been treated with intravenous amoxicillin and the consultant microbiologist has recommended 3 weeks of intravenous therapy. Miss Newman has made an excellent recovery and is now mobilizing off the ward, usually to go for a smoke. Unfortunately, Miss Newman now wants to discharge herself. Her reasons are that she has two young children at home being looked after by her sister, she does not like the attitude of some of the nursing staff towards her, particularly about the smoking issue, and she finds hospital food unpalatable. The ward sister has tried to discuss this with her. However, as she is, in part, the object of Miss Newman's unhappiness, she has asked you to speak to her to persuade her to stay to complete the course of treatment.

Your tasks are to: ascertain why Miss Newman wants to discharge herself, discuss why it would be best to stay and offer alternatives if she refuses to stay.

Subject/patient/relative information

Miss Stella Newman, aged 19, is a single mother of two small children under 5. She was admitted 7 days ago with neck stiffness and reduced consciousness. She was told that she had meningitis, which is being treated with intravenous antibiotics. She made an excellent recovery and is now well enough to go off the ward for a smoke. She has never settled on the ward as she is worried about her two young children at home, who are being looked after by her sister. She cannot understand why she has to stay when she feels so much better. She does not like the attitude of some of the nursing staff towards her, particularly regarding her smoking. She finds them snooty and they give her the feeling that they think they are superior. The hospital food is totally unacceptable – disgusting in fact! The 'needle' for the antibiotics is particularly irritating and the nurses are useless at putting new ones in, taking at least three attempts each time it needs changing. She has had enough and now wants to discharge herself. The ward sister tried to convince her to stay but she is as bad as the rest! The ward sister has now got the medical doctor (the candidate) to come and talk to Miss Newman to try and persuade her to stay. Despite the candidate's reasoning and concern that she stays to continue intravenous antibiotics, she is still keen to go. She is happy to compromise by continuing oral antibiotics at home but at the same time appreciates that the doctor does not feel she is ready to go and so the decision to self-discharge will have to be her own responsibility.

Thoughts and questions the patient/subject may have
- *Why can't I go home? I am being bossed about like a child!*
- *I am much better and don't need the needle in my hand any more.*
- *If you give me tablets I can take them at home.*
- *Can you stop me from going?* Or, if the consultation is difficult she may say *You can't stop me from going.*

Examiner information

1. Conduct of interview
- Introduce yourself to Miss Newman and explain why you are there.
- Ask her what her concerns are and show an understanding of the problems.
- Explain why it is wise to stay – maybe she is not aware of the importance of continued intravenous antibiotics. Explain all the risks so that she is fully informed about her actions and possible consequences.
- Aim to address her grievances by suggesting some solutions, e.g. ask if it would be practical for someone to bring food in for her, suggest that someone more experienced such as yourself will put in any further cannulae and that you will speak to the nursing staff about how she perceives their attitude towards her.
- She may say she is still determined to go and, if so, remind her that she would have to take responsibility for her own care in this situation and that she will be advised to sign a formal statement outlining that she has been advised that she is taking her own discharge against medical advice.
- If she is not willing to do so, do not make a fuss but explain that you will make an entry in her notes outlining what has happened, her reasons for leaving and the advice which she has been given (this should all be documented anyway).
- If she still insists then tell her that the consultant microbiologist needs to be contacted to discuss the possibility of changing her to oral antibiotics and that it would be helpful if she would agree to wait until this has been organized.
- Ensure an early follow-up, i.e. first available clinic.

2. Exploration and problem negotiation
The candidate should be able to:
- sit down and listen to the patient's grievances, showing understanding and empathy
- respond objectively and suggest an action plan to try and make it easier for her to stay
- inform her of the clinical reasons for wanting her to remain in hospital and potential consequences
- ensure she understands that a decision to go early is her right but also will be her responsibility
- provide an alternative antibiotic regimen as a compromise.

3. Communication, ethics and the law
- Health professionals, understandably enough, worry about patients who are intent on discharging themselves against medical advice. Often these worries are articulated with subjective irritation or frustration – this is never constructive in challenging situations where sophisticated communication skills are essential!
- Carefully exploring the reasons for self-discharge against medical advice is vital in case there is a poor understanding of the medical condition, or where practical measures could be put in place which might encourage the patient to stay. Sleep deprivation is a common motivator for self-discharge but is often missed.
- Patients cannot be kept against their will, especially if they do not show signs of psychiatric illness which could impair their capacity to make a decision. It is the doctor's responsibility to inform them of the importance of staying and that the patient will be taking full responsibility for their self-discharge against the advice of the doctors. If the patient is still

keen to go, it is important at least to make a compromise, i.e. suggesting a course of oral antibiotics as continued intravenous antibiotics would not be feasible after discharge.

- Patients choosing the option of self-discharge should not be punished for doing so. If they require medication then it needs to be provided (even if this means someone collecting it from the ward later if they insist on going immediately), and if follow-up is necessary then it needs to be arranged.
- It is advisable to inform a senior colleague, and the patient's GP should be notified promptly (particularly in the case of significantly ill patients) so that if the patient falls ill again then the GP will be aware of the prior situation.
- It is also prudent to try and advise the patient about what they need to do if they feel unwell or worse when they get home.
- However, it is important to first ensure that the patient has full capacity to make these decisions regarding their own healthcare and hospital stay. Failure to do this could mean that the clinician is negligent in not providing best care for the patient.
- Situations in which it is of particular importance to assess the patient's mental state before deciding that they have the capacity to self-discharge are:
  - patients under the influence of alcohol or other drugs
  - patients admitted with acute or chronic confusional states, including delirium
  - those with a diagnosed or suspected mental health illness which could impair their decision-making capacity
  - children under the age of 16, who are not normally allowed to make self-discharge decisions without parental involvement.
- However, remember that the capacity to consent to or decline healthcare is decision specific and time

specific. One must not make assumptions about an individual's competency based on their diagnosis, age, appearance or other such attributes.

- The competent patient's autonomy in these cases outweighs the ethical imperative of the clinician to do no harm and to do good – this can be hard to accept in reality.

Comments on the case

No-smoking rules on hospital premises are entirely rational and increasingly common. However, for a stressed, nicotine-dependent patient whose liberty is restricted, this can represent a real contention.

Patients who feel unable to accept rational compromise with medical staff on any issue are naturally going to elicit non-comprehension or frustration in clinicians who are, after all, trying to do their best for the patient.

Sadly, at times, physicians will find that despite all the considerations provided by them, some patients will not comply with any medical advice and so when it comes to leaving against medical advice, it is not surprising that any persuasive dialogue breaks down. In this type of situation, it is important for the physician to remain calm and objective to ensure that they fully inform the patient of the reasons why it is best to stay, and that self-discharge is taken against medical advice, so that the patient can make an informed autonomous decision and take responsibility for their action.

Case 57 | **Major incident exercise**

Candidate information

You are the medical registrar on-call.

Please read this summary and then continue with the consultation.

Re: Major incident exercise dry-run

As the medical registrar on-call during the weekend, you are part of the team participating in a mock emergency training exercise in your hospital. The scenario is a suspected terrorist attack in the region involving possible nuclear substances and your hospital has been selected as one of the centres to receive 'real victims' (played by staff and actors). It will require all hospital staff who are participating to wear personal protective equipment (including helmets and bodysuits) and ensure that 'casualties' undergo decontamination before being seen in specially cordoned-off areas in casualty. The purpose is to test your hospital's ability to deal with the casualties of a major incident involving chemical, biological, radiological or nuclear substances whilst causing minimal interruption to the running of the other services in the hospital. As you are likely to be busy for a couple of hours with this exercise, you need to organize your junior doctors to manage the medical on-call and the wards.

Your tasks are to: speak to your medical CT1 (junior doctor) about what this major incident exercise involves and arrange with him/her for the medical patients to be covered whilst you are occupied with this exercise.

Subject/patient/relative information

The hospital is participating in a mock emergency training exercise this weekend. The scenario is a suspected terrorist attack in the region involving possible nuclear substances and your hospital will be one of the centres receiving 'real victims' (played by staff and actors). As a result, areas of the A&E department will be cordoned off and the staff participating in the exercise will be required to wear special protective equipment (including bodysuits, helmets and eye and ear protection). The medical registrar on-call (the candidate) will be involved in the exercise for a few hours and therefore will be relying on the medical CT1 to manage the on-call and the wards. The CT1 doctor (the subject) is a junior doctor who will need to 'act up' to cover the team's responsibilities to its patients while the registrar is tied up with this major incident exercise. The CT1 doctor would also like to ask the registrar (the candidate) more about this major incident exercise because he has never come across one before.

Thoughts and questions the patient/subject may have

- *What do you want me to do?*
- *Why is the major incident exercise being carried out?*
- *What will it involve/how long will it go on for?*
- *What is the role of the registrar?*

Examiner information

1. Conduct of interview

- Start by saying that you would like to discuss the major incident exercise that is due to take place in the hospital this weekend and how this may affect the medical team on-call.
- The junior doctor may ask to know more about what the whole exercise consists of and how it works.
- Tell him/her that due to the high level of security alert in the UK with regard to global terrorism, increased vigilance and adequate preparation are required on everyone's part.
- Ensuring that the health services are prepared for dealing with a terrorist attack forms part of this. Therefore, from time to time different parts of the country hold major incident exercises such as this and the local hospitals/staff will be expected to participate too. The objective is to ensure that the hospitals test out their vital procedures and systems in the face of such an attack and that the hospital staff are adequately trained in them.
- The 'terrorist attack' will take place somewhere in the local area and your hospital will be receiving the 'victims'.
- The organizers do not usually reveal the details of the 'attack' until the end so as to simulate a situation as true to life as possible for the participants and emergency services staff (including police, fire services, ambulance crew and hospital staff). However, it is likely to be a situation where chemical, biological, nuclear, radiological or other hazardous materials are released. In some situations, the 'incident' might be a plane/train/multi-vehicle crash, bomb blast or natural disaster.
- Once the 'victims' arrive at the hospital, they may need to be decontaminated in special tents outside, then triaged based on the extent of their injuries and sent to the most appropriate place.
- All this should be done with minimal disruption to the running of the hospital and the care of the other patients – this needs to be stressed to the junior doctor.
- Tell him/her that there will be staff walking around in bodysuits and masks and the hospital may seem chaotic for a while. However, it is important that all patients and visitors are reassured that this is only a training exercise and there is nothing to worry about and the junior doctor has a responsibility to help with this reassurance.
- As the medical registrar on-call, you will be required to assist in the operation for a few hours and therefore will be relying on the CT1 to manage the medical team on-call (which will probably include two or three more junior doctors, including FY1s).
- Check that he/she is happy to do this.
- Tell him/her that you are still contactable for emergencies and you must ensure that you leave your bleep number with him/her. Also say that you will be informing the medical consultant on-call about this exercise as well.
- Make sure you tell him/her what time you expect to finish with the exercise and return to normal duty.
- Ask if he/she has any other questions.

2. Exploration and problem negotiation

The candidate must be able to:

- explain the purpose of a major incident exercise and the role of the hospital/health service
- describe in brief the process of the major incident exercise and what staff/patients/visitors might expect to notice around the hospital
- organize the junior doctors so that there is minimal disruption to the work of the medical team on-call during the exercise.

3. Communication, ethics and the law

- A major incident is defined as 'an event which threatens to cause serious damage to human welfare, the environment or to the security of the UK'.
- With regard to the health services, such a major incident is likely to result in more casualties than can be easily coped with by local hospitals, ambulance services and primary care organizations.
- All NHS organizations are required to have systems in place.
- A hospital has several key roles to play during a major incident:
  - to provide urgent medical care and advice to casualties
  - to liaise with the ambulance services, other regional hospitals and healthcare providers to manage the influx of victims
  - to communicate effectively with the casualties, their families, staff members and the media about the impact of the incident
  - to ensure that the care of existing patients, and the running of the hospital, continues during the exercise.
- All NHS organizations are required to have the following systems in place to ensure that their major incident contingency plans are robust: a 'live' exercise

every 3 years; a 'table-top' exercise every year; a test of their communications process every 6 months.

- Each NHS trust will have an emergency planning co-ordinator (usually an A&E consultant or other senior clinician) who is in charge of the plans in place in the hospital to deal with a major incident. He/she will be responsible for managing these major incident training exercises, evaluating the hospital's response to it and reviewing/rewriting the plans if necessary.
- All hospitals should have action cards detailing the duties of the departments and staff involved in a major incident. It is the responsibility of the heads of the different departments to ensure that all staff in that department are familiar with these action cards.
- The main areas of the hospital which are likely to be involved in such an incident are A&E, theatres, trauma wards, ICU, laboratories, etc.
- However, staff in other clinical areas that are less likely to be directly involved need to co-operate by, for instance, loaning staff where required, speaking to family, friends and casualties with minor injuries.
- An important component of such a major incident (or training exercise) is the debriefing required in the aftermath. This will consist of a 'hot' debrief that should occur immediately after it is over, followed by a more formal one later on to fully evaluate the event and identify lessons to be learnt.

Comments on the case

This might initially seem like a daunting scenario to tackle as many junior doctors will not have had much experience with a major incident training exercise. The important thing to remember is that the candidate will not be expected to know the fine details of what happens during such an exercise. A brief overview of how the hospital will be affected by the event and the candidate's organizational and leadership skills in terms of managing the junior doctors are what the examiners will be on the lookout for. It is expected that all NHS trusts will have policies for dealing with major incidents and therefore all clinicians need to have some familiarity with these documents when they start employment at their trust.

Further reading

Department of Health. *The NHS emergency planning guidance.* London: Department of Health, 2005.

Case 58 | A struggling team of doctors

Candidate information

You are a medical doctor (CT1) working in the Department of Medicine.
Please read this summary and then continue with the consultation.

Re: Staff shortage in the Department of Medicine

There has been a significant shortage of junior doctors over the last 6 months in the Department of Medicine at your hospital. As a result, the 30-bedded ward in which you work has only been allocated one FY1 doctor instead of two and the other ST1 doctor who is on your team is a GP trainee and only works part-time. There is a registrar but she is often busy in clinic. You are worried about the potential risk that this situation poses for your patients and you have been working extra hard to cover for the lack of your team members, often only finishing a normal working day at 7pm. This working pattern has affected your training because you have not had the chance to attend outpatient clinics and have even missed a couple of Grand Rounds and mandatory training days because ward work has been so heavy. You have some suggestions about what can be done to alleviate the situation. You recognize that the current situation is increasing your stress levels and you are going to speak to your consultant, Dr Cooper, about your concerns.

Your tasks are to: speak to your consultant, Dr Cooper, about how the staffing shortage is affecting your professional and personal life and to suggest some solutions to the problem.

Subject/patient/relative information

Dr Cooper is the consultant in charge of the candidate's team. He is aware that the Department of Medicine in the hospital has been struggling with staff shortages over the last 6 months due to several reasons such as maternity leave, some doctors working part-time and prospective FY1s not passing their final exams and hence being unable to take up their posts. As a result, his ward team which was meant to be covered by four full-time juniors now only has 2.5 doctors. His registrar is often busy with outpatient clinics. He realizes that the doctors have been working extra hard to cover the workload but until the candidate informs him, he was not aware that they were staying well past their rostered hours and missing out on the educational aspects of their training – this is a cause for concern. He wants to hear the junior doctor's (the candidate's) version of events and their suggestions about what can be done to improve the situation. He needs to reassure himself that the candidate realizes that the current working arrangements contravene European Working Time Directives (i.e. to be working extended hours on a regular basis). It is also essential that the junior doctor appreciates that they may not be indemnified if a clinical error occurs outside of their allotted hours of work. The outcome of the discussion should be that Dr Cooper agrees to speak to the Medical Director/Human Resources department to try to arrange locum cover for the ward.

Thoughts and questions the patient/subject may have

- *What impact is this having on you (as a junior doctor) and your colleagues?*
- *What impact is this having on the patients and have there been any adverse incidents?*
- *What have you done about the situation already and what support do you require?*

Examiner information

1. Conduct of interview

- Establish with the consultant that the objective of the meeting today is to discuss the staffing levels within the firm and the workload of yourself and the other junior doctors on the team.
- Ask the consultant what he knows about the current situation and go on to explain the issues in detail and the impact on patients and the team.
- In essence, say that there are only two full-time junior doctors on the ward team plus another ST1-grade GP trainee who only works 2 days a week. This is instead of the four full-time doctors that were meant to cover the firm.
- Provide details of the team's current workload – for example, how many patients the team covers in total, typical hours of working, etc.
- Indicate your concerns that this situation increases the risk for patient safety as it may potentially jeopardize clinical care.
- You should be asked what actions you have already taken to draw the situation to the attention of the organization. You should have recorded the details of your work pattern on a monitoring form to be submitted to the Human Resources (HR) Department.
- The consultant may ask you if you are getting sufficient senior support on the team (if not, you should outline your thoughts about this).
- Take the opportunity to highlight any clinical errors or near-misses that you or the FY1 have experienced, which may or may not be the result of the excessive overtime worked or high levels of stress due to the additional strains on the team.
- You should be able to articulate the situation and your concerns coherently, concisely and honestly.
- Provide details of how the educational aspects of your training have been compromised as a result of the heavy workload – for example, how many mandatory training days or departmental teaching sessions have

been missed, whether or not you are able to attend the stipulated outpatient clinic sessions, etc.
- You should assert that it is not acceptable to miss the mandatory training sessions and acknowledge that it is your responsibility to ensure that you get cross-cover to be able to participate in these sessions.
- Tell your consultant how your stress levels have been affected by the situation at work and what coping strategies you are using to deal with it.
- Outline what measures you have already taken to try and alleviate the situation, for example:
  - speaking to the HR department in advance to let them know about the team's on-call or annual leave days to request locum cover so that neither doctor is left on their own
  - provide support for the FY1 so that they are not professionally compromised into making decisions beyond their competency level.
- Present some suggestions to resolve the current situation, for example:
  - ask the consultant if he could request a locum doctor (or the loan of a junior from another team that is better staffed) to join your team
  - if the consultant rules this out due to financial restrictions, ask him whether he thinks leaner working practices within the department might be helpful (e.g. transferring some patients to another team)
  - you could also ask if the registrar's timetable could be reviewed so that she has a few more ward sessions to ensure that sufficient senior support is available if this is feasible without compromising the registrar's training commitments.
- Reassure the consultant that you will fill out an incident form if any situation occurs in which patient care was compromised due to lack of junior doctors on the team.
- Thank the consultant for his time and arrange another appointment to come back and see him in a week or so to review the situation.

2. Exploration and problem negotiation

The candidate must be able to:

- succinctly explain the difficulties faced by them and other members of the team due to the lack of prospective cover
- highlight any near-misses or clinical incidents caused by this, including the missed training opportunities
- suggest practical steps for how the problem can be resolved
- propose an action plan for ensuring that the HR department are aware of the situation.

3. Communication, ethics and the law

- Hierarchical professional relationships can be complicated. Personality differences can make team members less or more inclined to raise difficult or challenging issues within the clinical team structure and this can affect individual confidence levels. However, the over riding imperative in circumstances such as this case is that every health professional, whatever their level within the healthcare setting, recognizes and acts on the numerous obligations placed on them to communicate shortfalls in staffing levels as well as the potential impact of this on patient safety and staff well-being.
- In circumstances where we think we may have challenges in negotiating or asserting ourselves, it can be really helpful to make bullet point notes before the meeting to discuss issues which need to be addressed diplomatically and thoroughly.
- The moral obligation to provide safe care for patients is instilled in all healthcare professionals. Any shortfalls in staffing levels, and the concomitant risks which come with increased workloads, physical and emotional stress inevitably place patients at much higher risk of harm. This is why it is ethically unacceptable to avoid having such conversations and raising concerns formally, both verbally and in writing.

- Junior doctors should have a working knowledge of employment law and legislation in place in the UK.
- Since August 2009, the European Working Time Directive (EWTD) has applied to all doctors in training. This limits junior doctors to a maximum of 48 h a week (averaged over 26 weeks).
- Doctors are able to opt out of this but this must be agreed between the doctor and the employer and put down in writing. However, under the New Deal contract requirements, the overall hours worked by a doctor should not be more than 56 h a week (including all their employments and any locum work they do).
- It is important to remember that doctors cannot opt out of rest breaks or annual leave under EWTD regulations.
- New Deal legislation also states that all doctors are required to have their working hours monitored twice a year over a 2-week period and trainees are contractually obliged to record their hours accurately.
- If a junior doctor believes that they are continuously working beyond the hours of their rota, it is their responsibility to bring it to the attention of their employers.
- This involves first speaking to your consultant, clinical lead or medical director. Most situations will be resolved at this level but if it isn't then the HR department, college or deanery needs to be informed. Doctors can also seek advice from their union representative (e.g. BMA).
- Remember that junior doctors have an educational component to their training aside from service provision. Therefore, if they have reason to believe that their training is being compromised by their service commitment this should be brought to the attention of the consultant in charge as well as the educational supervisor/Royal College of Physicians tutor.

Comments on the case

Shortfalls in the staffing of medical teams, gaps in the rota and cross-cover arrangements are commonly faced by junior doctors and consultants alike.

Situations such as the above are not uncommon in clinical practice. Some of the reasons for this may include regulations on capping working hours for junior doctors, greater facility for doctors to go on flexible training schemes, more stringent criteria to ensure that trainees meet minimum competencies before being allowed to progress in their training and so on. All these measures are present whilst the staff's workload and hospital admissions are not decreasing in many places. All junior doctors need to be vigilant about problems arising from lack of prospective cover in their departments and they must flag up any potential or actual clinical incidents due to this.

It is essential that any regular deviation from the EWTD is recorded formally on a monitoring form and submitted to the Human Resources department. This is very important and is usually part of all junior doctors' contractual agreement with their trust. It also ensures that the extended hours you have been working have been reported formally to the trust so that the situation can be investigated.

Failure to report concerns or consequences can place the clinician in ethical, professional and potentially legal peril.

Further reading

EWTD Reference Group. *A guide to the implications of the European Working Time Directive for doctors in training.* London: Department of Health, 2009. www.dh.gov.uk/en/Publicationsandstatistics/ Publications/PublicationsPolicyAndGuidance/DH_ 110100

Case 59 | A colleague with hepatitis B infection

Candidate information

You are a medical doctor in a large district general hospital.

Please read this summary and then continue with the consultation.

Re: Dr Alikhan Fahad, aged 26

Your friend, Dr Alikhan Fahad, is a surgical FY2 where you work. He's a bright and career-minded young doctor who has recently been appointed to the local teaching hospital surgical rotation. He tells you that an occupational health hepatitis B test has found him to be hepatitis surface antigen (HbsAg) positive. He is from overseas and has never had hepatitis B immunization. He is clearly upset and cannot understand how he has acquired the virus. He wants to speak to you for more advice.

Your tasks are to: counsel him about his recent positive finding with an explanation of the results, advise on how this may affect his career and what he needs to do next.

Subject/patient/relative information

Dr Alikhan Fahad is a young surgical Foundation Year 2 doctor (FY2) who has trained overseas. He has shown diligent application and has got on to the local teaching hospital surgical rotation and he intends to take all his postgraduate exams. He had an occupational health hepatitis B test which has shown him to be hepatitis B surface antigen positive (HBsAg). The results also state that he has no HBe markers but that further tests are necessary. He is clearly upset by this news as this may well affect his future career. He does not know exactly where he has acquired the virus, possibly from needlestick injuries while carrying out surgery abroad. He is a good friend of the medical doctor (the candidate) and wants further advice. He wants to know the real implications of his blood test and what the effect will be on his career.

Thoughts and questions the patient/subject may have

- *How serious is it to have a positive HBsAg result? Does it mean I have active hepatitis infection?*
- *What does this mean for my surgical career? Will I be able to join the surgical rotation?*
- *Should I let my consultant know about this positive result? Will he stop me from operating straight away?*

Examiner information

1. Conduct of interview

- Show empathy and compassion, as he must be concerned for his health and career.
- Ask him if he has any idea where he may have acquired the virus from.
- Ask what type of surgery he has assisted with in the past and whether he has had any needlestick injuries.
- Does he have a partner and if so, is she known to have hepatitis B or is she immunized?
- Ask if he knows if he is HBeAg positive, anti-HBe negative or has no HBe markers.
- Explain that if he was HBeAg positive, then he would have restrictions imposed on his practice.
- If he is anti-HBe negative or has no HBe markers, he will need to have hepatitis B virus (HBV) DNA genome levels measured. If this is between 10^3 to 10^5 copies/mL, then he may still be able to carry out exposure-prone procedures whilst on antiviral treatment (see Department of Health guidelines below). If it is under 10^3 per mL, then he will have to have levels tested annually but no restrictions will be imposed.
- Tell him if HBV DNA genome levels are above 10^5 per mL, he will be restricted in carrying out procedures where there is a risk that injury to the healthcare worker could result in their blood contaminating a patient's open tissues. This would include where a worker's gloved hands may be in contact with sharp instruments, needle tips or sharp tissues (e.g. bone spicules or teeth) inside a patient's open body cavity, wound or confined anatomical space where hands or fingertips may not be visible at all times. This would obviously include open surgical techniques.
- Tell him that he must tell his consultant and that he must cease to perform any surgery until he has been properly assessed by the occupational health physician.
- Explain that he may have to retrain in a low-risk specialty if his practice does have to be restricted.
- Reassure him that confidentiality will be paramount but that the occupational health physician may have to decide on contact tracing of patients who may now be at risk.
- He would need to tell medical staffing at his future hospital.
- The occupational health physician may advise a referral to a hepatologist for a specialist clinical assessment.

2. Exploration and problem negotiation

The candidate should be able to:

- show empathy as his colleague is clearly devastated
- explain the meaning of the results
- explain what the occupational health physician will do next
- advise on the possible impact on his surgical career.

3. Communication, ethics and the law

Recommendations from the Department of Health.

- All hepatitis B-infected healthcare workers who are e-antigen negative and who perform exposure-prone procedures or clinical duties in renal units must be tested for viral load (hepatitis B virus DNA).
- Healthcare workers without the e-antigen, and who are refusing to have their viral load tested, should not be allowed to carry out exposure-prone procedures in the future.
- The latest guidelines from the Department of Health state that healthcare workers who are HBeAg negative but have HBV DNA levels $>10^5$ geq/mL should be stopped from performing exposure-prone procedures (EPP), whether they are on antiviral treatment or not.
- However, those who are HBeAg negative but have pretreatment HBV DNA levels of between 10^3 and 10^5 copies/mL can be allowed to perform EPP whilst on antiviral treatment provided their DNA levels fall to below 10^3 copies/mL after starting treatment. The recommendations are to monitor HBV DNA levels 3-monthly whilst on treatment to ensure that they do not rise above 10^3 copies/mL.
- If a clinician decides to stop antiviral treatment, he should also stop performing EPP immediately. If his HBV DNA levels remain $<10^3$ copies/mL a year after stopping treatment, he will be allowed to return to performing EPP, subject to further tests 6–12 monthly.
- The Department of Health guidelines clearly state that healthcare workers infected with hepatitis B should be entitled to the 'same right of confidentiality as any other patient receiving medical care'. Therefore, while the healthcare worker's employer may need to be informed by occupational health staff that a change in the employee's duties should take place, his/her hepatitis B status itself should not be disclosed without the individual's consent. However, where patients are, or have been, at risk it may be necessary in the public interest for the employer to have access to confidential information.

- Arrangements should be made to provide individual healthcare workers with access to a consultant occupational health physician.
- All hepatitis B-infected health care workers should be given accurate and detailed advice on ways of minimizing the risk of transmission in the healthcare setting and to close contacts.
- Employers should make every effort to arrange suitable alternative work and offer retraining opportunities. Postgraduate medical and dental deans also play an important role in retraining or redeploying doctors affected.
- The NHS Injury Benefits scheme and the Industrial Injuries Disablement Benefit scheme provide benefits where hepatitis B has been occupationally acquired.

Comments on the case

This case demonstrates the occupational ethical dilemmas facing a colleague with hepatitis B. One must show sympathy and treat the colleague with the utmost confidentiality. Any careless mutterings in the doctor's mess can be disastrous.

Further reading

Department of Health. *Hepatitis B infected healthcare workers and antiviral therapy*. London: Department of Health, 2007.

Case 60 | A colleague with a needlestick injury

Candidate information

You are the medical CT1 on-call with your recently qualified FY1.

Please read this summary and then continue with the consultation.

Re: Dr Alison Mariner, aged 24

Dr Mariner is your new FY1 and you are both on-call today. A patient with known HIV has been admitted with dyspnoea ?cause. Dr Mariner has clerked the patient and has arranged all the appropriate investigations, including blood tests which she took herself (using gloves). However, she comes back to you extremely upset as she has just had a needlestick injury whilst taking the blood.

Your tasks are to: calm the situation, to advise her about the management of a needlestick injury and to discuss the need for antiretroviral therapy.

Subject/patient/relative information

Dr Mariner is a recently qualified Foundation Year 1 doctor (FY1) working on-call with the medical CT1 (the candidate). She was asked to see an HIV-positive patient, well known to the infectious diseases department and who is already on numerous therapies including zidovudine, didanosine, indinavir and septrin. The patient has been admitted for dyspnoea ?cause, possibly *Pneumocystis jirovecii* pneumonia (PJP). The FY1 wore two pairs of gloves but after taking the blood and with the syringe full, she had a needlestick injury with the green needle entering about 0.5 cm into the pulp of her right index finger. She panicked and disposed of the whole syringe and needle into the sharps bin. She has done the correct initial procedure of washing the contaminated area with water and soap, avoiding scrubbing and allowing the injury site to bleed freely. She is obviously panicking because this is an injury involving an HIV-positive patient. She has only a vague idea about the possible risk of spread of HIV in such cases. She lives with her boyfriend and she is 4 months pregnant. She has been fully immunized against hepatitis B.

Thoughts and questions the patient/subject may have

- *Do I need to start prophylactic antiretroviral treatment straight away?*
- *Who should I go and see to get the tablets?*
- *What is the risk of me contracting HIV?*
- *I've recently found out that I am 4 months pregnant – could this injury, or the medications I have to take, harm my baby?*

Examiner information

1. Conduct of interview

- Ask the FY1 exactly what has happened. She also tells you she is 4 months pregnant.
- Firstly tell her *not to panic* because this will impair her thought processes.
- Tell her that her concerns for the baby will be dealt with and that you will speak to her obstetric consultant about this incident.
- Show empathy and reassure her that the risk of contracting HIV in this type of circumstance is low (around 0.3%). Also explain that there is a risk of contracting hepatitis B and C.
- Ask if she has been immunized against hepatitis B.
- Tell her she must immediately wash the contaminated area thoroughly with soap and water. Avoid scrubbing and allow the wound to bleed freely. She tells you that she has done this.
- Establish the type and size of needle in question, the depth of penetration, the amount of bleeding produced and the exact time of the needlestick injury.
- Establish who the patient is and confirm their HIV, hepatitis B and C status.
- If unsure what treatment to give to the house officer, tell her that you will ring occupational health immediately for advice on any established hospital guidelines.
- If this fails or the incident has taken place out of normal working hours, the senior nurse in the casualty department should know what the guidelines are and where the anti-HIV triple therapy starter pack is kept. This should be given within the first hour.
- Explain that treatment will be for 4 weeks and that she must watch out for side-effects such as sickness and a rash. The candidate must know of any medication that the house officer is on to assess potential drug reactions.
- Warn her of the potential risk of any drug interactions.
- She should be followed up regularly by the occupational health team.
- She should also watch out for symptoms suggestive of seroconversion (rash, fever, malaise, myalgia, lymphadenopathy).
- Tell the FY1 that the nucleoside reverse transcriptase inhibitors (NRTI) zidovudine and lamivudine are not contraindicated in pregnancy. In fact, zidovudine is shown to be particularly effective in preventing HIV transmission to the foetus due to its ability to cross the placenta. However, the non-nucleoside reverse transcriptase (NNRTI) inhibitor efavirenz is contraindicated. The preferred protease inhibitor (PI) and NNRTI drugs in pregnancy are ritonavir and nevirapine. It is likely that one of the two latter drugs will be added to two from the NRTI category as first-line therapy.

- Explain to the FY1 doctor that she should be encouraged to undertake an HIV test, explaining that without it, it would be difficult to claim compensation (Industrial Injuries Disablement Benefit) if she was found to be HIV positive at a later date.
- Counsel her for the HIV test, explaining what the test involves and give a reassurance of confidentiality (see Case 18 for further details).
- Explain that blood taken will also be tested for hepatitis B and C.
- Also tell her that you will explain to the patient what has happened and that you will counsel the patient for a hepatitis B and C test with consent.
- Explain that HIV retesting will be done again 6 months after stopping prophylaxis.
- Until then, she should decide how to tell her partner what has happened with consideration of practising safe sex using barrier methods, i.e. condoms.
- Ask the FY1 if there is anything that she is not sure about.
- Suggest she should go off duty and you will try and arrange some cover.

2. Exploration and problem negotiation

The candidate should be able to:
- assess, support and counsel the individual who has been put at risk with empathy and understanding
- know when to recommend postexposure prophylaxis (PEP): four factors increasing the risk of occupationally acquired HIV infection are deep injury, visible blood on the device causing the injury, injury with a needle that has been placed in the patient's vein or artery, and terminal HIV-related illness in the source patient
- know which PEP drugs are used (i.e. in pregnancy zidovudine 250 mg bd, lamivudine 150 mg and lopinavir/ritonavir 200/50 mg 2 tablets bd. In a non-pregnant person, tenofir and emtricitabine are the preferable NRTIs). Combination drugs have proven superior efficacy than NRTIs alone and are also more useful in drug-resistant strains
- initiate PEP drugs soon after the incident (within hours if possible, no later than 72 h); they should be continued for 28 days at least

- relay the importance of close follow-up by a senior occupational health physician with further counselling and postexposure HIV testing.

3. Communication, ethics and the law

Guidelines from the Department of Health.
- Confidentiality is paramount.
- If the HIV status of the patient is unknown but suspected, then HIV test counselling should not be undertaken by the individual exposed (in this case the FY1 doctor).
- Patients with unknown HIV status cannot have HIV testing without their consent and so an assessment of the likelihood of infection may have to be made.
- Pregnancy does not preclude the use of HIV PEP therapy. Zidovudine, lamivudine and lopinavir/ritonavir are not contraindicated in the second and third trimesters; such evidence for other drugs is limited.
- Healthcare workers exposed should be given the chance to discuss the balance of risks with appropriate psychological support, including information about the potential toxic side-effects and the risk of passing HIV to the baby, if pregnant, so allowing the individual to make an informed decision about whether or not to undergo PEP therapy.
- It would be wise to inform the FY1's consultant.

- Pending follow-up and absence of seroconversion, healthcare workers are not obliged to be the subject of work modifications, e.g. avoidance of exposure-prone procedures.
- All individuals exposed must be given advice on safe sex and avoiding blood donation.
- The occupational health physician is encouraged to report the case (in absolute confidence) to the Public Health Laboratory Service (PHLS) Communicable Disease Surveillance Centre (or Centre for Infection and Environmental Health in Scotland).

Comments on the case

This is quite a complicated case but one that can happen to anyone working in acute medicine. There are many ethical perplexities that the candidate must bear in mind which, unless adequately prepared, can lead to a badly conducted station. More guidance can be obtained from the Department of Health website.

Further reading

Department of Health. *HIV post-exposure prophylaxis.* London: Department of Health, 2008.

Case 61 | The improper doctor

Candidate information

You are the medical doctor in a cardiology department.

Please read this summary and then continue with the consultation.

Re: Dr Richard Morgan

The ward sister on the coronary care unit has complained to you that Dr Morgan, your Foundation Year 1 (FY1) doctor, whilst on-call last night, refused to take an urgent urea and electrolytes sample from an anuric patient. The sister also tells you that he was rude on the phone and that his excuse was that the phlebotomists would be coming round routinely later that morning anyway. Dr Morgan is a bright young man who has settled reasonably well into his job, but you do appreciate that support for him has been minimal. Your consultant is rarely seen except for one business ward round per week, there is no registrar available, and you are rushed off your feet doing clinics (which are on a different site), compiling discharge letters, seeing referrals, and presently covering another colleague who has taken indefinite compassionate leave for depression. You and your FY1 are never on-call together because of the shift rota system that the junior doctors follow and so it is impossible to have any 'firm' bonding. You approach the FY1 to obtain his version of the complaint and you appreciate that you ought to do more to support him.

Your tasks are to: obtain from your FY1 his story of the events, explain that there has been a complaint against him and generally counsel him to avoid any further similar occurrences.

Subject/patient/relative information

Dr Richard Morgan is a bright young FY1 4 weeks into his first post. He has settled into this job reasonably well but unfortunately support from senior staff is minimal. The consultant is rarely seen except for one business ward round a week, there is no registrar, and the CT1 doctor (the candidate) is too busy doing clinics (which are on a different site), compiling discharge letters, seeing referrals and covering another colleague who has taken indefinite compassionate leave for depression. There is never any time to ask for advice and quite simply he feels as if he is running the show single-handedly. He is never on-call with the CT1 because the shift rota system that the junior doctors follow does not allow this. He has to review sick patients on the coronary care unit (CCU) for which he feels totally out of his depth, and in the early hours of this morning he had an altercation with one of the night sisters who is notorious for insisting that everything has to be done by the book. The patient concerned was an elderly man with worsening heart failure who had become anuric late in the evening, probably as a result of hypotension and sepsis. The urea and electrolytes were deranged and the on-call registrar (who started the patient on intravenous dobutamine) wanted the tests repeated again at 6 am so that the results would be available for the 9.30 am ward round. Dr Morgan was up all night doing ward cover and when he was rung by the sister at 6 am to take blood samples, he felt quite exasperated because these could be taken by the phlebotomists in 2 hours' time and still be available for the ward round at 9.30 am. He felt that if blood was taken at 6 am, the registrar on-call was not going to alter his management as he was quite happily asleep in bed. So, he felt doing the blood test was inappropriate at that time, although he did have a go at the sister for not using any common sense.

Thoughts and questions the patient/subject may have

- *I can't believe the ward sister complained to you about me – can't she understand how busy I was all night running around from one ward to another!*
- *Why couldn't the nurses help out by taking the patient's bloods?*
- *I don't want to appear as though I'm complaining but sometimes I do feel out of my depth in this job.*
- *Will the consultant think I am incompetent or have a bad impression of me if he hears about all of this?*

Examiner information

1. Conduct of interview

- When speaking to the FY1, ensure that you show empathy, understanding and sensitivity, so that he feels you are on his side as a colleague.
- Tell him that you have received a complaint from one of the sisters on the CCU.
- Tell him what the complaint is about and the sister's version of the event.
- Ascertain his version of the story, acknowledging his feelings with empathy. Get the facts right.
- Make sure you appear to be listening with an open mind.
- Have there been any other clashes with other members of staff? Does he feel he is being targeted for criticism?
- Is he having difficulty in coping with his duties? Does he feel that he needs more support when he is on-call? Admit that support has not been adequate and show an appreciation of his hard work.
- Set out the broader picture by explaining that if a specific management plan for that patient has been set, then it is important that it should be followed. There is a chance that the phlebotomist would not have arrived, and so no blood would have been taken, leading to a delay in management decisions.
- Tell him that in these situations, politeness to other members of staff is very important to allow everyone to work as a team.

- Tell him that you will speak again to the sister so that the matter is dealt with but encourage your FY1 to apologize to her for any offence caused.
- Reassure him that if there are any other incidents similar to this or if he ever feels he is under any particular pressure then he should not be afraid to speak to you personally.
- Explain that you will try to be more supportive and you will also mention the problem with regard to support to the consultant.

2. Exploration and problem negotiation

The candidate should be able to:

- be diplomatic in the consultation without appearing to take sides
- take on board both sides of the story
- explain that medical practice is teamwork and that losing patience with nursing staff can be detrimental to team building
- be supportive of the FY1, with appreciation of the difficult job he has to do, and say that you will aim to offer a more supportive role on the wards with improved supervision.

3. Communication, ethics and the law

- The improper colleague tends to be clinically competent but rude and offensive to staff, often with poor time keeping as well.
- In contrast, the difficult colleague is clinically competent, fine with patients and staff but often

unco-operative and obstructive especially with managers with, for example, unorthodox ways of practising clinical medicine.

- One must get the facts right, particularly if there is an allegation of rudeness.
- Remain diplomatic without taking sides and always aim for an informal resolution by speaking to both parties involved.
- Aim to prevent a recurrence by, for example, altering practice, e.g. in this case ensuring better support and making the house officer feel that you are approachable with any problems.
- Seek advice from senior colleagues.

> **Comments on the case**
>
> The circumstances surrounding this case are unfortunately all too common in modern medicine. The candidate will have situations like this, whatever their seniority, and the importance of being able to handle them as a diplomatic manager cannot be overstated.

Case 62 | The incompetent doctor

Candidate information

You are a CT1 doctor on a medical firm.

Please read this summary and then continue with the consultation.

Re: Dr Andrew Stanton

Dr Stanton has been an FY1 on the team for the last 4 weeks. He has had a difficult start to his first job as his mother died 7 weeks ago with breast cancer and he is going through a stormy divorce after only 18 months of marriage. You have got to know him reasonably well and he is generally keen and career-minded. However, Sister Francis from your ward is not happy with his clinical performance. Dr Stanton is making numerous mistakes when writing up doses of drugs, he is never able to obtain intravenous access on the first attempt and when taking blood he has left needles on the bedside cabinet. Last week he put the wrong patient label on the biochemistry form. Sister Francis is not prepared to put up with any more mishaps and wants to speak to you about him.

Your tasks are to: discuss these mishaps with Sister Francis and provide suggestions on how the problems can be tackled.

Subject/patient/relative information

Sister Francis is a senior nurse on the medical ward. She has seen junior doctors come and go for over 20 years. She is quite a good judge of clinical competence and she does not think highly of Dr Stanton. He is very nervous with patients, has a low level of general medical knowledge and is constantly making silly errors with drug doses on the prescription charts. The FY1 on-call usually ends up rewriting the drug chart most evenings. Changing venflons is an agonizing event; repeated attempts are the rule, leading to patients becoming quite distressed. When taking blood, he has left needles on the bedside cabinet and last week he wrongly labelled a biochemistry form (using a different patient's identification sticker) but thankfully one of the nurses spotted this mistake. Sister feels that his performance must improve and she wants to speak to the CT1 (the candidate) to discuss a clear plan of action. She also wants the CT1 to speak to the consultant.

Thoughts and questions the patient/subject may have

- *He really is a liability to the patients, something has to be done about him!*
- *Will you please speak to your consultant and tell him what is going on?*
- *What plan of action do you have to ensure that Dr Stanton's competency is evaluated?*
- *I agree that the nurses on the ward, including myself, have been a bit hard on him. I will ensure that we are more supportive of him on the ward.*

Examiner information

1. Conduct of interview

- Discuss with Sister Francis what her main concerns are and ask her to give examples. Listen intently and with interest. She must have confidence in you otherwise she would not have asked for your advice.
- Be diplomatic and say that you are saddened to hear about these mishaps and that you will speak to Dr Stanton about them to get his side of the story.
- Be supportive of Dr Stanton (the last thing Dr Stanton would want is for everybody to take sides against him). Explain that the last few months have been unsettling for him but you agree that good standards of clinical competence have to be maintained whatever his domestic difficulties (you are not allowed to reveal the problems with regard to his mother or the divorce as these may be strictly confidential).
- Explain to Sister Francis that you will speak to the consultant as he ought to know.
- Offer a constructive plan for future training and say that you will try to improve matters by supervising his ward work more closely, constructively correcting any mistakes, improving his general medical education with regular teaching sessions and guarantee regular appraisals of his work with the consultant.
- Reassure Sister Francis that you will explore other alternatives after discussion with Dr Stanton and the consultant, such as leave of absence for a brief period for personal circumstances.

2. Exploration and problem negotiation

The candidate should be able to:

- listen to what Sister Francis has to say, respecting her concerns
- not take sides, and agree to speak to the house officer personally to get his side of the story
- have a plan of management to improve the house officer's clinical performance

- reassure Sister Francis that the consultant will be informed and all alternatives will be considered.

3. Communication, ethics and the law

- Doctors are not perfect and their clinical skills and human relationships may be suboptimal. However, some are so bad as to be dangerous and if the quality of medical care is to improve, these doctors need to be identified and given further training and education.
- To improve such doctors, it is important that they have the insight to understand that they need further training and education.
- Those aspects of clinical ability that need improving have to be identified.
- A plan of further training and education has to be contrived in a structured and systematic way after consultation with the consultant and the postgraduate dean — it is no good sending such individuals to more lunch-time grand rounds or audit meetings and in the end achieving nothing. A training programme has to be tailored to the individual's needs.
- The individual will need to be reappraised and reassessed regularly to see if the clinical performance has improved.
- Seek advice from senior colleagues.

Comments on the case

Underperforming doctors must be identified and counselled in the proper manner. There must be a sense of responsibility for these individuals and they should not be left to languish in ensuing jobs. So, senior doctors must be able to recognize such individuals and have a plan of action to deal with the shortcomings.

Case 63 | **The sick doctor**

Candidate information
You are the medical CT1 doctor.
Please read this summary and then continue with the consultation.

Re: Dr Stuart Pemberton

You suspect that Dr Pemberton, your Foundation Year 1 (FY1) doctor, has an alcohol problem. Rumours are rife that, when on-call, he disappears to have a drink in the on-call room. Recently he had a car accident in which he drove his car onto a motorway embankment without any other cars involved. You have noticed the smell of alcohol on his breath on a number of occasions. You are worried that his decision making may be suspect and that he has been forgetting to carry out certain jobs that he has promised to do. You feel he may pose a risk to patients so you decide to speak to him privately about the matter.

Your tasks are to: determine if Dr Pemberton has a drink problem and suggest ways of providing help.

Subject/patient/relative information
Dr Stuart Pemberton has been an FY1 doctor for 8 weeks. He has always had a reputation of being a 'lad who can take his ale' but behind this exterior he is quite an insecure young man, who lacks confidence and finds being a doctor extremely stressful. He is finding the hours particularly punishing and the on-calls very demanding. He was recently criticized by his consultant as being 'the laziest house officer ever' – this was particularly hurtful especially as he works as hard as anybody else. Many a time on ward rounds the consultant has ridiculed him in front of students with unprofessional foul-mouthed ripostes to sensible suggestions. He has not found anyone to confide in and as a result has turned to drink. On-calls are especially hard because of the fear of failure and escaping to 'the bottle' in the on-call room is the only way to achieve some form of relief. He has been drinking quite heavily over the last few weeks and recently was involved in a car crash when he drove off a motorway onto the embankment. The police breathalyzed him and he was found to be positive, so he is expecting a court summons. He does not believe he has a problem and probably lacks insight. He is not in any relationship at the moment and has not previously suffered from depression, although current events are resulting in a low mood and poor self-esteem. He does not take any illicit drugs.

Thoughts and questions the patient/subject may have
- *Why is everyone making a big deal about my drinking? Of course I have a couple of beers now and again but which doctor doesn't?!*
- *I suppose it has got a bit excessive lately, things at work are certainly not helping.*
- *Do you really have to tell the consultant? He already thinks I am useless!*

Examiner information

1. Conduct of interview

- When speaking to Dr Pemberton, be open without being threatening. Develop a good rapport.
- Explain that you are concerned that he may be drinking heavily.
- Ask if he feels he has a problem.
- If he denies there is a problem, give him the evidence why you and others suspect that there is a problem.
- Say you have heard that he was in a car crash. Ask if he had any injuries and if the crash was alcohol related. Were the police involved?
- Ask about the alcohol drinking and use the CAGE questionnaire.
- Ask if anyone else has hinted that there may be a problem or if he himself thinks he should reduce his drinking.
- Ask if there is a recreational drug problem.
- Explore if there is a reason behind the alcohol intake, e.g. break-up of a relationship, stress at work.
- Has he ever been off sick due to alcohol, e.g. due to a hangover?
- Explore any evidence of depression.
- Explain that you are concerned that continuing like he is may be putting patients at risk and you feel that he should seek help.
- Explain you are obliged to speak to the consultant. If he objects, he may agree to you speaking to someone else with authority, e.g. the medical director, but ensuring that confidentiality will be maintained throughout.
- Ask if he is registered with a local GP. The GP should also be involved.
- You can also suggest the BMA counselling helpline (0845 9200169). The Sick Doctors Trust (0370 4445163) is a confidential service for doctors which provides early intervention in chemical dependency and the Doctors Support Network (0844 3953010) is a self-help group for doctors with mental health problems.

2. Exploration and problem negotiation

The candidate should be able to:

- recognize and assess the problem
- determine if the individual has insight into the problem
- explain the importance of the situation, i.e. the risk to the individual and to the patients
- offer help
- seek advice from senior colleagues.

3. Communication, ethics and the law

- You must protect patients from any risk of harm posed by another healthcare professional's conduct, performance or health, including problems arising from alcohol or other substance abuse. The safety of patients must come first at all times. Where there are serious concerns about a colleague's performance, health or conduct, it is essential that steps are taken *without delay* to investigate the concerns raised to establish whether they are well founded or not and to protect patients.
- If you have grounds to believe that another healthcare professional may be putting patients at risk, you must give an honest explanation of your concerns to an appropriate person from the employing authority such as the medical director, nursing director, chief executive, director of public health or an officer of your local medical committee, following any procedures set by the employer. If there are no appropriate local systems, or local systems cannot resolve the problem, and you remain concerned about the safety of patients, you should then discuss your concerns with an impartial colleague or contact your defence body, a professional organization or the GMC for advice.

Comments on the case

Contrary to popular belief, doctors do become sick and these individuals must be attended to. Dr Pemberton's case could unfortunately be a real one in your own hospital and so the capability to recognize a sick doctor and to instigate appropriate management must be acquired by all doctors in training. Doctors who are sick tend to deny their illness, fail to seek advice early, self-diagnose, self-medicate and obtain unprofessional advice from colleagues who most likely possess no insight into the real problem. They resist the slightest contemplation of taking time off work.

Further reading

General Medical Council. *Good medical practice. Paragraphs 43–45. Conduct and performance of colleagues.* London: General Medical Council, 2006.

Case 64 | Consent for medical examination

Candidate information
You are the medical doctor on a general medical ward.
Please read this summary and then continue with the consultation.

Re: Mrs Edna White, aged 86

For once, time is on your hands and you have agreed to take the third-year medical students to see Mrs Edna White, an elderly lady who was admitted 2 weeks ago with a dense right hemiplegia. Presently, Mrs White remains unwell with global dysphasia and reduced consciousness, and is catheterized. She has no family and needs full 24-h nursing care. However, she has excellent neurological signs and the students have requested these signs to be demonstrated to them. You have seven students in your group but another group of seven appears on the ward complaining that their teaching has been cancelled. You feel charitable and so ask the second group to join you.

Unfortunately, the ward sister (Sr Brennan) is unhappy that you are taking 14 medical students to see Mrs White. She requests that you speak with her in the office.

Your tasks are to: discuss the reasons for her concerns and come to a compromise.

Subject/patient/relative information
Mrs Edna White is an 86-year-old lady who was admitted 2 weeks ago with a dense right hemiplegia, global dysphasia and reduced consciousness. She remains unwell with no signs of improvement, needing full 24-h nursing care, and she is catheterized. The consultant's impression is that her prognosis is poor. Mrs White has no family. The medical doctor (the candidate) has agreed to take 14 students to see Mrs White to demonstrate her physical signs. The ward sister (Sr Brennan) is unhappy that the doctor is taking so many students to see Mrs White because (a) she feels so many students would disrupt the running of the ward, (b) Mrs White would be unable to consent for physical examination, (c) Mrs White would be indecently exposed to the students as she has no undergarments on, (d) Mrs White would be unable to state whether she feels any discomfort during the examination and (e) most importantly, she feels that the teaching is not in the best interests of the patient. Sr Brennan feels quite strongly about this and wants to discuss this privately with the doctor. Sr Brennan does appreciate that students must learn and one possible solution is to have the students present in smaller groups during the junior doctor's or consultant's ward round which will allow them to watch an examination being carried out on Mrs White with her physical signs being demonstrated.

Thoughts and questions the patient/subject may have

- *Sorry to disappoint you and the students but as the ward sister, I have a duty to look after the welfare of the patients as well.*
- *Can you not find another patient who is less unwell and who is able to give consent for the examination?*
- *I can accept two or three students coming round but having 14 students crowded around Mrs White would certainly be too disruptive for her care and the running of my ward.*
- *Why don't you speak to your consultant and see if the students can come along on the ward round where you or your consultant can demonstrate the physical signs to them?*

Examiner information

1. Conduct of interview

- Sit and listen to what Sr Brennan has to say, don't be confrontational. Sister is senior and experienced and is not 'anti medical students'.
- She tells you that she is unhappy that so many students are around the bedside for the teaching; she feels this may disrupt the running of the ward.
- Sister also tells you that Mrs White would be unable to consent for any physical examination, would be indecently exposed to the students as she has no undergarments on, would be unable to state whether she has any discomfort during the examination and she also feels that the teaching is not in her best interests.
- Sister also tells you that she does understand that students need to learn and, in this case, one possible solution would be to observe the consultant or yourself examining her during a ward round when assessing her medical state/progress.
- You agree and decide that this is the best solution.
- Apologize to her for any misunderstanding.

2. Exploration and problem negotiation

The candidate should be able to:
- sit down and listen to what Sister Brennan's concerns are
- appreciate these concerns
- agree on a solution or compromise.

3. Communication, ethics and the law

- It is a general legal and ethical principle that valid consent must be obtained before starting treatment or physical investigation, or providing personal care, for a patient. This principle reflects the right of the patient to determine what happens to their bodies, and is fundamental to good clinical practice.
- For a person to have capacity, he or she must be able to comprehend and retain information and material relevant to the decision, especially as to the consequences of having, or not having, the intervention in question.
- To give valid consent, the patient needs to understand in broad terms the nature and purpose of the procedure. Any misrepresentations of these elements will invalidate consent. Where relevant, information about anaesthesia should be given as well as information about the procedure itself.
- Clear information is particularly important when students or trainees carry out procedures to further their own education. Where the procedure will further the patient's care – for example, taking a blood sample for testing – then, assuming the student is appropriately trained in the procedure, the fact that it is carried out by a student does not alter the nature and purpose of the procedure. It is therefore not a legal requirement to tell the patient that the clinician is a student, although it would always be good practice to do so. In contrast, where a student proposes to conduct a physical examination which is not part of the patient's care, then it is essential to explain that the purpose of the examination is to further the student's training and to seek consent for that to take place.
- Video recordings of treatment may be used as a medical record, a treatment aid and tool for teaching, audit or research. The purpose and possible future use of a video must be clearly explained to the person, before their consent is sought for the recording to be made. If the video is to be used for teaching, audit or research, then patients must be aware that they can refuse without their care being

compromised and that, when required or appropriate, the video can be anonymized. As a matter of good practice, the same principles should apply to clinical photography.

Further reading

Department of Health. *Reference guide to consent for examinations or treatment.* London: Department of Health, 2009. www.dh.gov.uk/en/Publicationsandstatistics/Publications/PublicationsPolicyAndGuidance/DH_103643.

Comments on the case

This case highlights the ethics of consent for examinations and treatment. Medical practitioners must be aware of the consent procedure and the Department of Health website provides useful guidelines.

Case 65 | Submitting an audit project

Candidate information

You are the medical doctor about to see the audit department manager.
Please read this summary and then continue with the consultation.

Re: An audit of the mortality rate for disease 'A'

Disease 'A' is a common acute illness which comprises nearly 5% of all acute
medical admissions at your hospital. Your hospital has approximately 40
acute medical admissions a day. The average national in-hospital mortality
rate for disease 'A' is 10%. You would like to know whether patients with
disease 'A' at your hospital have a better in-hospital mortality rate when they
are admitted under the care of the physician with an interest in this disease,
compared with other physicians. There is also some suggestion from a recent
survey undertaken by the Royal College that the mortality rate is better when
the patient is under the care of a physician with an interest in disease 'A'. In
order to undertake this project, you decide to embark on a retrospective
case-notes survey of all admissions of disease 'A' over a 6-month period. You
are about to see the head of the audit department, Mrs Norma Hunter, to
discuss this project and to obtain permission to have the notes retrieved. The
secretary has agreed to put the notes in one of the offices in the department.

Your task is to: discuss the audit project with the audit manager.

Subject/patient/relative information

Mrs Norma Hunter is the audit manager. She is about to see the medical doctor (the
candidate) who would like to submit an audit project looking at whether the in-
hospital mortality rate for disease 'A' is better when such patients are admitted under
the care of physicians with a specific interest in disease 'A' compared to when they
are admitted under the care of physicians without a special interest in disease 'A'. Like
all other audit submissions, she is keen that the medical doctor has a proper understanding of the principles of audit, with particular reference to (1) identifying the
problem, (2) setting the standards (e.g. from data elsewhere), (3) observing the
practice (i.e. the audit), (4) comparing the practice with the standards, (5) implementing change and (6) re-auditing to detect improvement in the standard of care.

Thoughts and questions the patient/subject may have

- *What background research have you done regarding the importance of this disease?*
- *What do you understand about the stages of clinical audit?*
- *Have you got an idea about the time period you want the audit to cover and when you hope
  to finish the work?*
- *How do you plan to disseminate the results?*
- *Do you have any idea about what sort of changes the hospital may be able to implement
  based on your findings?*

Examiner information

1. Conduct of interview

- Introduce yourself to Mrs Hunter.
- Tell her you would like to discuss an audit project which you would like to carry out.
- Start off by telling her what the aims of your audit are.
- She asks you how common disease 'A' is in the hospital. Tell her that 5% of acute medical admissions are due to disease 'A' and therefore, over a month, the average number of admissions with this is approximately 60.
- Tell her that the evidence from the Royal College suggests that the mortality rate may depend on who looks after these patients.
- Explain how you would undertake the audit and how long a period the audit should cover (6 months). Say you would like the coding department to give you a list of the names of patients admitted with disease 'A'. Ask if you can then get the audit department to retrieve the notes. Suggest where the notes should be sent.
- She asks you what you will do with the results. Say you will present them at the local audit meeting.
- She asks you what changes you will implement and when you plan to re-audit.
- Say this depends very much on the findings and that this will be discussed at the medical meeting. If changes are implemented then say that you hope your department would re-audit 1 year after implementation of the changes.
- When finished, thank her and say you will give her regular updates.

2. Exploration and problem negotiation

The candidate should be able to:

- understand the basic principles of audit
- understand how to set the standards
- know how to carry out the audit, i.e. notes survey
- appreciate that observed practice should be compared with the national standards
- decide how to implement change
- appreciate that an audit is not complete unless the subject is re-audited.

3. Communication, ethics and the law

- Audit can be regarded as the systematic and critical analysis of the quality of clinical care, including the procedures used for diagnosis and treatment, the associated use of resources and the resulting outcome and quality of life for the patient.
- Key principles of audit include:
  - maintaining and enhancing continual professional education and development
  - collaborative audit programmes to enhance integration across professions
  - incorporating audit into the quality strategy and involving general managers.
- Important features of audit are:
  - success and effectiveness are variable
  - audit is better established in a well-managed, supportive organization with good communication
  - developing clinical audit is a long-term commitment requiring real support from managers
  - costs of audit must be measured and justified as a large resource commitment has been made by the Department of Health
  - audit demands skills in teamwork, process analysis, data collection and problem solving.
- Audit departments provide general advice and support to professionals on any aspect of clinical audit and help plan and design audit projects. They offer assistance to collect and analyse data and produce reports and presentations. They help to identify ways in which quality improvements can be made and assist with the implementation of change identified by the audit.
- The above audit project is a typical project undertaken by a medical doctor. Practical problems faced by the doctor are as follows:
  - coding is never 100% accurate and so some patients will have been wrongly given the diagnosis of disease 'A', or some patients who had disease 'A' won't have had this diagnosis registered by the coding department (coding should be checked by the relevant physician on a weekly basis)
  - notes retrieval is never 100% successful. Some notes are inevitably missing. Notes retrieval of over 60% is excellent. Therefore, straight away 40% of the data are missing, which may skew the results
  - data from the notes are often unavailable, poorly documented or inaccurate
  - patients usually change consultants, which may hinder the data collection
  - collecting and storing notes can be a problem if space is unavailable. Confidentiality must be guaranteed, i.e. are notes going to be kept in the departmental corridor where other patients may come and go?

- data collection must be robust, i.e. using a computer database and not proforma sheets of paper
- comparing audit results with results in peer-reviewed journals can sometimes be difficult to justify as study designs are inevitably different
- implementing change may not be easy, i.e. if a difference in mortality rate is found, does the medical director insist that all future admissions with disease 'A' be transferred immediately to the physicians with an interest in disease 'A'? Will these teams be able to accommodate a further 60 admissions a month?
- finally, completing the return audit loop is not always successful. For example, the junior doctor moves on and, sometimes, if no changes are implemented, then the audit cycle has broken down even before the re-auditing stage.

Comments on the case

This case highlights the principles of audit and points out the common problems which affect audit projects undertaken by junior doctors.

Further reading

National Institute for Health and Clinical Excellence/ Healthcare Commission. *Principles for best practice in clinical audit*. Oxford: Radcliffe Medical Press, 2008.

Case 66 | Treating a prisoner

Candidate information

You are the medical doctor in a chest clinic.

Please read this summary and then continue with the consultation.

Re: Mr Tony Garrett, aged 27

Mr Garrett is a prisoner at the local high-security prison. He has been attending the chest clinic for the last 3 months for multidrug-resistant pulmonary tuberculosis. As he is a high-risk individual he comes accompanied by two prison officers and is handcuffed to one of them. His treatment is progressing reasonably well and he is due to come back in 6 weeks time. The clinic sister, Sr Rollinson, wants to speak to you concerning this patient. She feels it is inappropriate to have him treated in the chest clinic and wants him to be discharged back to the care of the prison doctor.

Your tasks are to: talk to Sr Rollinson to ascertain her grievances and to explain to her the importance of continued care at the chest clinic.

Subject/patient/relative information

Mr Tony Garrett is a prisoner at the local high-security prison. He was diagnosed as having multidrug-resistant pulmonary tuberculosis and he visits the clinic every 4–6 weeks. When he comes, he is handcuffed to one prison officer and closely watched by another. His presence makes all the staff very uncomfortable and none of them wants to undertake the routine clinic measurements such as his weight or blood pressure. Sr Rollinson is the senior nurse at the clinic and feels that the patient should have his tuberculosis managed by the prison doctor. She is keen to speak to the medical doctor (the candidate) to discuss the possibility of discharge for security and safety reasons.

Thoughts and questions the patient/subject may have

- *My nurses in the outpatient department are complaining that they don't feel safe when Mr Garrett is in the clinic.*
- *What is the risk to my staff and other patients by having Mr Garrett here?*
- *Since his TB seems to be improving, can he not be followed up by the prison doctor? That will be the most appropriate thing for him and everyone else involved.*

Examiner information

1. Conduct of interview

- Ask Sr Rollinson what her concerns are.
- Tell her that you understand how she and the other staff feel but that prisoners cannot be treated any differently from other patients.
- She asks why he cannot be managed at the prison by the prison doctor.
- Explain that as he has complicated multidrug-resistant TB, he has to be followed up closely by a physician with expertise in TB.
- Reassure her and explain that the risk of escape or threat to others has been assessed and that is the reason for the presence of two prison officers.
- Say that next time, you will discuss with her and the prison officers the current risk of escape or violence and decide how best to conduct the consultation.
- Reassure her that her concerns will be relayed to the consultant.

2. Exploration and problem negotiation

The candidate should be able to:

- ascertain why Sister Rollinson is not happy
- explain why you think the patient should continue to be managed at the clinic
- reassure that security and safety for all staff are of paramount importance, hence the presence of the prison officers.

3. Communication, ethics and the law

Guidelines from the BMA.

- Doctors have a duty to provide the best possible care for each of their patients. This includes respect for the patients' dignity and privacy. These issues are equally as important when treating those detained in prison, whether convicted or on remand, as when treating any other patient. Prisoners must have access to the same standards of healthcare as are available to the rest of the society.
- When prisoners are taken outside the prison grounds for medical care, the duty of the healthcare team to provide optimal care can often conflict with the prison authorities' duty to ensure that appropriate levels of security are maintained. Any measures which sought to remove all possibility of escape or violence would be so draconian as to lead to an unacceptable loss of the patient's dignity and basic human

rights. It is, therefore, necessary to reach a balance between the dignity of the patient and the security needs. Where there is a serious risk of escape or the prisoner represents a threat to themselves, the health team or others, then safeguards are required. However, these safeguards should be commensurate with the actual or perceived risk and should respect the patient's right to privacy to the maximum extent possible.

- There should be a presumption that prisoners will be examined and treated without restraints and without prison officers present, unless there is a high risk of escape or it is considered that the prisoner represents a threat to himself, the health professionals or others. It is important to assess the level of risk in each individual case and to tailor the safeguards to suit the circumstances. Where the level of risk is considered to be low then the prisoner should be treated accordingly.
- In cases where there is a high risk of escape or where there is a threat of violence, the safeguards should nevertheless respect the prisoner's right to privacy to the maximum extent possible. For example, where there is a risk of escape but no likelihood of violence, it should be possible for a prison officer to be stationed outside the consulting or treatment room with another in the grounds immediately outside. These precautions will allow the patient some degree of privacy, dignity and confidentiality whilst also ensuring that security is maintained. Occasionally, where there is a serious threat of violence or the prisoner is considered to be dangerous, it will be necessary to use restraints and it may also be necessary to have a prison officer inside the consulting room.

Comments on the case

It is not uncommon to have prisoners as patients and, despite any prejudice the physician may harbour, these patients still have the right to confidentiality, privacy and dignity as for any other patient. Delivering these rights is certainly influenced by the potential risk of escape, self-harm and threat to staff and so an assessment of these risks must be made between the doctor and prison officer before the consultation.

Case 67 | A violent and abusive patient

Candidate information

You are the medical doctor on-call.

Please read this summary and then continue with the consultation.

Re: Mr Thomas Jenkins, aged 43

Mr Jenkins is a man with type 1 diabetes mellitus who was admitted under your consultant's care yesterday with pneumonia, poorly controlled blood sugars and confusion. As a consequence of his confusion, he has physically assaulted one nurse and verbally abused another on the ward about 30 min ago. The security staff are with him at the moment trying to calm the situation. However, the senior sister (Sister James) wants to talk to you about the situation. She wants him removed from the hospital and threatens to call the police.

Your tasks are to: discuss the situation with Sister James, acquire full details of what has happened and discuss how to manage the situation.

Subject/patient/relative information

Sister James has been a well-respected member of the nursing staff for many years and she works on your consultant's ward. Mr Jenkins is a 43-year-old man with type 1 diabetes mellitus who was admitted yesterday with pneumonia, poorly controlled blood sugars and confusion. From the start of the admission, he has been quite agitated with constant wandering around the ward despite being told by the staff to stay in bed. There are no other obvious causes for the confusion such as toxic/alcohol, pharmacological, head injury, postictal, etc. and no reason for the acute escalation of misbehaviour. He pulled out all his drips, including his IV insulin, shouted expletives at the student nurse that cannot be repeated, and punched a male nurse in the face when he went to the aid of the student nurse. The male nurse now has a suspected broken nose. There are four security men by the bedside but they are not physically holding Mr Jenkins down. Sister is utterly disgusted by Mr Jenkins' behaviour and she wants to call the police to evict him from the ward despite his illness. He has an oxygen saturation of 91% on air and his blood sugars are still over 15 mmol/L. He has not been on any benzodiazepines or opioids and there is no evidence of any head injury.

Thoughts and questions the patient/subject may have

- *This is unacceptable behaviour – I cannot have my staff and other patients on the ward being put at risk because of this uncontrollable man!*
- *I agree that he is not medically stable yet but we need to come up with some way of managing him so that no one else on the ward gets hurt.*

Examiner information

1. Conduct of interview
- Sit down with Sister James and ask for the full details of what has happened, who has been attacked and what injuries have been caused. Make sure all details are officially written on an incident report and in the medical/nursing notes. Ask if any of the other patients have been harmed or distressed by the incident.
- Ask how Mr Jenkins has been since admission.
- Determine if there has been any particular reason for Mr Jenkins to be more unsettled.
- Ask if Mr Jenkins has a particular dislike for the two staff affected by this incident.
- Get an idea of how Mr Jenkins has been medically, i.e. oxygenation, blood sugars, temperature, etc.
- Ask if any benzodiazepines or opioids have been given and enquire about any history/evidence of a head injury.
- Ask if hospital security has been called and what they are doing now, i.e. restraining.
- Show that you fully understand Sister's concerns for the safety of her staff.
- Explain that Mr Jenkins is ill and such patients have a right for their medical treatment to be continued despite their lack of co-operation.
- Explain that you feel that Mr Jenkins cannot be removed from the ward by the police.
- Reassure Sister that you will first review Mr Jenkins medically to ensure that there are no reversible causes of his aggression. Then you will make an attempt to calm him and try to determine any particular reason for the bad behaviour.
- Explain that you will ask advice from the on-call psychiatrist with regard to controlling his violent behaviour.
- Explain that you will inform your own consultant immediately and that you will report the matter as a critical incident.

2. Exploration and problem negotiation
The candidate should be able to:
- listen to Sister's concerns
- take a careful account of what has happened and who has been involved
- determine if there are any medical causes for the worsening behaviour
- reassure Sister that advice from senior colleagues will be sought
- persuade Sister into understanding that the patient remains ill and that he cannot be removed from a hospital ward by the police and that it would result in a risk of further medical deterioration
- have a clear plan of management that Sister can agree with.

3. Communication, ethics and the law
- Such patients cannot be left without treatment.
- Hostility may be directed against a particular health professional, in which case he or she must not be further involved in the patient's care.
- Sedation may be considered if the violence is a symptom of the illness and when, in the interest of the patient, this is needed to prevent injury to themselves or others.
- Advice from a psychiatrist should be sought. He/she may be able to give advice on sedation and provide a nurse experienced in violent behaviour to work on the ward while the patient is in hospital.
- An experienced senior male nurse should be allocated to care for the patient, preferably isolated away from other patients.
- Antipsychotics should not be used to facilitate easier management.
- If the patient is physically violent then security must be called at once.
- It is not an acceptable request that a patient be removed by the police solely because they have behaved badly, when the patient needs medical care.
- Restraining measures may be required to prevent violent patients from hurting themselves or others, but restraint must always be the minimum necessary.
- Every case of restraint should be fully documented and reported as a critical incident (usually to the clinical risk department).
- Restraint should not be routinely used as an excuse for insufficient staff.
- Junior nurses or doctors should not make decisions regarding the medical care of such patients on their own and the consultant and hospital management must be informed.

> **Comments on the case**
>
> Unfortunately, this type of case is becoming more and more common. It is important that all doctors working in the NHS have some knowledge of how to deal with difficult patients, avoiding the temptation of taking the law into their own hands, and appreciating that there may be medical reasons to explain the bad behaviour.

Case 68 | Withdrawing treatment in intensive care

Candidate information

You are the medical doctor in intensive care medicine.

Please read this summary and then continue with the consultation.

Re: Mr Alfred Swallow, aged 80

Mr Swallow, an 80-year-old man, has cardiorespiratory and renal failure following an emergency aortic aneurysm repair 2 weeks ago. He remains intubated and sedated on the ICU and has been on maximum support, including inotropes and haemofiltration, for the last 8 days. You now strongly feel that the patient will not recover despite continuing with maximum therapy and you have been asked by the vascular surgeons for an opinion on withdrawing treatment. You approach the senior sister (Sister Green) to discuss the possibility of withdrawing treatment.

Your tasks are to: discuss with Sister Green the present medical condition of Mr Swallow, his most likely outcome and the possibility of withdrawing treatment.

Subject/patient/relative information

Sister Green is the nurse in charge of the ICU today and she and her other colleagues have been looking after Mr Swallow for the last 8 days. He was admitted to the unit after an emergency repair to a ruptured abdominal aortic aneurysm. His past medical history includes ischaemic heart disease and COPD. Since his admission, Mr Swallow has been intubated and sedated, has required inotropes (dobutamine and adrenaline) to maintain a decent cardiac output and 4 days ago he became anuric and acidotic which necessitated haemofiltration. He continues to be acidotic (base excess of -15), with a poor cardiac output (3.5 L/min) and needing a high FiO_2 (60%). There is one daughter who has been very supportive and understanding of the whole situation. She was always aware of the risks involved from the outset and she visits every day. The ICU doctor (the candidate) has been asked by the surgeons whether a plan should be made to withdraw treatment and whether he/she would like to discuss this with the ICU Sister. Sister Green does feel that a decision ought to be made regarding withdrawal of treatment as clearly the patient now has multiorgan failure and the outlook is very poor.

Thoughts and questions the patient/subject may have

- *Unfortunately the prognosis for Mr Swallow does not look good and we need to come up with a plan of where we go from here.*
- *I agree that withdrawing treatment is the next step but you or your consultant need to speak to his daughter first. She is very concerned about her father and visits every day.*

Examiner information

1. Conduct of interview
- Greet Sister Green and explain that you need to discuss Mr Swallow's condition.
- Firstly, confirm that there has been no improvement in the patient's condition over the last 8 days and obtain some objective evidence for this, e.g. vital signs, inotrope requirements, etc.
- Ask what Sister Green's opinion is on withdrawing treatment.
- Is there any family visiting the patient and how often?
- Have the family expressed any views on the patient's management and condition?
- Ask if she is aware of any wishes with regard to withdrawing treatment expressed by the patient (prior to illness) or the family.
- Ask if there is any member of staff known to her who would object to withdrawing treatment.
- Explain to Sister Green that you will be speaking to your consultant who will make the final decision.
- Ask her to call you when the family comes to visit the patient so that you can discuss the possibility of withdrawing treatment with them.
- Discuss with Sister Green which method of withdrawing treatment she feels is best for the patient and the family (withdrawing everything at once or gradually).

2. Exploration and problem negotiation
The candidate should be able to:
- recognize that the nursing staff are going to be more aware of the present condition of an ICU patient as they are the ones looking after the patient on a 24-h basis
- recognize that when a patient is in multiorgan failure and the outlook is poor, continuing treatment is not in the best interests of the patient
- appreciate the viewpoints of staff and family, including that of the patient before falling ill, if known
- acknowledge that withdrawing treatment is a team decision and not based purely on one individual's perspective.

3. Communication, ethics and the law
- The primary goal of medical treatment is to benefit the patient by restoring or maintaining the patient's health as far as possible, maximizing benefit and minimizing harm. If treatment fails or ceases to give a net benefit to the patient, that goal cannot be realized and the justification for providing the treatment is removed. Unless some other justification can be demonstrated, treatment that does not provide net benefit to the patient (ethically and legally) may be withheld or withdrawn and the goal of medical care should shift to the palliation of symptoms.
- Prolonging a patient's life usually, but not always, provides a health benefit to that patient. It is not an appropriate goal of medicine to prolong life at all costs with no regard to its quality or the burdens of treatment. Although emotionally it may be easier to withhold treatment than to withdraw that which has been started, there are no legal, or morally relevant, differences between the two actions. Even so, this is not to say that emotionally and psychologically the two are equivalent. Many health professionals, as well as patients, feel an emotional difference between withholding and withdrawing treatment. This is likely to be linked to the largely negative impression attached to a decision to withdraw treatment which can be interpreted as abandonment or 'giving up on the patient'. The BMA considers that where a particular treatment is no longer benefiting the patient, continuing to provide it would not be in the patient's best interests and, indeed, might be thought to be morally wrong. Greater emphasis on the reasons for providing treatment (including artificial nutrition and hydration), rather than the justification for withholding it may challenge this perceived difference. Treatment should never be withheld when there is a possibility that it will benefit the patient, simply because withholding is considered to be easier than withdrawing treatment.
- Developments in technology have led to a misperception in society that death can almost always be postponed. There needs to be a recognition that there comes a point in all lives where no more can reasonably or helpfully be done to benefit patients other than keeping them comfortable and free from pain.

Comments on the case

This case illustrates how important it is to make a team decision on the further management of the patient. Withdrawing and withholding treatment decisions involve many ethical issues, which the candidate must be aware of.

Further reading
British Medical Association. *End-of-life decisions: views of the BMA*. London: British Medical Association, 2009.

Section F
Experiences, Anecdotes, Tips, Quotations

'I know 'coz I was there.'*

---

*Max Boyce – referring to the victory of the Llanelli rugby team over the All Blacks, 9 points to 3, in October 1972. And then 'the pubs ran dry'.

These books exist as they are because of many previous candidates who, over the years, have completed our surveys and given us invaluable insight into the candidate experience. Please give something back by doing the same for the candidates of the future. For all of your sittings, whether they be a triumphant pass or a disastrous fail . . .

Remember to fill in the survey at www.ryder-mrcp.org.uk

THANK YOU

This section starts with full MRCP PACES *experiences*, written in the first person, of recent candidates since the change to PACES Station 5 in autumn 2009. There then follow some full PACES *experiences* from before the change in 2009. The aim is to give you an insight into the type of experience which lies ahead of you as well as, in the shorter accounts, to give a wider flavour of the type of combinations of cases that occur. Following this, we give further Station 2 and Station 4 *experiences* written in the first person. Then some miscellaneous anecdotes from our more recent surveys which have been referred to from Volume 1. Obviously, all these accounts represent the candidate's unchecked view of what the case was and what happened. Also they have not necessarily always remembered or bothered to record the exact wording of the written instruction, often preferring to just give us the basic 'Examine this patient's . . .'

This is followed by the majority of the experiences from the second edition of *An Aid to the MRCP Short Cases*, which are from the old-style examination. They span the last 10–20 years of the 20th century and, although the examination has changed from the 'short cases' which involved seeing six or more varied cases in 30 minutes with just two examiners, the later surveys have indicated that exactly the same cases are still appearing for the PACES format. The tragedies and triumphs do not seem to change with time.

We have placed the older extracts into specific groups. If an examiner spots a weakness, such as poor observation or examination technique, he or she is likely to explore this further before deciding whether to pass or fail a candidate. Consequently, some of the experiences are grouped according to which aspect of the candidate's clinical competence the examiner might have been probing most. A miscellaneous group of *anecdotes* follows the experiences. Although the outcome was not necessarily decided by the particular short case described, for additional information we have usually indicated whether the candidate passed or failed the overall exam.

A list of useful *tips* is given, and then the section finishes with a selection of *quotations* from successful MRCP candidates. At the end of the questionnaire, the candidates in our survey were asked if there were any comments they would like passed on to the candidates of the future. We felt that the consistencies and occasional discrepancies in the advice of such a large number of 'authorities' might be of interest to some candidates and so we present here a selection from those large number received. In order not to distort the force and intentions contained in these advisory comments, we have tended to offer them verbatim. Inevitably, some of the quotations are contradictory in their opinions – as with all examinations, individuals have different experiences and offer differing advice. Our views on these discrepancies are reflected throughout the book as far as they could be dealt with.* Ultimately, you will have to come to your own conclusion depending upon the circumstances of a particular case.

---

*For example, the discrepancies of quotations under the heading: 'Listen, obey and do not stray' – in general, we support extending the examination beyond the examiner's instruction, whenever necessary, so long as this is done with intelligence and discrimination.

Full PACES experiences in the first person (since 2009)

1. *I suggested then that an echo would be required to confirm the valvular problem causing the murmur, and was quizzed about the echo findings I'd look for, including the criteria for measuring a stenotic mitral valve!*

I spent about 10 weeks preparing for PACES, gradually increasing the practice time with colleagues and reading. I also attended the Hammersmith revision course 4 weeks beforehand.

Having been given a slot on the first exam rotation of the day, I travelled to London the day before with my fiancé (also revising for PACES at the time). There were several benefits of bringing him with me: firstly, we went out for a Chinese meal that evening (he paid!), and I even relaxed enough to have a glass of red wine!

As a result I managed to get some sleep and woke refreshed. Secondly, he made me eat breakfast! (a bacon sandwich, can anyone ever resist?), by reminding me of how incomprehensible I get if I don't eat. Thirdly, he helped me find the GUM department at St George's where the exam was to be held, a stress that I certainly hadn't thought about and wouldn't have desired just before the event.

We had to arrive about an hour before the exam actually started, and so there was quite a wait. Fortunately, there was coffee, water and even Danish pastries (but these had definitely lost their appeal by that point!). I knew one of the other candidates from the PACES course I'd attended 4 weeks previously, and so we chatted a little bit. There were five of us in total and all British graduates, a point which one of the candidates couldn't resist informing us meant that we were more competition for one another! I thought he was just trying to 'psych us out!'. I do wonder how he ever got on?

Finally we were brought to our first stations. I started with Station 3.

Station 3

Neurological: I was greeted by a very friendly, greying professor who introduced himself and his colleague. They then asked me to observe the lady sat in front of me and, to begin with, examine whatever I deemed most important!

Whilst this might have induced inner screams, the Asian lady had a clear asymmetrical upper and lower limb tremor. I therefore blew caution to the winds and went straight for it. I can't imagine how entertaining it must have been to see me trying to get a lady with

very little English to perform the tasks I wished her to, but she was quick (probably practised), and my smatterings of 'tikae?' made her smile (I think my accent was off). Despite this lack of an expressionless face, she demonstrated an asymmetric, distal, resting tremor (approximately 4 Hz), along with bradykinesia and a reduced amplitude of movement, whilst synkinesia increased contralateral tone. Her gait was not festinant, nor did she fall backwards and her eye movements were all present and normal. There was little else to detect on a fairly rushed normal motor exam, and consequently I failed to complete a full examination of sensation.

Having tried to target the examination, I realized I had elicited a hodge-podge of symptoms and therefore stated that a Parkinson's-like disorder would be at the top of my list of differentials. Before I could move on to list any other differentials, the Prof interrupted me and started to question me on what I would classically expect to find in Parkinson's disease. Whilst answering him the bell rang.

I still do not know what the diagnosis was, but from my breakdown it obviously wasn't Parkinson's. I got just enough marks to pass the examination but, interestingly, got full marks for communication!

Cardiovascular: I was ushered quickly into the next room, almost had alcohol gel squirted into my face before being asked to 'examine this gentleman's cardiovascular system'. He was Caucasian, of normal body habitus and elderly. He had no hand signs nor precordial scars.

His pulse was regular at both radial arteries, and of normal volume at the carotids. His apex beat was in the fifth intercostal space, mid-clavicular line, and on auscultation he had a pansystolic murmur audible across the precordium, but loudest at the left sternal border. There were no signs of pulmonary or peripheral oedema. At the time, I remember feeling annoyed that the peripheral signs did not add up with the quality and location of the murmur I had auscultated, and once again decided that honesty was the best policy. I was allowed to explain that I understood how a regular pulse and non-displaced apex beat do not go with a pansystolic murmur but that I would appreciate knowing the blood pressure in case the pulse pressure gave away any clues. I received my second smile and a reply of '120/80'. I suggested then that an echo would be required to confirm the valvular problem causing the murmur, and was quizzed about the echo findings I'd look for, including the criteria for measuring a stenotic mitral valve! Once again, I left feeling that I had done my best and tried to be sensible, but that once again had not got the diagnosis. My report confirmed that I dropped a few marks, but had still done enough to pass.

I think I had been lucky to start on that station and get my worst and most feared topics out of the way. I also had a few stations to compose again before the abdo and respiratory cases.

Station 4

I was given a few minutes to construct the plan for a counselling session with a gentleman newly diagnosed with HIV. He had contracted it following sexual indiscretions in Thailand whilst on business trips and had been informed of the diagnosis in a previous consultation. He was attending for further discussion and commencement of treatment.

This station flew by in a bit of a blur, but I concentrated hard initially to complete a good plan to direct my thoughts through it. It soon became clear that the gentleman did not wish to disclose his diagnosis to his wife, but was still having sexual contact with her. The consultation evolved to explain why this was necessary and to persuade him to do so, and explain to him the duties of the health services if he failed to do so. It was during this consultation that I realized how much I had got into the performance of it, and was treating it as a real encounter. I've always participated in drama, right up to graduation from university, and I think this really helped me to remain calm and 'perform' my way through it. The discussion at times was blunt, but always honest. As such I felt I created a rapport with the patient. The patient asked one question that I had to admit I did not know the answer to, but I ad libbed that I'd get the information for him for next time. I thought that would be an obvious hit for the examiners when we were done, but afterwards they asked me why I hadn't asked him about any other of his risk factors for HIV. I explained that as his mode of contraction had already been mentioned on the station information, I didn't think that was the best use of the time during this consultation when we came across such an important issue. I passed the station, dropping 1 mark.

Station 5

Once again, I tried to compose myself as much as possible between stations so as to think clearly for the dreaded station 5s.

Case 1: My first involved a gentleman in his fifties complaining of a painful left knee. In fact, he had a warm knee with a small effusion, which I demonstrated by dredging up the mantra of 'look, feel and move'. I certainly hadn't practised lots of knee examinations! He also had psoriatic patches on his extensor surfaces and telescoped fingers. I managed to take a history and examine at the same time, and picked up that he was on biological therapies to control his arthritis. I therefore explained that I was most concerned about him having a septic arthritis which should be ruled out promptly. My plan, therefore, included taking a full blood count to rule out lympho/neutropenia, tapping the joint for microbiology, and commencing antibiotics before investigating for inadequate control of his arthritis.

Case 2: My second station involved interviewing a gentleman in his 70s about his memory loss. This appeared to have occurred over a year and was progressive in nature. He scored 7/10 from an AMT10 and his main problems were with name finding and remembering to complete everyday tasks. I took quite an extended social history and established an unremarkable past medical history. A brief neurological and cardiological exam ruled out obvious deficits and atrial fibrillation so that my major differential included Alzheimer's dementia. I broached this by asking the patient what he was most concerned about and he agreed that he was worried about a dementing process. On questioning, I therefore suggested collecting a collateral history, arranging for a CT head (to rule out a subdural haematoma) and an ECG to confirm an absence of a cardiac arrhythmia. It was so hard to judge how I had done, especially with the severest-looking examiner, and quite a history-based station. I began to hope that I hadn't done too badly though after the patient chirped 'well done' to me as the bell tolled! Overall, it was just like being on MAU!

Station 1

Respiratory: Grateful to be back to the pure examination-based stations, I had to mentally shake off the preceding stations to stay focused, and this was getting increasingly difficult. My respiratory case involved examining an Asian middle-aged gentleman with clubbing, on 2 litres of oxygen and who, on auscultation, had end-inspiratory crepitations accompanied by scattered coarser crepitations. I diagnosed pulmonary fibrosis with evidence of type 1 but not type 2 failure (a normal PO_2). I started to offer differentials and was interrupted and requested to state how I'd investigate. I suggested chest X-ray, possibly followed by HRCT and pulmonary function tests. They then asked me what differentiated the clinical findings of pulmonary fibrosis and pulmonary oedema. I suggested that crepitations in oedema occur during both inspiration and expiration, and that there may be evidence of left-sided heart failure, including a loud P2.

Abdominal: I was then led to the abdominal station where I was asked to examine a young lady with abdominal pain. I groaned inwardly with the realization that one wince from the patient could end my chances! I was so careful and attentive during the examination and elicited spider naevi, abdominal striae and a 6 cm hepatomegaly in the absence of splenomegaly. There was no ascites and so I offered a diagnosis of compensated chronic liver disease to the examiners. I stated that the striae may have been due to previous ascites or steroid use and, given the plethora of spider naevi, I suspected autoimmune hepatitis, but that alcoholic liver disease and virally induced hepatitis were important and common differentials. I suggested an ultrasound scan of the abdomen after which I was asked what findings I would expect. I answered that I would look for confirmation of the organomegaly, any focal lesions, and the patency of the hepatic arteries, veins and portal vein. Reversed flow within intrahepatic vessels might represent the presence of a fibrosing process therein. Finally, they asked me outright whether I was sure there was no splenomegaly. It surprised me going back to my clinical findings so that I had to take a second to think, but then I remembered that the lady had a resonant left hypochondrium so I decided to be confident and said 'there was definitely no splenomegaly'.

I got full marks for the station!

Station 2

Almost heady to be near the end of the exam, I somewhat staggered into the final history station. I was introduced to a middle-aged woman complaining of tiredness. The scenario was set in a general practice. I got a 2-month history of proximal muscle stiffness in the mornings, such that she could not go to work for 9 am. There was no arthritis or arthralgia, rash or tender musculature. I completed the rest of a medical history, ensuring to rule out any evidence of giant cell arteritis. I asked her what her major problems and complaints were. The lethargy and stiffness came top. I explained

my suspicion of polymyalgia rheumatica and what that meant. I then explained that we would have to perform blood tests and start a course of steroids if there was evidence of inflammation. We then discussed steroids and the need for a protracted course, and the side-effects of them. As a postmenopausal lady, I therefore also decided to order a DEXA scan to assess her bone density pre-steroids. I explained that if the investigations did not indicate PMR then it would be advisable to perform a muscle biopsy to look for myositis. Further investigations might follow that. The patient was happy and understood all of the above, and I made a plan to meet the patient in a week's time to review the blood results. Following that, the bell still hadn't gone, so we discussed smoking cessation and I said I'd provide information about local smoking cessation services! I felt it went really well, and actually enjoyed the realistic interaction.

Comments

I left and pretty much instantly started remembering everything I hadn't done or said, and slept through the whole train journey home! Thankfully I passed first time. On reflection, I think it helped me to try and imagine that I was on MAU. In that way I kept my focus on the patient and always tried to be confident and relaxed with the patient if not the examiners! Then by being sensible and safe with my suggestions, I didn't dig any holes for myself on questioning.

---

2. *During the history taking it was obvious that the patient had a high BMI, a family history of premature cardiovascular events, osmotic symptoms suggestive of diabetes and also the classic symptoms of obstructive sleep apnoea.*

Station 1

Respiratory: This was a patient with bronchiectasis and rheumatoid lung disease. I was asked to examine the respiratory system and found evidence of left basal bronchiectasis. I also luckily noticed that the patient had florid rheumatoid changes in both hands. I was asked about the aetiology and management of bronchiectasis. I felt confident that this one had gone well and I scored 18 out of 20.

Abdominal: I was also very confident with the abdominal case. I had been asked just to examine the abdomen medically and there was no other information given with that request. The patient had a mid-line laparotomy scar but apart from that I could not find any other abnormalities. I was told later that the patient had had a fall from a height as an adolescent and I was asked for a differential diagnosis for the scar. I suggested splenic rupture with subsequent splenectomy and the discussion went in the direction of needing to give the indications for such a procedure, what the blood picture would be post splenectomy and any other precautions that would need to be taken postoperatively. I was really quite concerned that I had missed something in the examination but was reassured by the nature of the discussion. In fact, I scored 20 out of 20 for this case.

Station 2

In the history-taking station I was presented with a patient who had had an incidental finding of hyperlipidaemia discovered and the GP had referred in for further management. During the history taking it was obvious that the patient had a high BMI, a family history of premature cardiovascular events, osmotic symptoms suggestive of diabetes and also the classic symptoms of obstructive sleep apnoea.

Station 3

Cardiovascular: I was asked to examine the patient's cardiovascular system. I found that he had dextrocardia and aortic regurgitation. I also noticed that he had florid osteoarthrosis. I was asked about the investigations that I would perform to confirm dextrocardia and what the likely aetiology of the aortic regurgitation could be. I felt that I spent too much time looking for the apex beat and for evidence of situs inversus and was left with very little time to complete all the cardiac manoeuvres. I only scored 16 out of 20 for this case.

Neurological: However, I was then very confident with my neuro case. I was asked to examine the lower limbs of a patient who had difficulty in walking. I found that he had a symmetrical sensorimotor polyneuropathy and there was a bottle of glicloside tablets on the bedside table. I was asked about the differential diagnosis and the investigations I would do for a patient with mononeuritis multiplex and I scored 19 out of 20.

Station 4

For the communications station I had an elderly lady who had presented with delirium on a background of dementia. The main thrust of the scenario was to discuss the medical management and then the involvement of social services when the husband was very reluctant to accept any help.

Station 5

Case 1: For the first case I had a patient with atypical psoriatic arthropathy and I was fairly sure that there was some rheumatoid overlap here. I was asked about the appropriate management for this patient and I scored full marks with 28 out of 28.

Case 2: The next patient was a 50-year-old lady with polymyalgia rheumatica and giant cell arteritis. I had been informed that she had presented with new-onset, left-sided headache and blurring of vision and I found that she had a tender scalp in the left temporal area. I was asked what the indications for steroids would be and would I do a temporal artery biopsy. Again, I scored full marks with 28 out of 28.

> **Comments**
>
> I passed PACES at this sitting.

3. *This resulted in me attempting to exit my cardiovascular station via a cleaner's cupboard, much to the examiners' amusement.*

Station 5

I started at Station 5 and a resumé of my cases and questions is as follows.

Case 1: 'Poorly-controlled diabetic who had noticed problems with vision over the last fortnight'. I went into this case thinking cataracts or retinopathy and spent the first few minutes eyeing up the ophthalmoscope, wondering whether I was going to be able to switch it on. Fortunately, I did not jump straight to ophthalmoscopy but examined the eyes in the routine I had learned, and picked up a right homonymous hemianopia. This was followed by a rather hurried backtrack of the history, this time focusing on TIA/CVA symptoms whilst doing a quick power/sensation assessment. I was asked where the lesion was likely to be to result in this visual defect and the likely causes of it, and then about secondary prevention of stroke.

Case 2: 'This gentleman has come for review in the stroke clinic following a left MCA infarct. He now complains of a bad back'. The important part of this stem was the bad back, which turned out to be a very obvious ankylosing spondylitis, but when sat outside reading this scenario, I was thrown by the mention of the stroke follow-up, and had scribbled down to ask about secondary prevention, swallow problems, etc. I think the reason for this inclusion was that the patient obviously did have a dense hemiplegia. I was asked about management of ankylosing spondylitis and about the extra-articular features of the disease.

Station 1

Respiratory: This was a patient with a very straightforward upper lobectomy with otherwise normal lungs. They asked me for the indications for this operation, and confirmed it was a malignancy. Then they asked about how I would investigate a breathless patient and the possible differentials.

Abdominal: This was a patient with chronic liver disease with hepatomegaly. It was by no means a barn door case and I felt that the examiners could sense my hesitancy. They asked me about causes of hepatomegaly and how I would investigate the patient. I missed a Dupuytren's contracture which they then made me re-examine for, but I was actually very grateful for this because I felt they were helping me to be more confident about my diagnosis.

Station 2

I had a young farmer with breathlessness and a cough. As usual, there were many clues to tease out. He worked with hay, he had asthma as a boy, he had recently been put on an ACE inhibitor and there were, of course, all the social dilemmas to explore – his wife had MS and was deteriorating, there was nobody to man the farm, and money was tight, etc. Having said all of this, on the whole it was a nice station. I was asked to rank my differential diagnoses in order, with extrinsic allergic alveolitis the diagnosis they wished to discuss.

Station 3

Cardiology: The cardiac case was the toughest by a long-shot. It was a man in his forties who was absolutely covered in scars with a precordium like a music box and an absent left radial pulse. I think it was a corrected tetralogy of Fallot with a Blalock shunt, but what the examiners really wanted to get out of me was what the murmur was that I could hear. It was a VSD but it was like pulling teeth to get me there. The patient gave me a big thumbs-up sign when I finally got it!!

Neurology: The neuro case was a very straightforward case of peripheral neuropathy. I was asked about the possible causes. The examiner confirmed it was diabetes and then proceeded to ask me about how I would control this patient's blood sugar, and did I know of any new drugs on the market. We talked about the gliptins and DDP4 inhibitors, which I felt slightly off the point for a neuro station but the examiner was clearly a diabetologist!

Station 4

The communication skills station was about breaking the bad news to a young mother who had been diagnosed as having active TB and HIV as a result of her partner being unfaithful. There was so much to cover here including admittance to hospital for isolation, working out who would have her son, disclosing the information to her partner (she refused at first, but was easily persuaded), and screening her son for TB. She even asked me about the side-effects of the treatment which I really only went into very briefly as I was concerned about information overload. The discussion that followed was about breaching confidentiality to third parties at risk and the use of the Public Health Act to admit patients with infectious disease for treatment.

Comments

I sat my exam in Edinburgh and it was my first attempt. Overall, I would say it was far less of an ordeal than I had built it up to be, and the administrative staff were incredibly friendly which immediately put me at ease.

The most, and probably only, distressing part of the morning was the fact that I had absolutely no idea where I was. The outpatient department layout was very odd and I felt like I was being spun in circles in between stations and literally being herded through doors by the exam staff. This resulted in me attempting to exit my cardiovascular station via a cleaner's cupboard, much to the examiners' amusement. Fortunately, my sense of direction was not being assessed and they passed me anyway.

4. *I was given an ophthalmoscope to use.*

Station 1

Respiratory: I was asked to examine a patient's chest. I found bilateral crackles from the base to the mid zones on both sides and the patient was very thin. I was fairly confident that the diagnosis was of pulmonary fibrosis and I was asked what investigations I would do. I said that I would perform bedside spirometry and a peak flow and then would proceed to a CT thorax to confirm my diagnosis. They kept asking what other investigations I would do but I couldn't actually think of any.

Abdominal: I was then asked to examine a patient's abdomen. I found a palpable, ballotable mass in the right iliac fossa and I also noted a parathyroidectomy scar. I wasn't really very sure about this case but I assume that the abdominal mass was a transplanted kidney. I was asked about the cause of renal failure so I started to talk, and went on talking on everything I knew about renal failure and transplants but in a fairly structured way. I think that they had then run out of questions by the time I had finished! However, the last question was a bit more tricky because they asked me about calcium metabolism in renal failure and then I fell apart a bit but was saved by the bell.

Station 2

For my history-taking patient, I had a lady in her 40s with diarrhoea which sounded more like malabsorption in nature and I cannot really remember much more about it.

Station 3

Cardiovascular: I was asked to examine a patient's precordium and I found a pansystolic murmur, a mid-line sternotomy scar but no scars on the legs to suggest a bypass graft. I really wasn't at all sure about this one. I found it very difficult as I also couldn't hear any artificial valve sounds so I went down the route of coronary artery bypass graft plus aortic stenosis or mitral regurgitation and I couldn't make up my mind as there were hardly any other clinical signs. The examiner seemed surprised that I could not hear artificial valve sounds so I assumed I had probably missed something but I stuck to my decision, not wanting to back-pedal as I thought that would look worse.

Neurological: I was then asked to examine a patient's lower limbs, neurologically. There had been previous spinal surgery in the upper lumbar region and I found lower motor neurone signs in the left leg in L5 distribution. I was asked for a differential diagnosis and what investigations I would perform. I was pleased that I remembered to get him to walk and also looked at his spine before I started to examine the legs. However, I ran out of time before I could complete sensation and proprioception.

Station 4

For the communications skills, I had to discuss with the 'patient' about doing an HIV test as he had presented with PCP pneumonia and he had a male partner. The objective of the consultation was to discuss what his diagnosis meant in terms of the risk of HIV and the need for HIV testing. It was very difficult for the patient to take all the information in even though I gave it slowly and piecemeal. His main concern was that he didn't want to discuss it with his partner at all as he had had three affairs. I had to discuss the implications for a positive test for him and his partner when he had not been using condoms. During the questioning, I was asked how I felt the patient/actor had responded to the information I had given and how could I improve his understanding and retention of the information that he had received.

Station 5

Case 1: This was a young woman in her late teens/early twenties with known ulcerative colitis presenting with back pain and stiffness. I was asked to assess. It was obvious that they were expecting me to look for the symptoms and signs of ankylosing spondylitis. I was even given a measuring tape.

Case 2: This was a woman in her 40s who had presented to clinic with headaches. She was anxious for investigations to be done and was worried about serious intracranial pathology but clinically they were benign migrainous headaches. I was given an ophthalmoscope to use.

Comments

I passed PACES at this sitting.

---

5. *In retrospect, I think they were getting at secondary amyloidosis.*

Station 1

Respiratory: I was shown a male patient and told that he had presented with breathlessness and I was to examine his chest. I found the stigmata of regular BM monitoring, a right brachiocephalic fistula which was working and there was an IV cannula in place. He had an increased respiratory rate, cough, right basal dullness with overlying crackles and a few left basal crackles. I thought his main problem was of a chest infection with consolidation and probable pneumonia and there was dullness at the lung base. I was asked about the diagnosis (Light's criteria) and for a differential diagnosis of a unilateral pleural effusion and how would I investigate him.

Abdominal: The patient had hepatosplenomegaly and chronic liver disease. I was very confident about this case. I was asked to examine his abdomen and to report my findings. I found just about a full house of signs for chronic liver disease with hepatosplenomegaly but with no signs of decompensation. I was asked for a differential diagnosis of hepatosplenomegaly, how I would do a liver screen and how I would manage any hepatic decompensation.

Station 2

In the history taking I was faced with a man with bilateral leg swelling. It soon became apparent that his diagnosis was actually bronchiectasis secondary to measles that he had had at the age of 4. However, the leg swelling was new, bilateral and progressive. I diagnosed cor pulmonale secondary to bronchiectasis but it was obvious that the examiners were trying to get at something else which I couldn't fathom out. I suggested that one ought to do an echo to investigate his right heart and they asked what I would think if he had global hypertrophy. In retrospect, I think they were getting at secondary amyloidosis. They then asked me to summarize the whole case and we talked about differentials and investigations. Quite a bit of time was spent with the examiners pushing me towards the diagnosis of amyloid.

Station 3

Cardiovascular: I was only slightly confident about this case. I was asked to examine a man's cardiovascular system. I found an ejection systolic murmur with a loud S2 radiating to the back. He was a well-looking man with no scars and the murmur was heard best at the left upper sternal edge and exacerbated by inspiration. I said that he had pulmonary stenosis and was asked

about the differential diagnosis and the causes and management of pulmonary stenosis.

Neurological: The patient had Parkinson's disease and I was very confident with that diagnosis. I was asked to examine the upper limbs and found the classic features of Parkinson's disease. By now, there was little time left for many questions as I had been talked through the examination and I thought that that didn't go very well. The only question they did ask at the end was about the management of Parkinson's disease. I was actually a bit slow in picking up the Parkinsonian features and I think that they would have been really obvious if I had used my observational skills more cleverly.

Station 4

I had a scenario of an 18-year-old who was on the intensive care unit. He was postictal and the fit was secondary to the use of Ecstasy. I was asked to speak to his mother but the patient had asked me not to tell her about the cause of the fit. The instruction had been to tell the mother about his condition and the diagnosis and to talk to her about his driving as he was a van driver by occupation, whilst not mentioning anything to do with the drugs. I explained to her what had happened and that we were investigating him and I remained deliberately vague about the cause, saying that we didn't really quite know yet and that in 50% of patients like this, the probability was that they would not have another seizure. She asked if her daughter could be affected and if it could happen again and what the implications were, all of which then led on to a conversation about DVLA guidelines. They wanted me to justify not mentioning the drugs as a possible cause. I think they felt that I should have said we do not know the cause but that I had a duty of confidentiality to the patient whereas what I actually did was just to steer the 'mother' away from any discussion about the aetiology. They asked which ethical principles were important here and they seemed relatively happy with my answers.

Station 5

Case 1: My pre-case information was: 'this is a man who is blind in one eye and has had worsening vision in the other eye over the past month'. The diagnosis was Marfan's syndrome. The patient attributed his blind left eye to 'a lens problem'. He reported a family history of Marfan's and had his shirt open revealing a median sternotomy scar. In fact, he had nearly all the signs for Marfan's. On questioning, he asked if there was any link between his heart problem ('something to do with my valves') and his eye complaint. The examiners wanted to know about his gait and what I noticed about his hips (I didn't notice anything except kyphoscoliosis, although in retrospect I think his pelvis was tilted). They asked me several questions about Marfan's syndrome and wanted to know that the most important step in his management was an urgent referral to an ophthalmologist.

Case 2: The pre-case information was 'this woman presents with sore joints associated with dry eyes and mouth'. The patient gave a history of Raynaud's, Sjögren's and polyarthralgia. There was no history of other autoimmune disease. She had few signs – perhaps mild sclerodactyly. She also complained of tingling in Vb/Vc divisions of the trigeminal nerve but she had no objective signs. The discussion was around autoimmune profiles, diagnosis of rheumatoid arthritis, mixed connective tissue disease and the relevant managements. I suspect this was mixed connective tissue disease, but was not sure.

Comments

At the time of writing I have not had my results.

6. *I had no clue as to the diagnosis when I had finished my examination. Surprisingly, I did quite well on this station – it's not all lost if you don't have a definite diagnosis at the end! Just describe your findings, give a sensible basic differential and lay out how you'd go on to investigate.*

Station 3

Neurological: I was taken to the neurology case and basically asked to examine the legs. There was a wheelchair by the side of the bed and a written instruction on the wall said, 'This gentleman has difficulty walking. Please examine his lower limbs from a neurological perspective'.

I found the changes of peripheral vascular disease in the lower legs (loss of hair from shin down, neuropathic ulcer). There was peripheral sensory loss to mid-shin. There was no motor deficit. There was loss of vibration sense up to the hip and there was pain when testing sensation peripherally. They had actually hidden the vibration fork and only produced it when I said I would like to test vibration sense!

I gave the diagnosis of diabetic sensory peripheral neuropathy and I was asked for the differential diagnosis of sensory peripheral neuropathy and for the causes of a painful neuropathy. I was asked how I would investigate and which bloods I would send for in doing a 'neuropathy screen' (B12, etc.).

Cardiovascular: For the cardiac case I was shown a young lady and told, 'This lady had an operation as a child. Examine her cardiovascular system'. I found a mid-line sternotomy and an axillary scar. There were just loads of murmurs and a heaving apex. I had NO idea of the diagnosis when finishing the examination. It was in fact a Blalock–Taussig shunt and tetralogy of Fallot. I was asked about the findings and for a differential diagnosis. I said I had heard a pansystolic murmur – they asked me for the differential of a pansystolic murmur and how I would investigate. Then they went on to ask me what features I might expect to see on an echocardiogram in severe mitral regurgitation.

I had no clue as to the diagnosis when I had finished my examination. Surprisingly, I did quite well on this station – it's not all lost if you don't have a definite diagnosis at the end! Just describe your findings, give a sensible basic differential and lay out how you'd go on to investigate.

Station 4

I then moved on to Station 4 and the setting given was: 'You have planned to discharge an 83-year-old back to her own home after being admitted for a urinary tract infection and falls. She has had two recent admissions following falls at home. She has been assessed by the physiotherapist and occupational therapist, both of whom had done a home visit and instituted a package of care. After the acute delirium from the urinary tract infection the patient had been reassessed as having mental capacity. She had refused residential care, despite this being her third hospital admission in 6 months for falls. The daughter has arrived back in the UK from a holiday in the Caribbean and is angry about the fact her mum is being discharged and wants her sent to a residential home. Discuss her concerns and agree a plan of management'.

This was a common situation for any medical SHO! The best tip I had for the communication station was that you could offer whatever you want (scan the same day, consultant meeting that afternoon, clinic appointment next week) which makes agreeing a plan of action much easier than in the real world. Here we ended up arranging for a multidisciplinary team meeting the next day to include the patient, the daughter and the consultant to discuss the concerns regarding discharge and that we'd postpone implementation of the package of care until we'd had that meeting.

I was asked about what strategies can you use within hospital to plan for a difficult discharge? Why couldn't I send the patient straight to a residential home? Why did you think the daughter was angry? Is there anything you could have done differently during the consultation in retrospect?

Station 5

Case 1: The first patient had a foot drop and ulnar nerve palsy. I am sure it was a mononeuritis multiplex. There was a history of intermittent problems with typing at work and then difficulty walking. There were no other features of vasculitis or demyelinating disease. She had worked as a computer engineer so was finding it difficult at work due to the problems typing. There were no bladder or visual problems or stigmata of multiple sclerosis. I examined the gait and upper limb neurology and confirmed the foot drop and ulnar nerve palsy. I was asked about the causes of mononeuritis multiplex and how to investigate. I was then asked about the immediate management and would I admit the patient?

Case 2: The second patient was elderly and had presented with falls. He was a 65-year-old man who had been falling at home and this was always in the morning. There were lots of reasons! He had atrial fibrillation, was taking lots of antihypertensives, was diabetic taking a high dose of gliclazide just before bed, and had a history of previous TIAs. The hidden agenda was that he had to look after his disabled wife and didn't want to be admitted to hospital. I arranged a plan for ECG, carotid Dopplers, to reduce the dose of evening gliclazide and to see the diabetic specialist nurse that afternoon. I said I would check for postural hypotension and would adjust the antihypertensives accordingly. I also said I would refer to the social worker for help with his wife. Again – this is the perfect imaginary healthcare system where you can offer all of these services on the same day. This initially looked like a pretty simple scenario but turned out to be somewhat more involved!!

I was asked questions about the differential diagnosis, and the management and investigation of TIAs. They also asked if I thought I should have admitted this patient!

To pass the exam, you have to get good marks in the Station 5 scenarios as over one-third of the marks for the exam are based on this station due to the changes in mark distribution. Of my friends that failed, they invariably had messed up on this station, even when they did well elsewhere. I lost quite a few marks on the history station and Stations 1 and 3 but was spared having to sit the exam again as I had a strong showing in Station 5 which mopped up for mishaps elsewhere! There is very little time for the Station 5 scenarios and there is a lot to cover here. It's easy to run over and not get the marks allocated for addressing/managing patient concerns and explaining the management plan at the end. More than any other station, I think it's important to practise made-up scenarios with colleagues just to get an idea of how long 8 minutes actually is. Also, always revise with a mark scheme in your hand so that you can learn to tailor your approach to where the marks lie. It would be easy to spend your 8 minutes in Station 5 just doing an excellent history but you'd only get 2 points! Make it easy for the examiners to give you the points and make sure you learn an approach that will consistently cover all the bases on the mark scheme. Station 5 is the only one that tests EVERY skill.

Station 1

Respiratory: Again, there was an instruction on the wall, 'This patient has been complaining of shortness of breath. Please examine his respiratory system'. I found him to be tachypnoeic, cachectic and with a deviated trachea (I missed this but they took me back to it during questioning). There was an opioid patch in the left axilla. Other candidates heard reduced breath sounds in the left base but again I missed this!

In retrospect, I know he had a lobar collapse secondary to a bronchial neoplasm. I missed the clinical signs here and was punished accordingly with a low score for this station! As I hadn't got a very good list of differentials, they led the questioning down the route of the investigations of acute dyspnoea and pulmonary emboli. I think they were asking me easier questions than on previous stations as my performance had been quite poor during the examination and presentation.

Abdominal: I was told, 'This patient has been complaining of abdominal swelling. Please examine his abdomen'. I found a full house of signs of chronic liver disease together with massive ascites with a recent dressing from a possible ascitic tap. There was an encephalopathic flap. He had evidently been taken from the ward that day as he seemed quite unwell! I was asked, 'What are the causes of hepatic decompensation?', 'Why did I think the patient was decompensated?', 'What is hepatic encephalopathy and how is it graded?', 'What would you send an ascitic tap for?', 'How would you tell if the ascites was a transudate if the patient had low serum albumin (serum albumin ascites gradient)?', 'What are the indications for the use of terlipressin in hepatorenal syndrome?', 'What are the autoimmune and metabolic causes of hepatic failure?', and 'What is the important initial investigation in decompensated liver failure?'. I had finished the examination in 4 minutes, leaving more time for a thorough grilling! Being a budding gastroenterologist, I was quite confident on this subject. However, if I did the exam again I'd definitely try not to finish examining quite so quickly!

Station 2

I really messed up Station 2 as I lost track of time and so lost my structure – and (deservedly!) got slammed in the marking! In the 5 minutes before you go in, just make a list of subheadings (presenting complaint, history of presenting complaint, social history) so you don't lose your way in the heat of the moment. I thought I would nail the history section as we do it every day of our working life but the opposite turned out to be true! The patient was a 56-year-old diabetic

---

Comments

I can't remember being as nervous as this about anything else in my life! Almost as big a part of the exam as medical knowledge is having the ability to stay calm under pressure, give sensible (even if not necessarily correct) responses to questions and not to fall apart. Although its clichéd to say it, they are right about putting a bad station behind you and moving on to the next as being very important. Also, don't neglect Station 5 and practise well for this when revising. Of the group of us sitting PACES at my hospital, the performance at this station has seemed to make or break one's success or failure at the exam. If you mess up Station 5 you have to have an almost perfect performance elsewhere to make up for it as there is such a high proportion of marks allocated here (56 points for Station 5, 16 points for communication skills).

I passed. Good luck to you all!!

---

with hypothyroidism, weight loss and tiredness. There had been diarrhoea for 5 weeks and the bloods showed an iron deficiency anaemia. The patient was worried that this may represent cancer. However, the eventual diagnosis was coeliac disease but they had to lead me to this in the questioning. I was asked about the investigation of iron deficiency anaemia, the autoantibodies to be found and the associations with coeliac disease. I was asked why I didn't think it was inflammatory bowel disease.

7. *On examination the patient had obvious signs of Graves' disease. I was asked questions regarding the management of thyroid eye disease (prisms in spectacles, artificial tears, steroids, radiotherapy, surgery).*

Station 1

Respiratory: The case was interstitial lung disease and probably it was fibrosis. I had been asked to examine the patient's respiratory system and I had found bruising with thin skin and bilateral basal crepitations.

Abdominal: I was fairly confident also with the abdominal case. It was a patient with ascites and chronic liver disease. I had been asked to examine the man's abdominal system and found all the classic features of ascites. The examiner asked me what could cause this patient to present with an upper gastrointestinal haemorrhage.

Station 2

I had the following instruction: 'You're a medical SHO in clinic and please take a history'. I was presented with a lady with poorly controlled diabetes. The subsequent questioning centred on what my advice would be if this patient had asked me about becoming pregnant.

Station 3

Cardiovascular: I was asked to examine a patient's cardiovascular system. I was only slightly confident about this one but I found a collapsing pulse and I also thought that I could hear an Austin Flint murmur so I was more or less certain that this was lone aortic incompetence.

Neurological: I was then asked to examine the next patient's legs neurologically and found evidence of a motor and sensory neuropathy and all the visual features of Charcot–Marie–Tooth disease. There was symmetrical wasting and weakness of the distal muscles of the legs in the classic inverted champagne bottle distribution. The examiners pushed me on the differential diagnosis for these clinical findings.

Station 4

I just cannot remember what happened in this station at all!

Station 5

Case 1: My first case in Station 5 was a young woman (role taken by an actress) who had had an episode of headache followed by diplopia that had then completely resolved. There had been no previous similar episodes. There was no significant past medical history as far as I can remember. The MRI brain scan was normal as was a recent LP (the 'patient' freely volunteered this information). There was nil to find on examination. I was asked questions regarding the differential diagnosis. I'm not sure of the actual diagnosis they were looking for.

Case 2: This was a middle-aged woman (actual patient) presenting with dry, sore eyes. I can't recall if I was given any history of previous thyroid disease or not. On examination, the patient had obvious signs of Graves' disease. I was asked questions regarding the management of thyroid eye disease (prisms in spectacles, artificial tears, steroids, radiotherapy, surgery).

Comments

I failed PACES at this sitting.

---

8. *The discussion then centred around whether I can breach confidentiality and I said that in this case we ought to breach confidentiality and ask her husband and his contacts to be tested.*

Station 3

Cardiovascular: The cardiovascular case was a gentleman with a subclavicular scar on the left side but with no pacemaker *in situ*. He was definitely in atrial fibrillation. I couldn't feel the apex but there was a good going pansystolic murmur best heard at the 'apex' area. I described it as mitral regurgitation and was about to say how to investigate when they stopped me and asked me to present again the positive findings. I started with the irregularly irregular pulse and they interrupted again there and asked how I would deal with it. The discussion went on to the CHAD score and management of atrial fibrillation.

Neurological: For the neuro case I was next taken to a gentleman and the examiner said, 'This man has weakness on walking. Examine his upper limbs and explain the cause for the weakness'. I found unilateral upper motor neurone weakness with brisk reflexes and decreased power on the left side. All sensory modalities were impaired unilaterally up to the shoulder. I hesitated with the differential diagnosis and after some prompting I noticed the facial asymmetry. I said that he had a hemiplegia following a cerebrovascular event and the discussion then concentrated on the appropriate investigations.

Station 4

Apparently this scenario had appeared on a few occasions. A young housewife, whose husband is a long distance lorry driver, was diagnosed with sputum-positive TB and HIV. I was asked to explain the diagnosis and risk factors and agree on a management plan. I explained to her that she would need admission and that her son and other close relatives would need to be investigated for TB. I asked her whether there was anybody to take care of her son.

I told her very sensitively about the diagnosis of HIV and that actually she had AIDS but that there is treatment that will keep the condition under control and that we need to start this as soon as possible. I asked her about the risk factors. It seemed obvious that her husband was the source but he was currently abroad on work. I asked whether she would be agreeable for the Public Health department to contact him and request him to be investigated and treated. She was happy with this plan and she agreed to be admitted the same day. My impression was that she was very cooperative. It seemed that I did not say anything wrong to upset her or to blame anybody.

The discussion then centred around whether I can breach confidentiality and I said that in this case we ought to breach confidentiality and ask her husband and his contacts to be tested. They asked what I would do if the son was found to be HIV positive. In the scenario it was mentioned that the lady had a negative HIV test when she was pregnant. I said that in this case if he tested positive then I would suspect abuse and would need to inform social services. Thankfully the bell rang and I had to move to the next station.

Station 5

Case 1: This was an elderly lady with an obvious unilateral thyroid eye. She had noticed blurred vision for a few weeks. I asked about her past medical history and this included a partial thyroidectomy, palpitations and ischaemic heart disease that had required coronary artery bypass grafting. My differential diagnosis was either recurrence of the Graves' disease with thyroid ophthalmopathy or a stroke as she was an arteriopath with atrial fibrillation. I offered investigations for both diagnoses and there was not enough time for any discussion.

Case 2: This was a gentleman in his mid-forties with a few weeks' history of night sweats, weight loss and lethargy. From the history taking, he was known to have mitral valve prolapse and had had a recent dental procedure. On examination, there was a very loud pansystolic murmur. I explained to him that it was very likely that he had infective endocarditis and that he had to be admitted for blood tests and to be started on intravenous antibiotics. The examiners asked me whether I would wait for the ECHO results before starting antibiotics and I said, 'no'. Again, the bell rang immediately after the first question.

Station 1

Abdominal: The patient was a young lady in her thirties with jaundice and hepatomegaly. She was very cachexic. The abdomen was very distended but I could not identify any shifting dullness. There was a mildly enlarged liver but with no spleen palpable. There was a big tattoo on her back. I offered a differential diagnosis of hepatomegaly with chronic liver disease with possible hepatitis C as well in view of the tattoo. They asked if it could be a haematological malignancy. I said it was possible even without an enlarged spleen but that would be very rare. There wasn't time for more questions.

Respiratory: This was a patient who was mildly short of breath. There were bilateral coarse inspiratory and expiratory crackles at the bases with a widespread wheeze. I said that he had a background of obstructive airways disease with findings of pulmonary fibrosis. They asked me for a differential diagnosis and then I realized that I had actually heard bronchiectasis on auscultation. So I corrected myself and the discussion then was about how to investigate bronchiectasis and its management with physiotherapy, long-term oxygen and antibiotics. Although I couldn't answer every single question, I was getting enough positive feedback that the examiner was happy with my explanations.

Station 2

I have heard that this scenario was done by two other colleagues in different centres.

A gentleman presents with a haemoglobin of 8.9 g, microcytic, and is on warfarin for an aortic valve replacement. His father had died of bowel cancer.

I took a full history for the anaemia. He was asymptomatic without any bleeding and was maintaining a good diet. There had been no weight loss and he had no concerns. He was a lifelong smoker. I offered him smoking cessation advice and he was annoyed by that. I explained that there is a condition that can occur in people with aortic stenosis called angiodysplasia but that it is very rare.

I told him that we have to investigate with a sigmoidoscopy and explained what that was. I explained that if we don't identify a source of bleeding with that then we will do colonoscopy.

During the discussion the examiner said he was very pleased to hear that I would perform a rectal examination and that I would not give him a blood transfusion as he was asymptomatic.

Comments

With regard to Station 5, my impression was that although the time was just enough for taking a history and examining the patient, there was not enough time for making a proper plan and there was no time for a good discussion at all so the marks had to reflect what we had explained to our patients. Thankfully I passed.

9. *The examiners were friendly and the chief examiner came out to tell us all that it was going to be fun and not too difficult!*
This was my first attempt. The exam was set in the outpatient department and it was a Sunday afternoon in a 30° heatwave. The examiners were friendly and the chief examiner came out to tell us all that it was going to be fun and not too difficult!

Station 4

I started with Station 4 – communication and ethics. This involved counselling a young woman with diabetes who had poor compliance and had developed protein in her urine. She had a few issues at home. They asked me to summarize what we had discussed during the consultation and then asked a few questions about diabetic control.

Station 5

For Station 5 there were two young-ish men. *Case 1* had had a TIA-like episode and *Case 2* had presented with what sounded like a vasovagal episode. It felt very rushed and the examiner expected me to have asked a bit more about the past medical history than I did. He picked me up for not asking the TIA man specifically if he knew whether he had high cholesterol, even though I did tell him we would need to check it. In the second, they pressed me a little about whether I would arrange an ECHO. I said it depended on whether the ECG was normal.

Station 1

Abdominal: The case was situs inversus. The lady had some unusual keloid scars on her abdomen but otherwise I said that it was an essentially normal abdomen. The examiner did push me on this point. He said, 'Are you saying this is a *totally* normal abdomen?'. He then told me to go back and percuss the liver all the way up and of course this was resonant. He let me listen to her heart sounds. He asked me what I thought of the scars, which were very unusual. They were symmetrical, short scars in the upper abdomen, not suggestive of laparoscopy scars and too symmetrical for skin abscesses, though I offered both up as vague possibilities. As the bell went I said I would examine her chest and get a chest X-ray to look for bronchiectasis and mentioned Kartagener's syndrome which he seemed pleased with.

Respiratory: This was a man with a very small patch of pulmonary fibrosis at the right base. The discussion was around causes, investigations and possible treatments.

Station 2

This was a young woman with hilar lymphadenopathy and joint swelling. I was a little surprised that there wasn't anything else to elicit in the history – no symptoms other than what was written on the card and no major issues other than that she was worried she had cancer. I got very short sentences in response to open questions and a simple 'yes' and 'no' in response to a thorough systems review. I told her I thought cancer was very unlikely and that it was probably a condition called sarcoid. They then asked me about sarcoidosis and its management.

Station 3

Cardiovascular: This was a woman with rheumatoid arthritis and also aortic stenosis and mitral regurgitation, I think. I said a little bit about which was the predominant valve problem and was asked about severity and indications for surgery.

Neurological: My neuro case was a bit odd. He was a middle-aged man and I was requested to examine his legs. I asked him to walk. He used a stick and his gait was not normal but didn't really fit any pattern. I didn't get to finish my neurological examination but he seemed to have a mixed motor and sensory neuropathy, the motor element being global but the sensory being stocking distribution. I talked about the differentials for neuropathies and the examiner asked me some theoretical questions about what I would have thought had his plantar responses been up-going and if he had cerebellar signs (which he didn't). I wasn't sure if I had picked up all the signs for him and I didn't get to do all the sensory modalities in the legs.

> **Comments**
>
> My initial instinct when I left was that it had been all right, though I did think of a lot of things I could have done better afterwards and wasn't very confident by the time the results came out but in the end I did pass.

10. *'What did you think of her apex?' I said I was sorry but I forgot to palpate – then they said, 'Maybe you just couldn't feel it because it isn't there', at which point I shrieked, 'Kartagener's!'.*

I still can't believe I passed! My PACES exam was in the outpatients of a big DGH. Probably one of the worst parts was the waiting for it to start! Everyone was very friendly and gave us advice on where to find alcohol gel and who would show us round before it began.

Station 2

I started with history taking. There was a very long case summary, essentially progressive shortness of breath in an elderly gentleman. The patient was extremely verbose and had every relevant bit of history; he had cardiac symptoms, kept pigeons, had previous asbestos exposure, was a smoker with complex social circumstances, you name it! I got to summarizing what he had said and then ran out of time (having forgotten to ask about haemoptysis/weight loss). The examiners wanted a differential diagnosis (I think it was probably cardiac, i.e. angina/COPD/fibrosis) and what my management plan would be. They got cross when I started with 'I would consider doing . . . ' so I quickly changed to 'I WOULD do . . . '. I found writing down a differential/investigation plan on the basis of the lead-in sheet in the 5 minutes before you go in really helpful, as it gives you something to look back at when your mind goes blank.

Station 3

Cardiovascular: My cardiology case was aortic stenosis (the lead-in being chest pain on exertion). I thought I had it right as the examiner said, 'Yes, it's almost too easy, isn't it!'. I was asked about investigation, management, why patients with aortic stenosis get syncope on exertion, how the management would be different if the patient had no symptoms, and what drugs could be used.

Neurological: The neurology instruction was to examine the legs of a man who 'has noticed problems in his arms and legs'. He had orthotic implants in his shoes, walking aids, an abnormal gait (but I'm not sure what it was), and findings consistent with peripheral neuropathy. They asked me about causes and investigation of peripheral neuropathy (and then specifically about painful causes – all I could think to say was Lyme disease unfortunately!).

Station 4

In the communication skills I had to talk to the relative of a recently deceased medical patient who had been outlied and some of the antibiotic doses had been missed. It wasn't clear from the instruction whether the daughter knew he had died, so I asked the examiner to clarify before I started and they didn't seem to mind doing so. It was fine except when she said to me, 'Did missing one dose of antibiotics lead to his death?' and I was worried that the examiners might perceive 'no' as a lie. The questions were about managing complaints, why patients shouldn't be outlied, the ethical principles, and how to decide whether a patient should be for ITU care.

Station 5

My Station 5 was a complete nightmare.

Case 1: The first case was a lady with a photosensitive rash and some joint pains. On examining her, however, I couldn't actually find any physical signs. I ended up saying I would do bloods looking for systemic lupus and check her other medications for photosensitivity as a side-effect, but I really had no idea what was going on!

Case 2: This was a young man describing two episodes of palpitations associated with chest pain in the last few hours after taking cocaine. I thought he had a normal examination (I chose to examine cardiac/thyroid status) but I got unsatisfactory from both examiners so there must have been something else. I said I would admit him for ECG monitoring/troponin, etc., in case he had had a vasospasm/arrhythmia from the cocaine use. The examiners didn't seem very happy with this but then, talking to the other candidates, it was apparent that they didn't seem happy with those who didn't admit him!

Station 1

Respiratory: The patient had a thoracotomy scar and findings consistent with bronchiectasis. I told the examiners all the differentials I could remember and then they said 'What did you think of her apex?'. I said I was sorry but I forgot to palpate – then they said, 'Maybe you just couldn't feel it because it isn't there', at which point I shrieked, 'Kartagener's!'. Then they asked me about rheumatoid lung disease and hypogammaglobulinaemia and its treatment. I really didn't know the answer to what they were asking but they just kept asking anyway. I was very relieved when the bell went . . .

Abdominal: This was a patient with chronic liver disease – he had most of the stigmata but no signs of decompensation. They asked about causes, what I would advise the patient (I talked about diet, stopping drinking, signs of decompensation). The one who asked me about immunoglobulin deficiency before asked about why this patient might be immunocompromised – I think he must have been an immunologist! Then they asked me if I was sure he wasn't jaundiced – I didn't think so. They thought I should look again in daylight and brought him out from the dark corner he was in – he was definitely jaundiced!

11. *We discussed possible explanations for the association of aortic regurgitation and renal failure, including some pretty esoteric diagnoses.*

Station 3

Cardiovascular: My first station was cardiovascular. It was a middle-aged chap with a metal aortic valve and, incidentally, a fistula and a transplanted kidney. We discussed possible explanations for the association of aortic regurgitation and renal failure, including some pretty esoteric diagnoses.

Neurological: This was a woman with lower motor neurone left arm weakness, lymphoedema, and a left-sided mastectomy. We discussed radiation plexopathy and damage from surgical lymph node clearance, as well as possible axial recurrence.

Station 4

Communication skills was a woman with a new diagnosis of motor neurone disease who wanted to talk about prognosis and therapy, but mostly end-of-life issues including advance directives. A gift – she was most pleasant.

Station 5

Case 1: This was a woman who gave a classic description of Raynaud's, saying she had had it as a young woman. It had got better after a procedure and was recently returning. I probed for secondary causes of Raynaud's and noted her sympathectomy scars. The examiner asked what I thought was going on and I said sympathectomy for severe primary Raynaud's (she had

had digital ulcers) and that the nerves may have grown back. He asked me how I might confirm this and I replied that I believed that nerve activity can be measured directly, but didn't know any more. He asked me what I would do about it and I said the procedure may need to be repeated.

Case 2: This was a woman with long-standing type 1 diabetes who was having visual difficulties. Minimal questioning revealed that she had established retinopathy but the new visual disturbance was like a 'curtain falling over the eye'. I looked at her retinas (confirming retinopathy with maculopathy on the right), asked for the blood pressure and, for what it is worth, I listened to the carotids, then we talked about the investigation and treatment of amaurosis fugax and TIA.

Station 1

Abdominal: The abdominal station was a young woman with hepatomegaly and a splenectomy scar, and signs of chronic liver disease. We discussed the differential at length but I couldn't get the correct diagnosis. Finally, and cheekily, I asked the examiner for a clue, which he good-humouredly refused. In retrospect, I think it was a glycogen storage disorder (though there was nothing else phenotypically to suggest one) as this was pretty much the only thing I didn't say.

Respiratory: This was a man who very obviously had bronchiectasis and I said so, but also giving a differential. The examiner asked what I thought of the trachea (which I had said was central), and asked me to feel again. I prevaricated over whether it might be a bit deviated to the left. She clearly thought it was to the right. I couldn't fit this together particularly well with his bronchiectasis (he had no scars); this was my worst station.

Station 2

The history was of a man with unexplained weight loss, who was convinced that he had cancer. There was very little to go on after exhaustive questioning, apart from possible night sweats. I told him that there were many possibilities (and, yes, that included cancer, though it was not the most likely at the moment) and outlined a plan of investigation. The actor left unhappy, seemingly because I couldn't tell him he definitely did not have cancer. The examiners asked whether I felt I could be more reassuring about the possibility of cancer and I responded that, since he directly asked me, it would be unethical to lie, and that he would lose confidence if it turned out later to be true. They seemed reasonably happy with this and asked me for my differential. I felt very unsatisfied that I couldn't end the consultation well, but since the marks were good, I think the actor may have decided that he would not be talked down.

> **Comments**
>
> I passed with colours flying. The main thing I would like to comment on is that all my examiners were very friendly and that, listening to others' stories, people mostly fail by losing their nerve. Be confident (I know it's a bit of a trope, but it's true).

12. *On examination, he had yellow nails(!) and coarse crackles throughout the chest.*

Station 1

Respiratory: The patient had dullness at the lung base and I was fairly confident of my performance here and could give a reasonable list of possible causes.

Abdominal: This was definitely hepatosplenomegaly and again I was pretty confident about this case as well.

Station 2

The scenario in Station 2 was of a 41-year-old presenting with a collapse. It soon became evident that he was a working man who drank a lot at lunchtime and at home in the evening. However, he himself didn't think that he drank too much. I was asked about how alcohol can cause falls and then about the best investigations of this patient's collapse. I was specifically asked about the use of tilt table testing.

Station 3

Cardiovascular: I think the cardiac case was mixed mitral valve disease but I was only slightly confident about that. There was definitely a mitral valve murmur with a mid-diastolic plop.

Neurological: The neurology patient had a spastic scissor gait/ataxia, increased tone, up-going plantars, normal sensation, with no cerebellar signs. I guessed he had some kind of upper neurone lesion but I really did not have a clue!

Station 4

I had to break bad news to a young lady who we had found on a recent ultrasound scan to have features suggesting she had autosomal dominant polycystic kidney disease. Her father was having a horrid time on haemodialysis. She was just about to get married and would like to start a family. I broke the bad news and the patient/actress cried a lot. It didn't feel like I got very far and I was constantly being pushed as to how long it would be before she would need dialysis. I explained that this was difficult to answer and she wanted to speak to someone who could answer. It ended with me saying that I would get a renal consultant to see her.

The examiners asked me about the chances of her children having polycystic disease. Then we moved on to the management of polycystic disease, including the hypertension and the guidance about head scans looking for associated aneurysms, etc.

Station 5

Case 1: The first case was a middle-aged white man who was complaining of increasing breathlessness and sputum production. He was a non-smoker and worked in an office. There had been no weight loss. On examination, he had yellow nails(!) and coarse crackles throughout the chest. I gave a simple management plan as if I were in the medical admission unit, i.e. routine bloods, chest X-ray, arterial blood gases, sputum culture, etc. I cannot remember the examiners being too taxing on me!

Case 2: The second case was an elderly lady with unilateral lower limb swelling with no erythema. There was no examination couch and when I mentioned this to the examiners, I was told to just examine her in the chair. There was a measuring tape on the table next to her! It was just her calf that was mildly enlarged. There was not much else to go on so I asked questions relating to the risk factors for deep venous thrombosis (DVT), and for features that might suggest a Baker's cyst or a pelvic malignancy. I explored her concerns and discussed a simple management plan to initially exclude a DVT. The examiners asked about the other differentials. We discussed Doppler scans and that a D-dimer probably would not be that useful. We didn't get onto management.

> **Comments**
>
> Time goes very quickly in Station 5 as I think everybody has experienced so far!

13. *The examiners then asked me for the tests I would do. I completely forgot urine and sodium osmolality and they asked for more tests and I could not think of any more. The examiner looked astonished and went 'that is it?!'.*

Station 2

The case was a patient with tiredness referred by the GP for further evaluation who was noted to have low sodium secondary to SIADH from bronchial carcinoma. Unfortunately, the patient got extremely anxious when I told him the possibility of cancer as he thought he would get better by just taking more salt in his diet. So I could not wrap up the consultation properly and was thinking to myself I should not have gone down that path as it was not a breaking bad news station! The examiners then asked me for the tests I would do. I completely forgot urine and sodium osmolality and they asked for more tests and I could not think of any more. The examiner looked astonished and went 'that is it?!' I was then asked for the causes of SIADH and I went blank after small cell lung cancer and intracerebral pathology and they just asked for more. I thought I had failed that station but in fact I passed it!

Station 3

Cardiovascular: The patient was in a lot of pain every time she had to move and I was very wary of this. I heard a mitral regurgitation murmur and thought I heard AR as well but was not too confident so I did not mention this. The examiner asked me, 'Did you hear anything else?'. I said 'no'. Then he said hypothetically if she also had AR (!) – borderline.

Neurological: When I saw the neurology patient I knew she had CMT with the distal wasting and Charcot joints. Unfortunately, when I examined her I thought I elicited clonus and went down the route of spastic paraparesis! The examiner was kind and said 'but what did you find with her reflexes?'. I assumed they were trying to trick me and stuck with spastic paraparesis although I elicited no reflexes! The examiner tried to help me again and said 'how would you explain the reflexes?'. I still ignored it and continued my spiel for spastic paraparesis at which point the examiner gave up on me. It was only when I left the station that I came to my senses and realized what I had done – fail!

Station 4

I had to speak to a daughter who was unhappy as her mother was misdiagnosed with cholecystitis and there-fore the treatment for pneumonia was delayed by 2 days and she was now deteriorating. I had to apologize to her about that and gather further information to see if she was suitable for ITU. It was going well when, in the last 2 minutes, I asked her if she had any other concerns or questions so she asked about resuscitation. I said that is something we should address but I would need to discuss that first with her mother and then maybe arrange another meeting with the daughter as well if her mother consents. She was happy with this. The examiners asked questions around resuscitation and whether I thought she was an ITU candidate – clear pass.

Station 5

Case 1: The brief I got was of a lady with painful hands and as soon as I saw her I knew this was scleroderma. She had the classic ulcerations, sclerodactyly and facial features. Having got to the diagnosis relatively quickly, I asked her what her concerns were. She said, 'the pain in my fingers and I'm worried I will lose my fingers'. I explained to her that we will admit her, get advice from the rheumatologist and we would start her on a drip to improve the blood flow to her fingers and also explained things she could do to help as well. The examiners asked for the diagnosis, investigations and management and they seemed generally happy – pass.

Case 2: This was a lady who complained of a lump in her neck. I had a quick look at her neck when I introduced myself and it was clear that it was the thyroid. The examiner asked, 'What is your diagnosis?'. 'Thyroid goitre and clinically hyperthyroid' I said. He asked again – 'is she hyper- or hypothyroid?'. I said hyperthyroid assuming he had just misheard me and was not trying to guide me to the correct diagnosis! At the end they asked whether surgery was an option. I said 'No, unless it was causing respiratory compromise or swallowing difficulties' – pass.

Station 1

Respiratory: The brief was about a lady with rheumatoid arthritis and breathlessness. In my head I thought this should be pulmonary fibrosis and my findings confirmed it. I was asked about how I would manage her acutely and in the clinic setting. I forgot to ask her to cough to see if the crepitations shifted and the examiners prompted me to look at the sputum pot. Otherwise it went well – pass.

Abdominal: The abdominal case was of a patient who had hypertension at the age of 38. From the end of the bed it was evident he had a renal transplant with evidence of previous haemodialysis and peritoneal dialysis with cushingoid features (steroid use). I also mentioned 'he has a melanocytic naevus on his abdomen' at which point the examiners gave me a questioning look and looked at the patient. I then quickly said 'It is likely to be benign' and they nodded. The examiners asked about the causes of hypertension at a young age and how I would manage him at clinic follow-up and if he was admitted with sepsis – pass.

Comments

Overall I failed PACES on this attempt.

---

14. *For my neurology case I had to examine an elderly gentleman who had a wide-based gait and Romberg's was positive.*

Station 3

Cardiovascular: This was my first station and I had to examine an elderly lady all wrapped up in a surgical gown! I took my time to expose her and did manage to finish with plenty of time and the examiners offered me to listen again if I needed to. I only heard a mitral regurgitation murmur which I thought was possibly too simple for the MRCP so I listened again carefully and could not convince myself of another murmur. I presented my findings and the discussions actually went off on a tangent from what I had said so we never really got to the management of MR but eventually we were talking about anticoagulation because she was also in AF – clear pass.

Neurological: For my neurology case I had to examine an elderly gentleman who had a wide-based gait and Romberg's was positive. His motor function was normal but he had a sensory neuropathy. I did not have time to assess all modalities of sensation so I did pinprick and joint position sense. I presented my findings as a sensory peripheral neuropathy and was asked for differentials, investigations and management. I was also asked about what I would find on nerve conduction studies. It was 50/50 with axonal and demyelinating. I answered confidently yet gave the wrong answer (I later realized on checking the text), but the examiner seemed convinced by my answer and I didn't lose any marks! Clear pass.

Station 4

The case was straight from the Ryder 'gold' book about a healthcare worker (midwife) contracting hepatitis B and was I glad that I had read that! The layout of the room was odd. There was a desk in between myself and the actor. So as soon as I introduced myself to the actor, I realized that the table was too obstructive so after seeking the patient's (actor) permission, I brought my chair to the other side of the table. Note: I was not turning my back on the examiners either. I thought I probably should have done that before the start of the scenario. However, I felt much more comfortable to talk sensitively and empathetically once the chair was in the right place. After that it went well. I went through the diagnosis, consequences, treatment, then summarized and arranged a follow-up. The examiners asked what I would do if she was adamant that she would continue working and where I would get advice from and then about the modes of transmission of hepatitis B. Clear pass (I did not get marked down for the musical chairs!).

Station 5

Case 1: This was a patient with painful hands. The brief was that the patient was attending follow-up in the endocrine clinic and complained of painful hands. On inspection, it was obvious that he had acromegaly and I quickly established that the pain was secondary to carpal tunnel syndrome which he had had previously. I asked some questions and examined to look for recurrence of the pituitary tumour and explained to him the possible treatment options. The examiner asked for investigations and treatment; I forgot to mention steroid injections. Clear pass.

Case 2: This was a patient with a lump in the neck. Before the start of the station, the examiners told me not to concentrate on her past medical history as many candidates had spent too long on it so advised me to ignore it! So with the helpful hint, I started the station noticing the mid-line lump in her neck and took the history and then examined the patient to confirm a thyroid goitre and then assessed her thyroid status. She was euthyroid and had a smooth goitre. She was quite thin and had lost weight but at the same time had a hoarse voice. So I said it could be hyper- or hypothyroidism. Then the examiners asked for a specific diagnosis (she also had hypopigmented scars from pemphigoid, therefore autoimmune association). I said most likely diagnosis was Graves' disease (in retrospect, the hoarse voice could be secondary to compressive symptoms from the goitre) and they agreed and asked for investigations, management and indications for surgery. I also mentioned that I heard a bruit for which the examiners went 'oh really?'. It didn't seem like they had listened for one and now they had another sign (!). The patient smiled and gave me a thumbs up at the end – clear pass.

Station 1

Respiratory: I was asked to examine the respiratory system of a gentleman who had multiple cutaneous signs. There was an erythematous rash across his nose (?lupus pernio/?adenoma sebaceum) and he had multiple cafe-au-lait spots and patches of hypopigmentation. On examination, he had signs of pulmonary fibrosis although I gave the differential of bibasal crepitations either due to bronchiectasis or heart failure. I had time left at the end and they told me that I could examine again if I wanted to. So, I inspected the skin again and at that point I doubted myself as to whether I had done vocal resonance so I did it again. The examiner questioned me as to why I did this. He thought I must have heard a sign which I wanted to confirm but I had to confess that I wasn't sure whether I had found anything at all. They asked for the possible diagnoses for this gentleman. I said that with the cutaneous signs it could be sarcoidosis, neurofibromatosis or tuberous sclerosis and then they asked for more common causes! We then discussed investigations and management of pulmonary fibrosis – clear pass.

Abdominal: For my abdominal case I was asked to examine a middle-aged lady. She had swollen fingers with tight skin and also an ulcer on the middle finger. When I asked her to open her mouth, she couldn't open it very wide and she had some telangiectasia on her chest. So I thought 'ah, scleroderma'. As I proceeded to examine her, she had signs of previous haemodialysis (fistulae and scars from central venous access) and signs of peritoneal dialysis. There was also a fullness lateral to the umbilicus but with no overlying scar to suggest a renal transplant. When I asked permission to examine her legs, the examiner and the patient both giggled, which puzzled me until I found that she only had one leg and the other was a prosthesis. After I presented my positive findings and mentioned that she might have scleroderma, the examiners were not convinced and wanted me to point out all the signs of scleroderma that I had found. They agreed with the signs in the hands but then the patient let me down by opening her mouth very wide and then I realized that

the telangiectasiae were not very convincing. And then the examiner said, 'Well, it is obvious she has end-stage renal failure but what is the cause?'. I began to mention diabetes and vascular disease and then the bell rang – fail. I am still not sure what her diagnosis was and she may have had a renal transplant with a very faint scar.

Station 2

The brief was a GP referral letter for a young overweight female with weakness which the GP thought was all related to anxiety. She had also been found to have a high blood pressure. I had put on my differentials list all the causes of generalized weakness including hypothyroidism, anaemia, etc. When I went in and started taking the history, I discovered that she had had 'episodes' of weakness lasting 30 minutes to 8 hours (that one had occurred yesterday) with numbness of one arm and leg. Then she said, 'oh, I also have headaches . . . oh, and I suffer from indigestion . . . oh and doctor, I also have palpitations'. I could see the temptation to put it all down to a psychological cause but I took a detailed history of each symptom and assessed for risk factors. I told her we would need to do more tests for her heart and for her symptoms of headache and weakness, but I reassured her on the indigestion and gave some lifestyle advice and said I would prescribe antacids. The examiners asked for a summary and then asked for the differentials for the weakness. I said the main differential was TIA and then hemiplegic migraine, cerebral venous thrombosis, MS and BIH. They then asked for the relevant investigations (especially in a young adult) and treatment for TIA – clear pass.

Comments
I passed PACES at this, my second, attempt.

15. *The examiners went on to ask about renal failure and how I would be able to determine, through clinical examination, if the patient was on renal replacement therapy. I mentioned that I would look for vascular catheters or AV fistulae and, lo and behold, there was a fistula on the man's arm with fresh needle stab marks which had been hidden by the sleeves.*

Stress? I kid you not. The preparation period was so stressful. The exam itself was stressful. By the time I hit the exam, I was already so numb that I was devoid of all emotion. I just wanted to get it over and done with.

When the exam finally came around, it was nerve-wracking to sit in a room with 10 other doctors, all looking very smart and intelligent. I had my trustworthy Littmann cardiology stethoscope with me and I was wearing very smart clothes – black pencil skirt, black tights and a pin-striped shirt. I wanted to wear heels, but I thought they might be distracting, and I did not want to fall flat on my face in front of the examiners. First impressions DO count!

Station 4

I had to break bad news to a woman (an actress) regarding her husband. The scenario given was of a man who had had a fit at home. He was brought to the hospital and found to have a brain tumour which had bled into the surrounding brain tissue. I had to tell the woman what had happened, the diagnosis, the treatment options and the prognosis, i.e. the illness is terminal. Remember to be sympathetic and caring, and remember to tell the examiners that you would discuss a DNAR if you had time! **Score: 16/16**

Station 5

Case 1: I was given a referral letter asking me to see a patient who had watery diarrhoea. So, I took a history, examined the patient – at this point, I realized that the patient was actually an actor who did not have any abdominal problems because I failed to find anything abnormal. So, I came up with a plan – take blood, do microbiology investigations, do contact tracing, IV fluids for rehydration, endoscopy if it doesn't settle, etc., and I explained my plan to the patient. The quizzing was based on possible causes of the watery diarrhoea and the indications for endoscopy. **Score: 28/28**

Case 2: This time, it was a real patient. She had a history of thyroid problems, and she had now presented with swallowing difficulties. The history was vague, and I struggled to connect the dots. I got the diagnosis right, though – a multinodular goitre – but I was not convinced that the patient had systemic sclerosis although she complained of Raynaud's in her hands. Therefore, my management plan was to check the thyroid gland to make sure that it was not compressing the oesophagus, and if a trial of proton pump inhibitors did not do the trick, then the patient would be a candidate for upper endoscopy or a barium meal to rule out any intrinsic motility dysfunction. **Score: 28/28**

Station 1

Abdominal: I was brought to an elderly man who was wearing an unbuttoned long-sleeved shirt. The examiners instructed me to examine the abdomen ONLY. The patient had bilateral flank masses with a scar over the right iliac fossa. I could not detect a transplanted kidney although I would have expected to find one. Then, the examiners went on to ask about renal failure and how I would be able to determine, through clinical examination, if the patient was on renal replacement therapy. I mentioned that I would look for vascular catheters or AV fistulae and, lo and behold, there was a fistula on the man's arm with fresh needle stab marks which had been hidden by the sleeves. Therefore, the patient must have had a failed kidney transplant which had been removed, and was back on dialysis. **Score: 20/20**

Respiratory: The patient obviously had idiopathic pulmonary fibrosis with Cushing's syndrome secondary to long-term steroids. It was a really straightforward case, and I did not have any problems with it, except for the bit where I said the patient would need to have a bronchoscopy for prognosis and treatment planning, and the examiners just looked puzzled. **Score: 20/20**

Station 2

I was asked to take a history from a woman who the GP had referred for possible meningitis because she had a headache and was feeling unwell. The history sounded like a viral illness – headache, runny nose, fever, muscle stiffness with no red flags. I just reassured her that it was unlikely to be meningitis, but we would do some blood tests to make sure that there was nothing serious going on. Also, I told her that the diagnosis was likely to be a common cold, and it was not anything to worry about. **Score: 19/20**

Station 3

Neurological: I was asked to examine an elderly lady with a tremor of her hand. It turned out that the lady had parkinsonian features and also neurofibromas. I elicited all of the clinical features of Parkinson's, and went on to comment on the possibility of the patient having concurrent neurofibromatosis type 1. The examiner asked if there were any links between Parkinson's disease and neurofibromatosis. **Score: 20/20**

Cardiovascular: This was the only station which I did very badly on. To this day, the diagnosis still eludes me.

The patient was obviously in cardiac failure because of bilateral pitting pedal oedema. There were no scars and I could not hear any murmurs either. All I had found were signs of heart failure and an irregularly irregular pulse although, in retrospect, I think the patient probably had severe aortic regurgitation with a collapsing pulse. The examiners were busy pressing me for a diagnosis, and that was all I could give. Crashed and burned!
Score: 9/20

Comments

So overall, as you might see, it's a matter of luck on what sort of patients you get on the day of the exam. I came out of the exam feeling optimistic, bearing in mind that I totally bombed the last case. I was hoping that all of my other cases could make up for the one disaster, and they did! I passed the exam and now I don't have to worry about exams for a good few years! The stress was worthwhile because the skills that I have picked up have made me a much better clinician.

---

16. *Having failed to provide a satisfactory diagnosis in my neurology case and been openly given negative feedback in my communication skills station, I had to go through the rest of the exam believing everything was already over. This was the toughest part of the day and I really struggled to put my mind together and read through my Station 5 scenarios.*

Station 3
Neurology: I started the exam with neurology where I was asked to examine the lower limbs of a 30-year-old patient. My examination elicited increased tone on both sides with normal power, but with incoordination and impaired sensation (pinprick and vibration sensation) in a stocking distribution. I was having difficulties combining all these signs, and offered subacute combined degeneration of the cord as a potential cause, which didn't seem to satisfy the examiners. They asked for an acute cause to which I suggested acute disseminated encephalomyelitis. I never found out what the correct diagnosis was. (Scored 16/20)

Cardiovascular: My second case was cardiology, where I had to spend a good 2 minutes trying to find the hand gel, transfer the patient from a chair to his bed and help him to remove his shirt. I was told I had only 1 minute left just before I started my auscultation. Fortunately the patient had a rather straightforward, harsh ejection systolic murmur which was easy to detect in my remaining minute. This was followed by a discussion about the differential diagnosis of the murmur (aortic stenosis versus sclerosis), the severity of it, the management plan and the indications for chemoprophylaxis. (20/20)

Station 4
My communication skills station involved a consultation with a patient with newly diagnosed coeliac disease leading to fatigue, diarrhoea and iron/folate deficiency and who was not keen to comply with a gluten-free diet since her symptoms had improved with iron and folate replacement. In my effort to underline the risks of not complying with the diet, I mentioned the association between coeliac disease and bowel lymphoma, which seemed to surprise the patient and did not go down too well with one of the examiners who told me he thought I was 'too blunt' in mentioning this risk which is relatively small. I was also told that, in subclinical cases of coeliac, not following a gluten-free diet can be a reasonable option to which I replied that this is by definition not a subclinical case as the patient has developed clear symptoms of coeliac disease. The subsequent discussion was around the topic of patient autonomy. (10/16)

Station 5
Having failed to provide a satisfactory diagnosis in my neurology case and been openly given negative feedback in my communication skills station, I had to go through the rest of the exam believing everything was already over. This was the toughest part of the day and I really struggled to put my mind together and read through my Station 5 scenarios.

Case 1: My first case was a lady with a history of heartburn, dysphagia and breathlessness, which in PACES almost invariably indicates scleroderma. I asked all the relevant questions which confirmed my suspicion, but was only able to find debatable sclerodactyly (mild) and no facial features of scleroderma or crepitations on auscultation. I stuck to scleroderma as my working diagnosis with a differential of malignancy and suggested an urgent OGD and an autoimmune profile as the main parts of my management plan. The examiners looked satisfied and we had a brief discussion on the immunological tests that would support the diagnosis of scleroderma. (25/28)

Case 2: My second Station 5 scenario comprised a diabetic patient who had had a collapse. I took the relevant history and then auscultated the heart and examined the pulse. I offered to examine the retina but the examiners told me there was only background retinopathy. The patient (likely an actor) turned out to be a driver so I incorporated driving cessation and DVLA notification into my final plan. In my brief discussion with the examiners, I suggested a differential of hypoglycaemia, ACS, arrhythmia and vasovagal which the examiners seemed to agree with. (26/28)

Station 1

Respiratory: My respiratory case was an elderly lady wearing a hospital gown (likely to have been an inpatient) presenting with breathlessness. I noted arthritic changes in both hands but despite expecting to find fine crepitations on auscultation, the chest was clear with a prolonged expiratory phase. This and kyphoscoliosis were my only positive findings. Fortunately, I resisted the temptation of making up crepitations to fit the arthritic hand changes, and gave an honest account of my findings and suggested a diagnosis of obstructive lung disease. I was asked whether I thought emphysema or chronic bronchitis was more likely and opted for emphysema given the thin body habitus and absence of cyanosis. This was followed by a discussion on lung function tests and the current COPD guidelines. (20/20)

Abdominal: I was next asked to examine the abdomen of an elderly gentleman. I detected hepatosplenomegaly and some enlarged cervical lymph nodes, but I forgot to auscultate and did not examine for axillary lymphadenopathy which cost me a couple of marks. I gave a full differential of hepatosplenomegaly, advocating lymphoproliferative disease as the most likely cause given the coexistent lymphadenopathy. I was then asked how I would formally diagnose a lymphoproliferative cause in a case like this (excisional lymph node biopsy). (18/20)

Station 2

A young lady with arthralgia involving hands and feet was the case for my history-taking scenario. Raynaud's symptoms and polyarthralgia were revealed during the history taking, without any other features to point to a specific diagnosis. I gave a differential of connective tissue diseases supporting SLE as the most likely diagnosis given the patient's age. This was followed by a discussion on the autoimmune profile and antibodies that would support the diagnosis of SLE or other connective tissue disorders. (20/20)

Comments

I left the examination centre convinced that I had failed the exam, only to find out a few weeks later that I had in fact achieved a rather comfortable pass. This discrepancy between personal impression and actual performance as reflected in the final results seems to be quite common (if not the rule) among successful PACES candidates. I think it is important for one to remember that the actual exam will never run as smoothly as the evenings of PACES practice in the wards, but a pass doesn't require, or equal to, a flawless performance. The new marking system does allow for mistakes and imperfections, as long as one can get over them quickly without getting trapped in the catastrophic 'downward spiral syndrome'.

---

17. *I was asked about antibiotic prophylaxis for any dental procedures and what were the complications of valve replacement.*

Station 1

Respiratory: I was asked to examine the patient's chest. I noted clubbing and found fine basal crepitations. There was also a sputum pot on the bedside locker. I was fairly confident that the diagnosis was bronchiectasis.

Abdominal: I was asked just to examine the abdomen and I found hepatosplenomegaly and also a Dupuytren's contracture. I was asked for a differential diagnosis.

Station 2

In the history-taking scenario I was asked to take a history from a patient who presented with diarrhoea. There was a family history of bowel cancer. There was also a history of recent foreign travel but the diagnosis was probably going to be that of irritable bowel syndrome.

Station 3

Cardiovascular: I was asked to examine a patient's cardiovascular system and found a soft diastolic murmur in the aortic region. That was actually my best guess diagnosis as I wasn't entirely sure but I do think the patient probably had lone aortic incompetence. I was asked about antibiotic prophylaxis for any dental procedures and what were the complications of valve replacement.

Neurological: I was then asked to examine a patient's legs neurologically, having been told that the patient had had surgery to the feet. I found pes cavus and a distal symmetrical sensory loss. I was very confident that the patient had Charcot–Marie–Tooth disease.

Station 4

In the communications skills station I was asked to speak to the mother of an 18-year-old boy who had had his first seizure and who had been taking recreational drugs but didn't want his mother to know.

Station 5

Case 1: A patient with a right upper motor neurone facial palsy.

Case 2: A lady with dry mouth and painful joints. The diagnosis was Sjögren's syndrome associated with possible inflammatory arthritis.

Comments

I passed PACES at this sitting.

Full PACES experiences in the first person (before 2009)

The following full PACES experiences predate the change in Station 5 that occurred in autumn 2009.

18. *I said that the brachioradialis was weak and this was met with utter astonishment and 'What! Where is brachioradialis? Which nerve is damaged?'. I wasn't sure.*

Station 1

Examine this patient's respiratory system and comment on the positive findings as you go.

The clinical findings were of finger clubbing, nicotine staining of the fingers and fine, inspiratory crackles at both bases.

I was stopped at the hands and asked for my thoughts. I suggested that the differential diagnosis would be between a bronchial malignancy, suppurative lung disease and fibrosis unrelated to the nicotine staining. After suggesting these possibilities, I was asked about the causes of pulmonary fibrosis. I mentioned occupational dust exposure, extrinsic allergic alveolitis and drugs, but was not allowed to go on. They asked about investigations and I said pulmonary function tests which would reveal a reduced FEV and FEV_1 but with a normal FEV_1/FVC ratio, high-resolution CT scan and possibly bronchoscopy but they interrupted by saying that this was not often done now!

For occupational dust exposure I was pressed further so I said asbestos exposure, coal dust and beryllium. I was then stopped and the examiner said, 'Why did you say that – it just slipped out, didn't it?'. I agreed that I had not meant to say this but maybe I should have stuck to my guns as I knew that beryllium is used in the aerospace industry and does cause fibrosis. At the end, after asking about investigations, they smiled and said, 'And having diagnosed cryptogenic fibrosing alveolitis you can now go', just as the bell rang. I had never even mentioned this!

Examine this man's abdomen, commenting on what you are doing.

He had hepatosplenomegaly. I was not allowed (I was actually stopped when I tried) to examine for lymphadenopathy. There were no peripheral stigmata at all of chronic liver disease. I said he probably had a lymphoproliferative or a myeloproliferative condition and possibly portal hypertension but I pointed out that this was highly unlikely in view of the large spleen and the absence of any peripheral stigmata.

They went on to ask why it was not a kidney on the left and for some reason I do not think I answered this terribly well. I mentioned the inability to get above it, dullness to percussion and the splenic notch and they pushed me for more. They prompted me with, 'What about movement?' to which I replied that the spleen moves with respiration. They pressed on with, 'Does the kidney?'. I said, 'Yes, but less so'. They then asked for other causes of left upper quadrant masses and I said that other than the kidney it could be pancreatic but it was more likely to be gastric or adrenal. They looked happy and asked if I had ever felt an adrenal mass. One of the examiners said, pointing to his colleague, 'Dr X here sometimes feels them!'.

Station 2

This is a 36-year-old lady who has been diabetic for 2 years and is on insulin. She has recently been treated for a foot ulcer and wants to be more involved with her treatment and her diabetic control. Discuss her treatment with her.

She had had an ulcer on her right big toe for the last 3 months. It had healed once but had broken down again and for this second time she had needed intravenous antibiotics. The doctors had been worried about osteomyelitis but this had not actually occurred. The ulcer had now healed again. She had had three hypoglycaemic episodes in the past which had led to near unconsciousness but she had not been to the hospital. She had had laser treatment to the eyes and now had no visual symptoms. She complained of tingling in the right foot but of no weakness. She was a bank clerk and her place of work knew that she was diabetic. She only checked her BMs about 3–4 times a week and they normally ran between 8 and 15 mm/L. She was taking Human Mixtard 20 units bd using a syringe and needle. Her diet was poor. She ate anything and everything and had failed to attend her dietitian's appointment. She confessed to liking chocolate. In addition, she had never seen a chiropodist. I suggested there was a need for more home monitoring for a while until we had established a better pattern. I also suggested modification of the administration of insulin to using a pen (in fact, she asked for this) and that she should attend a chiropody and dietetic appointment. Overall, she appeared to be a woman who had not really taken on board the seriousness of her condition. She probably had not realized that the ulcer and the eye problems were caused by the diabetes and that tighter control was needed. I think this is what I failed to address with her. I discussed treatment and management with her, including more intensive BM monitoring so that we could modify her treatment. She did not like the testing and said it was painful so I asked how she did it and she told me that she pricked the finger pulps. I had read something specifically about this which said that the side of the finger was better as it had fewer nerve endings and I explained this to her.

The examiners asked me whether I thought she would be amenable to a more intensive regimen but I thought that she probably would not, given her dislike of needles. However, I pointed out that she may find the pen device more acceptable. (Unfortunately it was she who brought this up, not me.) The examiners also asked me how much chocolate she ate. I did not know because I had not asked. In the heat of the exam, I thought I might run out of time so I chose to move on to other things, although I would certainly have asked this in outpatients (and would probably have run well over the 14 min!).

I think the time limitation is difficult at this station. I failed this section during a mock exam because I did not get round to discussing the management side of the case. I thought I had taken a good history but did not feel I handled or even fully uncovered her concerns. At the end she started asking me about different types of diabetes. She plainly wanted to know more and at this point the bell rang. I think that I should have asked earlier on what she knew about the disease and the case would have fallen into my lap.

Station 3

This gentleman came in on the medical intake 2 days ago and he was breathless. Examine his cardiovascular system.
He had an irregular pulse and mitral regurgitation. There were no splinter haemorrhages. The apex beat was not displaced and by this stage he was no longer breathless.

The examiners wanted to know what I thought might be the cause of his breathlessness. I said that he could have a superimposed infection or he could have had a myocardial infarction, but I was told that his troponin levels were normal and that his ECG was OK. I mentioned the possibility of a pulmonary embolus but they said that he had no chest pain. I got stuck at this stage and the examiner said, 'I know you know this – forget it's the MRCP exam. What else did you say you had found?'. I then remembered the irregular pulse and said the atrial fibrillation might be acute. They asked what I would have done so I said I would have given him diuretics, controlled his rate with digoxin or amiodarone and that DC cardioversion would probably not be an option as the exact time of onset was not known. They asked for another drug and I foolishly did not think of warfarin!

Examine this lady's nervous system but concentrate on the legs.
She looked fairly normal and her gait also looked normal to me. There was no wasting or fasciculation and she certainly did not have champagne-bottle legs. She had pes cavus but I hedged a bit on that, saying I was not sure but I thought in the end that she did. Her tone was normal as was her power but she had mild

weakness of ankle dorsiflexion on the right. (They pressed me for other power abnormalities but I insisted that that was it.) There were absent ankle jerks, normal knee jerks and they would not let me check the plantar reflex or for sensation. Coordination, according to them, was normal.

The examiners asked me for my findings. I said that I had found pes cavus and distal weakness which led me to think about a hereditary sensory and motor neuropathy. Also I said that pes cavus occurs in Friedreich's ataxia but I said that, as her coordination was normal, this was unlikely. They did not press me for other causes of a peripheral neuropathy but they asked why pes cavus occurs and I tried to come up with something sensible but could not really explain the pathophysiology other than that the flexors must be stronger than the extensors. They requested that I ask the lady a question and so I asked about family history, which was positive. They asked me to examine her hands which had no wasting but there was mild weakness of the abductors of the fingers. Their final question was, 'We call this Charcot–Marie–Tooth but do you know any new terms?'. I just said, 'hereditary sensory and motor neuropathy'. I think they were fairly happy but it was not an easy case.

Station 4

You are asked to see the son of Mr JK who has metastatic carcinoma of the lung and has presented with shortness of breath and pain in his leg. It is thought that he could have a deep venous thrombosis (DVT) and a pulmonary embolus (PE). However, the patient does not want to be treated. The son agrees that he does not want his father to suffer and thought that 'he was on the way out'. The patient is very cachectic and unwell. Please discuss treatment, prognosis and resuscitation status.

The son was very aware that the cancer had spread, that we suspected a blood clot and that the outlook was poor. He wanted to know what we could do to treat him and I explained that we would need to confirm a clot and then give him blood-thinning injections which were not excessively painful but rather uncomfortable. I said that the treatment might prolong his life a little but that the prognosis was poor and that he would die sooner or later from the lung malignancy. I emphasized that I did not want to guess how long he might live. I said that if his father did not want treatment we would respect his wishes. The son wanted to know if he might get home following treatment of the DVT/PE and I said it might be possible. Then the son said, 'My mother

would never cope with him – she would have another heart attack and it would kill her'. I talked about pain relief and palliative care. He asked if we could give him something to end it all quicker to which I replied, 'We cannot deliberately end his life'. I said that we would discuss the resuscitation status with his father and the son thought he would almost certainly say 'No' to resuscitation. I said, 'My team would consider it appropriate not to resuscitate'.

The examiners asked me about how one would decide whether a patient is competent to give consent. At this point, it occurred to me that I did not know if the patient was compos mentis or not. I had rather assumed that he was but this was probably a fatal error. I wondered if they were giving me a chance to salvage things by asking what I would do if I thought he might be depressed and I mentioned that there should be a formal psychiatric review. I think this station was tricky because in real life I would have known the patient and would have already assessed whether he was confused/depressed or not. They also asked what I would have done if I discussed resuscitation with the patient and he had wanted to be resuscitated. I ran out of time on this but pointed out that the medical team can override his wishes but should discuss it fully and try to persuade him to agree.

Station 5

This man has a rash on his face. Please examine him.
There was a confluent, maculopapular, erythematous, lightly scaling rash over the whole face extending to the back of his neck and scalp. There were plaques on the anterior surfaces of the lower legs with thicker scales. Over the elbows there was some dry scaling but no erythema. There were no nail changes and the mouth and eyes were normal. There were no lymph nodes.

I said that this might be an atypical presentation of psoriasis and they looked pleased and asked why it was atypical. I said it was not on the knees/elbows and that there were no nail changes. I ventured that I would also consider a drug eruption. They asked the patient what it was and he said, 'Psoriasis'. I know I got a clear pass for this one – I saw the mark-sheet!

Look at this man's face and examine whatever else you think is necessary.
I found scant facial hair. There was no visual field defect and he looked normal in all other respects. In addition, his hands were normal.

This was a disaster! I said he had evidence of pituitary failure or gonadal failure and they asked why. I cannot remember what happened next but I found myself looking at his teeth and tongue in a vain hunt for acromegaly which clearly was not there. They said, 'Ask him to stand'. He was very tall as well as having what I thought was an odd-shaped chest but he was fully clothed in a room full of people! I am not sure why Klinefelter's syndrome popped out of my mouth but as everything I knew about this escaped me, I retracted it and, after much prompting, I figured out that growth hormone lack causes failure of epiphyseal fusion and therefore tall stature. I am sure this is all wrong. It is a gonadal failure that does it.

Examine this lady's eye movements.
There was no ptosis and the left eye was slightly down and out. There was some reasonable movement in the left eye but she had diplopia throughout except when looking down and out. She had a poor pupillary response.

The examiners asked me about pupillary sparing. I got this right but I was a bit flustered following the endocrine case and launched badly into my presentation, saying, 'The eye is deviated down and out' and did not even say which one was affected!

This man had an operation which is unrelated to the case and then woke up with a weak left arm. Why?
He had weak dorsiflexion of the wrist, weak finger extension and numbness and paraesthesiae over the first dorsal interosseus. I said he had a radial nerve palsy secondary to compression at a mid-humeral level.

The examiner asked me if any of the other muscles were weak and, 'Would you like to check elbow flexion again?'. I did so and there was mild weakness. I was asked why and I said that the brachioradialis was weak and this was met with utter astonishment and 'What! Where is brachioradialis? Which nerve is damaged?'. I was not sure. I knew I had got it all wrong and I still do not know what the examiner actually wanted.

Comments
I started at Station 4. Station 5 and the skin case was my first clinical case. I had thought it would be a good start. I felt confident about having passed the skin case easily in the mock exam that I had sat but I think it actually

turned into my worst case/station. My advice is 'Don't be nervous'. 'I was nervous,' said my friend who did PACES last week, 'and there was nothing to be nervous about'. To this end I bought a copy of *You and Your Wedding* from the hospital concourse newsagent (I am getting married in 6 weeks) which was better than anxiously pacing up and down and reading Dr Ryder's book right up to the last minute, which is what other candidates were doing! The magazine calmed my nerves and I spent the last 10 min of the waiting time reflecting on the months of work, how I had got right most of the cases I had seen on the wards in the last few weeks and really feeling that I could not possibly fail.

During the exam I found it was easy to forget one's previous stations' performance and start fresh with the next set of examiners – this is a good change in the format.

So why did it seem to go so wrong? I think I did some good things but made some fundamental errors. I can only say that if I was a consultant looking for a registrar then I would not choose me!

Result
I passed – to my surprise. Which all goes to show you can commit all sorts of real or imagined sins and still do OK.

19. *I gave a differential diagnosis of firstly pyoderma gangrenosum and they asked why it wasn't, and finally they told me he was diabetic so I suggested necrobiosis diabeticorum. They then asked me why it wasn't typical!*

Station 1
This man has become increasingly breathless over the past 2 years. He is a non-smoker. Please examine his respiratory system to determine a cause.
I only found a small area of bronchial breathing over the right upper lobe posteriorly. There were no peripheral signs of respiratory disease and I have to emphasize that the clinical signs of the bronchial breathing were very slight. There was no asymmetry of chest expansion, no scars and I did not detect any dullness on percussion or any increase in tactile vocal fremitus. I

wrongly reached a diagnosis of cryptogenic fibrosing alveolitis because there were some mild, bibasal, fine, inspiratory crepitations. The examiner asked, 'What was not in keeping with that diagnosis?' and I said that there was no clubbing and no cyanosis. He asked me to examine the chest again. I was not swayed about the percussion note or the tactile vocal fremitus but had to agree with the bronchial breathing. He asked me for a differential diagnosis for the cause of the bronchial breathing. I said, 'Consolidation', but at that point the bell went.

The case was an absolute nightmare. I had never been asked to re-examine a chest in all my practice teachings and I died inside when I was directed back. However, I was determined not to shrivel up and I just kept to being honest, I looked the examiner in the eye and carried on. I kept thinking that one nightmare does not fail the exam and tried to keep going. I also made a concerted effort to forget the respiratory fiasco as I was led to the abdominal case.

This 43-year-old man failed a routine medical examination for insurance purposes. Please examine the abdomen and suggest if you can find a reason why.
I found numerous spider naevi and lone hepatomegaly at about four finger-breadths. The examiner asked, 'What might be the underlying diagnosis; how would you investigate this man; what would an abdominal ultrasound scan show and what would his liver biopsy show?'.

Station 2
This 54-year-old man with a history of haemochromatosis, hypopituitarism and diabetes mellitus is now troubled with arthritis. He has previously been on voltarol but he had a perforated duodenal ulcer. He is now on meloxicam, testosterone injections and insulin. His HbA1c is 9.8%. His haemoglobin is about 14g with a ferritin of 40mg/mL. Please see and advise him regarding the painful joints.
I asked the patient to tell me what problems he was experiencing and he said impotence. He did not mention his joints and I was a wee bit thrown here! However, I kept going and gained some history of his main problems which were: (a) impotence; (b) his joints – in particular his hands were painful as a result of his part-time work as a fisherman; (c) heavy drinking of about 140 units/week; (d) marital disharmony secondary to (a) and (b) – he was unable to do any heavy work at home; and (e) poor diabetic control with lack of home monitoring.

We went through the whole standard history including past medical history, drug history, social history, family history, system review, etc. and then just ran out of time! I was feeding back to the patient a plan of action when the bell went. The examiner did agree with me that this was quite a complicated history so I think/hope that I was OK for not getting the whole plan over to the patient. I was asked what I was going to say and to summarize the main problems. We discussed the impotence, which was possibly secondary to his alcohol intake or to the poor diabetic control; the arthritis, and I was asked how to rule out other types of arthritis so I suggested by X-raying his hands and requesting a rheumatoid factor, antinuclear antibodies (ANA) and an erythrocyte sedimentation rate (ESR) test. We discussed whether he was a candidate for a COX-2 inhibitor and we discussed the role of physiotherapy, occupational therapy and joint protection. With regard to the alcohol, we discussed coping strategies and access to a counsellor, and for the diabetes I said that I would encourage him to keep a monitoring booklet and that we would need to review him fairly soon.

Station 3
This woman, who is about 60 years of age, is becoming increasingly breathless. Would you examine her cardiovascular system and see if you can find a reason for this?
There was a malar flush. There were no scars and she was comfortable at rest. The pulse was irregularly irregular at a rate of about 92/min, it was not collapsing and was of variable volume. The jugular venous pressure (JVP) was not elevated. The apex beat was in the fifth intercostal space in the mid-clavicular line but she was very overweight so it was hard to find. The heart sounds were loud and I thought I could hear a pansystolic murmur at the apex.

I found this really hard because of the atrial fibrillation and the fast rate and the patient's habitus. However, I presented the findings of mitral stenosis! The examiner raised his eyebrows and asked how that could cause breathlessness. I struggled through a discussion including uncontrolled fast atrial fibrillation, right ventricular hypertrophy, pulmonary hypertension, etc. I was asked what investigations I would do and I suggested a chest X-ray, ECG and echo and they asked what I would expect to see. I am haunted by the thought that she may have had a systolic murmur at the left sternal edge which could have been pulmonary stenosis. It was all very difficult.

This 84-year-old lady has been having difficulty walking and with her balance. Would you examine her neurologically to find out why?

I asked if I could see her walk and they said, 'No, just examine her neurologically on the bed'. My findings were of bilateral weakness of about grade 4/5 with the left side worse than the right. There was no difference between the distal and proximal muscles. No reflexes were elicited as the lady could not relax! I found a peripheral glove-and-stocking sensory loss to light touch with loss of vibration sense, and equivocal joint position sense. I was stopped because of time constraints and asked to present what I had found.

They asked what I thought could be the cause and I suggested a peripheral neuropathy and mentioned a few tests I would like to do, including a blood sugar and also to ask about drug history and then the bell rang.

Station 4

You are the SHO on the ward. A 50-year-old teacher, and mother of two children, has been admitted to your ward with hypercalcaemia and confusion, and a history of back pain. She now has a normal calcium and is lucid. She has a past history of a mastectomy 10 years ago with follow-up radiotherapy. Explain to her that you want to refer her to the oncologist for further treatment, probably chemotherapy and radiotherapy.

I introduced myself and asked the patient if she understood what had been happening in terms of the high calcium, which was now better, and her painful back. I asked about her family and who was at home. I explained the cause of the high calcium and of the back pain, which were both likely to be related to her previous breast cancer. The patient denied all of this by saying, 'I was clear at my check-up 2 months ago'. I explained to her that it was hard to tell if some cells had remained after the surgery and then she became angry and asked, 'Why wasn't I given chemotherapy 10 years ago?'. I said that it was impossible to comment on other doctors' treatment but I could get hold of the old notes and discuss it with the specialist. She did not want me to tell her family but I explained that the family could be a source of support and help and they would want to know in order to help her. I also suggested that it would be hard to keep the diagnosis hidden with repeated hospital trips and the side-effects of the treatment. She wanted to know exactly what treatment would be given and I explained the broad principles and said that I would arrange an urgent appointment with the cancer doctors who could answer her more detailed questions. She asked if it would be cured and

I had to say, 'No, the treatment would help the symptoms but would not cure the cancer'. I summarized the diagnosis and the plan of action and asked if she had any questions.

At this stage the examiners came over and asked me how I would cope with the patient's anger and what would I do if the daughter cornered me on the ward and asked what was wrong with her mother.

Station 5

This lady has had previous problems with her thyroid. Examine her to determine her thyroid status.

She had a pulse of 80 beats/min which was regular, there was no palmar erythema and no tremor. There were no eye signs but she had a small, smooth goitre. However, there was no water present to watch her swallow. There was no pretibial myxoedema. I said I would like to examine her reflexes to complete the examination. However, I thought that she was euthyroid.

The examiners asked me what her thyroid status was and I confidently said, 'euthyroid'. There were then lots of complicated questions involving her management and investigations and I think I mentioned thyroid function tests, an ultrasound scan and thyroid uptake scans.

Your House Officer has examined this lady's fundi. She is a 23-year-old nurse. He is concerned and has asked for your opinion.

I found a reduced red reflex in the right eye and myelinated nerve fibres on the right side. The examiner said to me, 'This lady presents with headaches, what would you say to her?'.

This 50-year-old lady has problems driving. Examine her arms to find out why.

She had a peripheral symmetrical arthropathy affecting the proximal interphalangeal joints and the metacarpophalangeal joints with a boutonnière deformity. She had a small mouth but there were no other signs of connective tissue disease.

They asked me for a diagnosis and I gave a differential between connective tissue disease and psoriatic arthropathy. I was told that she did not have psoriasis but that she had had a hemicolectomy for ulcerative colitis 10 years ago. What did I think now? I suggested arthritis secondary to ulcerative colitis. They said, 'Can you get this after a complete cure?'. Then they asked me what other types of arthritis can occur with ulcerative colitis.

Examine this man's leg.

I found a raised erythematous area over his left shin with old, atrophied scars. There was pigmentation over two of the scars on the inner shin/calf.

I gave a differential diagnosis of first pyoderma gangrenosum and they asked why it was not that, then I suggested discoid lupus erythematosus and again they asked me why it was not. Finally, they told me he was diabetic so I suggested necrobiosis diabeticorum. Then they asked me why it was not typical!

20. *She also did not want a letter to go to her GP until their return in case the GP told her husband.*

Station 1

This gentleman presented with a cough and shortness of breath. Please examine his respiratory system.

He had obvious weight loss and there was very marked asymmetry in his chest expansion with reduced expansion on the right side. There was a small scar from a previous chest drain in his axilla, stony dullness to percussion and a trachea that was deviated away from that side.

The questions centred on, 'What might be the causes of the dullness?' and 'What investigations would you like to do?'. We talked about investigations on pleural fluid for quite some time, 'What would you do if you couldn't aspirate any fluid?' and we discussed ultrasound guidance for aspiration or for premarking a specific point for aspiration.

This gentleman has lost weight and is experiencing fullness in his abdomen.

There was hepatosplenomegaly with axillary lymph nodes. There was no ascites but the patient looked very cachectic.

They asked me how I would best investigate this gentleman to make a diagnosis. We discussed lymph node biopsy and histology, and bone marrow examination. This led to a discussion about the Philadelphia chromosome.

Station 2

This 52-year-old lady has chronic active hepatitis initially treated with steroids and she is now quite stable on azathioprine. However, several other problems have emerged and the GP thinks it better if she is followed up by the hospital. You are the SHO in the general medical clinic.

She was a quiet lady who had obviously been told not to volunteer anything unless I specifically asked the right questions. She had had non-insulin-dependent

diabetes mellitus but was now on insulin. She had coeliac disease and was on a gluten-free diet. She had hypercholesterolaemia and was on a low cholesterol diet. She had chronic anaemia and had been treated with B12 injections and was now on iron supplements. She had osteoporosis which had been confirmed on a previous scan and she was on cyclical etidronate and calcium. She had had a hysterectomy at quite a young age for heavy and irregular periods. There was a possibility of primary ovarian failure or struma ovarii. She now had paraesthesiae in her fingers which was possibly caused by a peripheral neuropathy secondary to the diabetes. She was depressed, her husband was unemployed and they had financial difficulties. She was the sole carer for her young schizophrenic daughter.

The examiner asked me to summarize her main problems and he wanted to know what else I would have asked if I had had more time. He asked me what she might find most difficult to cope with and wanted a discussion about her dietary restriction of gluten, sugar and cholesterol. I had to outline what dietary advice I would give and the examiner also asked if I thought her diabetes was well controlled and how often I would test her haemoglobin A1c.

Station 3

This young lady presented with increasing shortness of breath on exertion.

I found aortic regurgitation but no stigmata of subacute bacterial endocarditis. They asked me for the causes of aortic regurgitation and how I would monitor her to determine when, and if, valve replacement was going to be necessary. They asked me what advice I would give her about preventing endocarditis and what prophylaxis I would choose for: (a) dental work and (b) a colonoscopy.

This elderly lady has had some falls and now has difficulty with mobility. Please examine her upper limbs.

I found dystonia and choreoathetoid movements mainly affecting her left side. However, I felt the need to perform a full upper limb examination and I also examined her gait. I was not interrupted at all.

They asked me for a likely cause and I plumped for the side-effects of anti-parkinsonian medication. They asked me how I would manage her and they expected a discussion of other therapeutic options. I remembered to say that I would include the patient in the discussion because most patients would prefer to be jerky and switched on than rigid and completely immobile. They asked me what other abnormal movements one might find in drug-induced dystonia and they were expecting me to say facial grimacing and orofacial dyskinesias.

Station 4

This is a woman in her fifties who has had a non-small cell lung cancer treated 2 years ago with radiotherapy. She now has extensive metastases in her spine causing pain down her right leg. You have the bone scan results which she does not yet know. Discuss them with her.

The patient was a very good actress. I asked her what she was worried about and she volunteered that she thought the cancer may have spread and at this stage she became tearful. She did not want her husband to know just yet because they were due to go to France on a holiday with all her family, including her grandchildren, and she did not want it to spoil the holiday. She promised she would tell him on their return because she appreciated that he needed to be involved as her main carer. She also did not want a letter to go to her GP until their return in case the GP told her husband. She desperately wanted to be able to go on the holiday as she thought it may be the last one she would have. I explained that I needed to see the films myself and to discuss with the radiologist to see if there was any evidence of cord compression, but on the whole I felt the right thing to do was to let her go on her holiday.

They asked me questions about holiday insurance and would the insurance company pay to get her treated abroad if her illness was already known? They asked me if she was legally obliged to tell her insurance company of her deterioration and would a fellow EEC country treat her anyway? Would the insurance company pay to get her back home if she deteriorated rapidly? Are you skating on thin ice if you do not notify the GP straight away?

Station 5

This middle-aged man complains of headaches. Would you like to assess him and tell me why?

He was acromegalic but with inactive disease. They quickly stopped me examining him any further when they were satisfied that I knew the diagnosis.

The questions included, 'How would you confirm the diagnosis?', 'What imaging modalities would you use and why?', 'What typical visual field defect do patients get?' (they did not ask me to demonstrate this).

Examine this man's fundus. Just the right one.

I found dot and blot haemorrhages with a normal macula. He had a bilateral corneal arcus and I said the diagnosis was background diabetic retinopathy.

They asked me why I wanted the light on in the room at the beginning and they said, 'Good for you!', when I answered that I was looking for a ptosis, arcus, pupillary irregularity and xanthelasmas. They then asked why I did not use the green light and suggested that I look again. They laughed when I said I never use it. They said, 'Nobody does, but don't the haemorrhages and aneurysms look much clearer?'.

Have a look at this lady's hands and talk me through your examination.

She had rheumatoid hands with no obvious skin thinning or purpura, but she did have a cushingoid face.

They asked me what treatments she might be taking and I suggested steroids. They asked what other investigations would be appropriate and I replied a DEXA scan. 'Good girl', they said.

Have a look at this lady who presented to the casualty department with acute shortness of breath and tell me why.

Comments

I sat the traditional format of the exam in October 2000. This new PACES exam was much fairer. It gave you time to compose yourself and collect your thoughts before moving onto the next case. I started with the history-taking station. This went particularly well and gave me the confidence to proceed. In this sense it tests what you do every day in a more realistic manner than the previous format. Candidates with good English skills definitely have an advantage in the history and ethics stations. The examiners never interrupted me in the main stations. There does seem more time for discussion and I would suggest that candidates need to have thought of the answers before they are asked, as the questions were really quite predictable.

A colleague of mine missed her first murmur so was taken to a second cardiovascular case. She definitely got this one correct and still passed.

The lady had adenoma sebaceum and subungual fibromas, so I diagnosed tuberous sclerosis. They wanted a spontaneous pneumothorax, caused by lung fibrosis and bleb formation as the cause of the acute shortness of breath. I did not get this!

Examine this man's neck.
He had definite pseudoxanthoma elasticum. They asked whether this was inherited or acquired and I said, 'acquired'. They then asked what drugs have been implicated and I said penicillamine. They wanted to know which condition(s) is penicillamine exclusively used for. I mentioned autoimmune 'things' but they specifically wanted Wilson's disease. Looking back, he was a young man with parkinsonian features.

21. *She was short in stature and had a large head with a hearing aid, so I immediately looked at her shins. They were a bit prominent so I said Paget's disease and felt very pleased with myself. Unfortunately, the examiners weren't pleased at all.*

Station 1
This gentleman is breathless on climbing stairs. Examine his respiratory system.
I found diminished chest expansion with intercostal retraction and the use of accessory muscles, the lung fields were hyperresonant with no audible wheeze and the liver dullness was obliterated. I completed my examination by saying that I would like to examine his sputum pot and look at his peak flow chart.

I was asked, 'What did you notice when you examined this patient from the end of the bed?'. 'Intercostal retraction,' I replied. I was asked what diagnosis I was considering and I replied that it was most likely chronic obstructive pulmonary disease (COPD). They then asked for the criteria for long-term oxygen therapy.

During my examination of the patient I was interrupted while I was assessing vocal resonance, with the examiner asking me, 'Why are you doing that?'. I said that I was looking for consolidation. The examiner said, 'Do you think there is any consolidation?', and my answer was, 'no'.

The moral of this is 'do not do something for the sake of completion'. Instead, show the examiner that you are thinking while you examine.

This gentleman was found collapsed. Examine his abdomen and give a differential as to the cause of his collapse.
I found mild jaundice, spider naevi, dilated veins, hepatomegaly but no splenomegaly and there was defi-nite ascites. There was no flapping tremor or any other stigmata of chronic liver disease.

I was asked for some possible causes for his collapse and I suggested encephalopathy, hypoglycaemia, alcohol intoxication/withdrawal, fits or anaemia. Then they asked me how I would manage the patient and how much fluid I would shift in a day. I said not more than 1 kg in weight with careful monitoring of his kidney function.

Station 2
This patient has a serum cholesterol level of 8 and triglycerides of 2 mmol/L. He has persistent symptoms of claudication despite previous vascular surgery. The surgeons have referred him to you for an opinion regarding the use of a statin.
This gentleman had no other risk factors for ischaemic heart disease or for a stroke apart from being a heavy smoker and the raised cholesterol. He had a previous alcohol problem but this was now under control. He had the classic symptoms of peripheral vascular disease (PVD) which seemed not to have resolved with surgery. I persisted with the idea of a recurrence of the PVD on the grafted vessel.

At the end of the discussion I was asked how I thought the interview went. My response was that I thought it went well (I was trying to seem confident even though I was not). I think I failed to entertain other causes of pain such as neurogenic pain. Consequently, I was failed by one examiner in my interpretation and use of the information but I made up for it with clear passes in obtaining data and in the discussion. I therefore passed the station.

I was also requested to answer the surgeon's question. The answer I gave was 'yes', but a more accurate answer would be that he should be on both a statin and a fibrate because of the increased triglycerides and that he needs a complete lipid profile. The triglyceride level of 2 mmol/L is at the top end of the normal range. The initial treatment would be with a statin alone.

Station 3
Examine this patient's cardiovascular system.
I found a regular pulse with good volume and a normal character. There was a displaced apex beat which was heaving. There was a pansystolic murmur at the apex and a mid-diastolic murmur best heard in the left lateral position. There was also an early diastolic murmur at the left sternal border.

The examiner asked for my diagnosis. I answered that there was mixed mitral valve disease and aortic regurgitation and that the predominant lesion was mitral regurgitation. The examiner asked, 'What investigation would you do?'. I said, 'Full blood count, urea and electrolytes, liver function tests and a coagulation screen'. The examiner was surprised. He asked me why I would do these. I had to think of reasons to justify what I would ordinarily do in a routine day's work. I said the patient may have infective endocarditis and I may wish to start antibiotics or to anticoagulate. He asked me, 'What is the definitive test?'. I replied, 'An echo'. He asked, 'When would you refer for surgery?'.

Examine this lady's central nervous system. She has difficulty in dressing.
There was wasting of the small muscles of the hands with a claw hand. The upper and lower limb muscles were wasted bilaterally. The tone was normal but power was reduced because of the wasting distally. The reflexes were intact.

The examiner asked, 'What is your diagnosis?'. I did not have a clue! The examiner then asked what else I had noticed. At this point I saw fasciculation, so I said the patient could have motor neurone disease. While examining the patient, I did the finger–nose test which was normal. I went on to look for dysdiadochokinesis and the examiner stopped me to say, 'Now what does that tell you?'. I think he was trying to point out that I had already established that there was no cerebellar lesion so why was I wasting time?

Station 4
A 28-year-old lady with a recurrence of Hodgkin's lymphoma, and who has refused further chemotherapy, presents in casualty with a deep vein thrombosis (DVT). She refuses warfarin and prefers to take herbal medication. Try to convince her to take warfarin.
The patient's point was that she had lost faith in doctors as they had failed to cure her Hodgkin's disease. She had therefore reverted to alternative medicine. She was very tearful as she thought that everyone felt that she was being difficult.

I started the conversation by assuring her that she was not being difficult and that it was perfectly normal to feel apprehensive. She wanted to know for how long, if she took the warfarin, should she continue with it and, once she stopped it, would the clot recur? I said there was no guarantee that it would not recur. To that she said, 'Why should I take something that is not going to cure me?'. I explained about the potential risk of further thromboembolic disease to which she said,

'Well, I am dying anyway'. I finally managed to convince her to come back to clinic the next week to speak to me again after she had talked it over with her husband.

I was asked what the ethical issues were and replied that the patient has a right to refuse treatment and that the medical staff must do what is best for that patient. He then went on to ask for my opinion as to what would be the best way to discuss this issue further with the patient. I said that probably it would be best to have a group discussion with her in the presence of her family and with senior members of the medical team and the palliative care team (case conference). I was then asked what I thought about her request to try alternative medicines. I replied that I could not endorse it but that I did not have any problems with it so long as there were no interactions or contraindications of any sort.

Station 5
This lady has had multiple fractures. What is your diagnosis?
She was short in stature and had a large head with a hearing aid so I immediately looked at her shins. They were a bit prominent so I said Paget's disease and felt very pleased with myself. Unfortunately, the examiners were not pleased at all.

I was told to look harder and I still did not have a clue. One examiner took pity on me and said, 'Look at her neck and elbow'. She had so much loose skin on her that I said 'pseudoxanthoma elasticum', which again was wrong. So I began to think, what has something in the neck and elbow and is short in stature? I started looking at her spine and one examiner cheekily said, 'You won't find anything there'. I took a shot in the dark and rather unconvincingly said, 'Turner's syndrome'. This was followed by, 'So, tell us the complications of Turner's syndrome'.

Examine the patient's fundus.
I found hard exudates and a circinate around the macula. I was asked the diagnosis so I said, 'There is background diabetic retinopathy with hard exudates'. One examiner passed me and the other one failed me. I should have said, 'There is a circinate maculopathy with background changes as well'. One examiner kept asking me . . . what else? . . . what else? I was too unsure to comment.

Examine the patient's hands.
I found swelling of the metacarpophalangeal joints, proximal and distal interphalangeal joints, ulnar

deviation and the surgical scars of previous tendon transplants. There were no psoriatic patches and there was some functional limitation.

I was asked the diagnosis and suggested rheumatoid arthritis. This was wrong! I was asked why I thought this. I said there was a symmetrical polyarthropathy. However, in actual fact there was one joint that was spared which I had failed to notice. And although there were no psoriatic patches, there was minimal nail pitting and onycholysis.

This time I was not so lucky and failed on this case.

Examine the patient's hand.
There was tight skin with minimal telangiectasia.

I was asked to give the diagnosis so I volunteered scleroderma. I was asked about the major complications, usual causes of death and treatment options. I was asked about other questions I could ask her. This was to determine the associated features.

Comments

By and large the examiners are very nice. They are stone-cold in expression and that often makes you feel that you are doing badly but it is not always true.

Do not feel obliged to complete or stick to your routines for the sake of it. Examiners prefer it if you think and show that you are able to change your routines and adapt as necessary. Do not do something for the sake of it when it is obvious that it is not going to yield any positive signs.

Do not lose hope even if you think you are doing badly. That only makes the rest of the stations feel worse.

---

22. *The 'son' was an SpR in medicine who was a dismal actor with no inflexion, actions or responses. It was very different from a real 'relative' or actor.*

Station 1

Examine this man's chest from the back.
There was a tender area on the anterior chest wall at about the third or fourth intercostal space just to the right of the midline, together with a deformity of the anterior chest at the apex. I found reduced expansion on the right side with reduced breath sounds and increased vocal resonance at the right apex.

I was asked about the significance of the increased vocal resonance and for the underlying diagnosis. The examiner wanted to know the significance of the tender area which also had a small scar over it. I assumed that there had been a previous biopsy. Both examiners gave me 1/4.

Examine this man's abdomen.
The patient was a middle-aged man who was obese and appeared cushingoid. He had multiple scars on his right wrist but there was no arteriovenous fistula. There was a thyroidectomy scar. There were at least six abdominal scars and some deep small scars which looked like healed fistulas or drain sites. There was also fullness in the left iliac fossa.

The examiner asked what else I noticed so I replied that he appeared cushingoid with muscle wasting. I was asked for a diagnosis so offered the possibility of a relapsing/remitting disease such as Crohn's. 'What else could it be?' he asked. I suggested a renal transplant. The examiner asked what all the scars were for. I thought that one of the scars in the right iliac fossa would be an appendectomy, the other two might be from a renal transplant that was later removed. The scar in the left iliac fossa was probably a later transplant which was still present. The mid-line scars could have been from peritoneal dialysis, infection, drains, etc. My marks were 1/4 and 2/4.

Station 2

This man has been losing weight. Please take a history.
This was a real patient, a man in his fifties who appeared quite cachectic and had a nasogastric tube in place. He had lost 2 stone in weight over the last year with reduced appetite and he had postprandial vomiting. He had had a partial gastrectomy and proton pump inhibitors (PPIs) had failed to eradicate multiple gastric and duodenal ulcers. His past medical history included alcoholic pancreatitis and a partial pancreatectomy in 1985 which then led to insulin-dependent diabetes. He had also had Henoch–Schönlein purpura. He had not drunk any alcohol since 1985. He had also been a heavy smoker until then and since had cut down to 20 cigarettes/day. He was unsure of his medication and had no known allergies. However, he was on ferrous sulphate which had given him black stools, and creon which had resolved the steatorrhoea. PPIs had had little effect. The family history revealed that his mother had died from cancer at the age of 48 but the primary was unknown.

He had retired early from journalism because of ill health and now lives alone. He was otherwise well and his diarrhoea seemed to be related to medical compliance.

I was asked to present his history and to say what I thought was contributing to his problem. I suggested that his smoking must be irritating any ulcers that are present. 'And his physicians!' was the reply. Then they asked what investigations I would like to do. I mentioned an endoscopy (OGD), biopsy and histology and was told that these were all normal. As he had multiple peptic ulcers which had not healed on high doses of PPI, they wanted me to consider the Zollinger–Ellison syndrome and to do a gastrin level. Marks: 4/4, 4/4.

Station 3

You are seeing this elderly lady in the cardiology clinic. She has been attending for some time.

She had a mid-line sternotomy scar, a displaced apex and a prosthetic first heart sound.

Before I listened, the examiner asked me what I thought, and then afterwards said, 'What's the diagnosis?', 'Is the valve functioning well?', 'How do you know?', 'If you were seeing her in clinic what would you ask her?', 'What causes for anaemia would you think of?'. Marks: 3/4, 3/4.

Examine this man's legs.

The patient was in his mid-thirties. He had an upper motor neurone weakness in the left leg with a normal right leg and an upper motor neurone facial nerve palsy.

The examiner asked me what else I noticed and I replied that the left arm was also paralysed. He said, 'What would you consider if the left arm had lower motor neurone signs?'. He wanted me to say, 'cervical myelopathy'. 'Why is this not the diagnosis?' He wanted to hear that the weakness was not symmetrical and that there was no fasciculation. 'Demonstrate his facial nerve signs', 'Why is this an upper motor neurone lesion?', 'What do you think has happened to him?' I suggested a differential of embolic disease, a haemorrhagic event and a space-occupying lesion. 'What do you think happened?' 'A subarachnoid haemorrhage.' 'Yes!' Marks: 3/4, 3/4.

Station 4

You are the SHO on-call at night. You have to see the son of a patient who you do not know. She presented yesterday with a fit and the CT scan today shows a large mass

consistent with a glioblastoma. She had a transient ischaemic attack (TIA) 4 months ago and the CT scan at that time was reported as normal and she was given aspirin. The son is irritated that he was told by the ward sister on arrival that his mother has a brain tumour.

The 'son' was a specialist registrar in medicine who was a dismal actor with no inflexion, actions or responses. It was very different from a real 'relative' or actor. As an introduction, I asked him what he knew already. He was angry at having been told by the ward sister in the corridor. I apologized. 'Don't you have mechanisms for this kind of thing?' Again, I apologized. The son asked me, 'What can we do for her?'. I said that this needs to be discussed with the team and with the neurosurgeons but that it was likely to be inoperable. He asked if this had been missed on the CT scan 4 months ago as his mother had never been right since that time. I said that I personally would not know and that the scan needed to be reviewed by the neuroradiologists. He wanted to know what might have been if it had been diagnosed 4 months ago. I did not know but explained that we needed to move on from where we were now. I discussed the complaints process.

The examiner asked me what I thought about his grievance that 4 months had made a difference. I answered that we needed to discuss this with the neurosurgeon. There was a possibility that a swelling was visible on the CT scan 4 months ago but even so we still need to discuss it with the neurosurgeon.

'Couldn't you have put him off from complaining? You told him about the complaints procedure.' I replied that, 'It's not my role. I need to set up an appointment for him to discuss with the consultant and his mother to have it explained, but if he wishes to complain he is entitled to do so and trying to put him off will only make things worse.' The examiner went on to ask me, 'What about the way he was told?'. 'One needs to apologize unreservedly,' I said. 'What should you do next about it?' 'I would next find the ward sister, ask for her side of the story and discuss it with her.'

Station 5

Examine this lady's thyroid status.

She was a middle-aged lady who was euthyroid. There was no lid lag or exophthalmos. She was in sinus rhythm at 80 beats/min. There was no tremor but there was a small nodule within the large goitre.

The examiner asked me what I thought. I said that she was euthyroid but that I would like to ask her some questions. He asked me what tests I would do to confirm. I said thyroid-stimulating hormone. He then asked me for my differential diagnosis.

Examine this lady's eyes.

Visual acuity was good on the left, even without glasses. On the right, she was unable to see the first line of the Snellen chart although she was able to perceive light. On examination of movements, initially I thought there was defective abduction of the right eye but then I thought it was normal. On examining the pupils, the right was dilated with no response but I was told that it was 'always like that'. The left pupil had normal direct and consensual responses, normal reaction to light and accommodation. On examining her fields, the acuity was poor on the right and on the left there was a nasal field defect. I was stopped before I could examine the fundi. The bell rang just in time as I did not know what the diagnosis was!

One examiner gave me a clear pass on this eye case and the other a fail – I am not sure what to make of this!

Examine this lady's hands.

I found normal nails, elbows and skin. There was a symmetrical, deforming polyarthropathy affecting the metacarpophalangeal and proximal interphalangeal joints.

I was asked for the diagnosis, what else I would like to examine, how to treat her and about the use of first-line disease-modifying drugs.

Examine this lady's skin.

There were lots of red plaques, particularly on the elbows. I felt that they may indicate psoriasis but there was no scaling.

'Where else would you look for psoriasis?' Answer: scalp. 'Go on then.' I found psoriasis on the scalp. 'What else would you like to look for?' Answer: arthropathy. I found an asymmetrical arthropathy involving the distal interphalangeal joints and was asked about treatment – both for the skin and the joints.

23. *What are the RCP guidelines for home oxygen and what is the evidence behind the guidelines?*

Station 1

This gentleman is short of breath, please examine the chest.

The patient was very cachectic and using the accessory muscles for respiration. On further examination I found clubbing and bibasal, fine, end-inspiratory crepitations.

The examiner asked me for my diagnosis and to give some possible causes. 'What investigations would you do?' he asked, 'and what would you expect to find on arterial blood gases, X-rays and CT scan of the thorax?', 'What is his prognosis, and how can one tell?'. The examiner carried on with questions, 'What are the RCP guidelines for home oxygen and what is the evidence behind the guidelines?' and 'How would you counsel the patient and what advice would you give him?'.

This lady presents with lethargy, please examine her abdomen.

My clinical findings were of a thin, pale lady with no stigmata of chronic liver disease but I did find hepatosplenomegaly. I thought the diagnosis could be myelofibrosis.

I was asked for a differential diagnosis, how would I investigate the patient, and then what would I expect to find on a full blood count, film, and bone marrow aspiration. He wanted to know what I thought would be the prognosis and how would I counsel the patient. 'What problems can occur with the platelets?' Then there was a discussion about platelet storage disorders and coagulopathies, and finally we touched on the treatment of disseminated intravascular coagulopathy.

Station 2

This 70-year-old gentleman has recently moved to our practice and has noticed worsening of his diarrhoea. He was diagnosed with ulcerative colitis 5 years ago at his local hospital and has been on mesalazine ever since. He has also had two pulmonary emboli in the past. I would welcome your advice.

The patient had concerns that he needed a colectomy as he had recently noticed a deterioration in his vision, and he had been told initially that if he had too many complications that a colectomy would be needed. He had originally been diagnosed following a colonoscopy and biopsy. However, he had been on mesalazine since diagnosis, with no problems. He was having about three bowel actions per day with no blood or mucus and was not concerned about the frequency despite the GP's comments. He had also seen an ophthalmologist who had reassured him regarding the formation of an early cataract which was probably steroid induced. He had had only three courses of steroids for flare-ups since diagnosis. He could not remember if he was on a calcium supplement but thought he did have 'weak bones'.

The first pulmonary embolus occurred during the initial illness following a deep vein thrombosis (DVT). He was treated with warfarin for 3 months and then it was stopped. Two years later, following a flight back from Australia, he developed another pulmonary embolus. He was aware that he is now on warfarin for life. He is fit and independent and lives with his wife. He visits his son in Sydney every year and has no problems with his bowels when flying.

The examiner asked me about the patient's priorities and concerns, and were they the same as the GP's or mine? They wanted to know what I would do next. I said that I would reassure him, arrange a routine colonoscopy and get his notes from the old hospital. 'Why do you want to scope him?' they asked, 'and what would you do regarding his warfarin if rectal bleeding should become a problem?' They asked me about the eye complications of inflammatory bowel disease and what evidence there is for the need for bone protection with steroid therapy.

Station 3

This gentleman has been more short of breath recently, please examine.
I only found a possible collapsing pulse and the early diastolic murmur of aortic regurgitation.

The examiners asked, 'Why do you think it is aortic regurgitation and not mitral stenosis?', 'What qualities are discriminatory?', 'How would you investigate?', 'What would you look for on the transthoracic echo?', 'What would you tell the patient?', 'If it was aortic stenosis what would you expect to find, what problems would you expect and what would influence decisions for surgery, etc.', 'How would you initiate warfarin, and what would you tell the patient about risks, etc.', 'Why don't you think it could be a ventricular septal defect (VSD)?'.

This gentleman is having difficulty reading his newspaper. Please examine his hands and proceed accordingly.
It was a Polish chap who was sitting with his wife and was fully clothed. He had a blank expression. I found a fine, resting tremor bilaterally and there was increased tone with lead pipe and cog-wheel rigidity. I was told not to focus on his hands (muscles, power sensation, etc.) as there would be nothing to find. I assessed his gait and it was hesitant and shuffling. I found a gross tremor on finger–nose testing but there was no dysdiadochokinesia. There were no other cerebellar signs and the speech was normal.

I was asked for a differential diagnosis and would I like to ask him some questions? I said that Parkinson's disease was above benign essential tremor in my list of possibilities but after asking how long he had had the tremor for, I was invited to revise my order! I was then asked how I would treat both of these conditions and what role physiotherapy has in the management of Parkinson's disease.

Station 4

You are the medical SHO in clinic and are about to meet Mrs X who is the daughter of the patient, Mr Y, who underwent an endoscopy (OGD) for dyspepsia last week. They have returned to clinic for the results of the investigations. Mr Y is hard of hearing so has asked you to speak to his daughter while he is next door getting changed. The results have come back, surprisingly, as gastric carcinoma. You are expected to inform the daughter of the results and discuss further options.

The conversation flowed easily as the lady was very understanding and calm. She took the diagnosis very well and then went on to ask some sensible questions. She was obviously upset and asked me questions about how long, how bad, should he cancel his holiday to visit his son and newborn grandson in the USA which was due in 2 weeks' time, should she tell her brother to come over, will her father be admitted, what treatment is there, will he be in pain, how will she tell him, how does she tell her mother, etc.

I addressed each question in turn, clearly explaining those that I could answer and those we would leave on hold until after the CT scan and the combined meeting, etc. We agreed to meet up next week with the CT scan results and the decision about surgical treatment options.

The examiners asked me how I felt the conversation went. They asked if I thought it was too harsh using the word 'cancer'. Then they went on to question me about the first principles of talking to relatives in terms of consent, autonomy, etc. 'What would happen if the family did not want him told or if they didn't want him to have an operation?' 'What would you do if the patient wanted treatment but the family were not happy?'

Station 5

This lady has headaches, please examine and proceed accordingly.
I found that the patient had acromegaly with a bitemporal field defect and carpal tunnel syndrome. The examiner asked me if I thought that the disease was

active and how I would investigate and treat. 'What would you tell the patient?' they asked me. 'What does visual field testing involve?'

Please examine this man's fundi.

My clinical findings were of the background changes of diabetic retinopathy with two laser scars visible just below the macula. The eyedrops were wearing off so I was unable to get a full view of the left eye. However, the examiners seemed satisfied that I tried!

They asked me for my diagnosis and would I be concerned if this gentleman was examined in clinic and these findings were detected? What would I suggest regarding follow-up? What is the pathophysiology of the lesion requiring coagulation? How would you manage the patient and what is the evidence for such treatment? Should he be driving?

This gentleman keeps dropping things. Please examine him.

He had severe, chronic, rheumatoid arthritis with fusion of the wrists and various joint replacements. There was obvious purpura so the patient was possibly on steroids.

I was asked for my management plan in terms of pharmacological and non-pharmacological methods. The examiner wanted to know how I would assess function and what impact would this have on his quality of life. What could I suggest to help with some of the household chores? He then said, 'Imagine you are a rheumatologist and this patient has been referred to you with rheumatoid arthritis that is resistant to all first- and second-line disease-modifying agents, what would you suggest, what are the side-effects of using TNF (tumour necrosis factor) and what are the contraindications of using such drugs?'.

This lady has had an episode of epistaxis, please examine and proceed accordingly.

She had telangiectasia over her face and around her mouth. There were no peripheral lesions to suggest CREST syndrome.

I was asked for the diagnosis and how I would manage the patient. What would you tell her? What would you expect to find if you were examining other members of the family? What would you do and what is the prognosis?

24. *I thought in my head that the patient had Cushing's syndrome but for some bizarre reason I said the patient had scleroderma!*

Station 1

This man has a cough. Please examine his chest.

He had coarse crackles over the right lower and mid zones but there were no other physical signs. I said that bronchiectasis was the most likely diagnosis.

The examiner asked what my investigation of choice would be. I suggested a chest X-ray, high-resolution CT scan, bronchoscopy and sputum analysis. There was a discussion of all of these.

This man has high blood pressure. Please examine his abdomen.

On examination, I found that he had a left arteriovenous fistula with a thrill. There were warts on his hands and he had a mid-line sternotomy scar. He had a right hernia scar, no organomegaly, and I forgot to auscultate.

I was asked what my concern would be in a patient with high blood pressure when performing an abdominal examination. I said that I would look for polycystic kidney disease and renal artery stenosis. 'Oh!' I said, 'I would have auscultated for bruits.' He asked me about the warts and we discussed immunosuppression but I could not palpate a transplanted kidney and the fistula was active. I was then asked for the causes of a failed transplant and I was shown the medication chart. He was on cyclosporin and prednisolone. Then the examiner said, 'What about the mid-line sternotomy scar?'. I said, 'Has he had a heart transplant?' and they said, 'Yes!'.

Station 2

You are in the outpatient clinic. Mr X is a 50-year-old man with a history of alcoholic cirrhosis and variceal bleeding. He presents with abdominal pain. Please review his medications.

The whole experience was awful. He had had about 15 previous hospital admissions with various degrees of cirrhosis and hepatic decompensation. I had no time to review his medications and when I finally did, the bell went and the examiner shouted 'Give it back!' at me as I was reading the prescription chart.

The questions I was asked by the examiner included, 'What were the main differential diagnoses?', 'Do you think that he has truly given up drinking?' and 'What precipitated him to give up drinking?'.

Station 3

This man has just returned from ITU. Please examine his cardiovascular system.

He had a mid-line sternotomy scar. There was gynaecomastia and a tracheostomy site which was covered with gauze. He had a right brachial percutaneous transluminal coronary angioplasty (PTCA) scar and there was peripheral oedema. He had prosthetic second heart sounds with no features to suggest a leaking valve. He was in congestive cardiac failure but there were no stigmata of subacute bacterial endocarditis.

The examiner asked me, 'What are the likely causes of gynaecomastia in this man?'. I replied that it could be a result of digoxin and spironolactone in a patient with a cardiovascular history. The examiner wanted to know, 'What else causes gynaecomastia on an ITU?'. I had no idea!

This man is unable to walk. Examine his legs.
He had an ulcer on the base of his right foot and there was a urinary catheter *in situ*. He had global reduction of tone, power, reflexes, coordination, vibration sense and proprioception and there was a stocking distribution sensory loss.

The first question was, 'Do you think that testing coordination in a patient with 3/5 weakness and who can't walk is helpful?'. 'No,' I said, feeling very stupid. Then the examiner asked me for a differential diagnosis and I said that he had a sensory motor neuropathy. I was asked why I included a motor element. I replied, 'Because of the weakness'. He asked me what could explain the need for a catheter and I wondered if he had a cauda equina lesion. 'What else would you want to do?' In retrospect I should have said, 'Ask about the timing of the onset'. Instead I uttered, 'Examine the remainder of the nervous system!'. The last question was, 'Would you expect signs in the arms with a cauda equina lesion?'. 'No,' I said.

Station 4

This is a middle-aged lady who has a top position in cosmetic sales and today she has had her first seizure. You are the SHO on-call. She is almost ready to leave the casualty department and you need to instruct her about the implications for driving, about possible treatment options and the need to avoid other dangerous situations.
We discussed the presentation of the seizure and that it may not necessarily be epilepsy. The patient was very concerned about why she had had a fit and what could be done to find the cause. She was extremely upset about the driving implications as driving was her livelihood.

The examiner quizzed me on, 'Would I, and when would I, inform the DVLA, what would I tell her boss

if he telephoned, and what might be important to mention about treatment if she requires it?'.

Station 5

This lady has uncontrolled hypertension. Please examine her.
I thought in my head that the patient had Cushing's syndrome, but for some bizarre reason (?microstomia) I said the patient had scleroderma! The examiner said, 'No, what are the causes of high blood pressure?'. I said that 90% were idiopathic, 10% were a result of endocrine causes such as Cushing's and Conn's syndromes and a small number had renal artery stenosis. The examiner said, 'One of those answers is correct'. Then she asked the patient to stand up and she had obvious proximal myopathy. We discussed the causes of Cushing's syndrome and then she said, 'The patient has a mass in the pituitary on an MRI scan. What would you examine to assess the size?'. 'Visual fields,' I said. Then she asked me to demonstrate.

This lady has had neurosurgery. Please examine her eyes.
I found a right upper homonymous quadrantanopia but I was not asked any questions as the bell went at this stage.

Examine this lady's hands.
I found a symmetrical deforming arthropathy with scars over the wrists. There were no nail changes. She also had scars over both elbows but there were no nodules and no evidence of psoriasis.

I said the patient had rheumatoid arthritis and the examiner asked if I was sure about this to which I replied, 'Yes'. The examiner asked me if it could be anything else. I replied that, 'If psoriatic plaques had been present then possibly this could be arthritis mutilans as there was evidence of telescoping of the fingers'. He then asked if I thought one had to have psoriatic plaques in order to have psoriatic arthropathy. I replied, 'Probably not!'. I was asked what drugs she could be on and I suggested non-steroidals. The examiner asked me, 'Would you take methotrexate?'.

This man has itchy skin. Please examine.
He had thickened skin with diffuse extensive erythema and multiple abrasions. I said I would be concerned about the drug history. 'What else?', they asked. 'I would consider infections such as herpes zoster but the abnormality is not in a dermatome distribution.' The examiner asked, 'What would give you extensive skin

thickening?'. I replied, 'repeated trauma and itching'. 'What diffuse processes?' he asked and I suggested, 'psoriasis or eczema'. 'Yes,' he said, 'this is eczema!'

Comments

The exam was horrible and extremely stressful. I felt like an idiot with things coming out of my mouth that I wished had stayed in.

Afterwards, I was full of disappointment that they did not see the real me, frustration about what did they really want when they asked a question and tears both of relief and a fear of failure.

---

25. *I was asked 'What is the diagnosis and what investigations would you do next?'. I said, 'A chest X-ray' and they produced one!*

Station 1

This man complains of shortness of breath. Examine him and find out why.

He had obvious finger clubbing with bibasal, inspiratory, fine crepitations.

I was asked, 'What is the diagnosis and what investigations would you do next?'. I said, 'It's pulmonary fibrosis and I would do a chest X-ray'. They produced one! 'Does this support your diagnosis?', 'What further tests would you do?', 'What causes pulmonary fibrosis?', 'Ask him some questions to find a cause'. I asked about his occupation and discovered that he was an electrician so they wanted me to ask about asbestos exposure. Finally the examiner asked, 'How would you treat him?'.

This lady has thrombocytopenia. Examine her abdomen and come up with a likely diagnosis.

The lady had purpura on her forearms. I found a small spleen but I could not feel a liver. She also had a lower mid-line abdominal scar.

The examiner asked me, 'What is the diagnosis?'. I suggested that it was likely to be a lymphoproliferative or myeloproliferative disease. 'Does she have any petechiae?' 'Is the abdominal scar relevant?' I said she may have had a hysterectomy because of menorrhagia and he seemed satisfied with that answer. 'Would you expect hepatomegaly with your diagnoses?' he said.

Station 2

You are the SHO in clinic. This 57-year-old man has had asthma since the age of 7 and was then diagnosed with pulmonary eosinophilia in 1960. Since January he has had recurrent chest infections including Haemophilus influenzae *pneumonia. Please see and advise.*

The patient had never smoked and had not been treated for the pulmonary eosinophilia. He had been asthmatic most of his life but for the last few months had noticed increasing shortness of breath and a cough with green sputum and this was now associated with sweats. He had had repeated courses of antibiotics from his GP. He had worked as a wood machinist for 20 years. He had used a mask but his symptoms always improved when off work. He was now a manager for a cleaning company. He was on inhaled steroids and had been on oral prednisolone 10 mg/day for the past 10 weeks.

I was asked to give an account of the history. The examiner said, 'What do you think is going on?'. I said it could be poorly controlled asthma or pulmonary eosinophilia but he may now have bronchiectasis secondary to allergic bronchopulmonary aspergillosis (ABPA). After offering this diagnosis, they asked, 'How do you diagnose ABPA?', 'What blood tests could you do?', 'How do you treat it?'. I mentioned postural drainage, etc. 'If the bronchiectasis is localized to the upper lobes how could you treat it?' 'Have you heard of a flutter valve?' I said, 'No!'.

Station 3

This man has a heart murmur. Please examine him.

He was in sinus rhythm with a non-displaced apex but with a pansystolic murmur best heard at the apex and radiating to the axilla. There was a mid-line abdominal scar.

The examiner asked me, 'What is the murmur?', 'What are the features that make you say mitral regurgitation?', 'Can you connect the murmur and the abdominal scar?'. I said, 'No' and he said, 'We'll come back to it at the end and I bet you get it!'. Then he asked me about the causes of mitral regurgitation and finally he asked about the scar again. I said he may have had mitral regurgitation secondary to ischaemic heart disease and therefore he may have generalized atheromatous disease with an abdominal aortic aneurysm repair. He said, 'Told you so!'.

This lady has difficulty walking. Please examine her legs.

She had a broad-based gait but was steady on her feet. There was lower leg wasting but with brisk reflexes and up-going plantars. I thought that she may also have a stocking distribution sensory loss.

The examiner said to me, 'You have described upper and lower motor neurone signs. What is the diagnosis?', 'How does the sensory component fit in?' I offered a combination of common diseases such as cervical myelopathy and diabetes. The examiner did not seem to be impressed! Thankfully, the bell went before he could grill me any more!

Station 4

A 75-year-old lady who had a stroke 1 year ago, now living alone with social services support, has presented with a gastrointestinal bleed but is stable. You have requested an endoscopy (OGD). There is no organic confusion but the patient has refused the investigation and says she wants to die. Her daughter has come from Scotland. Explain to her what is going on.
The daughter was very upset. She said, 'Mum isn't thinking straight, go ahead with the test, you must do everything. I'll sign the consent form'. I had to explain that her mother was not confused and we had to abide with her wishes. Then the daughter said that her mother had been depressed at home and that she is doing this to spite her as she has had little contact with her mother since moving to Scotland. I explained that I would ask my consultant to see her and that also I would get a psychiatric opinion to exclude depression.

The examiner said, 'What is the essential problem here?'. I said, 'A consent problem in someone who is refusing treatment and who is mentally competent and of sound mind'. The examiner said, 'What is the legal term for that?'. I didn't know. 'If she became comatosed would you do the OGD then?' 'Do you think the daughter will complain?' 'How would you prepare for this?'

Station 5

This man is followed up in the eye clinic. Have a look at him and tell me why.
I said the patient had exophthalmos. The examiner said, 'Go on to examine his eyes'. I found he had diplopia but I forgot to mention the lid lag. I ended up saying I would do fundoscopy. Somehow I then got confused and started thinking of diabetes. It was all a bit of a mess!

This man has trouble with his vision.
He was wearing yellow, plastic glasses. The right eye looked normal but there were black, pigmented lesions on the temporal part of the retina of the left eye.

The examiner asked, 'What is the diagnosis?'. I said, 'choroidoretinitis' and he replied, 'Where did you see it?'. He did not seem impressed and asked what would be my main differential. When I said retinitis pigmentosa he was satisfied. This diagnosis was confirmed by the registrar invigilator afterwards.

This man has had painful hands. Please examine him.
There were obvious rheumatoid changes in the hands with nodules at the elbows and evidence of previous surgery. I was asked, 'What is the diagnosis? List your findings', 'What could cause wasting of the small muscles of the hand in this man?'. I went through all the neurological causes, e.g. nodules causing ulnar nerve palsy, etc., but he just wanted me to say 'diffuse atrophy'.

This lady has a rash. Examine it.
There was an obvious, deforming arthropathy of the hands with a rash on the dorsum of the upper arms and upper chest, i.e. the sun-exposed areas.

The examiner said, 'What do you think it is?'. I said psoriasis at first but he asked, 'Is it the typical distribution, i.e. why is it worst on sun-exposed areas? What else could it be?'. I said, 'systemic lupus erythematosus (SLE)'. Then he asked, 'Would SLE cause this degree of arthritis?'. We eventually got around to mixed connective tissue disorders, which was the correct diagnosis.

> **Comments**
>
> The 5-min gaps between cases are great if it is a 'talking station' as you have time to prepare the given material. If it is a 'clinical station' it is too long to sit and become more nervous. They did supply us with drinks, though, to combat the xerostomia!
>
> I ended with Station 1. As I was leaving, the examiner said, 'If I were you, I would go and have a good drink now!'. I was not sure if this was meant to reassure me or not!

26. *The surgical registrar calls you and tells you that his SHO has been found collapsed in her room with syringes around her and with all the signs of diamorphine having been given.*

Station 1

Examine this patient's respiratory system.

The patient had a hoarse voice, a trachea that was central but there was a noticeable scar on the right side posteriorly with no other obvious chest deformity. He had, in fact, had a right-sided lobectomy.

The examiner asked me what I noticed about the voice and to explain my findings. I had to give some possible reasons why the patient had had a lobectomy. They asked me about the different types of lung cancer.

Examine this patient's abdomen.
The patient had bilateral Dupuytren's contractures which were more noticeable on the left side. There were lots of spider naevi on the chest wall and, on abdominal examination, there was hepatosplenomegaly. The examiner told me that the patient was anaemic and my diagnosis was of alcoholic liver disease.

I was asked for a differential diagnosis for hepatosplenomegaly and the examiner asked me if I thought the patient was anaemic. Then he changed the subject to questions about lymphadenopathy and hepatosplenomegaly, what investigations I would do and what would be my management plan.

Station 2
There was a GP letter regarding a 54-year-old lady who had moved from America 2 weeks previously. She presented with jaundice and pruritus to her GP who had carried out a blood test which showed abnormal liver function tests with an obstructive picture. She had a recent history of weight loss and had been using herbal medicines. She had now noticed swelling of her abdomen.
The history that evolved just clarified the information given in the GP letter.

I was asked for a differential diagnosis and what further investigations I would do and then what management I would instigate. I was asked for the causes of an obstructive picture in the liver function tests and I forgot to mention the important cause, i.e. gallstones (I was so preoccupied with the history of weight loss). Neither did I mention primary biliary cirrhosis!

Station 3
Look at this patient and describe what you see.* Then listen to the heart.
I found that the patient had a kyphoscoliosis with a wide arm span and a high-arched palate. On auscultation, it was obvious that he had had a mechanical aortic

---

*A clue to the diagnosis is in the instruction.

valve replacement but there was no evidence of a para-prosthetic leak.

The examiners first asked me to inspect the patient generally and to describe what I saw. I said he had the features of Marfan's syndrome but there was no obvious lens dislocation. Then they asked me to examine the heart. Next, they wanted to know how I would manage this patient in terms of anticoagulation with warfarin. I was expected to say that I would need to know the rest of the patient's drug history, especially with regard to any non-steroidal anti-inflammatory drug (NSAID) medication. Finally, they asked me to outline the problems that can occur with valve replacement.

Examine this patient's cranial nerves and check the reflexes in the lower limbs as this patient has had noticeable weakness of both legs.
The patient had obvious nystagmus – internuclear ophthalmoplegia and brisk reflexes. I also checked for clonus, although I was not asked to do so, and found that the patient had noticeable sustained clonus.

The examiners asked for my diagnosis and I suggested demyelination as there was evidence of an internuclear ophthalmoplegia and a spastic paraparesis. They asked me what internuclear ophthalmoplegia is and I named five causes for it. The examiners seemed very happy with this case and they stopped me as soon as I had told them the causes of the ophthalmoplegia.

Station 4
You are the medical SHO on-call. The surgical registrar calls you and tells you that his SHO has been found collapsed in her room with syringes around her and with signs of diamorphine having been given, such as pinpoint pupils. She has been given naloxone and has woken up. The surgical registrar would like you to talk to her.
I told her that the surgical registrar was concerned about her and that we suspected that she was abusing diamorphine. I explained to her the risks of hepatitis and HIV by using needles and this included explaining the risk to herself and to her patients. I had to tell her that her consultant would have to be informed. The SHO denied the use of intravenous drugs and said that she was a diabetic and was checking her blood sugars.

The examiners asked me who I would like to inform, and I said the GMC, and would I suspend her from work and I said, 'yes'.

Station 5
Examine this lady's neck.

She had a multinodular goitre with no bruits. She was euthyroid as she was not anxious or sweaty. There was no tremor, tachycardia or lid lag. I mentioned all of this to the examiner. He asked me what sort of goitre she had and I responded that it was multinodular. He asked me for the most likely cause and what my further investigations and management would be.

Look at the fundi and describe what you find.
There were bilateral cataracts and bilateral laser therapy scars. I initially forgot to mention the cataracts but managed to bring it into the conversation when one examiner asked me what else I could see. He asked me about the other complications of diabetes mellitus and about the use of ramipril and the HOPE study.

Examine this patient's gait.
He had a very protuberant abdomen and a kyphosis so I diagnosed ankylosing spondylitis. The examiner asked me for the possible complications and I listed anterior uveitis, aortitis, apical fibrosis, atlantoaxial subluxation and the risks during anaesthesia.

Look at the hands, look at the face and give the diagnosis.
I found evidence of hypertrophic osteoarthropathy at the wrists and bilateral periorbital xanthelasma. These findings were not connected in any way.

The examiner asked me what X-ray finding I would see in hypertrophic osteoarthropathy and then he asked me what I could see when looking at the patient's face. I mentioned the xanthelasma.

Comments

It is more likely that one will not score as highly in the ethics and history-taking stations but that one can make up for this if one knows the clinical examination routines well.

Read the instructions properly at each station as they usually give vital clues.

Pretend that you are a registrar presenting cases on a ward round.

---

27. *It was unusual to have a Marfan's syndrome as the respiratory case. The patient was not a typical Marfan's because the kyphoscoliosis made him look much shorter*

and the flexure deformity of the fingers obscured the arachnodactyly.

Station 1

This is a 56-year-old lady who has been dyspnoeic for a long time. Examine her respiratory system.
I found bilateral, fine, inspiratory basal crackles. I also noted the kyphoscoliosis and a scar over the back. I thought that there might be arachnodactyly and an arthropathy of the fingers.

I was asked to give my findings and to suggest the most likely diagnosis. I answered that it was likely to be ankylosing spondylitis with pulmonary fibrosis and that the dyspnoea may be caused by a chest wall deformity and a restricted ventilatory defect. After the exam, I met the patient in the car park and she told me that she had Marfan's syndrome!*

Examine this patient's abdomen.
The patient was moderately jaundiced with a possible parotid swelling and numerous spider naevi. The jugular venous pressure (JVP) was not raised. There was four finger-breadth hepatomegaly which was firm and non-tender. However, there was no splenomegaly and no oedema. I was asked for a differential diagnosis.

Station 2

This 36-year-old lady has had arthritis for 3 years. There is a history of bronchial asthma and she is on oral steroids, and Ventolin and Becotide inhalers. There has been an increase in the joint pains. Please ask her some questions.
I obtained a history of a progressive polyarthritis, mainly affecting the small joints of the hands, elbows and knees. There was significant early morning stiffness and Raynaud's phenomenon but there was no photosensitivity, fever or any other extra-articular features. There was ankle swelling but the asthma was stable. There had been no response to the steroids despite the side-effects of weight gain and hypertension. The chest X-ray showed possible fibrosis.

I was asked for the likely causes of both lung and joint disease. Finally, the examiner confirmed that it was rheumatoid arthritis with lung involvement and I was asked about the management in terms of drug treatment with disease-modifying agents such as

---

*For respiratory complications of Marfan's syndrome, see Vol. 3, Station 5, Locomotor, Case 9.

azathioprine and methotrexate. I then had to enumerate the side-effects of methotrexate.

Station 3

The GP has referred this 72-year-old lady with a murmur. Please examine her.

Examination showed that the patient was in atrial fibrillation although the pulse was strong and the carotid pulse was visible. There was a systolic murmur at the mitral area with no radiation. The murmur was also heard at the left sternal edge but not at the carotid root. Both heart sounds were normal with no other murmurs.

I was asked for a diagnosis and I offered a differential of mitral regurgitation and hypertrophic obstructive cardiomyopathy (HOCM). The discussion then centred on mitral regurgitation. I was asked again for a differential diagnosis and what I would consider if the patient's condition deteriorated. I suggested infective endocarditis and, possibly, pulmonary oedema.

Look at this patient and examine neurologically.

There was frontal balding with a bilateral partial ptosis. I also found weakness of the facial muscles and wasting of the small muscles. There was no gynaecomastia or myotonia.

The examiner asked me what I thought the diagnosis was, so I suggested myotonic dystrophy or myasthenia gravis. He asked how I would differentiate between the two and which did I think was the most likely? I was then asked how to confirm the diagnosis and for the investigation and management of myotonic dystrophy. He asked me, 'What is myotonia?' and 'What is the prognosis?'.

Station 4

You are the SHO in chest medicine. A 57-year-old lady was admitted about 5 weeks ago with pneumonia. She has small muscle wasting and diaphragmatic weakness. A neurologist has been consulted and thinks this is motor neurone disease. You plan to do an electromyographical (EMG) study but the patient wants to know what is wrong. Please tell the patient about her condition, the management plan and the prognosis.

I explained about motor neurone disease and that the diagnosis is by exclusion of other causes. I told her that the management is very multidisciplinary rather than with a specific drug treatment. She wanted a second opinion and to know the prognosis. She wanted to know about any feeding and respiratory difficulties. I explained that her pneumonia was probably a result of

aspiration because of difficulty with swallowing and that she might need a percutaneous endoscopic gastrostomy (PEG) in the future. I also told her of the poor prognosis but that we needed to exclude other possibilities.

The examiners asked about the fact that the patient lived alone. Would she need residential or nursing home care at some stage? 'Should the patient be allowed a second opinion?' 'Yes,' I said, 'she has a right to that.' 'Are there any newer treatments?' 'Yes, there is riluzole which improves the quality of life but does not improve survival.'

Station 5

Look at this patient.

I noticed the obvious features of acromegaly and I was asked about the investigations and management.

This elderly man has had a sudden onset of blindness in his right eye. Please examine him and explain why.

There was right-sided optic atrophy with attenuation of the vessels in the right temporal region but there was no cherry-red spot. I was asked for the diagnosis and suggested either central retinal artery occlusion or an ischaemic optic neuropathy.

This is a lady of about 80 years. Please look at her hands.

She had a bilateral symmetrical arthropathy with the distal interphalangeal joints involved as well. There were Heberden's nodes and gouty tophi and subluxation of the metacarpophalangeal joints.

I was asked for a differential diagnosis and then asked which features were in favour of rheumatoid arthritis and which were against this possibility. Also, which features were for and against osteoarthritis.

Look at this patient's face.

I saw lupus pernio and lots of telangiectasia. I was asked for the diagnosis so said, 'Lupus pernio,

> **Comments**
>
> It was unusual to have a patient with Marfan's syndrome as the respiratory case. The patient did not exhibit typical Marfan's syndrome because the kyphoscoliosis made him look much shorter and the flexion deformity of the fingers obscured the arachnodactyly.

and possibly hereditary haemorrhagic telangiectasia (HHT) as well'. I was then asked to outline how to investigate and confirm a diagnosis of sarcoid.

28. *I thought he was normal! But managed to persuade myself that he had short fourth and fifth metacarpals!*

Station 1

This lady is short of breath, please examine her respiratory system.

The patient was on oxygen, had central cyanosis and was clubbed. On auscultation, there were widespread crackles. I was asked about long-term oxygen trials (LTOT),* steroid trials and pulmonary function tests. I was also asked for the causes of pulmonary fibrosis and which questions I would ask the patient.

I was given some haematology results which were suggestive that the patient might have splenomegaly.

I could not find a spleen and I was sent back to have another look! I think he also had cervical lymph nodes. I was asked how I could confirm a spleen if I was not sure clinically. Then I had to list the causes of splenomegaly.

Station 2

This 30-year-old lady has had fits and needs to be started on antiepileptics. However, she is thinking of starting a family – please advise.

She had had about four grand mal seizures in the last couple of months. Her mother had a brain tumour. She was on the oral contraceptive pill but wanted to stop it and start a family. She was not keen to have any tablets that could be harmful to a baby. We talked about doing a CT scan and an electroencephalogram (EEG) to investigate for possible causes, about not driving, and about taking the contraceptive pill until all the investigations were complete. I explained that antiepileptics are teratogenic but that the risks are less if one takes folate supplements. I explained that having a seizure could be more harmful.

The examiner kept dwelling on the blood tests that would be useful to investigate the cause – I think he was

driving at systemic lupus erythematosus (she was Afro-Caribbean).

Station 3

This patient had a myocardial infarct 1 year ago. Please examine the cardiovascular system.

There was an ejection systolic murmur at the aortic area with no radiation. The pulse and blood pressure were both normal. However, there was also a pansystolic murmur at the apex. There was no overt cardiac failure.

The examiner asked me: 'What is the most significant lesion and the probable cause for it?', 'How would you investigate?', 'What would be a significant gradient across the aortic valve?'.

This patient has a 20-year history of weakness in the right arm and shoulder.

I found asymmetry, wasting and fasciculation over the right shoulder and some areas of the arm – I thought it could be a C5 radiculopathy.

'What are the causes?' I suggested motor neurone disease, polio and syringomyelia. 'Which is the most likely?' 'Which nerves/roots are involved and why?'

Station 4

A 55-year-old man has recently been admitted with an aspiration pneumonia. He is at the end-stage of motor neurone disease. His chest is now better and he is going home. You need to speak to his wife and discuss his resuscitation status, his suitability or not for ITU, withholding antibiotics and the use or not of non-invasive positive pressure ventilation (NIPPV) on future admissions.

I explained to the wife that he was at the end-stage of the disease and that it was probably unkind to prolong his suffering. We discussed whether he should stay at home when he gets the next chest infection and to arrange for different agencies to come in to help her, such as the GP, the district nurse and palliative care nurses. He could be given oxygen at home and be given a syringe driver to relieve unpleasant symptoms. By the end of the discussion she appeared quite happy with the above.

---

*Long-term oxygen therapy (LTOT) trials were carried out to look at the effect of oxygen given for over 15h/day on survival in patients with chronic obstructive pulmonary disease (COPD) – it did prolong survival and in fact is the only pharmaceutical treatment for COPD that has shown a benefit on survival. Inhalers that we all spend £ millions on do not. Oxygen therapy has not been shown to improve longevity in pulmonary fibrosis but

keeping saturations of oxygen above 92% obviously has other benefits, e.g. quality of life, prevention of polycythaemia and also mental/psychological parameters.

We suspect this case was a pulmonary fibrosis patient but LTOT trials questions would be more relevant in COPD patients as there are guidelines on when to prescribe these in COPD and the evidence is convincing.

I was asked to explain how I could be sure that she had got the message and who was going to follow this up if he is going home today.

Station 5

Please examine this patient's hands. He is a 15-year-old boy who presented with carpopedal spasm as a child.

I thought he was normal but managed to persuade myself that he had short fourth and fifth metacarpals! The examiner exclaimed, 'Isn't he a bit tall for pseudo-hypoparathyroidism?'. He went on to ask, 'How is it inherited?' and 'Could it be anything else?'.

Examine this patient's fundus.

There were bilateral cataracts and photocoagulation scars. The examiner wanted to know how I would prevent further retinal damage and asked what the ideal cholesterol level was. 'What tablets should she be on if she has high blood pressure and proteinuria?'

Examine this patient's hands.

There were multiple neurofibromas over the hands and also over the trunk. I had to discuss inheritance, complications and family screening.

Examine this patient's foot.

The patient had a diabetic foot ulcer. The feet were cold, with reduced sensation including vibration sense, and also the arterial pulses were absent.

The examiner asked me, 'How can you best prevent these ulcers?', 'What is the best method of treatment and what further investigations would you do?'. I talked about Doppler ultrasound and angiograms.

Comments

Everyone was nice. It was good to have a 5-min break between each station and to know that the next two examiners are totally objective and are not aware of how you did at the previous station.

---

29. *The examiner asked me why the patient was pale, what are the mechanisms of anaemia in renal failure and is there any condition in which the patients are not anaemic?*

Station 1

This man has a long history of breathlessness. Please examine his respiratory system.

On examination, there was no clubbing but he had fine, end-inspiratory crackles and so I diagnosed pulmonary fibrosis.

The examiner asked me for the causes of pulmonary fibrosis and what did I think was the significance of this patient having a parrot at home. He asked what tests I would perform and I had to explain what is meant by the transfer factor. He concluded by asking me what treatment I would give this patient.

This patient attends the renal clinic with hypertension. Please examine his abdominal system.

I found the patient to have an arteriovenous fistula with a scar in the lower abdomen. A transplanted kidney was palpable. However, I could not feel any polycystic kidneys.

The examiner asked me why the patient was pale, what are the mechanisms of anaemia in renal failure and is there any condition in which the patients are not anaemic? He then asked me why this patient was in end-stage renal failure and why had he had a transplant? He also wanted to know what medication he should be on post transplant, why is he hypertensive and what would be the treatment for the hypertension?

Station 2

This 30-year-old lady has a previous history of back pain which was thought to be renal colic. She now presents with further back pain. Her past medical history also includes amenorrhoea for which she is on bromocriptine and a recent abdominal X-ray shows nephrocalcinosis. Please take a history.

During the history taking, we discussed her back pain which was similar to her previous episodes. We discussed her amenorrhoea and associated galactorrhoea and the fact that she was now menstruating. Scans performed at the time had shown a pituitary 'problem' which I assumed was a prolactinoma.

The examiner wanted to know the overall diagnosis and I suggested multiple endocrine neoplasia (MEN) type 1 (see Vol.3, Station 5, Endocrine, Case 6). He asked me what the components of this were, what investigations I would perform and then we had a discussion about pituitary function tests.

Station 3

This man has been complaining of chest pain and palpitations. Please examine the cardiovascular system.

I was not very sure about my findings but thought he had an ejection systolic murmur so I thought the diagnosis should be aortic stenosis. At first I said he had mitral stenosis! We talked about an opening snap, the duration of the murmur and the loud first heart sound. The discussion then went on to the clinical indicators for the severity of aortic stenosis.

This patient has problems with his balance. Please examine his cerebellar system.

I found left-sided cerebellar signs with increased tone and hyperreflexia and a probable internuclear ophthalmoplegia.

The examiner wanted to know the causes of a cerebellar syndrome and what the likely cause was in this patient. I suggested multiple sclerosis and he asked me what investigations I would perform and what treatment I would give. He asked me who decides about who gets interferon.

Station 4

This is a young asthmatic who has had a recent severe exacerbation. He is due to go home but is worried about this happening again. Please discuss his concerns.

This patient's main questions were, 'Will this happen again?', 'How can I prevent it?', 'Can I exercise now?', 'This episode started while I was decorating my house, should I stop doing this?'. He was also confused about his inhalers and thought that they were making his cough worse.

The examiner asked me to summarize the situation and then asked me how I felt the conversation went. He asked if I thought that the patient was satisfied and whether he had understood about peak flow monitoring and the use of inhalers.

Station 5

This lady has had recent headaches. Please examine the appropriate systems.

The patient was obviously acromegalic and the examiner asked me why she was acromegalic and what else I would like to examine. He asked what investigations I would perform and what treatment I would give. He asked me what I needed to be worried about postoperatively in such patients.

This patient is blind. Examine his fundi.

I found he had cataracts and also retinitis pigmentosa. The examiners did not ask me any additional questions.

Look at, and examine, this man's legs.

He had wasting of the quadriceps and a scar from a muscle biopsy. I was asked for the causes of a proximal

myopathy and why he had a muscle biopsy scar. I was then asked for the associations of polymyositis, its treatment and prognosis.

Describe this lady's abnormalities.

She had sclerodactyly, telangiectasia and microstomia so I suggested limited systemic sclerosis as the underlying diagnosis.

The examiners requested that I ask the patient some questions, then they asked me what functional disabilities she might have and what problems one can get in diffuse systemic sclerosis.

Comments

In general, this exam was very fair and the examiners were nice. Often, I was looking for a hidden agenda but it was really just straightforward.

---

30. *They asked, 'What difference would it make in terms of the anatomical site of the problem whether the hemianopia had macular sparing or not?'.*

Station 1

This patient presented with worsening shortness of breath. Please examine his chest.

I found bibasal end-inspiratory fine crepitations. There was no clubbing and no signs of scleroderma. I was asked about the possible causes of pulmonary fibrosis and how I would investigate this patient.

Please examine this gentleman's abdominal system and comment on the findings.

There were multiple spider naevi over the chest. There was ascites with dullness in the loins and a caput medusa. I was not asked any additional questions.

Station 2

A 26-year-old bartender presented with a history of two episodes of tingling over the right side of the body each lasting 10–15 min. She has one daughter. She is a smoker and takes the oral contraceptive pill. Please take a history and discuss with the examiners. You are not expected to examine the patient.

She was a 26-year-old lady who smoked 10–15 cigarettes/day and had been on the oral contraceptive pill for 2 years. She presented as above. Both of the episodes were associated with tingling over the right side of the face, upper and lower limbs. There was no motor weakness and no loss of consciousness. On both occasions she had taken one tablet of 'speed' (she did not tell the GP about that, so it was not mentioned in the GP letter). Otherwise she was fit and well. She was on no other medication and no over-the-counter tablets. There were no symptoms of worsening weakness or general tiredness. There was no history of previous spontaneous abortions, nor of photosensitivity nor deep vein thromboses. She had no mouth or genital ulcers and no gait abnormalities.

The examiners asked me for a differential as to the most likely possibility and then we went on to a discussion about other possible causes. They wanted to know what the appropriate investigations would include.

Station 3

This lady has a heart murmur. Please examine her cardiovascular system.

On inspection, there was a left valvotomy scar and all the signs of a left hemiplegia. There was a tapping apex beat, an opening snap and the classic diastolic murmur of mitral stenosis. No questions were asked.

Examine this patient's cranial nerves.

I examined the cranial nerves and told them the patient had a right homonymous hemianopia with macular sparing. They asked, 'What difference would it make in terms of the anatomical site of the problem whether the hemianopia had macular sparing or not?'.

Station 4

This patient presents with chorea. His father died of Huntington's disease and his sister has the disease. He is in the neurology clinic to see the consultant who has had to leave early and you are left with him. Please counsel him about his chorea. You are almost certain that he has the disease. He is not at all happy that the consultant is not in the clinic.

I apologized for the situation. I then asked him if he had any idea as to what might be the cause of his symptoms. I asked him what he knew about the disease and I gave him time to express his worries. (His wife, who was not with him, was very concerned and he did not want to cause stress to his family, particularly as his 12-year-old son was taking exams.) He has two sons aged 12 and 4, and a 9-year-old daughter. I asked him if he thought that he might be willing to speak to his children regarding genetic testing. At the end I offered for him to return to the clinic with his wife to meet both me and the consultant.

The examiner wanted to know if I thought that offering genetic testing on the children was possible without the consent of the children. He then went on, 'As antenatal testing for Huntington's disease is possible, do you think that it is fair to put the 50% of foetuses who do not have the disease under the risk of amniocentesis?'. Then he said, 'At what age do the human rights of the individual start?'.

Station 5

This patient has a goitre. Please examine her.

I found exophthalmos and a homogeneous, non-nodular goitre but the patient was clinically euthyroid. There were no questions.

Examine the patient's fundi.

A 25-year-old man was sitting in a conservatory at 12 mid-day with the curtains open! However, I did manage to see background proliferative diabetic retinopathy with photocoagulation scars and flame-shaped haemorrhages. I had to explain how I would differentiate between old and new photocoagulation scars on fundoscopy.

Examine this patient's spine (patient sitting on a chair reading a newspaper).

There was ankylosing spondylitis and I listened to his heart and found aortic regurgitation. The examiners moved on without asking anything else.

What is the diagnosis?

I found a psoriatic erythema and no questions were asked.

31. *On this attempt (my fourth), I treated the exam as a ward round and did not feel the examiners could 'hurt' me any more. Perhaps in hindsight that is the reason I passed. With reaccreditation looming, I think it would be worthwhile getting MRCP examiners to actually sit the MRCP PACES exam under exam conditions – that would be fun!*

Station 1

This gentleman has been getting more breathless in recent months. Please examine his chest.

The patient was tachypnoeic and tachycardic. The trachea was deviated to the left. There was reduced air entry* on the left side with reduced expansion on that

*It is more accurate to say 'reduced breath sounds'.

side of the chest and there was also a left-sided thoracotomy scar.

The examiner asked me for my findings and then asked me to show him how I assessed the position of the trachea. 'What do you think is the reason for your findings and why do you think the patient is breathless?'

Examine this gentleman's abdomen.
This was a man with dark glasses and a walking stick. I found that he was jaundiced with spider naevi, hepatomegaly and ascites but he had no significant central or peripheral oedema.

The examiner asked me to give my findings and to tell him about the pathophysiology of ascites, what metabolic abnormalities might be present and to describe a management plan.

Station 2

Take a history from this business manager who is stressed at work and describes abdominal symptoms.
He described symptoms of difficulty with defaecation and passing pellet-like stools. He also described rectal bleeding and was concerned because his father had died in his fifties from colonic cancer. He was stressed at work but had no actual weight loss. He did not think he had haemorrhoids and had had no significant change in his bowel habit. He was very anxious about his condition as he had a wife and three children to support.

The examiner asked me what I thought this gentleman's main concerns were and what plan of management I would propose. He then asked me what I knew about heredity factors in colonic neoplasms.

Station 3

Examine this man's cardiovascular system.
The gentleman was elderly, fully dressed and sitting in a chair. I was required to get him onto the bed and into the correct position. I found that he had a slow-rising pulse with an ejection systolic murmur radiating to the carotids.

The examiner wanted me to give my findings and to demonstrate the position of the apex beat. I had to roll the patient over to do this. He asked me what features of the history might be of relevance, what investigations I would perform and, on a cardiac echogram, what gradient would concern me.

Examine the legs of this lady.
She was about 40 years of age and I found upper motor neurone signs with an element of a sensory deficit. I

thought she had hereditary motor and sensory neuropathy (HMSN) and I was asked to demonstrate all the methods of eliciting a plantar response, i.e. Babinski, Oppenheim, Gordon, etc., and then to demonstrate the presence of clonus.

Station 4

This 88-year-old lady has had a dense, completed stroke. She is extremely unwell and is unable to take adequate nutrition. The team have decided that her outlook is poor. Please talk to her daughter about the issue of 'not for resuscitation'.
The patient has two daughters, one of whom is in Japan. The daughter I was speaking to was keen that her mother be kept comfortable and that she was 'not for resuscitation' (NFR). However, the daughter in Japan wanted everything to be done for her mother in terms of active management. I had to delve into the daughter's assessment of her mother's health and her premorbid state and discuss issues regarding a living will. At the end of the discussion, an agreement was reached for her to be NFR.

I was asked about the scenario of the daughter leaving and the mother arresting; would we resuscitate? I was also asked about the issues of documenting the decision in the notes.

Station 5

Look at this patient's eyes.
The patient had bilateral exophthalmos and also had a frosted left lens in his glasses. No additional questions were asked by the examiner.

Please examine this patient's fundi.
I found background diabetic retinopathy and I was not asked any further questions.

Look at this patient's hand and legs.
The patient had sclerodactyly and an ulcer on the leg. The examiner asked me what type of ulcer it was and I suggested that it could be vasculitic.

Look at this patient's skin.
I found some weird-looking lesions that did not fit into any characteristic appearance of psoriasis but, because of the distribution, I plumped for that as a diagnosis.

I was then asked about the treatment, management and complications of psoriasis so perhaps I had been right with the diagnosis!

32. *This man's skin was really red. There were no plaques or scales but I said he had psoriasis. The examiners asked me how I would manage this man if it was a Friday at 5.30 pm and I was in the accident and emergency department and I could not get in touch with a dermatologist.*

Station 1

This lady is breathless. Please examine her chest.
The patient had simple emphysema. It was a ward patient who had been brought along at the last minute as the expected patient had not arrived. I was asked how to differentiate the different types of lung disease.

Examine this patient's abdominal system.
I found hepatosplenomegaly and the stigmata of chronic liver disease but the patient was not jaundiced.

The examiner asked me about the management of acute gastrointestinal bleeding in a patient with liver disease and the emphasis was on the 'ABC', etc.

Station 2

This 40-year-old lady has presented with a persistent cough and shortness of breath. Inhalers have not helped and a chest X-ray carried out by the GP has been reported as normal. Please take a history.
The patient was living in the East End of London surrounded by people with tuberculosis. She was a smoker and had a family history of thrombotic events.

The examiners asked me what investigations I would do and what I thought the likely outcomes of these investigations would be.

Station 3

This patient has had an acute episode of breathlessness. Please examine the cardiovascular system.
I found evidence of aortic stenosis. I thought it was clinically mild but I was subsequently told that the gradient was 70 mmHg.

The examiner asked me if I was surprised at the gradient. He told me that the patient was unfit for surgery and so how would I follow him up, and in which way might he deteriorate? The discussion covered ischaemic heart disease, left ventricular failure, Adams–Stokes attacks and subacute bacterial endocarditis.

This lady has difficulty doing the housework, especially with taking things out of cupboards. Look at her face and examine her hands.
She had the classic features of myotonic dystrophy. The examiner said to me, 'She wants to have children, how would you advise her?'. He then asked me how the condition might progress and what else might be affected.

Station 4

You see a heavy goods vehicle (HGV) driver in the casualty department who has had several funny turns in the past but today has had one that was definitely an epileptic seizure. Counsel him about the implications of this diagnosis.
I explained to him that he does have epilepsy. (He argued.) I explained to him that he must stop driving. (He protested.) I explained about the financial benefits that are available to compensate for the loss of earnings and that he could find other work. I explained that medication controls the epilepsy but that he still cannot drive. I emphasized that this was because of safety for himself and for other people on the road. I was unsure as to whether he would ever be able to drive HGV vehicles again but said that I would find out straight after the consultation and get back to him and that I would ring a social worker about any available financial benefits.

I thought the conversation went very well. The examiners asked me about any possible situations in which one can legally break confidentiality. We talked more about driving and epilepsy and I was asked how I would know whether he was continuing to drive or not.

Station 5

Examine this patient's neck.

The patient had a goitre but was euthyroid. I had to list the possible complications of a goitre including dysphagia, stridor, etc., and what could be some causes of a sudden deterioration, e.g. bleeding into a nodule. They wanted to know how I would detect stridor.

Examine this patient's fundi.

I found dot haemorrhages on the right side, with silver wiring and arteriovenous nipping bilaterally. The examiners wanted a classification of diabetic retinopathy but I cannot remember the rest of the questions!

Examine this patient's hands.

He had obvious psoriatic arthropathy although it looked somewhat like rheumatoid arthritis but there were psoriatic plaques. I am sure that I was asked some questions at this point but I cannot remember what they were.

Look at this patient.

This man's skin was really red. There were no plaques or scales but I said that he had psoriasis.

The examiners asked me how I would manage this man if it was Friday evening at 5.30 pm and I was in the casualty department and I could not get in touch with a dermatologist. I said that I would rehydrate, that I would treat any infection aggressively and that I would use simple aqueous creams. I passed the exam but on reflection, I realized that I should have said that he had a drug reaction because as I was walking away, the examiner said, 'Did you really think it was psoriasis?' and I said, 'No!'. They smiled.

Comments

I would definitely have benefited from more practice in history taking and in communication skills before the exam.

---

33. *I finished the history taking very quickly so had to sit in silence until time was up. That was awful!*

Station 1

This patient is complaining of shortness of breath. Please examine the chest.

I found a left-sided pleural effusion. I was asked what the important points in the history taking would be and for the further investigations and management. There was a discussion about pleural plaques.

This patient has been referred from the cardiology clinic with sweats and a mass in the abdomen. Please examine.

I found splenomegaly which was apparently secondary to infective endocarditis. I was asked for the differential diagnosis of splenomegaly, the treatment of chronic lymphatic leukaemia and the diagnosis and management of endocarditis.

Station 2

This man has had palpitations and has been started on amiodarone. He is now hyperthyroid and has been started on carbimazole 5 mg bd. The thyroid-stimulating hormone (TSH) is still very low.* Take a history.

I took a cardiac history and asked about the palpitations for which he had been started on amiodarone. He was sweaty and agitated, and the thyroxine (T4) was still high with a low TSH. He had been started on carbimazole but was not really any better.

I was asked how I would alter his drug management and about his social history. The examiners also asked me about the mode of action of amiodarone.

Station 3

This patient is short of breath. Please examine the heart.

I found mixed aortic valve disease. The examiners asked me to measure the blood pressure and to say which was the most serious lesion. I was then asked for the diagnostic tests and the management of aortic regurgitation and aortic stenosis.

---

*Amiodarone contains iodine and can cause disorders of thyroid function; both hypothyroidism and hyperthyroidism may occur. Clinical assessment alone is unreliable, and laboratory tests should be performed before treatment and every 6 months. Thyroxine (T4) may be raised in the absence of hyperthyroidism; therefore tri-iodothyronine (T3), T4 and TSH should all be measured. A raised T3 and T4 with a very low or undetectable TSH concentration suggests the development of thyrotoxicosis. The thyrotoxicosis may be very refractory, and amiodarone should usually be withdrawn at least temporarily to help achieve control; treatment with carbimazole may be required. Hypothyroidism can be treated with replacement therapy without withdrawing amiodarone if it is essential.

This patient has had weakness of the legs for 3 years. Please examine the legs and find out why.
The patient had a spastic right leg but the left was normal. I was asked to give the causes of a spastic paraparesis but then there was no time left for a discussion or any further questions.

Station 4

This man, with a long history of alcohol abuse, has had to wait 8 weeks for an outpatient appointment. The ultrasound scan of his abdomen has shown a 10 cm lesion in the liver. This has been biopsied and found to be a hepatocellular carcinoma. The patient is happy for you to speak to his wife. You have to break the bad news to the wife who does not want her husband to be told.
I explained the diagnosis and she definitely did not want her husband to be told. However, I explained the problems with this approach and she eventually relented. I explained about further treatment and management.

I was asked by the examiners how I thought the conversation had gone and did I think that I handled it as well as I thought I could?

Station 5

This woman has glycosuria. Look at her and examine anything that is relevant.
The patient was obviously acromegalic so I examined for, and demonstrated, xanthelasma and a bitemporal hemianopia.

I was asked how the xanthelasma could be associated with acromegaly and why there should be glycosuria.

This patient feels as if he is walking on cotton wool and has had recurrent Bell's palsies. Please examine his eyes.
There was a preproliferative diabetic retinopathy but no laser burns were visible. The examiner asked if he had had any treatment to his eyes and why he had altered sensation in his feet. He also asked me for a reason for the recurrent Bell's palsies and to explain what is meant by Bell's phenomenon.

This patient is tired all the time. Why is that?
There was koilonychia so the patient must have had an iron deficiency anaemia but there was no time for any discussion.

Examine the patient's hands and any other relevant joints.
The patient had CREST and also there were nodules at the elbows. I was asked how I would differentiate

between CREST and rheumatoid arthritis, what is the treatment for CREST and what further questions I would ask the patient?

34. *Despite being told how difficult it is to cope with the indifference with which some examiners treat you, when it actually happened it was far more devastating than I was prepared for.*

Station 1

Examine this man's respiratory system.
I cannot remember anything about the Station 1 respiratory case!

Examine this man's abdomen and tell me what you find.
I found most of the signs of chronic liver disease – liver palms, spider naevi and ascites, in a thin and wasted man. The examiner asked for possible causes and the investigations that are needed to make a diagnosis of liver disease.

Station 2

Please see this middle-aged lady who is feeling lethargic. The GP has performed some blood tests and has discovered abnormal liver function tests with a hepatitic picture. She is being referred for further investigations.
The patient was a 46-year-old married lady who is a teacher. She had noticed progressively worsening lethargy but she had very little in the way of other symptoms. It was probably all a result of alcohol consumption.

The examiner wanted me to give some possible causes for her symptoms and the abnormal liver function tests. He asked if I thought that the alcohol was a probable cause but I had not taken a very good alcohol history! He asked me about primary biliary cirrhosis and I thought that her symptoms could be caused by that. He finally asked if there were any other things that I should have asked her and I had to admit that I had also forgotten to ask about any intravenous drug usage.

Station 3

The GP has noted a murmur – can you tell me what you think?
I found the murmurs of mixed aortic valve disease. The examiner asked if I was sure and how would I judge the significance of the predominant murmur?

This man has had a collapse – please examine his limbs.
There was evidence of a facial weakness and a left hemiplegia. I was asked for possible causes and I had noted that he was in atrial fibrillation. I had to list the investigations that I would do (routine blood tests, ECG, CT scan of the brain, etc.) and they wanted to know my treatment plans. I talked about physiotherapy and anticoagulation.

Station 4

This gentleman has recently had a cardiac arrest. He has been left with severe marked cerebral damage and is in need of huge amounts of inotropic support. Please discuss the resuscitation status with his son.
The conversation that I had with the son included having to tell him how sick his father was and that any attempt at resuscitation was unlikely to be successful. I had to explain about the severity of the brain impairment and that I did not think that cardiopulmonary resuscitation would be in his best interest as he was unlikely to recover from this acute episode.

The examiner asked me if I thought that the son understood what I was trying to explain and I replied that I thought he had understood. I was then asked to discuss the prognostic indicators for a patient after a cardiac arrest.

Station 5

What do you think of this lady?
She was a cushingoid lady and I was asked for the possible causes and the complications of long-term steroid use.

Examine this person's eyes.
I found tunnel vision, and on fundoscopy there was retinitis pigmentosa although it was not very florid at all. The examiner did not ask me any questions – he just grunted and walked off!

Examine this man's hands.
He had rheumatoid hands and scars from what I assumed were bilateral decompressions for carpal tunnel syndrome. The examiner asked what I thought the scars were caused by and why he was on methotrexate.

Take a look at this lady's rash.
She had a widespread, macular, erythematous rash and the examiners told me that the dermatologists did not know the diagnosis! I described the rash and explained that I would take a full history, including a drug history, and if in doubt I would do some blood tests and biopsy the lesion. They did not ask me any questions.

Comments

Despite being told how difficult it is to cope with the indifference with which some examiners treat you, when it actually happened it was far more devastating than I was prepared for. This occurred in the first station and I felt dreadful but I remembered having been told that the next case is a new case and treat it as such otherwise one can fall into a downward spiral. It worked for me and I got into the 'swing' of the exam. I think it was the most dreadful experience of my life and I felt emotionally drained after it. Thank God I passed! The very best reason to pass the exam first time is that you never have to take the bloody thing again!

35. *In the ensuing questions I was asked about what ethical issues this scenario raised and to explain 'duty to act justly'.*

Station 1

This man has developed a productive cough. Please examine his chest and suggest a cause.
The patient had bilateral, upper lobe, fine crepitations and I suggested a diagnosis of pulmonary fibrosis.

The examiners showed me the chest X-ray and there was an opacity in both upper lobes. I suggested aspergillosis affecting old tuberculous cavities and they asked me what further investigations I would do. I suggested sputum for culture and sensitivity/cytology/acid-alcohol-fast bacilli.

This lady has been having abdominal pain. Please examine and suggest a cause.

I found evidence of polycystic kidneys and a polycystic liver. There were multiple scars from previous operations to drain the cysts. There were no arteriovenous fistulae. She had palmar erythema but was not jaundiced and the abdomen was generally tender.

The examiners asked me questions about polycystic kidney disease, i.e. chromosomal abnormalities and what possible complications could occur.

Station 2

The GP letter describes a history of funny turns and then subsequent development of a right hemiplegia. The letter asks for a review of the diagnosis of a stroke and then to suggest further appropriate management.

The patient was a 68-year-old lady who, 4 months previously, had noticed intermittent episodes of a dizzy feeling. She denied vertigo or any other associated neurological or cardiac symptoms. A month later, she developed a right-sided weakness which had been preceded by impaired coordination. There had been no headaches, no loss of consciousness and no visual disturbances. Now her function was improving although she still had difficulty with stairs, tired easily and was frustrated that she could no longer work in the family pet shop. Her risk factors included the fact that her father had ischaemic heart disease, there was no family history of stroke and she was found to have hypertension. She did not smoke and did not have diabetes mellitus. There was no other past medical history. Her drug history included antihypertensives and aspirin and she was unclear as to whether she had had her serum cholesterol level measured.

The examiners asked me what I thought about her presentation and the differential diagnosis of her funny turns. They asked if I thought she was depressed and what questions I would ask her to establish this.

Station 3

This patient presented with shortness of breath. Please examine the cardiovascular system.

The patient definitely had mixed mitral valve disease and was in atrial fibrillation. However, it was difficult to ascertain the predominant lesion. I thought there was also a murmur of aortic sclerosis.

There then followed a discussion about atrial fibrillation, its management and possible complications and the examiners wanted to know how I could clinically assess for the dominant valvular lesion.

This man has difficulty walking and has falls, especially at night. Examine his gait and then his legs.

His gait was very unsteady. It was broad-based and the Romberg's test was positive. There were definite cerebellar signs and I also thought there was a sensory neuropathy. The examiners wanted me to suggest possible causes.

Station 4

You are the resident medical officer and a 37-week pregnant woman presents to the casualty department with symptoms suggestive of a pulmonary embolus. Please discuss the likely diagnosis and outline management plans.

I discussed with her the possible diagnosis and important investigations. I then explained the benefit versus the risk to the baby of appropriate management and treatment and the reasons why pulmonary emboli occurred during pregnancy.

In the ensuing questions I was asked about what ethical issues this scenario raised and to explain 'duty to act justly'.

Station 5

This woman presents with painful eyes. Please examine her.

There was quite marked chemosis of the eyes and an obvious goitre. They also wanted me to examine her thyroid status.

This man had sudden onset of blindness. Please look at the fundi and suggest why.

He had glaucoma with marked cupping of the discs. I wondered if he had had a retinal artery occlusion as well and we discussed the possible causes of sudden blindness.

This man has a painful knee. Please examine his hands and suggest why.

He had an asymmetrical arthropathy with gouty tophi. The following discussion was about gout, its management, investigations and complications.

This lady complains of some abnormalities in her gums. Please examine her.

She had the classic features of lichen planus and I also saw a lesion of lichen planus on her skin. The examiners wanted to know if I knew any other causes of gum hyperplasia.

36. *I was asked about the mechanism of the reflex arc.*

Station 1

Examine this patient's chest.

I found a right-sided pleural effusion and was asked for the possible causes, the investigations that should be carried out in their order of priority and, finally, for the management of a pleural effusion.

This patient is complaining of tiredness. Examine his abdomen.

I found hepatosplenomegaly and clinical anaemia in a patient who also had rheumatoid hands. I was asked for causes of hepatosplenomegaly and the most likely cause in this patient. I was then asked for further possible explanations for the anaemia.

Station 2

This lady with Crohn's disease has recently had an ileal resection for fistulating disease. She now has abdominal pain and has noticed some hair loss. She was discharged from hospital on 6-mercaptopurine.

The patient had a history of Crohn's disease which had not settled with 5-aminosalicylic acid (5-ASA) and prednisolone. She subsequently had surgery and had undergone multiple operations. The pain had now improved but not totally gone and her main concern currently was the hair loss. The patient and I discussed the options of changing the therapy and of further investigations for the hair loss.

The examiners asked me, 'What is the most likely cause for her hair loss?', 'Do you think that her Crohn's disease is active?', 'What alternative therapy could be used?' and 'What would be your further management?'.

Station 3

Examine this gentleman's heart. He has been complaining of palpitations.

I found atrial fibrillation with a mitral stenotic murmur. There was no valvotomy scar and there was no evidence of cardiac failure. I was asked about the likely cause for the mitral stenosis, the treatment of atrial fibrillation and what was the cause of the opening snap.

This gentleman has noticed a tendency to drop objects. Please examine his motor system.

I found the patient to have a right hemiparesis and I was asked about the mechanism of the reflex arc.

Station 4

A patient under your care has been diagnosed with Huntington's chorea. Her daughter would like to discuss her mother's condition.

We discussed the need for consent to discuss her mother's condition with her. I gave an explanation of the diagnosis of Huntington's chorea and how it had so far affected her mother. We talked about the process of genetic screening, whether this was indicated for her, and how this may affect her life. I outlined the further support and treatment that would be planned to help her mother in the future.

I was asked about the problems of consent to test for Huntington's chorea if the patient refused and whether it would be beneficial for the daughter to be tested. I was asked how I thought the interview went.

Station 5

Examine this gentleman. What do you notice?

The patient had marked cushingoid features and I was asked the possible reasons for the patient being on steroid therapy.

Examine this patient's fundi.

The patient had unilateral optic atrophy and angioid streaks. I was asked for the causes of optic atrophy.

Examine the patient's eyes.

The patient had a unilateral III, IV and VI nerve palsy which was caused by a cavernous sinus thrombosis (see Vol. 1, Station 3, Central nervous system, Case 16 and Vol. 3, Station 5, Endocrine, Cases 1, 4 and Station 5, Eyes, Case 8.

Examine this patient's hands.

The patient had marked rheumatoid hands with nodules.

Examine this patient.

She had peripheral and central cyanosis with warm swollen hands and I was asked for the cause.

> **Comments**
>
> There is plenty of time to examine thoroughly and the questions are usually management based.
>
> At Station 5, I had two eye cases so I had a total of five patients at that station. This station seemed much more flexible than the others, with no written instructions.

37. *They asked for causes of dysarthria so I volunteered bulbar and pseudobulbar and of course they wanted causes for both!*

Station 1

This man has noisy breathing. Please examine his chest to find out why.

The man had no signs in his chest at all but I did notice that on his skin he had a very large (10–20 cm) psoriatic plaque.

The examiners asked me where I thought the lesion was likely to be and I said in his upper airway. They asked how I would confirm this diagnosis and I said by performing a respiratory flow loop test. They asked me what it would look like but at that point the bell went.

Examine this patient's abdomen.

I found hepatosplenomegaly with minimal ascites but there was no evidence of chronic liver disease.

They asked me why I thought the swelling on the left side of his abdomen was a spleen and not a kidney and then they asked if I had checked for a notch, but of course I had not!

Station 2

This 40-year-old lady has suffered from chronic intermittent diarrhoea and back pain. She took a holiday to India last year with her family. Please take a history.

I asked her for further details about the diarrhoea and the back pain and most of her history pointed to a diagnosis of irritable bowel syndrome. However, I tried to exclude inflammatory bowel disease. It was all very straightforward but I made sure that I included questions about her menstrual history and her social history.

Station 3

Please examine this patient's cardiovascular system.

The patient had a mid-line sternotomy scar and there was a systolic murmur which I thought could be a flow murmur or could be a result of mitral valve disease.

They wanted to know what I thought the scar was for and I suggested that it was either for a valve replacement or a coronary artery bypass graft.

This patient has difficulty in walking. Please examine him.

There was subtle, left-sided dysdiadochokinesis and he could not do the tandem walking test so I concluded that he had cerebellar signs but I was not that convinced about any dysarthria. I was then asked to examine the

facial nerve and found that he also had a left facial palsy which I thought was supranuclear.

I was asked to link all this together so I suggested cerebrovascular disease or multiple sclerosis. They asked for the causes of dysarthria so I volunteered bulbar and pseudobulbar and of course they then wanted causes for both! They asked for other causes of dysarthria and I suggested that a large tongue could be responsible for it.

Station 4

An elderly lady had a cerebrovascular accident (CVA) last year and is on aspirin medication. She lives alone and now presents with a gastrointestinal bleed. She is refusing to have an endoscopy (OGD) and is 'fed up'. The daughter still wants her to have the investigation against her wishes.

The discussion centred on the ethical implications of this. The examiner asked if the patient was mentally competent or was she depressed or demented.

Station 5

This lady has had headaches. Please examine her.

She had very subtle facial changes of acromegaly and, in addition, I noticed bilateral scars at her wrists from treatment for carpal tunnel syndrome.

This patient has rheumatoid arthritis. Please check the functional status.

The patient was unable to pick up a coin or to do up buttons. There was no pincer grasp at all. I had to discuss the treatment options for rheumatoid disease.

You must know the diagnosis of this patient.

I think the patient had the typical, multiple lesions of neurofibromatosis and as I gave this diagnosis, they jumped straight into the questions. They wanted to know the possible neurological complications and I gave them a satisfactory list. They asked, 'What can be the cardiovascular complications?'. I did not know the answer to that one at all!

Comments

I did not expect to pass but I did.

---

38. *This took me by surprise as I was prepared to take a history rather than to be asked questions by the patient.*

Station 1

Examine this gentleman's respiratory system.

The young man had a sternotomy scar. There was no clubbing and auscultation was normal. I was told that he had had a lung transplant and I was asked for the symptoms and signs of organ rejection. I was then 'grilled' on bronchiolitis obliterans!

Examine this lady's abdominal system.

She had hepatomegaly and inguinal lymphadenopathy and I was asked to offer a differential diagnosis.

Station 2

This gentleman attends the outpatient clinic referred by his GP with possible lung fibrosis secondary to methotrexate. Please proceed as necessary.

The patient immediately asked several questions including, 'Do I need home oxygen?', 'How long have I got to live?' and 'Is it secondary to the methotrexate?'. I proceeded to take a history about the background of the problems, i.e. rheumatoid arthritis, and about the symptoms and signs of the breathlessness.

I failed this station outright and my impression was that the examiners wanted me to answer the patient's questions rather than take a history, although it was the history-taking station. This took me by surprise as I was prepared to take a history rather than be asked questions by the patient!

Station 3

Examine this gentleman's cardiovascular system.

The patient was a young man who had clubbing, a sternotomy scar and a pansystolic murmur in the aortic region. I was asked for a differential diagnosis and in retrospect, I wonder if it was some form of cyanotic congenital heart disease and that perhaps he had a corrected Fallot's tetralogy.

Examine this lady's lower limbs.

I found pes cavus, ataxia and distal weakness. I was asked for a differential diagnosis and I offered Charcot–Marie–Tooth disease which I was told was incorrect so I then suggested Friedreich's ataxia.

Station 4

A 40-year-old man who had some coryzal symptoms was admitted to hospital following a collapse and an epileptic fit at work. A lumbar puncture has shown meningococcal meningitis. His Glasgow Coma Scale (GCS) is now 8/15. Please explain the situation to his wife.

I explained the diagnosis and the surrounding details. She asked about their child who was also exhibiting similar coryzal symptoms. I explained about the infection control department and the need for prophylactic antibiotics.

The examiners then asked me to outline the poor prognostic indicators in meningococcal septicaemia.

Station 5

Look at this patient.

The patient had obvious acromegaly and I was not asked any additional questions.

Examine this patient's eyes.

This patient had a complete third nerve palsy and I was asked to list the possible causes.

Examine this patient's hands.

The only abnormality here was squaring of the hand with no other signs. The patient must have had osteoarthrosis. The examiner asked me the name of the joint involved in 'squaring of the hand' and what was the differential diagnosis.

Examine this lady's face and hands.

The patient looked cushingoid and there were multiple warts on her hands. I was not asked any questions here but in retrospect, I wonder whether she had human papillomavirus following a transplant.

Comments

I felt that the cases were comparatively hard and unusual. The instructions were not always made clear, especially in the history-taking station. I had expected to examine some fundi but this was not requested at all in this exam.

39. *Lots of empathy was needed and I tried to structure the conversation into sections. I can't remember the details about the discussion with the examiners but I do know that whilst talking to the daughter, I got some of the details about the inheritance/penetrance/blood testing wrong but I came clean about this during the discussion. I still passed!*

Station 1

Examine this patient's chest.

I found all the features of bronchiectasis and was asked to give the details and significance of any investigations and what possible treatments there were for this condition.

Examine this patient's abdomen.
This was a young man who also had some 'chest problems'. I found him to have hepatosplenomegaly and ascites and the examiners wanted a list of possible causes.

Station 2
This man has paroxysmal atrial fibrillation. Please take a history.
It was a very complicated history and I cannot remember all the details. Quite a few of his different conditions meant that certain agents would be contraindicated in his management.

However, the examiners asked me to outline a management plan for him and would I anticoagulate him with warfarin or not? They asked me about the use of amiodarone and β-blockers, but the patient had asthma.

Station 3
Examine this man's cardiovascular system.
He had atrial fibrillation and a prosthetic mitral valve. The examiners wanted to know about investigations and possible complications.

Examine this man's neurological system.
He had a proximal myopathy, foot drop, a peripheral neuropathy and ulcers on his toes. I thought he probably had diabetes mellitus and the examiners asked me for my views on his further management.

P.S. Don't forget to examine the patient's gait!

Station 4
A lady has been diagnosed with Huntington's disease. Please discuss the implications with her daughter.
There was far too much information to fit into too short a time. However, we talked about the clinical features, the differential diagnosis, inheritance, support networks and discharge planning. The daughter was very concerned about whether her son – the patient's grandson – would get it. Lots of empathy was needed and I tried to structure the conversation into sections.

I cannot remember the details about the discussion with the examiners but I do know that while talking to the daughter, I got some of the details about the inheritance/penetrance/blood testing wrong but I came clean about this during the discussion and I still passed!

Station 5
Look at this man and examine him as you feel appropriate.
He had all the features of acromegaly and I was asked what investigations I would do.

Examine this man's eyes.
He had Graves' eye disease. He was supposed to have diplopia at the extremes of vision but not even the examiner could demonstrate it!

Examine the patient's hands.
The patient had a deforming arthropathy and I was asked to give a differential diagnosis and to give the differing features between each possible cause.

Examine this lady's skin.
This lady had neurofibromas (but not many of them) together with axillary freckling and café-au-lait spots. I diagnosed von Recklinghausen's disease (neurofibromatosis type 1). I was asked for the associations with this condition and the differing features from neurofibromatosis type 2.

Comments
Both the history section and the communication/ethics section are very rushed in the exam. It will feel very artificial because you will find there is too much to cover in 14 min (plus 1 min for reflection and then 5 min of questions) but persevere and be empathic.

If you do not know the answer to a question do not make it up but say 'I will find out the answer and we will talk again soon'. It worked for me.

40. *The examiners asked me what I would say to the patient if he had asked me to help him end his life.*

Station 1
Examine this patient's chest.
There was a chest drain on the left side with an effusion still draining. I was asked about the likely aetiologies of a pleural effusion.

This patient's abdomen has shown intermittent swelling – what could one cause be?

The patient had many of the signs of alcoholic liver disease with minimal ascites. He also had hereditary haemorrhagic telangiectasia. I was asked for the cause of the abdominal swelling.

Station 2

This patient has had a cough for some time. The chest X-ray last year was normal. There was some initial improvement with inhalers. Now nothing seems to work. Please take a history.

There was no shortness of breath on exertion and the only problem seemed to be the cough. There was a history of excessive smoking and the patient had no previous industrial exposure nor had he kept any pets. I was asked about the likely cause of the cough and what investigations were needed.

Station 3

This patient has been having palpitations – can you find a cause?

The patient was in atrial fibrillation but I could not hear a mitral stenotic murmur. We had a discussion about whether or not mitral stenosis was present and then on how to manage the atrial fibrillation.

This patient has a worsening tremor of his upper limbs. Please give some reasons.

There was an intention tremor which was worse in the right arm. There were no other cerebellar signs but there was a patchy peripheral sensory neuropathy. I was asked what the cause could be, given the above findings.

Station 4

This patient has been admitted with an aspiration pneumonia and it is now thought that he has motor neurone disease. He has seen a neurologist who is planning further investigations but he has already told the patient that this is the likely diagnosis. The patient has some questions to ask and you are the on-call doctor.

The patient was concerned about any cognitive decline and about any possible cardiovascular complications. The patient did not want to be a burden on his family and wanted to know if there were any treatments and whether there were any better treatment options in the USA where his daughter lived.

The examiners asked me what I would say to the patient if he had asked me to help him end his life.

Station 5

This patient has noticed a swelling in his neck – please examine.

There was a large goitre and the right lobe, in particular, was very swollen. I was asked what investigations were needed and whether the patient was euthyroid.

Examine the eyes of this diabetic patient.

There was evidence of panretinal photocoagulation with hard exudates near the macula.

Look at this patient.

She had scleroderma and I was asked about the CREST syndrome.

Look at this patient's hands.

There was rheumatoid arthritis but without any significant deformity. I was asked what treatments were available.

41. *This is a discussion about living wills, euthanasia, options for pain control and her anger at the 'delayed/ missed' diagnosis.*

Station 1

Examine this man.

There was a collecting bag on the right posterior chest wall containing fluid. Presumably a chest drain had fallen out. There was lymphoedema of the left arm. I was asked for the likely causes.

This man has pain on walking. Please examine him.

He had a ruddy complexion and hepatosplenomegaly. I was asked for the diagnosis which was probably polycythaemia rubra vera. I was then asked to describe the position and the anatomy of the spleen and the treatment for polycythaemia, for which I volunteered venesection.

Station 2

Take a history.

The patient had peripheral vascular disease, hypertension, diabetes mellitus, renal artery stenosis and impaired left ventricular function. There was a discussion with the examiners about renal failure and the role of ACE inhibitors in this patient.

Station 3

Examine the patient's heart.

There were the features of mitral stenosis. I was asked about the methods of treatment and I offered valvotomy, valve replacement, rate control of the atrial fibrillation and thromboprophylaxis.

Examine the patient's legs but omit looking at the gait.
I found a sensory neuropathy in a stocking distribution, upper motor neurone signs including brisk knee jerks, absent ankle jerks and up-going plantars. I was asked for the causes and I suggested probable subacute combined degeneration of the cord.

Station 4
The lady has metastatic carcinoma of the breast. Discuss the diagnosis and management with her.
This included a discussion about living wills, euthanasia, options for pain control and her anger at the 'delayed/missed' diagnosis.

Station 5
Look at this patient.
The patient had acromegaly with a bitemporal hemianopia, an old transfrontal scar at the right inner canthus and a carpal tunnel scar. We discussed replacement therapy and the different zones of the adrenal gland.

Look at the patient's fundi.
I found proliferative diabetic retinopathy with new vessels and photocoagulation scars. I was asked about the cofactors for eye disease (hypertension, lipids, etc.). The eyes were not dilated, the room was not darkened and the signs were very subtle!

Examine the patient's hands.
I found the signs of chronic tophaceous gout. I was then asked about the management and treatment of chronic gout.

Look at the patient's face.
The patient had obvious hereditary haemorrhagic telangiectasia. I was asked about iron deficiency anaemia in this condition and about the need to investigate with endoscopy to exclude any other coexistent bowel pathology.

Comments

The College still seems to have some aggressive, 'hawk-like' examiners who interrupted my examination routines at an early stage before I had finished a complete routine.

---

42. *I found very little and the whole case was just a nightmare!*

Station 1
Examine this lady's chest.
I found that she had had a bilateral lower lobectomy and there was fibrosis in the left lung. I was asked for a cause.

Examine this gentleman's abdomen.
The patient had alcoholic liver disease with many of the signs of chronic liver disease, encephalopathy and tender hepatomegaly. I was asked for all the other possible causes apart from alcohol.

Station 2
Take a history.
The patient had atypical chest pain which was probably pericarditis. I can remember talking about a rash and arthralgia and I was asked about the risks of systemic lupus erythematosus.

Station 3
Examine the cardiovascular system.
I found a jerky pulse, cardiomegaly and quiet heart sounds. I diagnosed hypertrophic obstructive cardiomyopathy.* I was asked about the causes, risks and treatment.

Examine the gait and anything else which is relevant.
I found very little and the whole case was just a nightmare!

Station 4
This patient possibly has hyperthyroidism. She is in atrial fibrillation.
Please discuss the diagnosis, the causes of atrial fibrillation, the risks and the management.

Station 5
Examine the patient's eyes and anything else appropriate.
The patient had Graves' eye disease and all the other features of Graves'.

Examine the patient's fundi. The patient has a central scotoma.
I diagnosed retinitis pigmentosa and diabetic maculopathy. The examiner wanted to know what questions

---

*These days the condition is referred to as hypertrophic cardiomyopathy.

I would ask the patient. I said family history, whether he was diabetic, smoked and had good or poor night vision.

Examine the patient's hands.
The patient had the signs of rheumatoid disease and was wearing a cervical collar. The examiner asked me about treatment, including the new advances, tumour necrosis factor α (TNF-α) and the risks.

Examine this patient's skin.
The patient had psoriasis and I was asked about treatment.

Comments
The exam seems much fairer than the old style.

---

43. *The examiners wanted to know which antiepileptic is the safest in pregnancy.*

Station 1

Examine this lady's respiratory system from the front.
About half a minute later I was asked to examine her chest from the back. I found that the patient had had a previous right pneumonectomy. The examiners wanted to know how common lung cancer was in women.

This 62-year-old man has a lymphocytosis. Please examine his abdomen.
I found him to have splenomegaly. The examiners wanted to know what further investigations were required and what one would see on a peripheral blood smear.

Station 2

Miss Green is a 30-year-old flower shop assistant with a history of two fits, one of which was associated with incontinence and was witnessed by her fiancé. She had been started on antiepileptic pills by her GP but she stopped taking them after 2 weeks as she wanted to conceive and she had heard that antiepileptic medications could have side-effects on the baby. Please take a detailed history and address the patient's concerns.
The history taking went quite well and the examiners wanted to know which antiepileptic is the safest in pregnancy.

Station 3

Examine the patient's cardiovascular system.
The patient was in her late seventies. There was a midline sternotomy scar and there was evidence of a prosthetic valve. The examiners wanted to know which valve had been replaced.

Examine this patient's upper limbs. There has been a weakness for about the last 5 years.
I found proximal weakness in the left upper limb with fasciculation over both arms and I suggested a diagnosis of motor neurone disease.

Station 4

This young lady with meningitis has three children at home. She wants to discharge herself. Please convince the patient that hospital treatment is essential.
We discussed why the treatment was important but I also empathized with the fact that she had three children and was relying on neighbours, friends and relatives to look after them. We eventually compromised on her staying in to complete intravenous antibiotics and that she could go home as soon as she could go on oral medication.

Station 5

Please examine this patient's eyes.
I found the patient to have exophthalmos and there was a discussion regarding the eye signs.

Please have a look at this patient's eyes.
I found a third nerve palsy and was asked for the causes.

Please look at this patient's ankles and feet.
There was an ulcer on one heel with a Charcot joint at that ankle. I was asked for possible causes.

Examine this patient's shin.
There was obvious neurofibromatosis and I was then asked for the possible associations.

44. *There was diabetic maculopathy and I was asked to draw my findings!*

Station 1

This young man is breathless. Please examine his chest.
I found evidence of chronic obstructive pulmonary disease. The examiners asked me about the likely forced expiratory volume (FEV) and what was a possible aetiology – in fact he had α1-antitrypsin deficiency. He also had a subcutaneous infusion running but I was not sure what it was although the examiners did try to get me to give an answer.

Please examine the abdomen of this man who is complaining of pruritus.

The patient looked unwell. He had a continuous ambulatory peritoneal dialysis catheter *in situ* and I could feel a right polycystic kidney. The examiners wanted to know what his glomerular filtration rate would be.

Station 2

Take a history from this young professional woman who is diabetic and who is having recurrent hypoglycaemic episodes.

She also had an infected foot ulcer and was driving a car on a regular basis.

Station 3

Please examine the cardiovascular system.
I found mixed aortic valve disease.

Examine this patient's legs.
There were all the features of a mixed upper and lower motor neurone disorder and they questioned me about the possible aetiology.

Station 4

I had to interview a patient with possible Huntington's disease and I had to discuss the implications for the family and for family screening.

Station 5

Please look at this patient.
He had definite acromegaly.

This patient has visual loss. Please examine the fundi.
There was diabetic maculopathy and I was asked to draw my findings!

Look at this patient's hands.
The only abnormality that I could find was a single, swan neck deformity. It was very difficult!

This patient is diabetic. Please look at the feet.
There was a unilateral sensory loss and absent dorsalis pedis pulses. There was a Charcot joint at the ankle.
    I was asked for a diagnosis.

Comments

It is good to prepare by going on a course, although the added fear factor and sweating makes the real exam very tough.

Additional Station 2 experiences

45. *You are the SHO in the department and you are told that you should present this patient at a regional haematology meeting. Take his history and summarize.*

The patient was a young man with multiple myeloma who had been treated with C-VAMP (cyclophosphamide, vincristine, adriamycin, methyl prednisolone), the treatment being complicated by infections. He was awaiting an autologous bone marrow transplant with high-dose melphalan. He was very anxious.

The examiners asked about the social aspects of the diagnosis. Would haematologists at a regional meeting really be interested and what was the evidence for an autologous bone marrow transplant in multiple myeloma?

46. *I was given a GP letter regarding a lady with worsening shortness of breath, who had a past cardiac, respiratory and thyroid history.*

She described increasing shortness of breath and fatigue. She had started smoking again and had had significant life events. I thought she could be depressed as well as having cardiac problems with being on amiodarone and the previous hypothyroidism. I was asked about further management and for a differential diagnosis.

47. *I was given quite a long letter regarding a lady on digoxin and carbimazole who had presented with episodes of fainting and nausea.*

It was a difficult case as the patient did not appear to have been primed that it was a role play and answered most of the questions about her fainting episodes by saying that they were months ago and now resolved. The essentials were that she had amiodarone-induced thyrotoxicosis (she was in atrial fibrillation) and so she had been switched to digoxin and was probably now experiencing bradyarrhythmias. She had therefore had her dosage reduced. Now her main complaint was of tiredness.

I was not helped by the examiners getting the timing wrong and stopping me after 10 min! The questioning centred on the differential diagnosis of faints and tiredness.

48. *I had to see a middle-aged gentleman with recurrent abdominal pains. He had had a recent admission for surgery when normal bloods and normal findings on OGD were obtained. The GP had referred him to the medical clinic.*

I obtained a history of recurrent abdominal pains over the last 20 years. There were lots of stress factors in his life, especially relating to his work. There was hardly any weight loss, no blood passed *per rectum* and only occasional mucus. There was no history of diabetes mellitus, heavy metal poisoning or porphyria. The patient had obvious concerns regarding a possible malignancy as he had a positive family history for colonic carcinoma.

The examiner asked me how I would write back to the GP, what invasive investigations would I do and what did I think was the most likely cause? I said, 'irritable bowel syndrome'.

49. *I was given a detailed GP letter. It was regarding a lady in her seventies with congestive cardiac failure. She was known to have ischaemic heart disease with a previous myocardial infarction. She had hypertension and chronic renal impairment. The GP requested advice on further investigations and management. She was taking atenolol, bendrofluazide (bendroflumethiazide), frusemide (furosemide) 40 mg and aspirin 75 mg. Her blood pressure was 160/90 mmHg and relevant blood investigations showed a urea of 20 mmol/L, creatinine 250 μmol/L and cholesterol 8 mmol/L.*

The history was quite straightforward. A 70-year-old lady with hypertension, hypercholesterolaemia and chronic renal failure who had had a small myocardial infarction several years ago, presenting now with shortness of breath on exertion and orthopnoea. She had been started on diuretics by the GP. She lived with her husband and had no social problems.

I was asked to give a problem list and to dictate the letter to the GP as if I had just seen the patient in clinic but, with the examiners and the patient watching this, it was not easy! I was asked what investigations I would do and what changes to her treatment I would arrange in the clinic. They really wanted to see what I would actually do if I had this patient in front of me in outpatients.

50. *I was asked to see a 50-year-old lady who presents to the clinic with diarrhoea which has lasted for more than a few weeks.*

The history evolved like a case of thyrotoxicosis with a past history of increasing appetite and loss of weight with a goitre. She even mentioned her staring appearance. I remembered to sum up my plan for investigations to the patient before time was up.

I was then asked about the investigations that I would do, the treatment that I would start her on and the management of thyroid eye disease.

51. *The GP requests a further assessment of a 63-year-old known diabetic who has had a coronary artery bypass graft in the past. He is now complaining of increasing frequency of angina. He has had a left, below-knee amputation and has methicillin-resistant* Staphylococcus aureus *(MRSA) in an ulcer on his right foot.*

There were many, many problems! I ran out of time on the social history. He had angina and reduced mobility as a result of this and his limb prosthesis. He was blind in the right eye and was still smoking and had numerous social problems!

The examiners asked me how I would investigate the angina and what was the feasibility of nuclear scanning. They asked me how I would treat his MRSA ulcer and, finally, they wanted to know what I thought his prognosis was.

52. *I was given a GP referral letter for a patient who had developed a 1-month history of chest pain and had a past history of multiple joint pains and backache.*

The 43-year-old lady had a 1-month history of tight, retrosternal chest pain which was worse on exertion and on lying flat and which was associated with shortness of breath on exertion. She had a past history of pericarditis diagnosed by the GP 9 years previously but this had required no treatment. She had a family history of ischaemic heart disease with both her mother and brother dying in their fifties. The pain was not like the pain of her pericarditis, there was no history of diabetes mellitus or of hypertension. She was a non-smoker and had minimal alcohol intake. She also had a flitting arthralgia which was not a true arthritis as there was no swelling. I finished the history taking by outlining to the patient the physical examination I would perform and the investigations I would request which would be looking into the possibility of ischaemic heart disease, peptic ulcer disease, systemic lupus erythematosus (SLE) and musculoskeletal pain.

I was then asked to outline my differential diagnosis and was asked what investigations I would perform, so I suggested an ECG, an exercise ECG and an echocardiogram. They asked me what would be the diagnosis if the ECG showed ST elevation in all leads. They briefly asked me about SLE but then the bell went.

53. *I had to take a history from a lady who presented with a 6-month history of a cough. She had been on ACE inhibitors for the last 18 months.*

She had a dry cough which was associated with panicking. There were no features of asthma or of left ventricular failure and the most likely diagnosis was a cough resulting from ACE inhibition.

They asked me what I would put in the GP letter so I said I would stop the ACE inhibitors and change her to an angiotensin II receptor antagonist and that I would do a peak flow rate and arrange for pulmonary function tests.

54. *There was a very long GP letter giving the patient's past history of ulcerative colitis. The main concerns of the GP were about recent* per rectum *(PR) bleeding and about the use of steroids.*

The history I obtained consisted of a recent onset of PR bleeding which was dark in colour. There was no weight loss or loss of appetite. She had long-standing ulcerative colitis but was stable with no increased frequency of bowel movements or diarrhoea. She was taking non-steroidals and steroids. She also had psoriasis but it was well controlled. The patient's concern was whether this was colonic carcinoma.

The examiners asked me what investigations I would do and how I would deal with the side-effects of steroids.

55. *I had to see a 36-year-old lady with insulin-dependent diabetes mellitus who had had a recent admission for a foot ulcer. All peripheral pulses were intact. The GP had referred her to the clinic because of the ulcer and was requesting measures to encourage the ulcer to heal. I was given the blood pressure of 130/80 mmHg.*

She had previous poor diabetic control and was unaware of any hypoglycaemic episodes. She was a non-smoker. She had two children and, as her family was now complete, her husband had had a vasectomy. She drank three glasses of wine every day. She had a low BM in the mornings and was on Insulatard and Actrapid tds. She had a painless ulcer and had not seen the chiropodist recently.

I was asked about the role of the diabetic nurse and the chiropodist. The patient did not drive but the examiners asked me anyway whether she should have been advised against driving and I said, 'Yes, the patient should not really drive'.

56. *There was a GP letter asking whether this 72-year-old lady with weakness of her right arm and leg had had a stroke and what should be the management.*

The patient was a real inpatient and was a very bad historian! She had a 6-month history of falls and now had weakness of the right arm and leg. She was virtually unable to stand unaided and was not able to give a clear

history of the duration or the onset or of any progression of her symptoms. She also complained of incontinence, unsteadiness and confusion – the triad of normal pressure hydrocephalus (NPH). She had no headaches and had had no social input as she 'hated' the social services, etc.

The examiners asked me the following questions: 'What differential diagnosis would you give in a letter to the GP?' and 'What action would you take?'. I said I would admit the patient but that made it a very confusing scenario. 'What investigations would you do?' and 'What differential diagnosis would you write on the CT scan request?' We then had a long discussion as I had not mentioned a space-occupying lesion which the examiner clearly had as the top priority in his own mind. I thought he was wanting NPH. This was a very frustrating station as the patient was not a good history giver.

57. *The patient was an elderly man with chronic obstructive pulmonary disease (COPD) and social problems. There was also a previous history of an operation for small bowel obstruction.*

I was asked for my management plans and the likely underlying causes of the small bowel obstruction.

58. *Speak to this 36-year-old lady with diabetes who is on insulin and who has recently been treated for a diabetic foot ulcer. Take a history from her and explain to her the important problems that she now has.*

She was a 36-year-old lady who looked healthy. She was on regular insulin but her home BM readings varied quite considerably. She had one daughter aged 3 years and she had no other past medical illnesses. She had had a recent foot ulcer which had now healed well. She complained of a tingling sensation over both feet. She had already been seen in the ophthalmology clinic for an eye check. She had had no hypoglycaemic episodes but was adjusting the insulin dosage herself according to her BM results. The GP had planned to check her HbA1c. She was not on any drugs for pain relief and the GP notes said that both her dorsalis pedis pulses were palpable.

I was asked several questions by the examiners. 'What is the cause of her leg pain?' I said it would be either neuropathic or ischaemic and as her dorsalis pedis pulses were palpable then it was more likely to be neuropathic. 'What is the treatment if it is indeed neuropathic pain?' I said I would try carbamazepine but the examiners asked if that really was the first line of treatment. 'Is there any history of claudication?' and 'What about her eye signs?' I explained to the examiner that the patient had told me that she had seen the ophthalmologist and had been told that her vision was normal. 'Is she driving now?' 'Yes,' I said, 'but she does have to inform the DVLA and she cannot drive heavy goods vehicles'. The examiner asked me, 'What is the main problem that you have identified?'. I replied, 'neuropathic leg pain'. 'So how will you manage that?' I replied, 'with strict BM control, and carbamazepine or gabapentin'. 'What will you advise in the letter to the GP about this patient and her diabetes?'

59. *I missed this station because I arrived late! It is not a good idea to miss one complete station! It is still possible to pass the exam but one would need to get 100% on the other four stations and also if you are late for the first station, you are likely to be flustered for the remainder of the exam. It is best to travel to the exam the night before and to be relaxed when you arrive.*

60. *The patient is a 60-year-old man with Parkinson's disease and on long-term medication. Recently, he has developed worsening of the tremor. He has a history of a myocardial infarction with a coronary artery bypass graft and also he has prostatism. Explore his Parkinson's disease and suggest any further intervention and medication.*

I took a history regarding the Parkinson's disease and the drugs that he had been on. He had recently been affected by worsening symptoms and I had to delve into the other features of his disease. I asked him how his symptoms affected him in different ways, such as physical/social. I also enquired about his myocardial infarction and took a history about chest pain/angina. I asked him about his prostatism and, in fact, he was due to have a repeat prostate operation. I included the other routine sections of the history taking, including family history, allergies, social history, etc.

The examiners asked me how I could improve his symptoms. I was not asked about any specialized drugs as the scenario was not centred on a specialist neurological clinic. They asked me how I would seek out further information if I was unsure as to what to give. I said I would refer to a specialist clinic or look up the literature. The examiner asked me about the risks of having a repeat operation for his prostate and, finally, how were his symptoms related to micturition.

61. *Take a history from this patient and think of how to reply to the GP.*

The patient was a 65-year-old with symptoms of a transient ischaemic attack with slurred speech and weakness. The patient also had Hodgkin's disease. The GP was worried about disease recurrence.

I was asked about the psychosocial factors and whether the patient could have a superior vena caval obstruction.

62. *I was given a GP letter regarding a patient with arthritis who had had recurrent falls and was not coping at home.*

The patient herself was not concerned but her family had gone to see the GP with their concerns for their mother. She had had recurrent falls and had burnt-out rheumatoid arthritis. There was no active disease and she was on no treatment. She had a regular home help.

I was asked whether I should be talking to the relatives without the patient's knowledge.

63. *A 57-year-old Chinese gentleman is referred by his GP, diagnosed to have hypertension about 18 months ago. He has been treated with β-blockers and hydrochlorothiazide but the BP has remained uncontrolled. He was subsequently changed to an ACE inhibitor but the patient has defaulted with his medication. His blood pressure is now 185/105 mmHg and investigations have revealed urinary glycosuria, blood sugar 8 mmol/L, blood urea 7 mmol/L and serum creatinine 145 mmol/L.*

I introduced myself and asked him how the hypertension was diagnosed. Apparently he had had a headache and saw his GP who noted the high blood pressure. He was not aware of any sweating or palpitations. I explored any possible complications of hypertension such as chest pain and he did describe atypical chest pain on effort but the ECG had been normal. There was no paroxysmal nocturnal dyspnoea or orthopnoea, he had no intermittent claudication but did have transient weakness of his limbs. There was no focal neurological deficit and he had no symptoms of diabetes with no polyuria, polydipsia or excessive nocturia. He understood his diagnosis so I then went on to assess his cardiovascular risk. He was a chronic smoker, previously smoking two packets/day for 18 years, but had now reduced to 10 cigarettes/day. He consumed three units of alcohol/day. He played golf twice a week and I suggested a brisk walk in addition. He was overweight with hyperlipidaemia and had an excessive salt intake. I asked why he was not compliant to the medication and he explained that he was experiencing side-effects with erectile dysfunction from the β-blockers and a dry, irritating cough from the ACE inhibitors. I asked about any family history of hypertension, diabetes or ischaemic heart disease and I enquired about his psychosocial history with regard to occupation, stress, family, etc.

His problem list was that he had hypertension which was not controlled because of poor compliance as experiencing side-effects from the medication. I also said that I would have to rule out a secondary cause for the hypertension. He had atypical chest pain which needed to be followed up by an exercise stress test. He had glycosuria which needed to be further investigated with a fasting blood sugar. I listed his risk factors for ischaemic heart disease in terms of age, sex, hypertension, smoking, alcohol, weight and hyperlipidaemia. I told him that he needed some lifestyle modification.

64. *You are asked to see a 20-year-old with a headache. The GP wonders if he has had a subarachnoid haemorrhage. He was seen by the neurosurgeons as a child.*
He had had a ventriculoperitoneal (VP) shunt inserted in infancy for hydrocephalus and this had been revised at the age of 10. The history was clearly not of a subarachnoid haemorrhage and there was a positive family history for migraine. He had no aura before the headaches, which were focal on the right side, although he was under considerable stress as he was studying and also working part time. I felt the differential diagnosis here was of migraine.

The examiners asked me for a differential diagnosis for the headache and what were the complications of a VP shunt and expected me to include a subependymal abscess! I was asked how to investigate headaches and how to treat migraine. They asked me what percentage of patients get an aura.

65. *Please see this 50-year-old lady with type 2 diabetes diagnosed 1 year ago. She takes gliclazide. She developed watery diarrhoea while on holiday in Greece and this has persisted for 4 weeks after her return. She has had one negative stool sample. Please advise.*
She had had weight loss, polyuria and polydipsia, all of which had begun before her holiday and had continued subsequently. There were no symptoms suggestive of inflammatory bowel disease. Her home BM checks had been acceptable and no other family members who were on holiday with her had been affected.

I was asked about the causes for the symptoms and the signs of poorly controlled diabetes such as infection. 'What investigations would you like to do?' We returned to the possible causes and eventually I mentioned hyperthyroidism which appeared to be what they were looking for!

66. *Please could you advise on this 60-year-old man with chronic respiratory problems.*
He had had bronchial asthma for 50 years. For the previous year he had had recurrent chest infections, which had improved with steroids given by his GP. However, his chest X-ray now showed a lesion. I thought the diagnosis could be bronchopulmonary aspergillosis.

Additional Station 4 experiences

67. *A retired nurse, who had worked in Hong Kong, had an elective hip operation cancelled because she was hepatitis C antibody positive. She was told this without any explanation and just sent home. She found out more about hepatitis C herself and was concerned about the possibility of either a hepatoma or cirrhosis developing. She comes to casualty very upset.*
The discussion centred on her concerns regarding 'Have I got HIV?', 'Have I got cirrhosis/hepatoma?', 'Will I ever have my hip operation?', 'Why did they do the test without telling me and why did they not explain anything?'. It was probably because they were surgeons!

The questions were 'Was their attitude ethical in doing the hepatitis screen without informing her?' and how would I have investigated her?

68. *A lady has come back to clinic and you are the only doctor there. All the others are away. She has recently been investigated for multiple sclerosis and you have to give her the diagnosis.*
The conversation centred on the above and she wanted to know about the diagnosis and whether she could work. She asked if she could still drive, if she could have children and were there any treatment options.

I was asked what I would do if her boyfriend telephoned me and asked me to tell him about the consultation because she would not discuss it with him.

69. *Breaking bad news – multiple sclerosis. You have come to clinic early today and you are the only person available.*
The patient did not know much about multiple sclerosis and so I had to go back to basics. The patient asked me very limited questions and I finished by asking her to come to an appointment the following day with her partner. The examiner said to me that her partner telephones you at 5 pm demanding to know what she has been told. What would you do? The examiner also says that the patient has asked about interferon. How would I manage that?

70. *I was given a clinical scenario of a man with recently diagnosed carcinoma of the lung. I was asked to tell the patient his diagnosis and to ask for his consent for a bronchoscopy.*

I went over with the patient the symptoms he had presented with and then broke the bad news. I paused frequently, which I felt was very important, and I listened to his concerns. He did not want his wife to know so I explored why and managed to convince him that I should see them together. He was happy about that. We discussed the prognosis and he thought he was going to die in the next few weeks. He was concerned about having the bronchoscopy as a friend of his had had a bad experience with a rigid bronchoscope. I explained to him that the modern procedure uses a thin, flexible tube and that sedation is given. However, I did not have enough time to tell him about the dangers of bronchoscopy.

The examiners asked me about these dangers and about what I would do if his wife wanted to know the diagnosis and the patient was not there, which raised the issues of confidentiality, etc.

71. *A 55-year-old lady who had had previous radical radiotherapy for carcinoma of the lung had recently been for her 6-month check-up which was OK. She now presents with back pain, and both a bone scan and a CT scan have shown bony metastases in her spine, pelvis and ribs with an unstable L2 vertebra. Explain the results of her tests.*

She was a nurse but played a good patient. She was 'in denial'. The family did not know anything and she did not want them to until they had been on their holiday to France. I explained the situation and offered support and suggested that I could talk to her husband with her. I said that she was free to go on holiday but that she should really see the orthopaedic surgeon and the radiotherapist to get an opinion on the stability of her spine before she went.

I was asked about her rights.

72. *You are about to see a 24-weeks pregnant lady who has swelling of her leg. She has taken antibiotics which did not help. Discuss with her the methods of investigating for a deep vein thrombosis.*

The patient was worried about the risks from any radiological investigation and we then discussed methods for anticoagulation. I was asked about the dilemmas of investigation and treatment with low molecular weight heparin.

73. *Explain to this lady that her mother probably has Huntington's chorea with a recent relapse.*

The 'relative' appeared well educated and was asking many questions. She wanted to know about investigations, prognosis, any possible cure and future implications. It all went very well and the examiners looked pleased.

74. *You are the SHO on-call and you have been asked to talk to the daughter of a patient who is being tested for Huntington's disease. The genetic tests are not back yet but the daughter is very concerned.*

I asked her how much she knew already and what provisional diagnosis she had been given. I explained about Huntington's disease in relation to the patient having choreiform movements. She wanted to know all the implications for the family and I explained these. She was concerned about if her mother did not want the family to know then could we tell her the diagnosis as it may affect her and her children. Confidentiality was discussed at length and we also briefly touched on genetic counselling.

The examiner asked me if we could break confidentiality here and could I outline any diseases where confidentiality could and should be broken. I needed to be prompted with a scenario of a teacher being diagnosed with tuberculosis before I mentioned that notifiable diseases was an area where confidentiality had to be broken. I was then asked to define a notifiable disease.

75. *You have to see a heavy goods vehicle driver who was diagnosed 3 months ago with insulin-dependent diabetes mellitus and you have to advise him that he cannot drive HGVs any more.*

We discussed the history of his diabetes and his recent review at which he had been started on insulin. He had not been told that he must stop driving at that review although I explained to him that he was legally required to renounce his HGV licence. He was unwilling to consider this as he was the only wage earner in the family and it would affect his livelihood and that of his family. We discussed the legal position and whether the police would need to be informed.

I was asked who I would discuss this with and I suggested that his GP should be informed as well as the DVLA and my senior colleague.

76. *A young woman is admitted to the casualty department with a hypoglycaemic episode. She has type 1 diabetes mellitus and is a heavy goods vehicle driver. You* have to ensure that she informs the DVLA and stops driving HGV vehicles.

The whole conversation was very difficult! The actor performed as a stubborn patient. She was not listening to any of my arguments. We tried to establish the cause for the hypoglycaemic episodes and I tried to suggest that we get the GP and the diabetic nurse involved/informed.

The examiner asked me what I would have done next if the patient persisted in driving.

77. *You occasionally attend the neurology clinics and are called to outpatients as a lady has arrived without a clinic appointment wanting to know the results of her investigations. She has had internuclear ophthalmoplegia and investigations have shown an oligoclonal band in the cerebrospinal fluid and an MRI scan is suggestive of multiple sclerosis. Please tell her that she has multiple sclerosis and that the consultant neurologist is busy elsewhere.*

It was awful! There was a large table between us so I moved my chair closer to the patient and then had the examiners right in front of me and I also had difficulty in seeing the clock. The 'patient' was obviously neither a patient nor a good actress and showed very little emotion. I did not want to get into the finer details of multiple sclerosis so I established early on that the patient ought to return with her fiancé and she had no further questions. We finished early and then had 2 min of complete silence!

The examiner asked me how I thought the patient would feel when she got home and should she have been given some warning before the investigations were carried out that she might have multiple sclerosis. One examiner gave me a clear pass on all aspects and the other just on the conduct of the interview.

78. *This lady's father has recently been diagnosed with Huntington's disease. She has some information about the condition from the internet but wants to discuss the inheritance risks and her concerns about starting a family.*

I started off by ascertaining her understanding of her father's condition and what her main concerns were. I explained that the inheritance was autosomal dominant, i.e. 50% risk of passing the condition on to any child. I asked her if she had discussed this with her husband and suggested that she bring her husband in to discuss these issues. We also discussed what support had already been given to her father. The 'relative'/actress appeared well informed and was, I think, an SpR in medicine who appeared to be totally unemotional.

The examiner asked me what her husband's views were likely to be. Would I have informed her of the 50% inheritance risk if the husband had been present? We then went on to talk about the ethics of advanced directives and how often advanced directives needed to be updated.

79. *You see an 18-year-old girl who is newly diagnosed with insulin-dependent diabetes. She had presented with ketonuria and hyperglycaemia. Explain the diagnosis and its implications to her.*

She was a typical teenage girl with diabetes who refused to know about her diagnosis and kept changing the subject. She asked about driving but then moved to the next question before I was able to say anything about notifying the DVLA. I was able to bring it up again later and I then noticed the examiners were changing their mark-sheets!

The examiner asked me what I would do if the patient decided to leave without accepting insulin therapy.

80. *You must speak to the son of a 76-year-old man who has bronchogenic carcinoma and who is refusing to undergo treatment. You must discuss with the son your management strategy and his father's resuscitation status.*

The son was keen for no further treatment as his father was suffering quite a lot. I told the examiner that if the patient is mentally fit and not depressed then we cannot force treatment. If he is not mentally fit then the consultant has to decide the management after consulting with the relatives. Regarding resuscitation status, I needed to talk to the patient in order to make a decision.

81. *You are about to see a young lady with lymphoma and you have to break the bad news to her.*

The patient was very emotional and I was unable to control the situation. I felt that I did really badly here and in fact I had a clear fail.

82. *I had to see a 30-year-old lady with probable multiple sclerosis. She was working full-time and this was her first consultation after having been referred from the GP after an episode of loss of vision in one eye which had now resolved. She had problems with shaking/tremor in her hands and diplopia. She had been advised to come in for further investigations. A previous CT brain scan was normal.*

I was asked to speak to the patient about the possibility of multiple sclerosis but to explain that we needed to confirm the diagnosis by doing further investigations in hospital and this would require admission. I was asked to explain about an MRI scan and a lumbar puncture. The patient had some social concerns about going to work, the probable chance of having multiple sclerosis and the implications for her teenage daughter.

83. *You have to see the daughter of a lady who is very unwell and likely to succumb to a severe pneumonia. Please counsel the daughter regarding resuscitation status.*
The whole counselling, with a very agreeable and cooperative 'relative', lasted a mere 7 min! The examiners asked me about the principles of ethics in terms of autonomy and paternalism.

84. *You are about to see a patient with atrial fibrillation who is taking amiodarone. Talk to the patient about starting warfarin.*
We discussed the pros and cons of warfarin therapy and discussed risk versus benefit.

85. *This 27-year-old lady was diagnosed as having migraine. She has a strong family history of migraine, including her sister and mother. She has expressed her concern regarding worsening headaches and requests a CT scan. She is also concerned about the renal complications following prolonged analgesic ingestion. One of her friends has just died of a brain haemorrhage. On a previous occasion you have examined her and found no serious pathology.*
I explained to the patient that I had been asked to explain to her the plan of management. I asked her to tell me more about her concerns and then tried to address these. I attempted to evaluate the headache, enquiring about the site, nature, frequency and duration of the pain and about whether there were any sinister symptoms and signs. I asked about recent changes in lifestyle and in particular about any recent precipitating foods, stress, poor sleep, etc. I enquired about the medication she was on in terms of type and frequency of medication. I explored any occupational stress, interpersonal relationships with staff at work and regarding her family support. I explained to her that both the history and physical examination had not revealed any serious pathology in her brain. I tried to reassure her and provide support. I explained about avoiding precipitating factors, e.g. tyramine-

containing foods, and to take her migraine prophylactic drugs and then we discussed any possible side-effects. I touched on stress management with breathing exercises, yoga and meditation and arranged a follow-up appointment for 1 month's time. I explained that if she had improved by then that all would be well, but that if no improvement was obvious then one would have to consider a CT scan. Meanwhile I explained to her that a CT brain scan was not required as it was costly and may pick up minor abnormalities which would further worry the patient. I addressed her concerns regarding kidney function and reassured her that the frequency and dosage of tablets would be minimal and that one can assess renal function by investigations. I said that if she had any serious symptoms she was to return to clinic sooner than the given appointment.

86. *A young female patient who had had her first fit returns to clinic. You must discuss the implications of this with her. She is a keen sportswoman and drives a car, having just passed her test. Her occupation is in computing.*
The patient asked me lots of questions including, 'Is this epilepsy?', 'Will I fit again?', 'Why can I not drive?'. The patient was upset at having had this fit and was very concerned about the stigma of epilepsy.

87. *A 55-year-old lady, who had had a mastectomy 10 years ago for carcinoma, now presents with hypercalcaemia and back pain and is found to have metastatic recurrence. You are the SHO on the ward and must tell the patient the diagnosis, the need to refer her to the oncologist and the likely treatment options.*
I broke the news early on. The patient was very shocked and then became angry, particularly stating that she was not told 10 years ago that the disease could return. She asked me if I thought it was wrong not to have told her. I did not agree or disagree with her but merely expressed my regret and sorrow. We discussed chemotherapy and radiotherapy and I tried to emphasize the seriousness of the condition and the fact that this was unlikely to be curable. I asked her about her other concerns. Her mother had recently died an 'undignified' death and the patient asked me about the possibility of euthanasia. I explained that this is illegal in this country and then went into the specifics of palliative care in an attempt to address her particular concerns of pain, etc.

The examiner asked me what one should do when a patient criticizes another doctor and then about whether the decision to resuscitate should always be discussed with the patient.

Invigilators' diaries – Stations 2 and 4

Poor start
On starting the consultation, the candidate's first sentence was, 'Sorry, but I have forgotten your name'. Another first sentence was, 'Right then, how can I help?'.

First impressions
On approaching the patient, the candidate sneezed into his hands and then shook the patient's hand.

Keeping eye contact
The candidate was so involved in taking notes during the history taking that he missed how the patient described her chest pain, a sweep of the hand from the epigastric area to the throat mimicking her heartburn.

In a rush
A candidate mistimed the whole station; he raced through the history of the presenting complaint in about 1 min, proceeded to briefly take the rest of the history, and then realized he had 9 min left. The silence was broken by, 'OK then, tell me about these palpitations again'.

Interruptions
A patient with a previous history of ischaemic cardiac pain, angioplasty and coronary artery stenting was describing her present chest pain (resulting from oesophageal reflux) and just about to say that this present pain is different from her previous chest pain, when the candidate interrupted and said 'So, tell me more about your angioplasty'.

Specific questioning
When asking about the smoking history, the candidate could not keep the questioning as open as possible and asked, 'How many cigarettes do you smoke a day, 10, 20, 30 or 40?'.

Ignoring the past medical history
A patient presents with breathlessness and is on amiodarone for atrial fibrillation. She has had a coronary artery bypass graft in the past. The candidate asks the patient 'Have you had any operations in the past?'. 'Yes, a heart operation,' was the reply. The candidate followed this by saying, 'Oh, that's interesting. Moving on, tell me, do you smoke?'.

Inability to pick up hints of emotions and lacking tact
The consultation revolved around a patient with blurred vision. The young patient was worried she may have multiple sclerosis. The patient says to the candidate, 'I'm worried this may be something serious'. The candidate replied, 'That doesn't surprise me'.

Any questions?
After a consultation with a patient presenting with haemoptysis, the candidate asked the patient, 'Any questions?'. The reply from the patient was, 'So, what is the problem?'. The candidate then said, 'I don't know but I will refer you on to a respiratory specialist'.

End of station 2
A candidate, after seeing a patient with funny turns, gave no indication of any tests to be performed, any follow-up or any thoughts about the possible causes for the funny turns, and ended the consultation by saying, 'Thanks, we've finished now'.

Some anecdotes from our most recent surveys

88. I was asked to examine the chest of a patient who had a history of chronic productive cough. On examination, I found bilateral thoracotomy scars. The examiners then pointed me towards the marfanoid features which I hadn't really noticed because it was the respiratory station and it was a patient with a productive cough. I felt it was an unfair case as I was not aware that the bilateral thoracotomy scars were because of pneumothoraces. I was thinking of lobectomy for bronchiectasis. The patient had Marfan's syndrome and bilateral thoracotomy scars because of bilateral pneumothorax.

89. I was asked to examine the respiratory system. I did a full examination including the hands so I was thankful that I spotted the yellow nails. I also found evidence of bronchiectasis, VATS (video-assisted thoracoscopic surgery) scars, a nephrectomy scar, and there were pressure stockings on the legs because of obvious lymphoedema. The patient had yellow nail syndrome with bronchiectasis. I was asked about other complications associated with yellow nail syndrome and then about the treatment of bronchiectasis.

90. I was asked to examine a man's respiratory system and I completed that satisfactorily. I found the classic signs of bronchiectasis and also noticed he had yellow nails. The examiner pointed to the bedside locker and I was asked what the piece of equipment was. I answered that it was a tidal volume incentive device. I was asked about the role of surgery in bronchiectasis. It was all quite straightforward.

91. I was told that the patient had come to clinic for assessment of shortness of breath. I found severe kyphoscoliosis and reduced chest expansion. The patient had Klippel–Feil syndrome and the kyphoscoliosis was congenital. I was asked about what diagnostic work-up I would do and what would be the indications for NIV. They also asked an additional question about the skin condition that he had. Luckily I had noticed the ichthyosis!!

92. This gentleman presented with breathlessness, please examine the chest and tell us why. I found kyphoscoliosis, reduced expansion, but with normal percussion and auscultation. He had congenital kyphoscoliosis and there then ensued a discussion about type 2 respiratory failure. Examiner 1 asked 'Why might he present to a neurologist?' and 'What would you do in a neuro clinic if he presented?' and 'What tests would you do in an MAU situation?' and finally 'What would you expect the pulmonary function tests to show?'. Examiner 1 then told me he was a neurologist!

93. This patient had a collapsed lung. I knew that was the answer as a friend of mine was in the same carousel and she got a 4 with this answer. I had had no clue whatsoever! The gentleman had presented with a cough. I had found decreased air entry at the lung base with dullness and a shifted trachea. I was asked the causes of pulmonary fibrosis.

94. I was asked to examine a man's abdomen. There were lots of scars everywhere and a PEG tube *in situ*. I did not have a clue what it was all about. I was asked about the reasons for the PEG, what else could it be for, the uses for it, and the causes of scars (the surprising thing was that it was not Crohn's disease).

95. 'This gentleman has a chronic condition affecting his abdomen, could you examine him and tell us what you find.' There were multiple scars on the arms, and several abdominal scars. There was a PEG tube *in situ* and a feed in progress. There was no organomegaly. I suspect that he may have had inflammatory bowel disease, but the examiners did not confirm or refute

this. Some candidates just looked at the tube and scars on the arms and said this was CAPD. The feed was covered up in a backpack, but they didn't stop me unzipping it and looking.

96. 'This patient has abdominal pain, please examine.' There was a PEG tube in place and I was asked about the indications for PEG feeding.

97. 'Examine this man's abdomen.' There was a feeding tube with multiple laparotomy scars. I was asked about the possible reasons for the PEG/feeding tubes, and about the types of motor neurone disease! I went off on a tangent about motor neurone disease being an oesophageal cause for a PEG!

98. The patient had hepatomegaly from pernicious anaemia. I was asked to 'examine this patient who has a peripheral neuropathy'. He had yellow skin but the sclerae were white. There was hepatomegaly present. I certainly didn't get the diagnosis right as I thought it was alcoholic liver disease!

99. I was asked to examine the abdominal system and then the eyes and then the shins. There were multiple surgical scars, Argyll Robertson pupils and pyoderma gangrenosum. I diagnosed Crohn's disease. I was then asked to suggest the operations that the lady had had and I was asked to put the scars and the other signs together. I suggested steroid-induced diabetes. They seemed happy with that.

100. I was told that the patient had diarrhoea and was asked to examine the abdominal system. There was no clubbing/jaundice, there was a upper mid-line abdominal scar and 2 cm scar across left clavicle, one radiotherapy tattoo upper abdomen. The diagnosis was oesophagectomy and radiotherapy scar. I was asked the cause of the diarrhoea.

101. I was asked to examine a patient's abdomen. There was a parathyroidectomy scar and a palpable ballotable mass in right iliac fossa. I thought it was a transplanted kidney. I was asked about causes of renal failure. I tended to talk and talk about what I knew about renal failure and transplants, but in a structured way, and I think this meant they'd run out of questions by the time I'd finished! Apart from the last question, asking about calcium metabolism in renal failure when I fell apart a bit, then was saved by the bell!

102. 'Please examine this patient with back pain and shortness of breath.' I found the signs of an aortic valve replacement in a patient with ankylosing spondylitis. To be precise, I found a prosthetic S2, abdominal protuberance, a fentanyl patch, a sternotomy scar, a hunched-up posture and was then asked about the different type of valves, why patients with ankylosing spondylitis need an AVR, the complications of valve replacements, what is the best analgesia for ankylosing spondylitis. It had said on the curtain outside that the patient had back pain and shortness of breath so it gave me the opportunity to think of the most likely things you'd see in a PACES exam that would fit with that. I guessed it would be ankylosing spondylitis with valvular heart problems and was relieved to find that it was.

103. I was asked to 'examine this gentleman'. It was a young gentleman with 'v' waves, a pansystolic murmur and quiet heart sounds. The questions were mainly about the diagnosis, of which I did not have a clue. I said there were signs of tricuspid regurgitation. However, I was sure it wasn't an ASD or VSD. I suggested doing an echo. I asked the chap after the examination what his diagnosis was and he said 'Ebstein's anomaly'.

104. I was asked to examine the CVS. I said I had found an irregular pulse and prosthetic heart sounds. There was a systolic flow murmur and a mid-line sternotomy scar. I was then asked to look at his hands again and consider the diagnosis. I had completely missed the rheumatoid hands! It was obviously a connective tissue disease causing AR with subsequent tissue valve replacement.

105. I had to examine a lady's heart. She had trisomy 21, early clubbing and a systolic murmur. I was asked for my clinical findings (I said ventricular septal defect in a patient with Down's syndrome), what investigations I would do and why I thought it was this diagnosis. I passed with 4/4 from both examiners.

106. I was asked to examine the lower limbs and I found signs of a peripheral neuropathy and a Charcot's joint. I was asked for the causes of a peripheral neuropathy and I made the best guess of a diagnosis for this particular patient.

107. My educational supervisor always emphasized the importance of being at the MRCP venue at least 2 days before the exam if there was any suggestion that there was likely to be bad weather, especially if travel-ling to Scotland. I never took that suggestion too seriously. I arranged to fly up to Dundee the afternoon before my exam. It was snowing heavily that day. After an agonising wait, my flight finally took off and was all of 5 hours late!! I landed in Arctic-like conditions. My luggage went missing and couldn't be traced anywhere. I had no suit, no tools, just plain fear. I didn't sleep that night. The next morning I bought a suit at 9 am and took the exam a few hours later. Needless to say, I failed miserably!

Experiences

These accounts from the pre MRCP PACES short cases start with four detailed experiences followed by a medley of short scenarios of individual cases. These are relevant to the current PACES format; because the same short cases are presented, albeit in different stations, a competent performance is expected and the examiners ask the same sort of questions. Important learning points emerge from each experience, which should be incorporated in your examination technique. We have highlighted some key points in the footnotes.

'The examiners let him realize that he had missed coarctation of the aorta.'

108. In his first case (first attempt) a candidate was asked to: 'Examine this man's heart'. He found a short systolic murmur in a hypertensive patient and diagnosed aortic sclerosis. He did not look for radiofemoral delay because he had been asked to examine the heart and not the cardiovascular system.

The examiners let him realize that he had missed coarctation of the aorta. Filled with anger and dismay at this injustice, he was taken to the next case where he was asked to listen to the back of a woman's chest. He had a quick look at the front (was not asked to) and spotted the radiation marks (he felt that the examiners were trying to hide this clue from him). He looked purposefully at the back and noted pleural aspiration marks. He therefore suspected a pleural effusion and performed the relevant clinical steps to confirm this impression. He was asked the probable cause and without hesitation gave the diagnosis of bronchial carcinoma along with the supportive evidence.

He was then asked to examine a man's cranial nerves. He performed a rapid, efficient screen and reported left VIth, VIIth, XIIth nerve palsies and left lateral nystagmus but he was not asked for a diagnosis. For his fourth case, he was asked to look at a man and he gave the spot diagnosis of acromegaly. When asked how to diagnose the condition, he suggested imaging of the pituitary fossa, glucose tolerance test (GTT) with growth hormone levels, etc. Next, he was asked to look at a patient's arm and he instantly recognized the 'plucked chicken skin' appearance of pseudoxanthoma elasticum in the antecubital fossa. Finally, he was asked to look at a woman's face where he saw nothing obvious until he spotted a small left pupil and slight ptosis. He immediately diagnosed a left Horner's syndrome and was asked for, and gave, the possible causes.

Although his performance in all but the first case had been impeccable, he was convinced, until the result arrived, that he had failed because of that first case. In retrospect, his reaction to the first case may have had a positive effect on the subsequent performance. Instead of going to pieces (e.g. Experience 109 below, and Quotations 383 and 385) he felt angry at being asked to examine the heart when the key finding was at the femoral pulse. He conducted the rest of the exam with ruthless efficiency and avenged himself by looking for more than he was asked to. The parting words of the examiner were: 'You'll never miss radiofemoral delay again, will you?'. (Pass)

'He looked down on two thin legs, imagined two inverted champagne bottles, and before he could stop himself, heard himself saying "Charcot–Marie–Tooth disease".'

109. On his second attempt, another candidate was asked first to, 'Examine the abdomen'. Without looking anywhere else, he coned down on the abdomen and felt the liver edge. After a long time, and some persuasion, he noticed the palmar erythema, anaemia, gynaecomastia and decreased body hair. These signs, in particular the gynaecomastia, together with the diagnosis of cirrhosis, had to be dragged out of him by the examiners. The candidate had been nervous before the start and now, realizing that he had performed badly on the first case through lack of proper inspection, was already becoming engulfed in the 'downward spiral syndrome'.

At the second case the examiner said, 'We haven't much time so just quickly feel the pulse and listen over the apex and base'. He was confused as he did not know where the base was so he listened at the lower left sternal edge and the apex. He did not look at the neck or at the precordium. He felt a collapsing pulse, heard a systolic murmur and diagnosed mitral incompetence. In retrospect, he thought that he must have missed mixed aortic valve disease.

On the next case he was asked to examine the patient's legs. He realized that things were going very badly and that he had to score highly from then on. He looked down on two thin legs, imagined two inverted champagne bottles and, before he could stop himself, heard himself saying 'Charcot–Marie–Tooth disease'. The examiner, who was apparently becoming increasingly doubtful about the candidate's capability of performing a competent clinical examination, had to drag a hesitant, unstructured examination out of him which revealed spastic paraparesis. A discussion followed on the possible causes.

In the next case the candidate looked at a fundus with whiteness around the disc and diagnosed myelinated nerve fibres. In his last case he examined a patient's hands with swollen metacarpophalangeal and proximal interphalangeal joints, tapered fingers, wasted intrinsic muscles and papery, thin skin. With his morale gone, it took a long time before he saw any of the abnormalities and longer still to suggest rheumatoid arthritis (?on steroids). (Fail)

'He was side-tracked into saying that she could have hereditary haemorrhagic telangiectasia.'

110. After an indifferent start in the short cases, a candidate was asked to examine a man's pulse. He found it regular and the rate was 40 beats/min. He was then asked to listen to the precordium but he failed to comment on the variable intensity of the first heart sound which could have led him to the diagnosis of complete heart block.

He was next asked to look at a woman's face. There was perioral tethering and telangiectasis, but as he had not performed a visual survey and his presentation was loose, he was side-tracked into saying that she could have hereditary haemorrhagic telangiectasia. It eventually became obvious to him (he was asked to look at the hands – sclerodactyly) that the patient had scleroderma. The examiner then asked him: 'On which part of the tongue would you say the telangiectasia would most likely be found in hereditary haemorrhagic telangiectasia, if you were teaching a class of medical students?'.

Having been unable to impress the examiners so far, he was asked to look at a man's neck. (The bell went almost immediately signalling the end of the exam.) The patient was lying down and his neck movements were completely restricted. The candidate diagnosed cervical spondylosis. The typical 'question mark' posture of ankylosing spondylitis only became recognizable when the patient sat up!

In his second attempt, this candidate was asked to examine a middle-aged woman with a goitre – he felt it was really quite straightforward. The goitre was asymmetrical but he annoyed one examiner by using the term 'slightly asymmetrical'. He also let out the word 'tumour' in front of the patient when asked to discuss management. (Fail)

'During the examination he was interrupted at various times.'

111. A candidate on his first attempt was asked to look at a man's legs (the examiner pulled the pyjamas to the lower end of the patella, leaving a lateral scar covered – which the candidate did not see until the end). He found a swollen, warm left leg and diagnosed a deep venous thrombosis. He was asked for other possibilities and said ruptured Baker's cyst. The examiner said he would not ask who Baker was but wanted an explanation of the term. The examiners probed for further possibilities such as cellulitis, muscle rupture and also asked about ruptured plantaris muscle.

On his next case he was asked to look at the patient's hands and describe them. He diagnosed rheumatoid arthritis and was asked to explain the reasons for ulnar deviation, subluxation and boutonnière deformity. The examiner asked: 'Why is it called boutonnière? Have you ever seen a button hook? Why is the wrist like that? What are the important functions of the hand?'. He was then asked to look at the knees of the same patient. He found a swollen, painful right knee which he thought resulted from synovial swelling. He said he had been about to say 'Charcot's joint' but realized it was painful. He diagnosed rheumatoid arthritis of the knee and was then asked how he knew it was synovial swelling.

At the next patient the examiners said: 'I think we would be interested in this lady's precordium'. During the examination he was interrupted at various times: 'What do you think of the pulse?', 'What do you think of the jugular venous pressure?' and they stopped him before he had finished and asked for the findings. He diagnosed mixed mitral valve disease but had missed the mitral valvotomy scar.

The examiner then handed him an ophthalmoscope and said: 'We would like you to use this on the next patient'. The candidate noticed that this patient showed some incoordination and a spastic leg so he expected to find optic atrophy. When he mentioned this diagnosis, the examiner asked him if he knew what sort of

visual field defect he would expect and then asked him to test the visual fields.

On the last case he was asked to feel the patient's abdomen. He found an inguinal hernia, a palpable aorta and a palpable liver edge at about 2 cm below the right costal margin. He said he did not think it was hepatomegaly. The examiners asked what signs he would look for if the patient did have hepatomegaly! (Pass)

In the following examples the examiner seems to be probing the power and range of the candidate's observations

112. A candidate was asked to examine the motor system of a man's legs. She found global weakness, wasting and loss of reflexes. She gave a differential diagnosis of lower motor neurone paralysis that included a disc lesion, spinal canal problems, degenerative disorders and motor neurone disease. The examiners asked her to look at the patient's tongue – it was fasciculating. She was then able to narrow the differential diagnosis to the last-mentioned possibility. (Pass)

113. A candidate was asked: 'Look at this man's chest and then examine his respiratory system'. The patient had a right mastectomy scar and the skin changes of previous radiotherapy. There was dullness to percussion and reduced breath sounds at the right base. The candidate diagnosed carcinoma of the breast with a right pleural effusion. (Pass)

114. A candidate was asked to listen only to a patient's heart. No other cardiovascular examination was expected. She found the features of mitral stenosis but did not notice the valvotomy scar. The examiner pointed this out to her. (Pass)

115. A candidate was asked to look at a woman's hands. He found the changes of rheumatoid arthritis. A description was not wanted, only the diagnosis. The examiner then asked him: 'Why is she wearing a cervical collar?'. The candidate, who had noticed it but not mentioned it, said that it could be because of atlantoaxial subluxation. (Pass)

116. After mistaking a malar flush for SLE in a patient who had mitral stenosis, a candidate was asked to examine a woman's hands. She diagnosed acromegaly. Although the patient had wasting of the thenar eminence, she missed this, and the diagnosis of carpal tunnel syndrome, until the examiner told her about the patient's symptoms. The candidate diagnosed optic atrophy, splenomegaly and hepatosplenomegaly successively in three other short cases and was then shown a patient and asked: 'On general appearance what is wrong with this man?'. She thought that he had a myopathic facies and diagnosed dystrophia myotonica. The examiner asked why she thought he had a hearing aid. She looked at the head again and realized that the patient had an enlarged cranium, rather than wasted facial muscles, and diagnosed Paget's disease. (Fail)

117. A candidate was shown a patient and asked: 'On general appearance what is wrong with this man?'. She thought that he had a myopathic facies and diagnosed myotonic dystrophy. The examiner asked why she thought he had a hearing aid. She looked at the head again and realized that the patient had an enlarged cranium, rather than wasted facial muscles, and diagnosed Paget's disease.* (Fail)

118. A candidate was asked to examine a man's abdomen. She found an enlarged, knobbly liver and diagnosed hepatic secondaries but forgot to test for ascites. She was asked if there was any free peritoneal fluid. The examiners watched intently as she demonstrated the presence of ascites. (Pass)

119. A candidate was asked to examine the patient's abdomen. He found bilateral masses in the loins and diagnosed polycystic kidneys. The patient also had a craniotomy scar from a repair of a ruptured berry aneurysm. On another case, he was able to diagnose hypothyroidism by looking at a woman's face. The examiner asked why she was in a surgical ward and he suggested severe constipation as a reason. (Pass)

120. A candidate was asked to, 'Examine this lady's cardiovascular system, commenting as you go'. He diagnosed mixed mitral valve disease but missed the cardiac cachexia and the left mastectomy scar. The examiners wanted him to comment that she was very ill and to suggest why. They also asked for comments as to whether the mitral stenosis or mitral incompetence was dominant. (Fail)

121. A candidate was asked to, 'Comment on this patient's appearance. Pretend he is sitting opposite you on the underground train and perform one clinical test'. The candidate noted frontal bossing, bilateral ptosis,

*It may be that in PACES such a case would be less likely to occur.

deafness, missing fingers on the right hand and a saddle-shaped nose. Initially, the candidate thought he had congenital syphilis and wanted to do a Romberg's test. The examiner manipulated the discussion and got him round to thinking about myotonic dystrophy. After this, the candidate suggested a handshake as the one clinical test.

He was then asked to examine the abdomen of the next patient. He found bilateral, enlarged, 'lumpy' kidneys which were easily palpable and he diagnosed polycystic kidneys. The candidate was shown the patient's left forearm and, having worked on a renal unit, he immediately recognized the presence of an arteriovenous fistula for haemodialysis. The examiners seemed quite impressed with this. (Pass)

122. Another candidate was shown the same patient with myotonic dystrophy and asked: 'What observations do you make?'. He commented on the bilateral ptosis, wasted sternomastoid and temporalis muscles and, after demonstrating myotonia in the hands, was able to make the diagnosis. There then followed a brief viva on cardiomyopathy in this condition. (Pass)

123. A candidate was asked to listen to a patient's heart. He found mitral incompetence and noted that the patient's face looked acromegalic. However, he did not mention the acromegaly until he was directly asked about it. (Fail)

124. A candidate was taken to a patient with a recent laparotomy scar and asked to examine his neck. He noticed a biopsy scar and, on palpation, found matted glands. He diagnosed Hodgkin's disease and the examiner just asked him for a differential diagnosis. (Pass)

125. 'Look at this patient from here. What would you like to do now?' The candidate noticed a man with long extremities, muscle wasting, a pustular rash, paronychia, nicotine-stained fingers and pectus excavatum. He had to be prompted to the diagnosis of Marfan's syndrome. He was then asked to look into the patient's mouth (high-arched palate) and to listen to his heart (aortic incompetence). He found both of these but did not mention the hyperextensible joints. (Pass)

126. For the cardiovascular case, a candidate's instruction was: 'This lady is breathless – listen to her heart'. He diagnosed mitral stenosis but the examiners pointed out that he had not noticed that the lady had rheumatoid arthritis as well.

Later on, for his respiratory case, he was told: 'This patient is breathless – examine the respiratory system'. He found crepitations and basal dullness so he diagnosed pulmonary fibrosis with a pleural effusion. Having learned from the earlier case, he was able to relate both to the rheumatoid arthritis which he had already observed in this patient. (Pass)

127. After having difficulty deciding whether a patient had diabetic or hypertensive retinopathy, a candidate was asked to examine another patient's neck. He diagnosed a small multinodular goitre but the examiners remained dissatisfied. They asked if the patient was thyrotoxic or not. While he examined for a tremor, he noticed the gross rheumatoid arthritis in the hands. He reported that the examiners were looking for the diagnosis of autoimmune thyroid disease. (Fail)

128. A candidate was invited to look at a patient's face. The face was normal when looking straight ahead but on further examination, he discovered weakness of the lower part of the right side of the face and he diagnosed a right upper motor neurone VIIth nerve palsy.* He missed the surgical scar just below the jaw on the right side and, in retrospect, felt it was a partial right lower motor neurone VIIth nerve palsy. (Fail)

129. A candidate was asked to look at a patient's face. He said: 'acromegaly'. The examiner asked if he was happy with that in such a way that he implied to the candidate that he should look for more physical signs. At once, the candidate said that he would like to look for complications such as a bitemporal hemianopia, hypertension, cardiomegaly or evidence of treatment already given. The patient did, in fact, have a hemianopia. (Pass)

In the experiences that follow the spotlight seems to be on the candidate's examination technique

130. A candidate was asked to make a neurological examination of a patient's legs. He found bilateral upper motor neurone signs and was then asked the level of the lesion. The candidate proceeded to examine the arms and found upper motor neurone signs in one

---

*The correct expression would be 'upper motor neurone facial muscular' palsy, because the lesion has to be above the nucleus of the VIIth cranial nerve.

arm. He then tested the jaw jerk, which was normal. No further questions were asked. (Pass)

131. A candidate was asked to examine a patient's abdomen. He found an enlarged organ in the left hypochondrium and thought that it was a polycystic kidney but he admits that his examination was 'cack-handed'. In retrospect, he thinks it was a spleen. For his eye case he was asked to look at a patient's fundi. He diagnosed choroiditis but, in retrospect, he feels that it was probably a diabetic retinopathy with laser burns. (Fail)

132. A candidate was asked to examine a woman's fundi, to look for pyramidal signs in her hands and to elicit her plantar responses. He found early papilloedema on the left, an increased finger jerk and supinator jerk on the right and a right extensor plantar. He admitted that he had made a mess of doing the finger jerks and did not know the two ways of eliciting these; the examiner had to demonstrate the tests. He was about to test the plantar response with the end of the patella hammer when he was stopped by the examiner who gave him a thin wooden orange stick! (Pass)

133. A candidate was asked to look at, and then examine, the legs of a man who complained of unsteadiness. He found ataxia, pyramidal weakness with clonus in both legs and bilateral extensor plantar responses and he diagnosed multiple sclerosis. However, the examiner was not at all happy with his neurological examination technique and, in fact, showed him how to do it! (Fail)

134. A candidate was asked to watch a patient walk and to examine his lower limbs. He could see bilateral foot drop with wasted anterior compartments but did not make the diagnosis of Charcot–Marie–Tooth disease. The examiners criticized the way in which he examined the reflexes. (Fail)

135. A candidate was told: 'This man has gone off his feet. Examine the legs and say why'. He found gross wasting, fasciculation, absent ankle jerks and flexor plantar responses and he diagnosed progressive muscular atrophy (motor neurone disease). He commented to us that he had to wait for what seemed to be 3–4 min before any fasciculation was seen, although when it did come it was very obvious. (Pass)

136. A candidate was asked to examine a patient's eyes. He was almost blind in the left eye with a left VIth nerve palsy. He commented that he might well have failed the examination had he not tested visual acuity and thus found the explanation for the absence of diplopia. (Pass)

137. A candidate was asked to examine neurologically a man's hand. The patient had gross wasting and weakness of the small muscles of the hand. Although the candidate diagnosed a T1 lesion, he admitted that he looked very confused examining the hands.

A little unsettled by this experience, he was later asked to examine another patient's abdomen and jugular venous pressure. He found a pulsatile liver and giant v waves. He diagnosed tricuspid incompetence but admitted that he lacked confidence and this showed in the way he carried out the examination.

For the respiratory case, he was asked to examine the chest of a patient who had a thoracotomy scar, stridor and clubbing. He did not notice the stridor and also missed the pleural effusion. (Fail)

138. On being asked to examine the abdomen of a patient, a candidate found bilateral subcostal masses. He gave the findings and said the diagnosis was probably polycystic kidneys. The left-sided mass could have been a small spleen moving diagonally across the abdomen from under the rib cage on inspiration but it was bimanually ballottable. He gave the findings and persevered with the diagnosis of polycystic kidneys. The examiners persisted in discussing the possibility that the mass was a spleen but the candidate stuck to his diagnosis which he thinks was right. (Pass)

139. A candidate was asked: 'Examine this man's chest. Is there anything else you would look for?'. He found ankylosing spondylitis with poor expansion of the chest, but commented that he had to get the patient out of bed before he appreciated the typical 'question mark' posture of ankylosing spondylitis. There was no evidence of aortic regurgitation or upper lobe fibrosis. (Pass)

140. A candidate examined the abdomen of a 35-year-old Afro-Caribbean woman and found a 6 cm spherical mass in the left upper quadrant. He commented that he was allowed to 'go through the routine' – nodes, mouth, hands, etc. He said it was not a spleen or a kidney and he explained why. He gave a brief differential diagnosis. 'Expressionless and without comment, they led me away.' (Pass)

141. A candidate was asked to: 'Show me how you examine the reflexes in the legs'. He found absent knee and ankle jerks and extensor plantar responses. He offered the differential diagnosis of tabes dorsalis, subacute combined degeneration of the cord and a hereditary neuropathy such as Friedreich's ataxia. He was asked what else he would like to examine and he suggested the pupillary reflexes. He found small, irregular pupils which reacted to light and accommodation, but more to accommodation. He was asked if these were Argyll Robertson pupils and he answered: 'no'. The other examiner said: 'You said that this picture in the legs may be caused by tabes dorsalis. How do you explain the extensor plantars?'. He answered that this indicates pyramidal tract involvement. The examiner pointed out that this is called taboparesis, not tabes dorsalis. The candidate felt that his unfamiliarity with the different manifestations of neurosyphilis let him down, and he had failed to recognize Argyll Robertson pupils. (Fail)

142. A candidate was asked to: 'Examine the abdomen'. He found an enlarged liver of three finger-breadths and a spleen of four finger-breadths and diagnosed hepatosplenomegaly. The examiner's parting comment was: 'It is no good only making a diagnosis;* there is a proper method to examine the patient!'. (Fail)

143. A candidate was asked to examine the back of a young man's chest. He diagnosed* bilateral pleural effusions and he felt that these probably resulted from nephrotic syndrome. He believes the examiners agreed. However, he had forgotten to test for vocal resonance or tactile vocal fremitus. (Fail)

144. A candidate was asked to examine a patient's heart. He went through all the correct examination steps except that he forgot to lift up the arm and feel for a collapsing pulse. He diagnosed mixed mitral valve disease. One examiner proceeded to listen to the heart while the other examiner asked if the candidate had felt for a collapsing pulse. The candidate now wonders if he missed aortic valve disease. (Fail)

145. A candidate was asked to examine the eyes of a young woman aged about 20–30 years. He went comprehensively through the routine, checking visual acuity and visual fields before testing eye movements.

*The purpose of the examination is to demonstrate the difference between a guess and the diagnosis.

He felt that the examiners were impatient at the delay in finding the nystagmus that was present. The examiners asked what he wanted to examine next. The candidate, thinking that the diagnosis was likely to be multiple sclerosis, and assuming the presence of cerebellar signs, said he wanted to look at the fundi (for optic atrophy). He could not understand why the examiners seemed so irritated by this. They wanted him to demonstrate the cerebellar signs that were present. The candidate felt that this was an easy case on which he had made no great errors and yet the examiners seemed to have been unimpressed by his performance.* (Fail)

146. A candidate was asked to examine a patient's legs neurologically and then to ask him some questions. He found global aphasia and a profound right-sided spastic hemiparesis. He diagnosed a dominant hemisphere vascular lesion. He was asked: 'What might be the cause? The patient is 40' (pause); 'Feel the pulse'. He was in atrial fibrillation. 'What do you think the cause is now?' (Pass)

147. A candidate was shown a woman with a spastic paraparesis which she correctly diagnosed. After she had been taken to the next case, the examiners said: 'By the way, which side of the fire does that previous lady usually sit by?'. Luckily, she had noticed the erythema ab igne on the legs. (Pass)

A lack of polish and fluidity may make the examiners reflect on the clinical competence of a candidate. In the following examples, the examiners seem to be endeavouring to find the real clinical depth

148. The instruction in a patient with typical rheumatoid hands was: 'This lady had a fit 6 months ago, examine her hands'. During his examination the candidate found no skin rash or nodules. He diagnosed systemic lupus erythematosus in view of the fit. However, in retrospect, he still wonders if the diagnosis was just rheumatoid arthritis. (Pass)

149. A candidate was asked to examine a patient's cardiovascular system. He found a slow rising pulse, an ejection systolic murmur and an early diastolic murmur.

He diagnosed mixed aortic valve disease with predominant aortic stenosis. The examiners asked him to guess the patient's blood pressure. (Pass)

150. In the neurological case, after correctly diagnosing a spastic paraparesis, a candidate was asked to give the differences between upper and lower motor neurone lesions. In the cardiovascular case he was asked to feel a man's pulse. He suggested slow atrial fibrillation but, in retrospect, he thinks it may have been complete heart block as there then followed a discussion about the differential diagnosis and the management of complete heart block, including a discussion about the different types of pacemaker. (Fail)

151. A candidate who was taking the examination for the fourth time was taken to his cardiovascular case and asked: 'Feel this patient's pulse and apex beat, and listen to the base of the heart'. He was required to give a full description of the findings and the probable diagnosis at each stage. He found pulsus bisferiens, a displaced apex, an ejection systolic and an early diastolic murmur. (Pass)

152. A candidate, who was unhappy with his examination technique and the mistakes he had made in an easy first case, was asked to examine the right arm of a 40-year-old man. He reports finding a 'flail' arm with increased reflexes. He thought his method of examination was poor and he was unsure of the diagnosis. He was then asked to examine the same man's abdomen and reports finding bilateral, large, smooth, more or less symmetrical masses in the lumbar regions which he diagnosed as bilateral hydronephrotic kidneys.† (Fail)

153. A candidate was asked to: 'Examine the eyes from a neurological point of view'. He found bilateral ptosis and a homonymous hemianopia and he said to the examiner that he could not explain the findings by one lesion. The examiner said: 'Examine the hands'. The candidate became preoccupied with the obvious rheumatoid arthritis and came up with the suggestion of rheumatoid arthritis associated with myasthenia gravis, which would explain the ptosis but not the hemianopia. The examiner said: 'Feel the pulse'. The candidate found an irregular pulse and diagnosed atrial fibrillation causing a cerebral embolus. (Pass)

*Having noticed the nystagmus, the examiners probably wanted him to move on to demonstrate cerebellar signs with little or no prompting.

†We wonder if this patient had polycystic kidneys and an old cerebrovascular accident (ruptured berry aneurysm/hypertension).

154. A candidate examined the back of a patient's chest and found a pleural effusion. He had to go through the full examination and was asked what he was doing at every move, what each finding was caused by and how he interpreted it, e.g. breath sounds, crepitations, etc. (Pass)

Common errors

155. A candidate was asked to give a running commentary as he examined a patient's cardiovascular system. He commented on a collapsing pulse and on a mitral valvotomy scar but found no murmurs. He diagnosed mitral stenosis and became involved in a long discussion on the causes of a collapsing pulse. (Fail)

156. A candidate was asked to listen to a woman's heart. He found systolic and diastolic murmurs maximal at the base of the heart, to the left of the sternum. He diagnosed mixed aortic valve disease. In retrospect, he is sure that he missed the typical machinery murmur of a patent ductus arteriosus.* (Fail)

157. A candidate was asked to examine a man's chest, commenting as he went along. Although he thought the patient had chronic obstructive airways disease, he was not actually asked for a diagnosis, but instead became caught up in a discussion on the distinction between a wheeze and stridor. (Pass)

158. A candidate examined the fundus of a patient whose pupil had been dilated. He could not find much wrong and wondered if there was some vascular abnormality. He made a wild guess at diabetic retinopathy and wonders, in retrospect, if this was a branch retinal vein or artery occlusion. His comment was: 'I was totally lost by this time!'. (Fail)

159. A candidate examined the fundi of a patient and diagnosed bilateral optic atrophy and background diabetic retinopathy. He told us he had blurted out his impressions before stopping and thinking. Even in retrospect he does not know what the diagnosis was. (Fail)

160. A candidate was asked to examine the fundi of a patient (dilated pupils, dark room). He saw haemorrhages, exudates and some whiteness around the disc.

*Confusing a continuous murmur of a patent ductus arteriosus for systolic and diastolic murmurs of aortic valve disease is a sin not easily forgiven. Paul Wood, a famous British cardiologist, is reported to have remarked that the two sets of murmurs are so distinct from each other that there should be no confusion in recognizing them (see Vol.1, Station 3, Cardiovascular, Case 29).

He was put off by the examiners talking in the background and by his paranoia that the examiners were thinking that he was taking too long so he stopped before he had finished. He offered the diagnosis of diabetic retinopathy and myelinated nerve fibres. One examiner looked in the fundi while the other enquired if any microaneurysms had been seen. The candidate was not sure. There was then a discussion about the treatment of diabetic retinopathy and when photocoagulation was mentioned, the examiner asked if there was any evidence of this. In retrospect, the candidate felt diabetic retinopathy was probably right but wonders about the possibility of having missed hypertensive retinopathy and papilloedema. He felt that if only he had continued examining longer to elicit the exact findings present, he would have saved himself the cost of another attempt at the exam. (Fail)

161. A candidate was asked to feel the pulse of a patient. She was unable to feel it and guessed that atrial fibrillation must be present. (She failed.) Another candidate was taken to the same patient and admitted that she could feel neither the radials, brachials nor carotids (the patient was in low output cardiac failure). Afterwards she was told by the examiners that they had re-examined the patient and agreed with her. (Pass)

162. A candidate was asked to examine the back of the chest of a patient with bronchiectasis. During auscultation, the patient, in her enthusiasm to cooperate, breathed deeply and expired forcibly, generating upper airways wheeze.† The candidate, who already had his stethoscope in his ears, was unaware of the racket the patient was making. He reported the finding of widespread wheeze (the basal crepitations were completely drowned) although there was no wheezing at all when the patient was asked to breathe deeply in and out in a relaxed fashion.

Look first

163. A candidate was asked to listen to the back of a lady's chest. Although only asked to listen, she

†You can generate upper airways wheeze yourself by expiring hard at the same time as voluntarily narrowing your upper airways. If in doubt in the hysterical asthmatic, ask the patient to purse his or her lips as he or she breathes. This manoeuvre will abolish factitious wheeze. Although the wheeze of such a patient may be heard down the corridor, the pulse is not significantly elevated in the absence of true severe asthma (unless the acute asthma is caused by the inappropriate prescription of a β-blocker!).

examined expansion, percussion, palpation and finally auscultation, thinking that they would stop her if all they wanted her to do was to listen. They did not interrupt. She presented her findings of bilateral mid to late inspiratory crackles up to the mid zone and her diagnosis of fibrosing alveolitis. The examiners asked: 'Look at the patient and tell us what you think is the cause in her case'. At first the candidate could see no obvious cause from the face and therefore looked at her hands and immediately spotted the changes of systemic sclerosis. She then looked at the face again and the telangiectasia and tight skin were evident. (Pass)

164. A candidate was asked to examine a lady's neck. The candidate started off looking at the patient generally. No jugular venous pressure was obvious. She started feeling for lymph nodes. The examiners said: 'What are you doing?' so she explained that she was looking for lymph nodes – they asked why. She explained that she could not see anything else abnormal and then spotted the glass of water on the window sill and 'twigged'. She then started a thyroid examination and found a left thyroid nodule which was both visible and palpable on swallowing. A discussion followed about the possible causes. (Pass)

165. A candidate was asked to examine a patient's legs. He initially noticed gross ataxia, nystagmus and dysarthria when he introduced himself and shook the patient's hand. However, he still managed to fail to make a diagnosis of Friedreich's ataxia ('youthful ignorance' was his own comment about this!) and also ignored the examiner's prompt when he offered him a tuning fork and a patella hammer! (Fail)

Double pathology

166. A candidate was asked to examine neurologically a woman's legs. She found absent ankle jerks, increased knee reflexes and equivocal plantars. She was told that the patient was a diabetic and she noticed that she was wearing a cervical collar. Her mind was alerted to the possibility that there was a combination of a peripheral neuropathy and cervical spondylosis. (Pass)

167. A candidate was asked to look at the face of a woman who had presented with melaena. In retrospect, he felt the patient had acromegaly and Peutz–Jeghers syndrome (!) but he had not spotted the latter condition quickly enough. He was asked to examine the visual fields and, having mentioned the presence of

greasy skin, was drawn into a discussion on skin function. (Fail)

168. A candidate was asked to comment on the appearance of a patient. She had proptosis and a prosthetic eye. In addition, there was a thyroidectomy scar, evidence of thyroid acropachy and pretibial myxoedema. She had also had a recent amputation. He was asked to examine the fundi and it was obvious that she was also a diabetic. (Pass)

169. A candidate was asked to examine the legs of a man whom he was told had diabetes mellitus. He found a peripheral neuropathy and peripheral vascular disease. He also spotted that the patient had coexistent facioscapular dystrophy. (Pass)

170. A candidate was asked to examine just the heart of a patient. He found mixed aortic valve disease. He also suspected mitral stenosis but did not mention it as he had 'not expected to find double valve pathology'. (Fail)

Tell them of the expert that told you

171. A candidate was examined on a patient with acromegaly and feels that he performed reasonably well. In the discussion as to why he had used a red pin to test visual fields, he told them that a neurologist whom he had worked for had recommended it for the peripheral fields. The examiners seemed happy with that explanation. (Pass)

Apologies accepted

172. A candidate was asked to look in the eyes of a patient. He thought the disc margins were blurred and said so. The examiners asked him if he could see venous pulsation. The candidate pointed out that he would not recognize it if he saw it! He said that the examiners appeared to like this response and went on to grill him on the different causes of blurred disc margins. The diagnosis was apparently hypermetropia. (Pass)

173. A candidate was asked to examine the fundi of a patient who was diabetic. She explained that she could not see with her left eye and could only undertake ophthalmoscopy with her right eye. The examiners responded: 'As long as you are competent, we do not care how you do it'. (Pass)

174. A candidate was asked to examine the precordium of a 55-year-old female patient. He found atrial fibrillation and mitral stenosis and a long discussion followed about 'How do you know it's atrial fibrillation?'. He forgot to mention the variable first heart sound. He reports that he made a big blunder when he said that the tapping apex was caused by a big left atrium. Thirty seconds later, he said: 'Sir, I was wrong earlier. The tapping apex is not caused by a big left atrium'. The examiner looked relieved and went on to ask where the candidate would feel for a big left atrium.* Luckily, the bell went at that moment and the candidate was not required to answer. (Pass)

175. A candidate at his fourth attempt was so nervous as he went into the viva that when the examiner asked the first question, though it was easy, he found he could not speak. After a pause, both examiners started writing on their pads which further increased the tension in the atmosphere. Eventually the candidate found his voice and gave a faultless performance for the rest of the viva. At the end, he was still very concerned that the exam was overshadowed by a bad start so before he left he apologized for it, saying that it was because he was so nervous. The examiners smiled and said that it was very understandable in a way which made him feel that his bad start had not had much effect on their overall judgement. He was glad he brought this up and obtained their reassurance because otherwise he feels he might still have been worrying about the viva when he went into the long and short cases. (Pass)

'Even though I didn't mean to say it – I did; I opened my mouth and all this rubbish came out'

176. A candidate, nervous on his first attempt, was asked to palpate the abdomen. He found bilateral masses in the upper quadrants but states that he was interrupted before he could examine them properly. He thought they were polycystic kidneys but in the stress of the moment he found himself saying hepatosplenomegaly before he could stop himself! (Fail)

177. A candidate was asked to examine a woman's abdomen. She found a deeply jaundiced woman with cachexia and a hard, craggy liver. She did not detect ascites nor, convincingly, a spleen. However, when asked to give her findings, she found herself saying 'and she has a 2 cm spleen'. She reports that she heard herself lying but was unable to stop herself. The examiner was

not convinced either and the candidate then started talking about 'a difficult to define mass in the left hypochondrium which could be splenic'. She said the examiner seemed happier with this but did not ask how to differentiate left hypochondrial masses. (Fail)

178. A candidate was asked to examine the cardiovascular system. He reports that he was stopped after examining the precordium before feeling the carotids and that although the signs had fitted with aortic stenosis, he was unsure whether the murmur was classically crescendo–decrescendo and he found himself giving the diagnosis of ventricular septal defect. The examiners made it obvious that they disagreed with this diagnosis. (Pass)

179. A candidate was asked to examine the fundi of a 19-year-old asymptomatic girl. On looking at the right fundus, she could not see the disc but the vessels and background were normal. She assumes now that there must have been papilloedema but it was the first case. She was in a complete panic and found herself saying that she did not know the diagnosis. She was told that she must know the diagnosis and then said: 'hypertension'. The examiners walked out without comment. (Pass)

180. A candidate was told that a female patient was breathless and he was asked to examine her abdomen and to explain her breathlessness. He found massive hepatosplenomegaly plus anaemia but instead of coming out with myelosclerosis as the diagnosis, he said sarcoidosis! At this stage the examiners, who had been very pleasant until then, began to look impatient! (Fail)

181. 'Examine the heart.' Having done so, it would have been easy to start by saying, 'This chap, who is comfortable at rest with a mid-line sternotomy scar, has mitral regurgitation'. However, my mouth went into action before my brain and a load of verbal diarrhoea came out. The diagnosis was correct but the delivery was awful. (Fail)

Invigilators' diaries

182. A candidate was asked to examine the legs of a patient. He was allowed to carry out a large proportion of a full neurological examination before he became aware, with prodding from the examiner, of the large skull, hearing aid and the bowed tibiae of Paget's disease. The examiner commented that if he had looked

*First heart sound is palpable; left atrium is not palpable.

at the patient first he might have saved himself the time wasted on the unnecessary neurological examination. (This would not happen now as this patient would be in Station 5 for a spot diagnosis.)

183. A candidate was asked to examine the eyes of a patient. He had examined the eye movements before he noticed the obvious blue sclerae of osteogenesis imperfecta. The examiner was irritated by this and commented that the candidate had wasted several minutes of the examiner's time by not looking at the eyes properly and noticing an obvious physical sign.

184. A candidate was asked to examine the fundi of a patient with diabetic retinopathy and laser photocoagulation scars. It was the end of the afternoon and the tropicamide drops, which had been put in that morning to dilate the pupil, had worn off. The candidate said she could see nothing and asked to take the patient into a darkened room. A side room was found but it was only semi-dark. She still said she could see nothing. The examiner was very unimpressed that she had missed what he considered to be a very easy case of diabetic retinopathy. When the invigilator tried to help save the candidate by apologizing that the drops had worn off, the examiner retorted that 'the pupils would not be dilated in the casualty department'.

185. A patient in the examination had a 'full house' of mixed mitral and aortic valve disease. The examiner commented that candidates kept failing to hear all the murmurs. He suspected that having heard one or two loud ones, candidates stopped listening for the others which were less obvious.

186. A candidate was asked to look at a lady's hands. He described Heberden's nodes, spindling of the fingers and proximal joint swelling, all of which the patient had. He suggested combined osteoarthrosis and rheumatoid arthritis. When the examiner asked about conditions associated with rheumatoid arthritis, the candidate looked beyond the hands and noticed the generalized pigmentation and then the palmar crease pigmentation of Addison's disease. The latter condition was the reason for the patient's inclusion in the examination – the joint changes had not been noted before!

187. A patient known to have Behçet's disease was included as a fundus case with optic atrophy. On fundoscopy, he had optic atrophy, choroidoretinitis and also sheathing of the vessel walls. All the examiners agreed that they had not seen a fundus like it before and that it was a 'museum' case. The underlying cause was not discussed with any of the candidates, who were only expected to see what was there and describe it accurately. Calling the vessel sheathing 'silver wiring', as one candidate did, was considered unacceptable.

188. A candidate was asked to examine the heart of a patient with mitral valve prolapse. Unfortunately, the backrest collapsed while he was examining and could not be repaired so the patient could only be examined lying flat or sitting upright. Although the examiners accepted that this was off-putting, they did not feel that it justified missing all the signs and getting systole and diastole the wrong way round!

189. An MRCP examiner was heard telling a group of students that many candidates fail to recognize atrial fibrillation. Furthermore, in his experience, about 20% of candidates cannot accurately demonstrate the second left intercostal space. He had also noticed that candidates were often poor in their technique of examining ankle jerks.

190. A candidate was asked to examine the fundi of a patient with diabetic retinopathy and obvious laser scars. She diagnosed diabetic retinopathy but when asked if she had seen any microaneurysms or photocoagulation scars, she was not sure.

191. A candidate was shown a euthyroid diabetic patient with necrobiosis lipoidica diabeticorum and he had been given some of the patient's symptoms which were vaguely suggestive of hyperthyroidism. He was then asked to assess the girl's thyroid status. Despite the normal pulse rate and lack of other supportive signs, the candidate apparently managed to diagnose hyperthyroidism!

192. An examiner was watching a candidate feeling for the apex beat of a female patient. The rough handling of the patient's breast irritated the examiner who later commented: 'That sort of behaviour brings a candidate immediately to the pass/fail borderline'.

193. After observing some candidates examining a patient with rheumatoid hands, a 'fly on the wall' advised: 'Don't give too much prominence to the possibility of psoriatic arthropathy in an obvious case of rheumatoid. If you are considering psoriatic arthropathy then look particularly for nail changes. If there are boutonnière and swan neck deformities, say so rather than spending ages describing what's happening at each metacarpophalangeal and interphalangeal joint'.

194. A flustered and overanxious candidate marked himself out by spending an inordinate amount of time fixing the patient's blanket and putting the patient's pyjamas back on rather than following the examiners to the next case – they had to come back for him twice. 'Oh heck!' he remarked at their second return for him. On another occasion he was still shaking hands with the last patient when the examiners were trying to get him to start on the next! After forgetting to listen to the neck in a patient with a systolic murmur in the aortic area, he elected to draw the examiner's attention to this without prompting: 'I'm sorry, I didn't listen to the neck!'. He was generally slow and took ages describing, hesitantly, peripheral and unimportant things, digging holes when it would have been better to come out immediately and say confidently: 'I think this patient has aortic stenosis'. On the rheumatoid hands case he spent ages trying to describe what was happening at each metacarpophalangeal and interphalangeal joint, struggling in his panic to find the right words when it would have been better to get straight to the diagnosis with just a few key extras such as 'boutonnière', 'swan neck', 'ulnar deviation', etc. The examiner commented: 'He looked as though he was going to fall apart at any moment; he didn't seem to be used to examining people; I wonder if he is in public health!'. It was estimated that during the 30 min he had said 'sir' about 84 times!

195. A candidate was taken to see a patient with one leg that was slightly shorter and wasted compared to the other. The candidate did not think of polio and the examiner had to admit that: 'A lot of young people won't have seen it'.

196. A candidate was asked to examine the hands of a patient with gross, generalized wasting and frontal baldness. The candidate carried out a long, detailed examination of the hands before reaching the diagnosis (myotonic dystrophy) after finally being prompted to shake hands with the patient.

197. A candidate on her first case had a patient with lymphoma presenting with a right iliac fossa mass, splenomegaly and generalized lymphadenopathy. The candidate missed the spleen, got bogged down in standard lists of causes of a right iliac fossa mass, including irrelevant ones such as an appendix abscess!

198. Before one examination session all the examiners gathered around a patient to be shown his signs, which were said to include splenomegaly. Two or three of the examiners felt the abdomen and agreed that they could not feel the spleen. After these had moved on, another of the examiners examined the abdomen and called the invigilator over, saying: 'Put your hand here, like this – the spleen is palpable – can you feel it?'.

Fly on the wall – complete accounts

In the same way that later in this section we have some complete first-hand accounts of candidates' experiences during the short cases, the following are two fuller accounts from one sitting, followed by two more detailed accounts from the same morning of another sitting – these are the notes of a 'fly on the wall'.

The second examiner chipped in: 'Can you have an opening snap in the presence of atrial fibrillation?'. The candidate looked nonplussed, hesitated and could not come up with an answer.

199. The first patient had hepatosplenomegaly and polycythaemia. He had a red face that was not noticed, or mentioned, by the candidate. Asked to look at the abdomen from the end of the bed while the patient breathed, the candidate did not notice the liver moving up and down. The fact that the liver was palpable was dragged out of her slowly. The examiner asked the candidate to mark the position of the spleen on the skin with a finger so that the size of the spleen could be verified.

For the next case, the examiner said: 'Check the pulse, jugular venous pressure and precordium'. The candidate proceeded to irritate him by examining the fingernails. The patient had loud mitral stenosis. The examiner instructed: 'Give me your diagnosis or findings – whichever you choose'. The candidate said mitral stenosis. Examiner: 'Why mitral stenosis, was there an opening snap?'. The candidate was unsure, asked to listen again and then said that there was an opening snap. The examiner asked: 'What is an opening snap, what causes it?'. As they were leaving the patient the second examiner chipped in: 'Can you have an opening snap in the presence of atrial fibrillation?'. The candidate looked nonplussed, hesitated and did not come up with an answer. The examiner said afterwards he thought this was a very relevant question which the candidate ought to have been able to answer.

The next patient had hereditary haemorrhagic telangiectasia and congenital nystagmus. The candidate moved hesitantly to the first diagnosis. She was asked why there was a scar on the left side of the chest. The candidate suggested an arteriovenous fistula. The examiner asked if there was a better, more commonly used term. The candidate was very slow to answer 'arteriovenous shunt and arteriovenous malformations'. She was slow to get congenital nystagmus as the cause of the nystagmus and was asked how she could tell it was congenital and not brought about by any other cause. She did not really know, but the fact that it was present in all directions was dragged out of her. The examiner (a neurologist) explained that the nystagmus was coarse, in the same plane as the eye movement, of variable frequency, with the fast phase sometimes in one direction and sometimes in another! She was asked if she knew of another condition that went with congenital nystagmus and she did not. The examiner explained that there were little nodding movements of the head that the patient sometimes exhibited which are called 'spasmus nutans'!

The next patient had psoriasis of the soles of the feet which the candidate got and also gave the differential diagnosis, when asked, of keratoderma blenorrhagica in association with Reiter's syndrome.

The next patient had rheumatoid hands with swan neck and boutonnière deformities. The candidate was asked about the cause of the swan neck deformity and she started talking about the small muscles of the hand. The examiner said: 'I wouldn't have said that but as you mention it, what small muscles of the hand?'. The candidate was very hesitant and eventually said: 'flexor digito . . . '. 'You are talking rubbish,' said the examiner, 'it is the interossei and lumbricals'. As the examiner moved on to the next case, the candidate said that there were also boutonnière deformities.

The examiner was about to ask the candidate to look into the eyes of the next patient when he stopped, reached in his pocket and pulled out an instrument and asked the candidate what the instrument was. She did not know it was a two-point sensation discriminator. 'Can be very useful in testing sensation,' said the examiner. The candidate's next case was diabetic retinopathy which she got right, including the fact that there were hard exudates near the macula.

In view of the previous, fairly disastrous, abdomen, the candidate was taken to look at the abdomen of another patient, who had hepatosplenomegaly; she got it this time and, when asked the cause, suggested 'a myeloproliferative disease' which was correct. She was asked to draw the edge of the spleen again. (Bare fail)

Other candidates in the same sitting had diagnosed the old choroiditis and not called it papilloedema; had diagnosed the retinopathy and not called it optic atrophy; had identified the palpable kidney and marked the correct size of the spleen, etc.

200. The first case was hepatosplenomegaly with the right kidney easily palpable. The candidate started off with: 'I would like to examine the patient from nipples to knees'. He was asked to concentrate on the abdomen. He said that he had found hepatosplenomegaly. He was asked to show the edge of the spleen and said it was 6 cm and marked it as such, when in fact it was just a palpable spleen tip. It was interesting to note that when he had actually been examining the spleen, one could see where he was feeling and he must have felt just the spleen tip with the patient turned on the right side, yet he went on to describe it as 6 cm enlarged. He did not mention the bimanually ballottable right kidney which presumably he thought was the liver.

After this bad start he did reasonably well on the patient with mitral stenosis. He was asked to examine the pulse, the jugular venous pressure (JVP) and the precordium. After feeling the pulse, looking at the JVP and palpating the precordium, the examiner stopped him and asked his findings. He gave them as those of mitral stenosis and said he expected to hear the auscultatory findings which he subsequently did. However, he got into a mess when asked to describe the venous pressure and said that it was a single wave and when asked about the relevance of this, started talking about atrial fibrillation and mitral stenosis. He said: 'cv waves'. The examiner raised his eyebrows at this. The candidate did not mention tricuspid incompetence which was the cause of the pulsations in the neck. The examiner then asked if there was anything else he had noticed about the patient (this was not on the official documentation about the patient but the examiner was an endocrinologist) and after a struggle the candidate said that there was a chest deformity and after a further struggle he mentioned kyphosis. There was more delay and struggling and then the examiner showed him the patient's axillae which had no hair. The candidate suggested that maybe the patient shaved and she said that she had not had hair for many years. The examiner asked if the candidate could tie up the absent axillary hair with the chest and spinal deformities and the candidate was unable to do so. It turned out that the patient had had an early menopause and had been oestrogen deficient for many years.

The next case was a patient with a fundus with a patch of old choroiditis superior and just temporal to the macula. The candidate diagnosed papilloedema.

The next patient had polyarteritis and bilateral carpal tunnel syndrome. The candidate diagnosed rheumatoid arthritis and bilateral carpal tunnel syndrome. The examiner said: 'If she had a patch of numbness on her right leg here (pointing below the knee), what would you say?'. The candidate answered: 'mononeuritis multiplex'. This was accepted by the examiner.

The next case involved examining the visual fields in a patient with widespread cerebrovascular disease who presumably had a right homonymous hemianopia. The candidate found a defective temporal field in the right eye but also a defective nasal field and said that both nasal and temporal fields were diminished. The candidate was asked, without comment, to go on and examine the legs and he said that he had found 'pyramidal weakness of the right leg'. He was asked what this meant and responded 'weakness of flexion at the hip, the knee and dorsiflexion at the foot'. This was accepted. He also said that he felt the reflexes were brisk bilaterally. The examiner (?a neurologist) asked what other reflexes could be tested – in cases of doubt about the briskness of reflexes ('How can you tell if reflexes are brisk if they are bilaterally brisk?'). The candidate said, and tested, the adductor reflexes.* The examiner asked what it is that causes the brisk reflex. The candidate struggled and was unable to describe the reflex arc. He was then asked what causes increased tone and started talking about muscles being perpetually in contraction, and was then asked if he meant that the muscles are contracting all the time, to which he replied: 'no'. He was asked why there could be discordance between tone and jerks.

The last patient had grade III hypertensive retinopathy. The candidate said there was no retinopathy but that the discs were pale. (Fail)

The candidate was asked to demonstrate with his finger exactly where the spleen and liver edges were.

201. His cardiology case was a youngish woman with mixed aortic valve disease and mixed mitral valve disease, although the mitral incompetence was debatable. He diagnosed mixed aortic valve disease but did not notice the mid-diastolic murmur, although the examiner did not seem perturbed by this. The candidate, when asked about whether the pulse was collapsing or not, said that it was not. The examiner then asked him for the peripheral signs of aortic incompetence and the discussion moved to the nail-fold sign. The candidate was asked what this was called and he said: 'Quincke's sign' and he was asked to see if the patient had this. The candidate thought he had and the examiner answered: 'I thought so too'.

The respiratory case was a patient with bronchiectasis and the candidate was asked to examine the chest. He examined first from the front and he was about to move to the back when the examiner said: 'Time is at a premium, could you discuss your findings so far?'. During the examination the patient had given a rattly cough on several occasions. The candidate thought that the diagnosis was bronchiectasis but then went on to say that he thought the patient looked cushingoid and wondered if he was on steroids for obstructive airways disease (he was not on steroids). The causes of bronchiectasis were asked for.

The candidate was then requested to look at a patient with Parkinson's disease and he spotted the diagnosis correctly and said he would like to examine the gait; he was allowed to do this. The only parkinsonian feature in the gait was that one arm swung less than the other and he exhibited a slight tremor. When the candidate said this, the examiner asked what features he might have had. In the ensuing discussion the candidate was asked what 'festinant'† meant. He said he did not know. The examiner told him that it meant 'dancing' and asked him why he thought this word should be used to describe the parkinsonian gait.

The next case was a patient with diabetic fundi, multiple laser burns and debatable new vessels on the disc. The candidate, during the discussions, said that the discs were normal and when pressed on this stuck to his decision that they were normal.

The next case was a patient with CREST syndrome and he was asked: 'What is your spot diagnosis?'. The candidate immediately answered: 'tophaceous gout'. When the examiner was obviously unhappy about this, the candidate explained that he was sorry that he had rushed to that diagnosis. The examiner told him that he should never rush to a diagnosis. The candidate

---

*Probably the examiners were expecting him to say abdominal reflexes and clonus.

†Festinant comes from the Latin verb *festinare* meaning 'to hurry'.

then discussed systemic sclerosis and CREST syndrome and a discussion took place about difficulties with swallowing.

The next patient had neurofibromatosis and the candidate was asked to: 'Look at the hands and tell me what you see – spot diagnosis'. The candidate got the diagnosis at once.

The next patient had hereditary haemorrhagic telangiectasia and the candidate got this diagnosis at once. He was then asked if the patient had anything else and he answered to the effect that the patient had gross nystagmus. On being pressed on this, he said that there was also a squint and when being pressed further for a diagnosis, he suggested that the patient had congenital nystagmus (which was correct).

The next patient had had a cerebrovascular accident, with cerebellar signs and a carotid bruit. The examiner told the candidate that the patient had difficulty with walking and asked him to perform a neurological examination of the legs. The candidate started off with observation and after a brief pause the examiner asked him to 'move on if you want to finish on time'. He examined power and reflexes and found the reflexes diminished at the right knee compared to the left, so he started discussing an L3/4 root lesion as the cause. The examiner told him to leave sensation and what else would he like to examine. The candidate did not come up with a suggestion. Eventually, the examiner suggested that he should check coordination in the legs and the candidate was then led to examine for cerebellar signs in the arms. Cerebellar signs were found on the right. When asked about the possible diagnosis, the candidate suggested cerebellar syndrome and a lower motor neurone lesion at L3/4. The examiner suggested that this was a bizarre collection of physical signs and asked the candidate to listen to the patient's neck. A right carotid bruit was found. The candidate then offered 'cerebellar infarction' as the cause, to which the examiner said: 'What about a middle cerebral artery stroke?'. In the ensuing discussion the examiner said: 'Do you disagree with me? You can, if you want to, you know'.

The next patient had hepatosplenomegaly and the candidate started his presentation by saying that the patient was pigmented. The examiner said: 'Do you really think he is pigmented? Actually, he's tanned; he's just been to Cyprus for his holiday'. The candidate was asked to demonstrate with his finger exactly where the spleen and liver edges were. In the discussion about the cause, myeloproliferative disease was first suggested, to which the examiner responded by saying that the

patient had had the spleen for 30 years. The candidate then suggested an 'ethnic anaemia' and a discussion took place about why it was not thalassaemia minor or thalassaemia major, and when the candidate suggested sickle cell disease the examiner said to him: 'You didn't mean that, did you?'. After the bell went he told the candidate that it was haemoglobin H disease but that the candidate need not worry because he was on the right lines. (Pass)

She got the patient to open his mouth and put his tongue out. The inside and outside of his mouth were covered with telangiectasiae – how did she not see them?

202. The first short case had systemic sclerosis which at first (on examining the hands) she called psoriasis, and then dermatomyositis, before coming to the right diagnosis.

The next patient had hepatosplenomegaly and she got it right without problems.

The next case was hereditary haemorrhagic telangiectasia and she was asked to examine the back. She found a thoracotomy scar and evidence of a lobectomy (presumably from removal of an arteriovenous shunt). Then, in a discussion which led to the fact that 'some lung had been removed', she was asked to discuss the possible reasons. (She was told the operation had been many years previously.) She suggested tuberculosis and this possible cause was accepted. 'Anything else?' She suggested there might be rheumatoid changes in the hands and this was accepted. 'Why would this lead to a thoracotomy?' The candidate started discussing pulmonary fibrosis before she realized that this would not lead to a thoracotomy. The examiner asked if she thought the patient was cyanosed. She got the patient to open his mouth and put his tongue out. The inside and outside of his mouth was covered with telangiectasiae – how did she not see them? She said she did not think there was cyanosis. Did she know why the patient might have had a thoracotomy? 'No.'

The next patient, she was told, was unsteady on the feet and she was asked to examine the arms. The patient had cerebellar signs following a cerebrovascular accident. She initially started discussing Parkinson's disease and cog-wheeling and then retracted this. She was asked to examine the eyes for nystagmus and soon after she began she was asked: 'Has she got it?', to which the candidate immediately answered: 'yes'. 'Tell us about the nystagmus.' She was asked to examine speech and eventually got the patient to have difficulty saying, 'West Register Street'.

She was asked for a spot diagnosis on a patient with neurofibromatosis and she got this. She was asked for a spot diagnosis on a patient with exophthalmos and got this too. When asked where else to look, she eventually said the shins for pretibial myxoedema which the patient had (debatably).

The next patient had a small to moderate multinodular goitre which the candidate said was a big goitre; initially that it was diffuse, although she later said it was nodular. The next patient had mixed aortic valve disease and mixed mitral valve disease. The candidate confidently diagnosed aortic stenosis but nothing else.

The next patient had diabetic retinopathy with laser burns and the candidate got this. The next patient had Parkinson's disease which she got. A discussion then took place on the causes of Parkinson's disease and when she ground to a halt after giving several possibilities, she was asked for any others. 'Have you heard of the expression "mad as a hatter"?'*

The next case was coarctation of the aorta. The examiner said that he wanted to put her in the area of the circulatory system but not to do a full examination of the heart because she had already done this. He led her to listen to the precordium and she heard something of a systolic murmur but the bell went before discussion could take place. She mentioned 'patent ductus' as she left the room. (Fail)

Ungentlemanly clinical methods

203. A candidate was asked to examine a patient's respiratory system. He found clubbing and basal crackles and diagnosed bronchiectasis. He confessed that he was helped along with this diagnosis as he could see it on the examiner's clipboard!

204. A candidate was asked to examine the fundi. The examiners were several yards away so as he was examining, he quietly asked the patient if he was a diabetic, to which the patient answered, 'Yes'. The candidate diagnosed proliferative diabetic retinopathy

---

*Chronic mercury poisoning (persistent involuntary movements, fatigue, insomnia, neuropathy, etc.) was probably the examiner's bee in the bonnet! Mercury was used by hat makers and chronic exposure caused poisoning with widespread manifestation in some of them. Although mercury is mentioned among the toxic causes of parkinsonism, most neurologists admit that they have never seen a *bona fide* case of parkinsonism attributable to mercury.

with photocoagulation scars in one eye and a vitreous haemorrhage in the other. He was asked why it was difficult to see one of the fundi well and replied that it was because of the vitreous haemorrhage. (Pass)

205. A candidate reports: 'I was asked to "look at this lady's right eye". I saw a cataract, retinopathy and laser scars. I said "diabetic retinopathy" – which was what I saw printed on the examiner's sheet!' (Pass)

206. A candidate reports: 'My last short case really made my day. Having arrived at the examination ward with little time to spare, I happened to meet an elderly woman going in the same direction who obviously was not a candidate and too polite to be an examiner! She asked if we were going to the same place and volunteered that she always came up for the examinations. She told me that they always looked at her eyes and shins, and then at her neck, volunteering that she had no scar but had "drunk iodine"! Sure enough, I was led to this same woman who smiled when I was told to examine her legs which showed pretibial myxoedema. I went on to demonstrate the exophthalmos with lid lag, a multinodular goitre and no scar!'. (Pass)

Miscellaneous 'pass' experiences

'The examiner said: "First class". This was the nicest remark made to me in the last 2 years!'

207. 'Would you examine these hands? This chap has a weakness in his hands.' He had obvious bilateral *ulnar nerve palsy* and I was asked for the causes.

'Examine this patient's abdomen. He came in with anaemia.' There was obvious hepatosplenomegaly and I was asked for a differential diagnosis. I included *myelofibrosis* and was asked why it could be this condition. I said because of the large size of the spleen.

'Examine this patient's fundus.' There were haemorrhages and exudates with arteriovenous nipping. I suggested diabetic eye disease but the examiner then said: 'What if I tell you that the other eye is normal?'. I then suggested a *retinal branch vein occlusion* to which the examiner said: 'First class'. This was the nicest remark made to me in the last 2 years!

'Listen to this lady's heart.' Before I went any further I checked to see if I was allowed to palpate, etc. 'No,' said the examiner, 'auscultate only'. I found a *mitral diastolic murmur* with an opening snap and ?presystolic accentuation. The examiner asked if the patient was in sinus rhythm.* I said I could not tell just by auscultating, but he went on: 'What do you think?'.

'This lady has a rash on her thighs'. It looked like purpura but then they showed me her shins. There was no lesion visible here. 'Does this put you off a diagnosis of purpura?' 'Yes,' I said. 'Quite right,' said the examiner. 'What if I told you she had pains in her joints and trouble with her kidneys?' I suggested polyarteritis nodosa. 'No,' said the examiner, 'but don't worry. I have only seen it once before!' (Apparently it was *Fabry's disease*.)

The next patient was in a side room which gave me a clue. I was told, 'This young man has lost weight and noticed these lesions on his chest. What are they?'. They were definitely *Kaposi's sarcomas*. I was then asked the mechanism of diarrhoea in *AIDS*. (Pass – sixth and final attempt)

'On leaving the room the patient commented loudly on what a nice young man I was and how I had said it all so nicely!'

208. I was asked to look at the fundi of an elderly lady with widely dilated pupils. I tested her pupil reactions to light but not to accommodation and elicited a light reflex. I then examined the right fundus. It was obviously *background diabetic retinopathy* and after approximately 20 sec I looked up and asked if they wanted me to specifically look into the left fundus. He said: 'Not if you are ready to present your findings'. I did present the findings, gave the diagnosis and emphasized that there were no proliferative or hypertensive changes or laser burns.

I was taken to a young woman with a mitral valvotomy scar, atrial fibrillation and the murmurs of *mixed mitral valve disease*. She was not short of breath or cyanosed. I presented the findings and continued to give my reasons why I believed the stenotic component was predominant. I was asked if the murmurs were haemodynamically significant. I replied that they were not and again gave my reasons.† The examiners and the patient all appeared pleased. In fact, on leaving the room the patient commented loudly on what a nice young man I was and how I had said it all so nicely!

I next saw a patient with obvious severe *rheumatoid arthritis* and evidence of previous joint replacements. I was asked to describe what I saw and then to look for additional evidence of rheumatoid arthritis, i.e. nodules. There were none present so they asked me where else they might be found. I replied: 'I would look on a chest X-ray'.

The next patient had pronounced *exophthalmos* and the examiner began by asking me to describe what I could see, saying: 'You can be as rude as you like about Mr L', to which the patient laughed. I demonstrated the examination of exophthalmos and lid lag and said that I could feel a goitre (which I think was present although not large). The examiner did not appear completely convinced but acceded to my observation. I was asked to assess the thyroid state clinically. He was *euthyroid* and I gave my reasons for this.

I was then taken to a patient who was in bed with a cervical collar on. I was asked to examine his legs neurologically because 'he has difficulty in walking'. He had a smaller, wasted, areflexic left leg suggestive of *old polio* and a very brisk set of reflexes in the right leg. I suggested that he had old polio of the left leg with superimposed *cervical myelopathy* affecting the right leg.

I was then asked to examine the back of a man's chest. There was dullness to percussion and reduced chest wall movement on the right side, but the air entry‡ was not diminished greatly in comparison to the left side. I gave a tentative diagnosis of a right *pleural effusion* but added why I was uncertain. I was then asked to examine his abdomen 'because my houseman informs me that he has *hepatomegaly*'. The liver margin was in fact easily palpable. However, on percussion it appeared low lying and I therefore suggested this and the examiner appeared to agree.

For my last case I was asked to palpate the precordium only. There was a systolic apical thrill. I was asked to give a differential diagnosis but at this point my concentration was somewhat flagging and I could only mention mitral regurgitation and forgot *ventricular septal defect*. He asked again if there was anything else of note on palpation! I had nearly missed his bilateral *gynaecomastia*. I was asked what drugs might be the cause in this particular case. I gave a reasonable list but

---

*The question was prompted by the candidate's mention of presystolic accentuation, which would not occur if the rhythm had been atrial fibrillation. The examiner was exploring whether the candidate threw in 'presystolic accentuation' without realizing its significance.
†The question of predominance of either lesion should not arise if the murmurs are not haemodynamically significant.

‡'Air entry' is not a good expression. It is better to use the terms 'breath sounds present/absent/diminished'. Breath sounds are not caused by the air entering into that part of the lung where they are heard, but rather generated in the major bronchi and conducted to the periphery.

could not think of spironolactone. He repeated the question but somehow mixed up his words and actually said: 'What are the spiros . . . '. I began to laugh as did both the patient and the other examiner who had been observing at this point. As the bell had now sounded they said that they would let me go. I thanked them and shook hands – phew! (Pass)

'I was then taken to see a gentleman who had a white stick and the examiner said: "This man is almost blind, please examine his eyes".'

209. 'This lady came in to have her varicose veins done and something else was noted incidentally. Please examine her abdomen and tell us what you find that is abnormal.' On examination, there was gross, visible splenomegaly with mild anaemia. I was asked the causes of massive splenomegaly and the definition of splenomegaly. She had *myelofibrosis*.

'This man has a cough and fever. Examine the respiratory system.' He was an Asian gentleman who was dyspnoeic at rest and had clubbing of the fingers. He had superb signs. There was dullness to percussion with increased breath sounds (bronchial breathing) and there was increased vocal resonance at the left apex. I was asked for a differential diagnosis and, because he was Asian, I said tuberculosis and, because he was a smoker as detected by the discoloration of his nails, I also suggested carcinoma of the lung. The examiner told me that he did not like my technique for testing for tracheal deviation (thumb to each side separately) and he showed me his way of doing it and asked me to try it. I had to admit that the trachea probably was deviated to the left. There was then a long dissertation from the examiner regarding the physical findings in the left upper lobe, i.e. collapse versus consolidation, and I was not really asked to contribute at all to this conversation!

I was then taken to see a gentleman who had a white stick and the examiner said: 'This man is almost blind, please examine his eyes'. I found no cataracts or corneal problems but there was gross choroidoretinitis. I desperately tried to find evidence of diabetic retinopathy to make this into laser therapy but I could not. Therefore, I thought it could be retinitis pigmentosa although I had never seen it before. I said this honestly to the examiners who agreed that the treatment of diabetic eye disease would be the most common cause of this type of thing but that (a) it was a bit different, and (b) this is the MRCP exam! It was in fact *retinitis pigmentosa*. I wondered if it could have been *Refsum's syn-*drome as the Whittington Hospital does have a patient with this.

My last patient was a lady and the examiner said: 'Tell me about her hands'. I had to be very quick as the bell had gone but she had gross *nodular rheumatoid*. I described the features as I was examining and I was also expected to perform a functional assessment. The examiners at the end said: 'Very good' and let me go. (Pass)

'I know this patient well, sir, this is Mrs L. and I biopsied her liver last year!'

210. I was asked to examine the precordium. She had *mitral stenosis* and atrial fibrillation. I was criticized for not actually counting the apical rate and only giving a 'guesstimate' of 130/min. I was then asked about the complications of mitral stenosis.

'This girl was admitted with an acute asthmatic attack. Can you find a cause for it?' After some prompting, I noticed a slight excoriation on the flexor creases and this was the only physical sign. I thought it was probably *atopic eczema*. The examiners then asked me what I would tell the girl's mother about her prognosis.

'Look at this patient's skin'. There were *café-au-lait* spots on the forearms and *neurofibromas* on the abdomen.

'Examine this patient's legs.' I recognized this patient so I said: 'This is Mrs G. and she has *Charcot–Marie–Tooth disease*!' 'Examine this patient's abdomen.' 'I know this lady as well, sir. This is Mrs L. and I biopsied her liver last year!' The examiner said: 'Have you worked in this hospital before?' and I replied: 'Well, er, yes!'. 'Palpate this patient's chest. No, feel again, there!' There was aortic stenosis with a systolic thrill which I missed initially. I was asked for further investigations so I mentioned echo and Doppler followed by cardiac catheterization.

'Look at this man's face.' He had definite facial flushing and we then discussed the features of the *carcinoid syndrome* and its treatment. The patient had had hepatic artery embolization.

I had been allocated to a hospital in which I had worked the previous year. My consultants advised me not to change as the examiners would not be prejudiced and I would not be at any disadvantage. However, I recognized two of the patients and I admitted to this. Although I was given credit for honesty it meant I missed out on the examination of two very good cases. The examiners told me afterwards that they had sat on the fence for the clinical but that I had passed comfortably in the other sections.

I would advise any candidates finding themselves in a similar position to inform the College and to ask for a reallocation. Events such as this might easily upset one's whole performance. (Pass)

'Just because you are cool, it doesn't mean that you know the answers. But perhaps it helps convince the examiners that you do!'

211. *Gross acromegaly.* 'Examine this lady's hands. What do you notice?' The diagnosis was easy. He asked me to enumerate the features found in the hand in an acromegalic patient. 'And what else do you notice?' I listed all the facial features. 'What would you find in the other systems?' Again I gave a nice list. 'What are the treatments for this condition?' This was the perfect start to the short cases. I felt the examiners had warmed to me and it was all quite easy from here on.

Ventricular septal defect. 'Listen to this boy's heart.' He looked like a healthy teenager. Inspection of the apex was normal and his pulses were normal; however, palpation revealed a systolic thrill and on auscultation he had a systolic murmur only. I listened to his back. 'Why did you do that?' 'Because if he has a patent ductus the murmur would be loudest at the back.' (The real reason was that I am terrible at interpreting murmurs and it gave me an extra few seconds to think.) Afterwards the examiner went back to listen.

Choroiditis. 'Look in this woman's eye. What do you see?' As I started to inspect her eye he said, 'No, just look at the fundus'. To begin with I could see nothing wrong but just as I turned to look away she changed her direction of gaze and I saw the grossly abnormal lesion. The moral must be to look everywhere in the retina.

Clubbing of the fingers. This was easy. I was allowed to ask some questions so I enquired how long the lady had had fingers like this. She was healthy and the answer was familial clubbing. I was then asked to recite the causes of clubbing.

Classical dermatomyositis. I had never seen this except in photographs and I almost missed it. She looked 'autoimmune' with white hair, pale skin and purplish eyelids and knuckles. I pointed this out but could not give a diagnosis. I was then asked to examine her arms where she had a small, healing, surgical scar over the triceps. Once I had 'clicked' that this was a muscle biopsy the diagnosis was easy. By now I was thoroughly enjoying myself and I turned to one of the

examiners and said, 'I almost missed that'. 'Yes,' he said, 'but you didn't!'

Paget's disease. This was bizarre. It was a lady of about 70 years whose radius and ulna of the right forearm were bent at 90°. I asked her if she had broken the arm and had a poor result from healing but the answer was no. I knew that there is a congenital cause of forearm deformity (Madelung's deformity?*) but this was not it so that left Paget's which I was told was the correct diagnosis.

IIIrd nerve palsy. It was a complete IIIrd nerve palsy. The examiner asked me to give the likely cause and the visible craniotomy scar gave me the answer.

Malignant melanoma with metastases. I was asked to examine this man's abdomen. He was deeply jaundiced and had a big, knobbly liver. I was then asked to describe the surface anatomy of the normal liver because his extended across to the left subcostal area and at first I thought he also had splenomegaly. However, the examiner demonstrated to our mutual satisfaction that he had hepatomegaly only. 'Now look in his eyes.' One was in the light and one was in shade so I looked at the one in the light. 'He is deeply jaundiced,' I said. I was then asked why and instructed to look in both eyes. One had a white sclera! On asking the patient how long he had had his glass eye, he said about 10 years and that he had had a tumour at the back of the eye! At this point the examiners did not ask me the diagnosis but simply thanked me and wished me good luck in the rest of the test. (Pass)

Afterwards the attending registrar said to me that I looked remarkably relaxed and cool under fire. I replied: 'Just because you're cool it doesn't mean that you know the answers'. But perhaps it helps convince the examiners that you do!

'The first thing I noticed was a puncture mark over the right lower chest suggesting a recent pleural aspiration.'

212. My first patient was introduced to me as a lady who was short of breath and would I do a cardiovascular examination to find out why. Just as I was about to listen to the lung fields at the end of my cardiovascular 'routine' I was stopped. My examiner asked if I had finished. I said: 'Yes'. And then I realized that I had not listened for an aortic diastolic murmur, but the examiner kindly allowed me to go back to do this. I was then

*In Madelung's deformity the arm is bent over the radial side as a result of the developmental overgrowth of the ulna.

asked for the diagnosis and I offered *mixed mitral valve disease* with a previous valvotomy. I was then asked which valve lesion was dominant. I plumped for stenosis by virtue of the loud first heart sound and was then pushed as to whether I wanted to change my mind. I did not so we passed on to the next case.

This was a lady whose neck I was asked to examine. It was obvious that she had a *goitre* but I tried to stop myself saying this before checking for other abnormalities. I showed them that I was examining for retrosternal extension and for bruits and then I was about to look for signs of hypo- or hyperthyroidism when they stopped me and asked me to describe my findings. As with the other cases, they let me start to show that I would extend my examination further and this seemed to impress but they always then stopped me in midflow. I told them I had found a smoothly enlarged thyroid goitre and they then questioned me as to whether I was sure it was smooth. I was about to go back and re-examine but then realized that this would not look impressive. I did think it was smooth and so stuck to my original findings. I later discovered another candidate had been pushed on the same point and had also stuck firm.

I was then taken to a gentleman with frontal balding, mild ptosis and some facial muscle wasting and I was asked to hazard a diagnosis. I suggested *myotonic dystrophy* and was asked why. I explained my findings and made the mistake of saying 'myopathic facies'. My examiner looked puzzled and asked me what I meant. I explained about the muscle wasting that I could see although retracted my description of 'myopathic facies' as an unhelpful statement so he did not push me further.

I was then taken to a young lady with a large intravenous cannula in her right antecubital fossa and was asked to examine the back of her chest. The first thing I noticed was a puncture mark over the right lower chest suggesting a recent pleural aspiration. I quickly found a right *pleural effusion* and was asked to explain what brought me to that diagnosis and what was the most likely cause. In view of her age and the intravenous cannula, I suggested pneumonia and was then asked the most likely microbiological cause for this lady and the most suitable antibiotic treatment.

I was then taken to another lady and was asked to examine her fundi and to describe my findings. I found early cataract formation, indistinct disc margins, arterial narrowing and patchy black *pigmentation* particularly in the *macular* region. I was asked where in the left eye was there a particularly dense black deposit. Unlike my first attempt, I did not try to pull the wool over their eyes with bluffing my way out. I was honest in saying I did not know where the densest deposit was and they allowed me a second look. I was then asked to hazard an attempt at putting all these features together and I was utterly stumped. However, my examiner just asked the cause of black pigmentation and we passed on to the next case.

I was asked to look at, and examine, a lady's hands. There was obvious *osteoarthrosis* but I did not want to be put off by this so I quickly checked for muscle wasting, clubbing and for a sensory loss. I was about to examine the elbows for gouty tophi and rheumatoid nodules when I was stopped and directed to discuss my findings. I was asked what were the eponymous names for the swellings of the proximal and terminal interphalangeal joints.

I was finally taken to a middle-aged lady with a complete left *ptosis*. I was asked what I saw from the end of the bed and for the possible causes. I was then asked to examine further. I made a bit of a mess of this case. I examined the pupils and then proceeded to examine for diplopia which I was very ham-fisted about. I was desperately trying to keep the left eyelid open and examine visual movements by asking her to follow my finger and I got my arms all in a muddle! The examiner quickly intervened and asked me what I had found. I mentioned the pupillary reactions and the down and out position of the left eye and so he asked me for a diagnosis. I told him it was a *complete IIIrd nerve palsy* and he then requested me to ask the lady some questions to elucidate the cause. I asked about headache, thinking of a posterior communicating artery aneurysm, and that seemed to cause some surprise in the examiner. I then asked about diabetes. The lady was diabetic but I was told that in her case this was irrelevant and asked to hazard one more question. Fortunately, I was inspired to ask how long she had had the ptosis and discovered it was congenital. I was pushed on the difference between a complete and partial IIIrd nerve palsy and after describing the probable findings was asked the anatomical difference in the lesions. I thought I was being asked something esoteric and was somewhat annoyed when it transpired that all he wanted me to say was that in a partial nerve palsy only some of the IIIrd nerve fibres are affected!

My advice is to keep your head even when you have made a mistake. If you know you have made a mistake be quick to say so before your examiner has a chance to capitalize on it. If your examiner challenges, do not assume it means you have said something wrong. He may just be testing to see if you will stick firm to your diagnosis because you are absolutely certain of it. Practise, practise and practise, particularly in front of people who make you nervous. I also found it helpful to regard some of my outpatients as potential short cases. I think some of them had never been so thoroughly examined! Make every effort to show the examiner you can put the patient at ease. Introduce yourself and ask their permission to examine them and tell them exactly what you are going to do. Do not forget to thank them afterwards. It gives you time to calm down and think – and also it impresses the examiners. (Pass)

'The patient sounded most alarmed and said she hoped her daughter wouldn't get it.'

213. The first patient was an elderly, rather slow lady. 'Examine this lady's heart and chest.' (It'll take hours, I thought!) I was almost panicked into combining my examination but then started doing the cardiovascular system alone. She was deaf and I felt I was not being very slick. I distinctly remember a wave of panic/fear that this was it! Anyhow, I found *mixed mitral valve disease* (MR>MS) and *aortic regurgitation*. I stood back and said this. The examiner nodded and said we would not bother with the chest. (My hands were cold when I started and the patient jumped which did not help my composure!)

The next patient was a young man with widespread psoriasis and a moon face. 'What do you think of this man?' I asked him if he had had any treatment, then stood back and said he had widespread psoriasis and could have been on systemic steroids. The examiner nodded, pointed out his palms and soles and asked what I would call this type of psoriasis. I answered: 'pustular'. They agreed and moved on.

There was an ill-looking, jaundiced, old lady in a rather dimly lit bay. 'Examine this abdomen.' The examiners listened intently to my percussion but otherwise did not hassle me. I said I should like to go on to test for shifting dullness and to do a rectal exam, but did not attempt to move her for the former because she looked so ill. They accepted this and moved away from the bedside. I said I had found *hepatosplenomegaly* in a jaundiced patient and that I had noticed inguinal and supraclavicular nodes and a node biopsy scar in her groin. I suggested chronic myelocytic or lymphocytic leukaemia/non-Hodgkin's lymphoma, or metastatic carcinoma as the differential diagnosis. They asked how I would tell a student to examine the spleen and what

its characteristic features were. (I wondered had I done it all wrong or felt a kidney instead!)

A lady with dilated pupils. 'Examine this fundus,' they said and then wandered away a little. I looked in one eye and then asked if I could look in the other and got a rather non-committal 'if you must' expression. But I did anyway. I said I'd found *grade II hypertensive retinopathy* with silver wiring and arteriovenous nipping but no sign of haemorrhages, exudates or papilloedema. The examiner just said: 'Yes' and moved on.

A lady with florid *hereditary haemorrhagic telangiectasia* (HHT). 'What's the diagnosis?' When I got my tongue round it, I said the diagnosis in full! They said: 'What question would you like to ask?'. I asked if anyone in the family had it. She said: 'No' and the examiners asked if I was surprised. I said it was an autosomal dominant trait and tended to run through the generations, at which the patient sounded most alarmed and said she hoped her daughter would not get it. The examiners placated her, saying there was a 50% chance. I felt annoyed that it reflected badly on me upsetting her but surely the patient must have heard of it running in families before!

A lady with *neurofibromatosis*. They asked for a diagnosis and then for any neurological complications. I replied: 'Epilepsy, cord compression, carpal tunnel syndrome, tumours'.

A grossly *acromegalic* man. 'What's the diagnosis and what features would you like to demonstrate?' I described his facies, jaw and hands. They led me on to *carpal tunnel syndrome* and got me to demonstrate wasting and to try to show any sensory loss (intact!) and to talk about testing for median nerve motor function.

An old lady with denuded blisters and mouth lesions. The diagnosis was *pemphigus*. He asked me: 'Where's the split in the skin?'. I said it was at the intraepidermal level.

Overall, my short cases went quite fluently. My worst moments were when I surprised a patient with my ice-cold, stress-induced hands, and when I apparently upset the lady with HHT for mentioning that it ran in families. One examiner questioned my use of 'He/she probably has . . . ' when the diagnosis was obvious from just looking. By the end I was being more dogmatic which seemed to go down better. Even with no disasters it was hard to treat each case afresh but I am sure that is the knack of scoring highly. (Pass)

'Yes,' said the examiner, 'tell me about the precursors of bilirubin.'

214. 'Examine this man and shake hands with him.' The diagnosis was obviously *myotonic dystrophy*. The examiner asked me what else I would like to ask the patient. I suggested asking about family history and the examiner said: 'Good'.

'Look at this man, what is the diagnosis?' He had *pseudoxanthoma elasticum* and the examiner again said: 'Good'. He asked me what the description of the skin was and I replied: 'plucked chicken skin' and again he said: 'Good! What would you expect to hear listening to his heart? That is what he is really here for'. I replied mitral valve prolapse. 'That's right,' said the examiner.

'Look at this girl, what do you think? She is 25 years old.' I said: 'If she will forgive me, she is rather short'. 'That's right,' said the examiner, 'what would you like to ask her?'. I asked her how tall her parents were. 'Anything else?' said the examiner. I asked her when her periods started, if at all. The examiner said: 'That's a good question, what do you think of her face? She has *Crohn's disease*'. I replied that she had a cushingoid moon face, and that steroids had probably been the cause of her short stature. 'Yes,' said the examiner, 'in association with the malabsorption'.

'What is the diagnosis?' The patient had obvious *hereditary haemorrhagic telangiectasia* so I looked in the patient's mouth, which pleased the examiner. The examiner asked me what the other name of the condition was and I replied: 'Osler–Weber–Rendu syndrome'.

'What do you think about this man's feet?' He had definite *pustular psoriasis*. 'That's right,' said the examiner, 'look at his hands.' He had the worst onycholysis that I have ever seen. 'Yes,' said the examiner, 'that's the third time this has happened to this poor chap.'

'Look at this woman. What strikes you about her?' I replied that she appeared green in colour. 'That's right,' said the examiner, 'why do you think that she is this colour?' I replied that I did not know but that perhaps it was very severe *jaundice*. 'Yes,' said the examiner, 'tell me about the precursors of bilirubin.' I replied that it was biliverdin.

'Look at this woman's rash – this part in particular.' Some parts of the rash looked bullous and others appeared to have target lesions. I looked in her mouth. My first thought was that it was pemphigoid but eventually I came out with the right diagnosis of *erythema multiforme*.

'Look at this patient's hands.' I rolled up her sleeves that had been left down to her elbows and this revealed many *neurofibromas*. There was also partial amputation of several of her fingers. (Pass)

'The other examiner, who seemed annoyed at his colleague, took over and took the bull by the horns!'

215. The first examiner dithered and was an irritatingly slow 'dove'. He asked me to examine the respiratory system. I introduced myself, stood at the end of the bed and thought of the Newport course! He allowed me to examine fully both the anterior and posterior chest. I found an area of posterior consolidation on the right, with what I felt to be an area of anterior effusion. He mumbled something about 'overdiagnosing' but agreed with the *consolidation*.

The next case was a nightmare. I was asked to examine a man's legs neurologically. Again, I introduced myself and observed. I examined extensively and only found loss of proprioception. The examiner agreed and told me that was correct and other sensations were normal. He asked me to look at the man's face. He had a left-sided eye patch and underneath was a partial ptosis. No further examination was allowed and I was asked for my thoughts on a possible diagnosis. This really stumped me and there was an embarrassing pause of several seconds. My only thought was of luetic disease but he was not satisfied. Again, a number of long pauses. In the end he just wanted polyneuropathy! I was told subsequently by the registrar running the exam that this was the *Guillain–Barré Miller–Fisher variant*. Most neurologists I have talked to since have disagreed with this!*

The other examiner, who seemed annoyed at his colleague, took over and took the bull by the horns! At the next cubicle I was asked to look at a man and to say immediately if I had a diagnosis. It was clear from the patient's expression (or lack of it) that he had *Parkinson's disease*. We quickly left the room.

The fourth case was again a spot diagnosis. The lady had glasses, a *marfanoid appearance* and a high-arched palate. I gave the diagnosis and he agreed.

I was then asked to: 'Listen only' to a man's heart. I palpated the carotid but that was not much help. There was a very, very soft ejection systolic murmur at the left sternal edge with no radiation to the neck. I got up and he asked specifically for a diagnosis. I told him (quickly) my findings and plumped for early *aortic stenosis*. He said nothing but hurried me to the next case.

*This patient probably had external ophthalmoplegia (part of Miller–Fisher variant; see Vol.1, Station 3, Central nervous system, Case 19) and the eye patch was used to obviate his diplopia. It would seem that the patient was in the recovery phase and some of the signs (areflexia, ataxia, etc.) had improved.

I was asked to look at the fundus of a lady doing some knitting close to her face. She had no cataracts and on inspection of the fundus she had what I am sure was *retinitis pigmentosa*, albeit not as typical as I had seen before.

With glee he then gave me the same instruction for the lady sitting next to her, also knitting but showing no family resemblance. She too had a very pigmented retina but this time it was *panretinal photocoagulation* scars.

For the next case I was asked to examine a lady's conjugate eye movements. She had a *bilateral VIth nerve palsy*. He agreed and asked me for the possible causes. I said the causes of mononeuritis multiplex and he seemed happy.

My next case was an elderly man with striking jaundice and firm irregular *hepatomegaly* with no spleen. He asked the most likely cause and I said malignancy. He agreed.

I cannot believe anybody comes out of the short cases thinking they have passed. My second case, in my own mind, was a disaster. I think it all comes down to how you look and the air of confidence you give. I heard them commenting on my good examination technique (learnt in Gwent) and I am sure this was the overriding factor that passed me. Finally, if disasters occur early, it is not all over. I survived and now have 'MRCP' to tell the tale! (Pass)

'*"What else would you like to examine?" The patient started winking at me. "I'd like to examine his eyes, please." He had small, irregular pupils which did not react to light.*'

216. The first patient was an elderly lady who was sitting upright. She was breathless at rest and quite cachectic. The examiner said to me: 'This lady is not very well so could you examine her chest from the back only?'. I looked quickly at her hands and she had gross clubbing. The left side of her chest did not move on inspiration and it was dull to percussion. The examiner stopped me at this point and asked for a diagnosis so I said there was a large left *pleural effusion* but it could be consolidation. He agreed and asked the most likely cause. I replied: 'NG', as the patient was listening, and he agreed with me.

The next patient was a woman who was lying flat and I was asked to examine her abdomen. I looked at her hands, eyes, mouth, neck and axillae quite quickly and then moved on to the abdomen. She had *hepatosplenomegaly* but there was no ascites on testing for

shifting dullness. The second examiner said that I should not bother to do shifting dullness if she was not stony dull in the flanks to percussion. I nodded. 'What do you think the diagnosis is?' I said that it was probably a lymphoreticular problem such as chronic lymphatic leukaemia or chronic myeloid leukaemia in view of the patient's age (she was about 60–70). 'What else could it be?' I suggested lymphoma but there were no nodes or it could be cirrhosis, malaria or another infection. The examiner said: 'No', to all of these suggestions so I have no idea what they were really after!

The third patient was another elderly woman sitting upright. The examiner asked me to feel her pulse. It was about 100 beats/min in atrial fibrillation. 'Is there anything else?' asked the examiner. 'No,' I replied. 'OK,' he said, 'then feel her apex beat'. Again, it was about 100 beats/min in atrial fibrillation and forceful. 'Forceful?'* asked the examiner. 'Yes,' I said. 'OK, carry on and listen to her heart.' I started to position the patient correctly at 45°, etc. but the other examiner said to me: 'Don't bother with that, it wastes time'. So I just listened. My findings were that she had *isolated mitral stenosis*. I told them this and they nodded.

The next patient was a young boy about 20 years old who was grossly overweight. I was asked to look at his abdomen and to say what I thought the scar was caused by. It was a horizontal scar mid-way between the umbilicus and the groin. If he had been older I would have said it was for an aortic aneurysm but it was a bit too low so I eventually told them that I had never seen a scar like that before. The examiner said that it was for an *apronectomy* and he asked me why I thought he had had it performed. The patient did not look cushingoid so I said it was probably for obesity as I did not think a surgeon would perform such an operation for a reversible metabolic cause. He laughed and said that was one way of looking at it! He asked if I thought he had *gynaecomastia*. I felt for breast tissue and said that there was. He then asked me to examine his testes which were very small. They took me outside and asked what I thought the diagnosis was. I said: 'Was it caused by alcoholism?'. They said: 'No'. I explained why I thought it was not Cushing's. They nodded. 'What else?' I suggested *Klinefelter's syndrome* because he was very tall. 'Yes,' they said.

The next patient was sitting in a darkened room. 'Look at his fundi,' they said. I thought he had proliferative diabetic retinopathy with extensive laser burns.

---

*The examiner must have been surprised to be told that the apex beat was forceful in a patient with lone mitral stenosis.

However, there was no reply from the examiner. 'What else could it be?' I said it could be retinitis pigmentosa but explained how it looked different as the vessels were not usually traversed. 'Yes, but what else?' '*Choroidoretinitis* is another possibility but it isn't usually circumferential.' 'OK,' they said.

For the sixth patient I had to 'Examine his visual fields'. I pulled up a chair and sat opposite the patient at arm's length. I started to examine his visual fields but the examiners were walking about and talking and generally distracting the patient. I kept asking him to ignore them and to look at my nose! He had a *left homonymous hemianopia*. They asked me for the site of the lesion. He had no other gross signs of facial weakness or hemiplegia so I said it was probably a right middle cerebral artery cerebrovascular accident but that the lesion could be anywhere along the optic radiation and they agreed with this.

The next patient was a man about 50 years old who was lying in bed. 'Examine this man's legs,' they said. He had a grossly deformed right ankle joint. I asked him if it was painful. He replied that it was not and never had been. I then said that it was a *Charcot's joint*. 'Caused by what?' they asked. 'Probably caused by *luetic disease*.' 'Yes, OK, what else would you like to examine?' I started to test the legs for sensation which was normal and for joint position sense which he did not allow me to do. 'What else?' The patient started to lift one of his feet and wiggle it about. 'Coordination,' I suggested. 'Yes, OK.' I found that he was ataxic. 'What else would you like to examine?' The patient started winking at me. 'I'd like to examine his eyes, please.' He had small, irregular pupils which did not react to light. 'Does that confirm your suspicions?' I replied that it did and that was the end of the exam. (Pass)

'I would advise candidates that, whenever they are on-call, to practise examining patients. I had the clinical on a Monday and was on-call all weekend. As it turned out, this was very good practice.'

217. My first patient was a cyanosed, elderly man with clubbing and basal crackles. I said that *fibrosing alveolitis* was the most likely diagnosis. The examiner said: 'What else could it be?', so I suggested occupational lung disease and this seemed to suffice. The examiner then showed me the chest X-ray and expected me to describe the reticular pattern. He asked me for the Latin name for lacy! I did not know the word so the examiner moved on quickly.

The next patient was a young Asian man with an old ulcer on his shin. I was asked to say what had caused this so I suggested *sickle cell disease* and this was correct.

The next patient was an old, pale man with *hepatosplenomegaly*. The examiner asked how I knew that it was not polycystic kidney disease. I initially bluntly replied that I had not formally examined for the kidneys (which I had in fact forgotten to do) and the examiner looked a bit taken aback. However, I went on to say that he had no evidence of dialysis (shunts or peritoneal) and I could not get above the masses, etc. I feel that although I had forgotten to formally examine the kidneys, he had obviously not noticed and my straightforward admission got me off the hook.

The next patient was a young lady and I was asked to examine her right hand. I noticed that both forearms seemed wasted distally. The right hand had both hypothenar and thenar wasting with clawing. I was asked first to describe this and then for what I thought it could be caused by (having briefly gone through a neurological motor and sensory examination and demonstrated the most likely nerve lesions). I felt that it could be a *hereditary motor* and *sensory neuropathy* extending to the arms and said that I would want to see the legs. In retrospect, I think that this must have been correct. The examiner did not seem displeased but then asked for other possibilities. We got on to peripheral nerve lesions, brachial plexus lesions and syringomyelia, each of which I had to justify.

The next patient had *proliferative diabetic retinopathy*. The examiner asked me where the microaneurysms were so I said between the vessels. He then asked me why they were not right by the vessels. Seeing me struggle, he asked about Harvey's theories at which I realized that they must be aneurysms of the capillaries!

The next patient had complicated heart murmurs including *aortic regurgitation* and *mitral stenosis/Austin Flint murmur* plus *mitral regurgitation*. She had had previous surgery and we got into a discussion about the indications for warfarinization with artificial pig valves.

The last patient had a straightforward *psoriatic arthropathy*.

I would advise candidates that, whenever they are on-call, to practise examining patients. I had the clinical on a Monday and was on-call all weekend. As it turned out, this was very good practice as when seeing patients I would just concentrate on one particular system. (Pass)

'There was a loud stenotic murmur so I didn't mention that I had heard the regurgitant jet.'

218. 'Examine this man's abdomen.' I started with the hands and was told (not unkindly) to move on. As soon as I had demonstrated the *spleen*, they stopped me. 'What is your finding?' I said a large spleen. 'What is the cause in this man?' He was about 70–80 years and I had to modify my list accordingly, which I did rather poorly.

The second patient had a *diabetic retinopathy* with laser scars. The examiner asked me about his visual fields and whether the scars involved the macula. 'Yes,' I said, 'so I expect a scotoma and a constrictive field defect'. 'Examine for this'. Of course, I found the patient had a completely normal blind spot and full fields!

The next patient had *optic atrophy*. It was an old man with hydrocephalus. I was asked what had caused his underlying optic atrophy and I replied that it was probably caused by chronic raised intracranial pressure. I had the impression that this was a case that they were not sure about including as they seemed pleased that I had made something of it.

For the next patient I was asked to feel the pulse. It was a collapsing pulse and I then had to examine the precordium. I heard the regurgitant murmur in the aortic area only. There was a loud stenotic murmur so I did not mention that I had heard the regurgitant jet (I do not know why!). I said he had *aortic stenosis* but why the pulse? 'I would like to see the blood pressure,' I said. This was 190/40. 'He must have *aortic regurgitation*'. The examiner said: 'Uhuh. Listen again', which I did and heard it again. (This time it was very loud!) However, I had been allowed to relisten to this patient. I felt that I could have done much better here in summing up the signs more sensibly.

The next patient was an elderly lady with a resting tremor, an intention tremor, titubation, a mini tracheostomy and clasp-knife tone. The examiner said: 'What do you notice?'. I said: 'She has a mini tracheostomy'. 'Yes,' said the examiner, 'the last candidate missed that'. My brief examination demonstrated all the above findings. The examiner said: 'What nerve supplies the larynx?'. There was then a brief discussion on brainstem syndromes and I discovered afterwards that the eventual diagnosis here had been the *olivopontocerebellar degeneration syndrome*! (Pass)

'I said "Infectious mononucleosis" before I could stop myself.'

219. I was asked to examine the language function of a patient. This went well as she had an *expressive dysphasia*. I was then asked to examine her visual fields and she had a *homonymous hemianopia*. I was asked about the general management of stroke patients and the factors involved in their prognosis. They seemed happy with my answers.

I was then asked to examine the next patient's heart. I therefore listened and felt the carotid pulse at the same time. There was a plateau pulse plus aortic stenosis. I gave my findings and asked for the blood pressure. I was told it was 120/80. I made a diagnosis of *aortic stenosis* and had to explain why it was not aortic sclerosis. I was told that the patient had presented as a collapse so we talked about syncope secondary to aortic stenosis. I then got on to arrhythmias and Adams–Stokes attacks. I know that they were trying to change my mind about the diagnosis but I said clinically my diagnosis was of aortic stenosis and that an ECG and an echo and possibly catheter studies would help confirm this. I am sure I would have failed if I had changed my mind.

We went on to the next patient and I was asked to examine the abdomen, to explain what I was doing and to give my findings as I went along. They stopped me after I had found *hepatosplenomegaly* and then asked me for a differential diagnosis. I gave alcoholic liver disease with portal hypertension as the most likely cause and infection. 'What sort of infection?' they asked. I said 'Infectious mononucleosis' before I could stop myself and the examiner laughed and said: 'Is it likely?'. I said: 'No, because the patient is in the wrong age group' and they seemed satisfied. I mentioned chronic myeloid leukaemia and they asked me about enzyme markers and that went OK.

For the next patient I had to examine the neck. There were large pulsating masses on both sides which were possibly *carotid aneurysms*. I examined the neck and then the examiner handed me my stethoscope! I presented my findings but was not asked for a diagnosis.

We moved on to the next patient: 'Examine these fundi'. The right fundus was normal but the left fundus had optic atrophy plus a small area of choroidoretinitis. They seemed surprised when they heard me describe what I had seen. Then they asked for the diagnosis.

I thought they meant of the *optic atrophy* and the *choroidoretinitis*. So I said: 'Toxoplasmosis!'. They laughed and said: 'No, the patient went suddenly blind'. I then offered a diagnosis of temporal arteritis. The examiner obviously did not know about the choroidoretinitis. I saw the patient afterwards and he told me that they had had another look. I hope they saw it!

The examiners were very pleasant. I know my examination technique was fine but sometimes I was a bit hesitant when answering their questions. (Pass)

'I thought the examiners were probably a little the worse for lunch but don't be fooled by their jovial attitude (if they are like that) into becoming frivolous yourself.'

220. The first patient had bilateral *polycystic kidney disease* and I was asked to examine the abdomen. I went straight to the hands and the examiners asked what I was looking for. They wanted to know if I had found any of these features and before I could say that they were in fact normal I was jovially accused of not having really looked but I firmly stated that I had! When I asked the patient if he had any pain in the tummy, they said: 'He soon will have!'. I was then told: 'We have to get our entertainment this afternoon somehow'. There was eventually a discussion on how polycystic kidneys present.

I was then asked to: 'Examine this woman's chest from the cardiovascular point of view'. She had *mitral stenosis* and *aortic regurgitation*. Again the examination was interspersed with quips from the examiners. They expected me to have felt the trachea to check the position of the mediastinum. I had not and was told: 'Naughty, naughty'. A look of horror must have crossed my face as they said: 'Don't worry, you're doing very well'.

The third patient had *diabetic retinopathy*. It was fairly uncomplicated except that the examiners fell around laughing when, having asked the patient if I could look in the right eye, I then asked if I could look in the left eye. The instruction had been: 'Examine this patient's eyes' (while they were handing me an ophthalmoscope), so I had asked if they only wanted fundoscopy and they had said: 'Yes'.

The next patient had *titubation* and *nystagmus* in all planes. The instruction was: 'Examine this patient's eyes'. I had the Snellen chart from this book and they were delighted, clapping their hands and saying: 'Bonus points for that!'. The rest of the examination of this patient was unremarkable and there was a brief discussion on possible causes.

The fifth patient had a *spastic paraparesis* and I was asked to examine the legs. It was uneventful until just before the plantars. I was asked which way they were likely to go and I said: 'Up'. He said: 'OK, make them go up like a real neurologist'. They went up and at that point I could not resist a broad grin! There was a brief discussion on possible causes.

The last patient had *clubbing*, *pigmentation* and *kyphosis* and we talked about a possible aetiology.

I thought the examiners were probably a little the worse for lunch but do not be fooled by their jovial attitude (if they are like that) into becoming frivolous yourself. When I started the exam they said: 'What are you good at? Don't tell me, everything'. I said: 'Well, I have been practising' and they roared with laughter. (Pass)

'The delayed fundal question ploy, I thought – I was ready for that!'

221. 'What do you think the skin lesion is on this leg?' (discoloured, purple/pink with marked scaling). 'Psoriasis,' I said, 'but there are no other plaques.' 'No – think again.' 'Drug reaction?' 'No,' said the examiner who appeared exasperated. 'How about infection?' 'Well, it could be *cellulitis*,' I said. 'Yes, at last. Well, perhaps you'll do better on the others.' (I had never imagined they would put a case of cellulitis in, especially an atypical one.)

'Examine this man's leg and talk as you go through it. You may ask him questions.' I grappled with demonstrating a *paraplegia* while speaking (which was difficult). 'What do you think of his speech?' (Heck! I realized it was not the content but the speech character they wanted me to note.) I asked a question and noted his *dysarthria*. 'Would you like to demonstrate the plantars?' I said that I would normally do them and showed they were up-going. (By this time I was despondent but determined.)

'Examine this girl's cardiovascular system quickly.' It went smoothly. I presented it clearly and discussed the *ventricular septal defect* (VSD) or mitral regurgitant murmur. 'Do you think the VSD is significant?' 'Well, no, because there . . . ' I said. 'Don't say why, just say yes or no' (exasperated examiner). 'No.' 'Fine,' he said.

'Look at this man. Perhaps it is easier if he stands up. Tell me what you think.' 'He has a *marfanoid appearance*, sir.' 'Yes, what would you look for?' 'Aortic and mitral regurgitation,' I replied. 'Which valve is most likely to be affected?' '*Aortic regurgitation*.' The examiner pulled back the shirt triumphantly to demonstrate the aortic valve replacement scar (Bingo!).

'Examine this fundus.' There was background *diabetic retinopathy*. I confidently presented my prepared speech. 'Yes,' he said and we walked away. Then he said: 'And were there any laser scars?'. 'No,' I said. 'And were there cotton-wool spots?' 'No.' 'Correct.' (The delayed fundal question ploy, I thought – I was ready for that!)

'Examine the abdomen of this girl.' There was a palpable liver and spleen so I gave these signs succinctly. We moved away and the examiner, noticeably relaxed, was filling time. 'What do you think is the cause?' 'Hodgkin's disease is most likely,' I said. 'Yes, anything else – how about biliary cirrhosis?' 'There are no signs of chronic liver disease and the palpable spleen goes against this,' I said. 'Yes, but it is *biliary cirrhosis*' and he shrugged his shoulders! (Pass)

'I have already made a diagnosis. Do you want me to continue?'

222. I was asked to examine the arms of a man who was complaining of weakness. He had the facial appearance of *myotonic dystrophy*. I shook hands with the patient and said: 'I have already made a diagnosis. Do you want me to continue?'. I then had to demonstrate how to examine power in the arms. I was asked if I wanted to ask the patient any questions. I asked him about family history and the effects of cold.

I was then asked to examine a patient's fundi. He had grade II *hypertensive retinopathy* with marked arteriovenous nipping.

The instruction for the next patient was 'Examine the respiratory system'. He had dyspnoea, cyanosis, clubbing and the fine, inspiratory, basal crackles suggestive of *fibrosing alveolitis*. I was asked to give the causes and differential diagnoses of fibrosis of the lungs. I was then shown the patient's chest X-ray and asked to comment. It showed bilateral lower zone fibrotic changes.

Next, I was asked to examine a patient's abdomen. There were bilateral *polycystic kidneys* and an arteriovenous fistula in the arm. I was asked to demonstrate one of the kidneys. The examiner seemed satisfied, and asked me the single most useful investigation. I answered: 'Ultrasound' and he nodded.

I was taken to the next short case and asked to examine the heart and to tell the examiner what the diagnosis was. The pulse was of normal character and there was a long *systolic murmur* all over the precordium, maximal at the left sternal edge. I said I was unsure of the diagnosis and gave a differential of mitral regurgitation and aortic sclerosis. He asked me what the heart sounds were like. I could not remember them clearly and said 'Normal'. He then said he thought the second sound was quiet. I wondered whether I had missed aortic stenosis. We then got into a discussion between aortic sclerosis and stenosis. I admitted that I thought aortic sclerosis was a bad term and wished I had never mentioned it! He asked me what I would do in the clinic if presented with such a murmur, so I said an ECG, chest X-ray and an echocardiogram. He nodded.

My advice is to stay as calm as possible and hope that the first case goes well. Always look at the patient's surroundings and general appearance before starting your specific examination. It is impressive if you can make the diagnosis, for example, of myotonic dystrophy from the end of the bed. (Pass)

'What they really wanted me to notice were the old-fashioned controls of a wheelchair.'

223. I was asked to examine a patient's abdomen. I thought I could get over the mass in the left hypochondrium and so I said the diagnosis was of polycystic kidneys. I then looked for dialysis marks on the arms. In retrospect, it was so clearly *hepatosplenomegaly*. In fact, I can still feel my fingers jumping over the sharp edge of the liver. I really do not know why I said polycystic kidneys. If I had been the examiner I would certainly have failed myself!

We then moved on to the next patient. The examiner said: 'What do you notice about this woman?'. There was half a minute's pause. 'She's in a wheelchair,' I said. 'What does that tell you about the chronicity of her disease?' 'If it's an NHS wheelchair then she will have been waiting some time!' (They liked this.) What they had really wanted me to notice were the old-fashioned controls. They went on: 'Examine her fundi'. She had the whitest discs that I have ever seen. 'What would you like to test next?' They obviously thought I was not extending my examination quickly enough. What they really meant was: 'Examine her gait', which I eventually did and she was grossly ataxic. 'What is your diagnosis?' '*Multiple sclerosis.*' It had taken a long time to drag me through this case! (Pass)

'She must have had cystic fibrosis presenting with a cerebral abscess.'

224. For my next case I was asked to examine a lady's abdomen. She was about 40 years old. I performed a standard abdominal routine and found that she had a large mass on the right side which I could get above. It moved with respiration and was hollow to percussion.

I thought it was most likely to be a polycystic kidney but, because I could not feel one on the other side, I suggested that I would investigate it further. The examiner said: 'Well it is a *polycystic kidney*, and I wouldn't worry too much about not being able to feel one on the other side'.

The next short case was a 30-year-old lady. I was told that she had come to casualty last week having had several fits. She had papilloedema and the examiners told me that she had had a CT scan. They then asked me to examine her chest. She had clubbing with a Hickman line *in situ* and she also had a left thoracotomy scar. There was a left pleural effusion with thickening and a right pleural rub. The examiner said: 'Can you piece it all together?'. I went: 'Um, um, um' and then the bell went. The examiner said: 'Come on'. I went: 'Uhh . . . uhh . . . '. He said: 'OK, forget it!'. I think she must have had *cystic fibrosis* presenting with a cerebral abscess.

One must look interested in the cases themselves and take time to be nice to the patients. I said: 'Excuse me' to one of the examiners while pointing to an open curtain behind him before examining a young lady's chest. He said: 'Sorry' and closed the curtains! (Pass)

You never know you've failed until the list is published

The following examples illustrate the extent to which the candidate's assessment of what is happening can be very different from that of the examiners. Although the examiners may appear rude and hawkish, and you may feel that you are doing badly, you may in fact be performing well enough.

'They then both walked off muttering, "Well, I would never employ this woman, would you?". If I had been nervous before, I was even worse now and felt certain that I had failed.'

225. For my first case I was asked to examine the abdomen of a 60-year-old woman. I found a large *mass on the left side of the abdomen*, there was no anterior notch, I could not get above or below it. I thought it was probably a kidney or a spleen but to this day I do not know what it was. I told the examiners I thought it was probably a renal mass and gave good reasons why, but I think I was probably wrong. They said nothing and looked displeased.

For the next case, they took me to a 70-year-old man and asked me to 'Listen to the back of the chest only'. There were bilateral, basal, fine, expiratory crackles and

clubbing. I told the examiners that there was pulmonary fibrosis and that it was probably idiopathic. This was followed by: 'For goodness sake, woman, calm down! What is the diagnosis?'. I told them the same diagnosis again. 'What does he have?' I told them again! 'What is the cause?' I told them again and got upset and said, 'I'm sorry but . . . '. The examiner said: 'Look at him again'. I looked and could see nothing so I said that. He eventually hinted at connective tissue diseases so I asked the patient to open his mouth – he had *scleroderma*! In retrospect, I feel that this was not obvious and that the examiner was unduly harsh in his attitude.

The next patient was a 35-year-old woman and I was asked to examine the cardiovascular system. I heard some sort of murmur. I noticed a sternotomy scar and a funny pulse. I was still shaking from my experience in the second case and was by now even more nervous. It was either mitral valve disease or combined aortic valve disease – I obviously got it wrong as the examiner listened and looked cross. The examiners muttered between themselves and I felt completely useless by this stage. The only saving grace was that I had examined the cardiovascular system of the patient efficiently.

The next patient was a 50-year-old man and I was asked to look at his fundi. The room was light and the pupils were not fully dilated. I used my own ophthalmoscope which was a great help. I reported early background *diabetic retinopathy* in the left eye only and they moved on. In the meantime, in a loud voice, the first examiner said: 'Well, I would never employ this woman, would you?'. If I had been nervous before, I was even worse now and felt certain that I had failed.

The next patient was a 60-year-old man with a harsh *pansystolic murmur* at the left sternal edge and a displaced apex. I again examined thoroughly and described what I had heard in response to the instruction, 'Feel the pulse, listen at the apex'. I was asked the diagnosis and said ventricular septal defect because of the apex and the harsh quality of the murmur. He wanted to know the differential diagnosis and how I would differentiate them clinically. The examiner was still unhappy. I think it must have been mitral regurgitation.

The next patient was a 60-year-old woman. I was asked to: 'Look at this face – what do you see?'. 'Cushingoid,' I responded. 'Name three causes in a woman of this age.' I gave three. 'Anything else you notice?' 'Basal cell carcinoma.' 'What else?' I could see nothing else so I pointed out a second basal cell carcinoma which I had already seen. They then both walked off muttering.

The examiners were rude and unpleasant. My only advice to future candidates is to pretend you are in the casualty department and ignore the examiners. (Pass!)

'The examiners looked surprised when I said the tone was increased. I was asked to demonstrate and therefore withdrew my rash and foolish remark and finally concluded with possibilities for combined upper and lower motor neurone lesions.'

226. 'Examine this lady's *legs and gait*': a disaster! Gait: partly obscured by a long nightgown – steppage or right foot drop? Examination on the bed: tone (patient nervous) seemed increased but reflexes and plantars could not be elicited, the power was reduced, and the testing of sensation was laborious and inconclusive. I was uncertain when to say I had finished. There were pitying looks from the examiners. I blurted out some findings. The examiners looked surprised when I said the tone was increased. I was asked to demonstrate and then withdrew my rash and foolish remark and finally concluded with possibilities for combined upper and *lower motor neurone lesions*.

We passed on with much relief but scarcely more success. 'Examine this patient's knees.' On inspection, the knees were clearly swollen, left more than right, and the quadriceps were wasted. On palpation, the knees were warm but I failed to elicit fluid even though effusions were obviously present. The examiners raised their eyebrows as I recounted my findings. 'Please show me how you look for fluid.' On this second attempt, I clearly elicited the patella tap sign. Causes for the *swollen knees* were not discussed. We passed on with increasing confusion on my part.

'Listen to this man's heart.' I heard and reported *aortic incompetence*, having noted the cannula in the patient's arm. I was asked for the aetiology and suggested subacute *bacterial endocarditis* which seemed to be what they wanted – at last (!) but surely I was beyond redemption.

'Look at this lady's neck.' I inspected the plucked chicken skin and gave the diagnosis of *pseudoxanthoma elasticum*. I was not asked any further questions.

'Examine this man's chest.' On inspection he was blue, bloated and very breathless and I proceeded with palpation, percussion and auscultation although the examination was punctuated by bouts of severe coughing which I thought would lead to his death at any moment! The examiners seemed understanding as I asked if he wished me to continue. My diagnosis of exacerbation of *chronic obstructive airway disease* was accepted.

I was grateful to get to the next patient. 'Examine this man's abdomen.' I was going through my normal procedure when the bell sounded, which is always off-putting and I sought to reach a hasty conclusion. I suggested that there was a non-tender 2 cm *liver edge* and then hazarded that there was a mass in the right iliac fossa. The examiners' eyebrows were raised again in response to this. I am not sure whether there was a mass. A colleague who also saw this patient told me later that he had only felt a liver edge. The short cases ended with ears ringing and I was convinced of failure.

Of my six short cases, two went smoothly, two were barely mediocre (not least because the bronchitic patient threatened to expire at the end of every breath) and two were terrible and I had to repeat the parts of the examination which I got wrong. So, I strongly emphasize that the odd calamity need not mean failure. The candidate is probably very poorly placed to decide how he or she is doing. (Pass)

'The examiners were continually unnerving me and making me feel that my answers were wrong.'

227. I was asked to examine the hands of a patient. They looked rheumatoid but the patient also seemed to have tophi. There were no nodules at the elbow and I eventually said it was inactive rheumatoid arthritis. One examiner asked what I would think if told that his uric acid was 0.6 mmol/L. I said that was because he had *gout* as well! On walking to the next case, they asked me about treatment and I managed to discuss this satisfactorily.

I was asked to talk to an elderly man with a nasogastric tube *in situ*. He had dysarthria. They stopped me before I got any further and asked what I thought. I said that with dysarthria and nasogastric feeding, which was probably as a result of dysphagia, that he had a bulbar palsy. They asked me how I would differentiate pseudobulbar from bulbar palsy – I said I would look at his tongue – it was small and fasciculating. I therefore decided on *bulbar palsy*. As they moved away, they asked me the cause – I could only think of multiple cerebrovascular accidents. I forgot this would not do for the bulbar palsy I had just diagnosed!

For the next case, I was asked to look at the fundi. I could see lots of *laser burns* but no signs of diabetic retinopathy and so I said so. They asked me what I thought of the vessels. When I was looking, I did think there was arteriovenous nipping but thought that I would be better not to mention this. However, as they were actually asking me, I said that there was arteriovenous nipping which I had not mentioned before because I thought it was a 'soft sign'. They did not seem to like this. I then said that there may be hypertension as well. They did not respond. I was beginning to get unnerved!

I was then asked to look at a lady's eyes. She had gross *unilateral exophthalmos* and ophthalmoplegia. They soon stopped me and asked me what I thought. The only thing I could think of was thyrotoxicosis. They said she was euthyroid and pointed to a scar just above the nose and eye. I did not have a clue what it was. They asked me what was directly behind the centre of the forehead. I told them the pituitary and that the exophthalmos might be caused by a space-occupying lesion. They asked me what type. I noticed the patient was quite hirsute but by this stage the examiners had walked away and, as I could not think, I did not say anything.

They showed me a man with a *large mole* on his left arm. I did not know what it was. Although it did not look like a melanoma, this was the only thing I could think of so I said that the lesion should be excised and biopsied. They told me that the patient had had the lesion for years and that he had another one on his leg and they asked me what I thought about this. I said that I did not know and that I would still biopsy the lesion! It seemed that I was arguing with the examiner and, as I realized this, it made me feel even worse!

I was then asked to examine the cardiovascular system of a middle-aged woman. She had both a midline and a lateral thoracotomy scar with *prosthetic heart sounds* but with no murmur at the apex – he stopped me before I could listen further. I said that she had a prosthetic valve without any murmurs and with the two scars she had probably had a mitral valvotomy and later a valve replacement. One examiner asked me if this was likely in view of the fact that she was in sinus rhythm. I said that one expects atrial fibrillation but that the sinus rhythm was possible. The examiner laughed! They asked me about the aortic area – I said I had not listened there as I had not had time. The bell went and I was allowed to go. I felt like walking out and giving up.

I thought I did very badly. The examiners were continually unnerving me and making me feel that my answers were wrong. I was made to feel very unsure and I felt that it was very difficult to keep going. By the third and fourth case, I had half given up. As I was told time and time again prior to the exam, I am sure the main thing is to keep going despite what happens – you never know whether you have passed or failed until the letter comes through the door! (Pass)

'I felt like going home there and then but I am glad I didn't.'

228. 'Listen to this man's heart – no, go straight to the precordium.' I was not given any history. I was so completely confused by the murmurs which were systolic and diastolic that I could not make head nor tail of them. Some findings were eventually coaxed out of me and a conclusion forced upon me. I felt like going home there and then but I am glad I did not. I was forced into saying that this was *aortic valve disease* with dominant regurgitation. I have not got a clue if I was right or wrong.

I was then asked to look at a man's hands. There was gross *clubbing* with no apparent cause, i.e. he was not cyanosed and there was no Horner's syndrome, etc. I was asked for more possibilities – they eventually told me that this was pachydermoperiostitis – I admitted that I had never seen it before!

'Look at this man's fundi.' I thought I saw a *pigmented lesion in the choroid* which was well demarcated and single. I was asked for more possibilities and to say what it actually was. I plumped for a melanoma.

I was then asked to look at another man's hands. He had *gouty tophi* but there was nothing on the ears or the elbows. They seemed satisfied with this.

The next patient was an 'Examine this man's abdomen'. I felt a *4 cm liver* and they asked me if I could feel a spleen. I said: 'No'.

I was then taken to a lady and asked to look at her – 'What do you see?'. She was pigmented and mildly jaundiced with leuconychia and xanthelasma. She also had hepatomegaly and ascites. I was then shown her hands again as I had missed her liver palms – but that was after I had already given the diagnosis of *primary biliary cirrhosis*!

My last short case was another 'Look at this man's hands' and he was another case of *gouty tophi*. The examiners told me that I was correct. I was absolutely convinced that I had made an irretrievable mess of the short cases. I still cannot understand how they passed me! (Pass)

Survivors of the storm

'I found hepatosplenomegaly and told the examiner this. He then turned to the patient and said: "What

operation have you just had?" and he answered: "A splenectomy!"'

229. 'What's the diagnosis in this patient?' I noticed he had both *neurofibromatosis* and finger *clubbing*. The examiner asked me if I could relate the two conditions. I said: 'No' and the examiner said: 'Neither can I!'. I was then asked to examine a fundus. I found *optic atrophy* and *resolving papilloedema*. The examiner suggested that I should look at the patient's neck and I found a ventriculoperitoneal shunt present.

The next patient had an abdomen to be examined. There was a recent mid-line scar. I found *hepatosplenomegaly* and told the examiner this. He then turned to the patient and said: 'What operation have you just had?' and he answered: 'A splenectomy!'.

I was then asked to examine a patient's cardiovascular system. I found atrial fibrillation, *mixed mitral valve disease* (it was a restenosis as there was an old valvotomy scar), *pulmonary hypertension* and *tricuspid regurgitation*. There were pronounced cv waves in the neck and a pulsatile liver. I am sure I scored extra marks by feeling the abdomen. I was then asked to discuss the waveforms of the jugular venous pulse and I even had to draw a diagram! (Pass)

'*The examiners appeared irritated by all my answers and when we had finished the female examiner shook her head scornfully!*'

230. The first two patients were in a dark room. Both had dilated pupils and I was asked to look at their fundi. I did not get the diagnosis with the first patient. I said that the vessels looked thin and the retina was dark and wondered whether it was *optic atrophy*.

The second patient definitely had a *diabetic retinopathy* and the examiner asked whether there were any hypertensive changes as well.

The third short case was a female patient with a small, smooth *goitre* and eye signs. I was asked to examine the patient and say why I was performing each action. I was then asked if the patient was *euthyroid* or not.

Next I was taken to a 30-year-old patient and asked to feel her abdomen. There was a *mass in the right loin*. I was asked what a horseshoe kidney would feel like, and I was then asked to give my findings before I had finished palpating the kidneys. So I just carried on feeling until I had finished.

I was then asked to examine another patient's heart and again I was asked for the findings when I had only

listened at the apex and the left sternal edge. The patient was a lady in her eighties. She had peripheral cyanosis, atrial fibrillation and *right ventricular hypertrophy* but I could hear no murmurs. I said that the diagnosis was probably tight pulmonary stenosis but I should really have said tight mitral stenosis or an atrial septal defect. I was really taken to task on the following points: Was the patient cyanosed? What other signs of cyanosis do you know? How common is pulmonary stenosis in this age group? What is the most common cause of pulmonary stenosis? The examiners appeared irritated by all my answers and when we had finished the female examiner shook her head scornfully!

The last patient was a lady aged about 30. I was asked to examine her pulses and to comment on them. She appeared to have *peripheral vascular disease* and *aortic stenosis*. (Pass)

'*I found that if my first answer was incorrect, the examiners continued questioning until I got the right answer; if my first answer was correct, then they took the questioning a little further.*'

231. 'Look at this patient. What do you notice?' There was pallor, mild jaundice and bruising. I thought the diagnosis could possibly be *pernicious anaemia* and the examiners asked why. 'Because it looks like it,' I replied. (Stupid answer!) I tried again and said: 'The patient is of the right sex and age'. The examiner went on to ask me to examine the fundi. There were haemorrhages present which were obviously secondary to the pernicious anaemia but I said it was probably diabetic retinopathy!

My second short case was a *ventricular septal defect* in a 25-year-old but I said I thought he had hypertrophic obstructive cardiomyopathy and we discussed the symptoms and findings, and finally the examiner said: 'What else could it be?'. I said a ventricular septal defect and then he seemed happy!

The third patient had *rheumatoid arthritis* with *subluxation of the cervical spine* causing a *spastic paraparesis*. I was asked to examine the legs neurologically. I found this difficult as all the patient's joints were incredibly painful. Therefore, tone and power were hard to test. I had noted the rheumatoid arthritis and the upper motor neurone signs in both legs but failed to put two and two together to come up with subluxation of the spine.

The fourth patient had a complete left *IIIrd nerve palsy*. I demonstrated the findings and suggested all the causes for this but unfortunately failed to see a scar which indicated that she had had an aneurysm clipped!

The fifth patient had finger clubbing and a marked tremor. I noted these findings and suggested *thyroid acropachy*. I was then asked to find whether she was in fact hyperthyroid. I concluded she was euthyroid and found out later that this was correct.

My last patient had *psoriasis* of the hands with an *arthropathy*. I described the nail changes and the skin changes but in my panic forgot to demonstrate the terminal interphalangeal arthritis.

I found that if my first answer was slightly incorrect the examiner continued questioning until I found the right answer; if my first answer was correct then they took the questioning a little further. (Pass)

'I was harassed continually by the examiner saying: "Why are you doing x, y, z?" despite the fact that I was trying to tell him!'

232. 'Examine this man's cardiovascular system and talk us through it. You've no need to do the BP.' I was harassed continually by the examiner saying: 'Why are you doing x, y, z?', despite the fact that I was trying to tell him! For example: 'Why did you roll him on to the left side?'. My final diagnosis was of *tricuspid incompetence* in a patient with right heart failure. I told the examiner that I would like to look for a pulsatile liver and he said: 'Show me'.

'This gentleman is from Mauritius. Examine his chest.' My findings were of clubbing with bronchial breath sounds at the left upper zone. I said that the most likely diagnosis was a mitotic lesion in the left upper zone. Examiner: 'Tell me where the trachea is'. Whoops, I had forgotten to feel, so I said I had forgotten to look for it. 'Would you like to do so now?' I said: 'OK, yes, it's displaced to the left'. Examiner: 'This gentleman has had these signs for 20 years'. I suggested that the most likely diagnosis was of *post-tuberculous bronchiectasis with collapse of the left upper lobe*. 'Correct. Why, if the upper lobe collapses, do you get bronchial breath sounds but if the lower lobe collapses you only get reduced breath sounds?' I said: 'It depends in either case on whether there is patency of a major airway'. Examiner: 'No, it is because the upper airways are less dependent'. All I could say was: 'Oh!'.

I was then taken to a side room with the lights put out. Examiner: 'Examine this lady's eyes with the ophthalmoscope'. I did so and found background *diabetic retinopathy*. Examiner: 'Tell me about the pupils'. (We were in a pitch black room!) I had to tell him that I had

not examined the pupils properly as he had asked me to look at the fundi. Examiner: 'Put on the lights and have a look'. I did so. 'The right eye is dilated and the left eye is constricted,' I said. Examiner: 'Look at the eyelids'. I was staring in desperation. Examiner: 'Do you think she has a left-sided ptosis?' I said: 'No'. Examiner: 'Well, she has. She has a left *Horner's syndrome* and midriatics in the right eye'. What a case to end on! (Pass)

'Two stone-faced, non-committal, silent, disapproving examiners! Despite expecting this, it still threw me a bit.'

233. Two stone-faced, non-committal, silent, disapproving examiners! Despite expecting this, it still threw me a bit. The first case was *hepatosplenomegaly* in a patient with *polycythaemia rubra vera*. I got the signs, then was asked for a differential – was then told he had polycythaemia rubra vera and then asked the symptoms. This unnerved me.

I was then asked to look at a patient's right fundus. At first, all I could see were a couple of haemorrhages. They said: 'Would you like another look?'. I was convinced I had failed. I then asked if I could use my own ophthalmoscope (with a beam just down from a laser!) and found a *branch retinal artery occlusion* which I described, although I had never seen one before. This satisfied them and they asked me to test his visual fields which was easy and I demonstrated the *unilateral left lower quadrantanopia*.

Still convinced I had failed, I was taken to another patient and told to examine the legs as quickly as possible. I checked the foot pulses, then did a neurological examination. I demonstrated a mixed motor and sensory distal neuropathy, but the plantars kept going up! I said this was probably *subacute combined degeneration of the cord* in an elderly lady, and said why it was not motor neurone disease or Friedreich's ataxia but that syphilis was also a possibility. They asked how else I could demonstrate a plantar response. I did Oppenheim's test but they still looked vexed as the toes went up. They asked how else I could demonstrate plantars but I could not think of another answer.

Even more convinced I had failed, we went to a lady with a malar flush. I was asked to examine the pulse and I found slow atrial fibrillation. I described the face and then they asked me to auscultate. I picked up *mixed aortic* and *mixed mitral valve disease*. They asked me the cause, and I said rheumatic heart disease. They gave no impression that I was right but asked if she was in heart failure. I replied that they had not allowed me to listen to the lung bases or to look for ankle oedema, but that her pulse was not fast and there was no third heart sound. I looked at the jugular venous pressure and pointed out the systolic waves of *tricuspid incompetence*. Then the bell went.

Presumably I passed because I had my routines completely 'off pat', so I did not hesitate while examining; I got the signs because I had been to so many practice sessions and had seen everything except retinal artery branch occlusion before. Also, I had always practised presenting cases in a loud, clear voice on the grounds that if I was wrong, I might as well sound good and that if I was right I would come across as being confident in my diagnostic ability! (Pass)

'Nothing else was said and they didn't introduce themselves.'

234. At the start, the examiners said very little and they did not introduce themselves.

The first patient was a young woman with a long laparotomy scar, which was pointed out to me, and a distended abdomen. I was asked to examine the abdomen and to suggest an explanation. She had a *palpable liver*. I suggested it was a staging laparotomy but in fact it was a splenectomy scar. They wanted to know the reason so I suggested haemolytic anaemia.

I was then asked to examine the cerebellar system of a man who was unable to sit up. He had nystagmus, past pointing, dysdiadochokinesis and internuclear ophthalmoplegia. They wanted a cause so I gave *multiple sclerosis*. They wanted to know what one would look for in the lower limbs so I suggested pendular knee jerks but only after they had discarded my original suggestion of looking at the gait.

The next patient was a young woman with a *palpable thyroid* and a nodule at the isthmus (it was also diffusely enlarged, according to the examiner). She was clinically euthyroid with exophthalmos. However, when I examined her I thought she had a staring appearance without exophthalmos. The examiner wanted to know the histology of Graves' disease!

I was then asked to examine a man who was short of breath, and to look particularly at the cardiovascular system. He had a collapsing pulse, was in sinus rhythm, had a carotid pulse, a displaced heaving apex beat with an early diastolic murmur and an ejection systolic murmur at the aortic area radiating to the carotids. So I suggested *mixed aortic valve disease* with predominant incompetence. They did not say anything and moved straight to the next case.

I was asked to examine the man's abdomen. He had *hepatosplenomegaly* and they asked me how big the spleen was. I said it was eight finger-breadths but they made me go back and measure it. I made it 15 cm but they made it 8 cm! (Pass)

'For some perverse reason, my mouth said pseudobulbar palsy.'

235. The first case was a young lady with *multiple sclerosis*. I had to examine her legs, gait and fundi. The examiners interrupted me continuously and wanted firm, quick decisions and some common sense. The case was easy and went well.

They then gave me a little case history. 'This gentleman was admitted as an emergency with newly diagnosed diabetes mellitus. Would you feel his abdomen?' I was given all of 30 sec to feel his abdomen and they wanted to know what I would put my money on as the cause of the firm *mass in the epigastrium*. I do not think they really cared if it was correct but just that I had logically reached a reasonable differential.

We then went on to the next patient. The examiner said: 'This is a quick one. Just look at this fundus'. In retrospect, he had *senile macular degeneration* but I did not get it at the time. The chap was very restless indeed, thus making the examination tricky. I described what I had seen but said that I could not make a diagnosis.

I was then shown a gentleman with an *axillary vein thrombosis*. This was easy as he had a heparin pump. The examiners laughed about this when I came straight out with the diagnosis. They then wanted a few investigations that I would do and this was really quite straightforward.

The next case was a disaster! They gave me a short history of the man's symptoms. He had classic *bulbar palsy* because of the nasal regurgitation and dysphagia, etc. However, for some perverse reason, my mouth said pseudobulbar palsy although I immediately corrected myself. I then got mixed up over which way the uvula deviates with a unilateral palsy. The examiner then corrected me and I just kept smiling!

The last case was my redemption. We only had a few minutes left so I was asked to 'quickly auscultate' a patient. She had *mixed aortic* and *mitral valve disease* which I diagnosed almost immediately. They slowed me down and asked me to explain which murmurs I had heard. Looking back on it, I am sure that I had got them right. I actually overheard the examiners discuss me as I walked away (I have very acute hearing!). They were agreeing that my general performance was

OK and excusing the pseudobulbar disaster as nerves! (Pass)

Some 'fail' experiences

Examiners rarely let the candidate know whether their diagnosis is right or wrong, or whether their clinical examination technique is professional. In the same way that candidates may perceive they have performed poorly and yet pass, as illustrated above, candidates may also think that they have performed well and yet fail. Such candidates may feel that the exam is unfair without being aware of the imperfections in the performance they gave, or that some of their diagnoses were wrong. In the following accounts, some of the candidates recognized that they should have failed but some did not.

'If she had Huntington's at that age, would she be doing the crossword puzzle in the newspaper?'

236. The first patient that I was taken to see was an elderly woman. The examiner said: 'This woman came to the thyroid clinic. What would you write in the notes after examining her eyes?'. I tried to test visual acuity but was told to examine the eye movements. I thought she had a left VIth cranial nerve palsy but the examiner seemed unhappy with this. I then said that she had a thyroid ophthalmoplegia. He asked whether it bothered me that the *proptosis* was in the other eye? I was not sure!

The next patient was a middle-aged woman with *eruptive xanthomas* over the elbows and knees.

We then moved on to the next case. This was an elderly woman who was constantly fidgeting with either choreiform or athetoid-type movements. I was asked to have a few words with her. She sounded a bit dysarthric. I was asked for the diagnosis and I wanted to say Huntington's chorea but did not wish to say so in front of the patient. So I tried to say a hereditary chorea. The examiner said: 'Like what?'. So I said: 'Huntington's'. He said if she had Huntington's at that age, would she be doing the crossword puzzle in the newspaper? I said: 'No'. I had not actually noticed that she was doing this beforehand. He asked me for another diagnosis. I hesitated but eventually got *drug-induced dyskinesia*.

I was then shown a man with very *deformed arthritic hands*. I pushed up his sleeves and showed the *psoriatic plaques* on the forearms and elbows. The disease looked burnt out so when she asked me what I would treat this man with, I said non-steroidals. She looked irritated and said: 'What else?'. I suggested coal tar or dithranol

for the skin. She was still not satisfied and walked off to the next case.

'Examine the cardiovascular system.' I examined the patient in silence and she then asked for my findings. Initially, I just said *mitral incompetence*. So she said: 'As manifest by . . . ?'. I then gave her my findings. The other examiner asked me if the pulse was in atrial fibrillation and I said it was not.

The next patient was a respiratory system case. I thought the percussion was a bit dull at the left base and said that there was a small, left, pleural effusion. They made me examine the *trachea* again but I still did not think it was *displaced*. She then told me to percuss out the chest again. By this time the bell had gone. They did not seem at all pleased about this last case. The senior registrar who led me away said: 'Don't worry about the chest – it's a tricky one'. (Fail)

'If I were examining the examiner, he would have failed!'

237. The examiner asked me to look at a woman's neck. She was sitting in a chair and she had obvious *proptosis and a goitre*. I went straight to the neck and told the examiner that she had a visible goitre. He seemed irritated by this, but I thought he was just trying to put me off my stride, so I continued with what I thought was a faultless presentation.

The same rotten examiner, who was young and abrasive, then asked me to examine a woman's cerebellar system. I asked for her address and he shouted: 'What are you doing?'. 'Examining her speech, sir,' I replied. 'But we have quotes for that,' he retorted. Again I thought he was just seeing if I would crack up. So I replied: 'Yes, sir, but I can hardly walk up to the lady and say, "Hello Mrs J, I am Dr S and can you say hippopotamus?"'! I moved on to finger–nose testing which demonstrated *gross ataxia*. I looked for nystagmus which I could not find but was asked about vertical nystagmus. I also demonstrated dysdiadochokinesis. He asked me to examine her legs so I began with: 'May I see the lady walk?'. He gave me a curt reply: 'She can't walk'. I then tested power, tone, heel–shin test, and he stopped me again abruptly. 'This lady has had some injections years ago, what other system do you want to examine?'. I confessed that I had no idea as I thought that I was looking at the cerebellar problem. He then said: 'Posterior columns'. I still do not know what the connection was. First I examined joint position sense – I thought I would get some extra marks here as I had demonstrated the technique to the patient and she complied well. Then I tested vibration sense – I examined sternal sensation first and then the sensation peripherally. 'What else?' he said. I retorted: 'Two-point discrimination, sir'. 'Yes, yes, what else?' He was obviously irritated and I said I did not know what he meant. So he said: 'Deep pain' and then he grabbed the woman's heels. If I were examining the examiner, he would have failed! However, I still felt he was trying to rile me so I continued, still believing I was doing well.

The next two cases were a *mixed mitral valve disease* and *psoriatic arthropathy* and I had no problems with either of these.

The final case was a patient with *hepatosplenomegaly* and nodes, which was possibly chronic lymphatic leukaemia and again I had no problems here.

Overall, I felt that I had coped with the examination and I went home feeling fairly confident that I had passed. However, I failed. I wrote to the College and they told me that I had failed on my neurology case. I talked to a local examiner and when I told him what had happened he said that the examiner must be new and that it all sounded very unfair. I still feel that he was unfair and now having passed the exam on the fifth attempt without doing anywhere near as well as on this attempt, I still say that the whole exam is very unfair! (Fail)

'I was asked about the severity of the lesion (aortic incompetence), how long it had been present and whether an operation was indicated. I was totally unprepared for this.'

238. I was initially taken to a young, well-looking patient and was asked to listen to the heart. He had a systolic murmur at the apex, normal heart sounds and no click. I volunteered a *mitral valve prolapse*. The examiner asked about the heart sounds which I said were normal. I think I was right on this case.

I was then asked to look at a patient's fundus having been told that he was completely blind. I found a *cataract* and *retinitis pigmentosa*. I stood up and the examiner asked if I had a diagnosis. I told him my findings and he asked about *optic atrophy* – I had not even looked! I said the discs were normal but they cannot have been.

The next case was: 'Please examine this man's chest from the front'. There was a slightly red patch on the right side of his chest. I watched him take a deep breath and was stopped and asked for my findings. All I had found was the red area which I suggested might be caused by radiotherapy for a bronchial neoplasm. I then found that the trachea was deviated to the left. Also the left hemithorax expanded poorly and the percussion note was impaired. I was then stopped and asked for the diagnosis. For some reason I said neoplasia. I am sure he had *old tuberculosis* at the left apex, and the mark on the right was incidental.

I was then taken to the next patient and was told that his GP had referred him to the clinic because he had a heart murmur and wondered about mitral incompetence. I found signs of lone *aortic incompetence* and thought that the diagnosis alone would satisfy the examiners. The signs were so straightforward that 99% of candidates would get them right. I was asked about the severity of the lesion, how long it had been present and whether an operation was indicated. I was totally unprepared for this and answered badly.

I was told that my next patient had been referred with anaemia and that I should examine her abdomen to find out why. The examiners 'tutted' as I looked at her hands, mouth, neck glands, etc. and impatiently hurried me on. She had *hepatosplenomegaly* and, although I was exceedingly gentle and explained what I was doing, she winced repeatedly. I appealed to the examiners – should I carry on? – but they remained impassive! I gave a list of different lymphoproliferative disorders to the examiners as I had also found numerous *lymph nodes in her axillae*.

I was taken to my last patient and was instructed to ask her some questions. I asked her for her name and she replied with a *cerebellar dysarthria*. I was asked for one other sign that I would like to look for and I proceeded to demonstrate that she had finger–nose ataxia. I volunteered cerebellar disease and suggested demyelination as the cause. One examiner grunted and the other wandered off! (Fail)

'The last patient had polycystic kidneys which I called hepatosplenomegaly. This was probably the final nail in the coffin.'

239. For my first patient I was asked to look in the eyes and I found *optic atrophy*. It was the first time I had ever seen it and I nearly said so! However, I had failed to notice the white stick and the aphakic spectacles.

I was then asked to look at a lady's face. I found a *Horner's syndrome* and again it was the first I had ever seen. I just managed to give a few causes.

For my third patient I was asked to examine a chest. I had no idea what the diagnosis was so I re-examined the front. There was dullness to percussion with reduced expansion and *coarse crepitations at the right upper zone*. I suggested fibrosis, tuberculosis or asbestosis. However, the patient also had an *ataxia*. I was hampered by the examiners asking for my findings at 10-sec intervals!

I was then taken to a patient and asked to: 'Listen here' (they pointed to the left sternal edge, fifth intercostal space). There was *mixed aortic valve disease* and I had been asked to auscultate only. There were no problems here and I was not asked for any causes or investigations or treatment.

The last patient had *polycystic kidneys* which I called hepatosplenomegaly. This was probably the final nail in the coffin. (Fail)

'I felt it was tapping and said so. This was a big error as it wasn't.'

240. 'This man has been referred by his GP because of a heart murmur. Examine his cardiovascular system and say what you think.' I was allowed to make a full examination and diagnosed *aortic stenosis*. They did not seem happy and asked: 'Did you hear any other murmurs?'. I had not and said so.

I was given the same history for the second patient. I was only allowed to feel the pulse briefly before being told that it was normal and to proceed to feel the *apex beat*. This was abnormal and slightly *displaced*. I felt it was tapping* and said so. This was a big error as it was not. On auscultation I had to amend my diagnosis. There followed a discussion about the different types of apex beat. I was able to answer all their questions quite well but I knew I had done badly on the first two cases.

I was then asked to look at a man's hands. He had classic *dermatomyositis* and I described it as such. However, I had to be prompted to test for muscle power which was much reduced.

For the next patient I was asked to examine the abdomen. It was a young man with *massive splenomegaly* and no other abnormalities. I was asked for a possible diagnosis so I said that it was possibly a myeloproliferative or lymphoproliferative disorder. They told me that it was not and asked for other diagnoses. I started to say: 'In a tropical country . . .' but was stopped. The examiner suggested that hepatic disease might cause such splenomegaly. I answered that it would be unusual to cause such massive splenomegaly and they agreed. I subsequently found out that the diagnosis was *sarcoid*.

I was then asked to examine a patient's fundi. The first retina showed scarring that did not really look like laser burns. I gave a differential diagnosis of diabetes with laser treatment or choroidoretinitis. They asked me to look in the other eye but not to take so long about it this time. The second retina showed similar scarring but also small haemorrhages, giving the diagnosis of a *diabetic retinopathy*. I was asked what I thought of my differential diagnosis of choroidoretinitis and answered that I thought it had been a mistake!

The last patient was a complicated one with heart failure, a raised jugular venous pressure and a pleural effusion. I know now that the diagnosis was *constrictive pericarditis* (from my college tutor). I badly muddled this short case and knew that I had failed the short cases outright. (Fail)

'They asked for a diagnosis. I tentatively said subacute bacterial endocarditis (I later found out it was hereditary haemorrhagic telangiectasia).'

241. Probable *diabetic fundus*. The patient had very thick glasses on and the examiners asked me to take them off. The ophthalmoscope was one I had not come across before and I could not focus it. I was too nervous to remember I had brought one with me in my handbag! (Incidentally, I would advise all female candidates not to take a handbag – they are just a nuisance.) I saw a few exudates and haemorrhages but was very unsure. This was a very bad start.

Then I was asked to examine a young man's chest. In retrospect, I found that it was *ankylosing spondylitis*. However, I managed to convince myself that he had unilateral signs consistent with an effusion and so I presented them. The examiners just said: 'Umm . . .' and moved me on!

I was asked to examine a man's cardiovascular system. He had atrial fibrillation, *prosthetic heart valve sounds* and also I thought he had a systolic murmur. However, I was very unsure what it all was. They said: 'So you don't think there is a diastolic murmur?'. I said:

---

*The expression 'tapping apex beat', commonly used even by some cardiologists and sadly in some books, is a contradiction of terms. The apex beat is a distinct, localizable impulse caused by the recoil of the left ventricle during systole, whereas the tapping impulse is the sharp, indistinct and non-localizable palpable first heart sound caused by the forcible closure of the mitral valve and the rocking of the left atrium. In fact, in severe, lone mitral stenosis with a pronounced tapping impulse (in the left parasternal area), the left ventricle is underactive and the apex beat impalpable.

'No' and we moved on (in retrospect I found out that he had *aortic valve disease*!).

I was asked to examine a man's abdomen. They did not let me look at the hands (see Vol. 1, Section B, Examination *Routine* 4), etc. and I found that he had *hepatomegaly*. However, I could not palpate a spleen although I did not turn him over or palpate bimanually. In retrospect, he was deathly pale and presumably had a myelo- or lymphoproliferative disorder. They then showed me what I thought was senile purpura – they dragged out of me that he might be on steroids and asked the mechanism for the discoloration. I talked about capillary fragility but he said: 'No, no, it's all to do with macrophages', in a tone of voice that made me feel really stupid for not knowing.

I was asked to examine a frail-looking lady with *ascites* and *deep jaundice*. I was asked just to assess what I thought was the most important sign from a practical point of view. So I looked for a *liver flap*. They asked about other causes for a flap.

I was shown a lady with cyanosis, clubbing and multiple petechiae and splinter haemorrhages (I thought!) and they asked for a diagnosis. I tentatively said subacute bacterial endocarditis and they gave me another chance but I could not come up with anything else so we moved on. I later found out it was *hereditary haemorrhagic telangiectasia*.

I was shown a young woman with a burn on her hand and an amputated finger. I suggested a sensory problem but they then gave me a clue by telling me that she was unable to move her hand away from trauma in time. I then asked her to grip my hand and she had obvious *myotonia*.

The next patient was a young boy with a *Horner's syndrome*. I was asked what question I would like to ask him and I enquired if he had had any neck surgery. (Fail)

'I said: "Demyelinating disease". The examiner asked me what I meant by that so I said: "Multiple sclerosis". The other examiner who was just approaching us at that moment said: "Never say that, say demyelinating disease!".'

242. My first patient looked as if she was of Mediterranean origin but I thought she had *polycystic kidneys*. The examiners asked me why it was not a large spleen and had I thought of thalassaemia as she looked Greek. I was uncertain after this but said to the examiners that I thought I could get above the masses. Most of the candidates who I spoke to afterwards thought this was polycystic disease but the registrar on duty would not comment.

The second patient was a young, fit man who had a corrected *Fallot's tetralogy*. There was a mid-systolic murmur loudest all along the left sternal edge. Initially, I said it was aortic stenosis despite the fact that there was an easily visible sternotomy scar. I was asked if it was usual to have a stenotic murmur after a cardiac operation and the penny eventually dropped!

The third patient had *diabetic retinopathy*. It was a simple background retinopathy and the pupils had been dilated.

The fourth patient had *rheumatoid hands*. I was just asked to describe the findings and not to examine. I began saying that she had a symmetrical deforming polyarthropathy and was then dragged off to the next patient who had pulmonary fibrosis.

I was asked to list the possible causes and what was the most likely cause in this patient. I said idiopathic *fibrosing alveolitis*. The patient was a fit, middle-aged woman with no other problems. 'What one question would you ask?' I suggested asking what her occupation was and they said that would be more appropriate if the patient was male. 'Anything else?' they said. I asked her if she kept any animals and they led me away.

The next patient had a *spastic paraparesis*. I was asked to examine the legs and the examiners were very pleased when I asked to see the patient walk first but I then got myself into a discussion about the various types of gait. 'Would you like to do anything else?' they asked. 'I would like to examine the fundi and the spine,' I replied. 'Good,' they said. They asked me what the most likely cause was, so I said: 'Demyelinating disease'. The examiner asked me what I meant by that so I said: 'Multiple sclerosis'. The other examiner who was just approaching us at that moment said: 'Never say that, say demyelinating disease!'.

Once again the short cases were late. The examiners seemed very fed up and annoyed right from the start. I was questioned *en route* between patients while I was trying to keep up with them. At one point the examiner in the front turned abruptly to look at the examiner coming up behind me and said: 'What did she say?'. The examiner behind me (who was really fed up) said: 'How should I know?'. I said: 'Shall I start again?' and they both roared: 'No time!'. (Fail)

'During auscultation one examiner pulled me from the patient by the back of my suit!'

243. 'This patient is breathless, find out why as quickly as possible.' I did not spot the *flattening of the apex on the right* and was asked to look again. I thought that the trachea was central, even on re-examination, but then said that I would not argue with the chest X-ray! The examiner seemed displeased.

The next case was: 'Examine the patient cardiovascularly'. There was fast atrial fibrillation at a rate of approximately 120 beats/min together with *mitral facies and a thoracotomy scar*. There was also a median sternotomy scar. The jugular venous pulse was difficult to see and I was told to move on. During auscultation one examiner pulled me away from the patient by the back of my suit! I described the findings and said that I did not know what the underlying diagnosis was. I was told to give a diagnosis: 'Come on – three, two, one, going, going, gone!'.

The next patient had a large spleen with no lymphadenopathy or hepatomegaly. The diagnosis, I thought, was *myelofibrosis*. The examiner wanted a list of the other possible diagnoses which I gave him.

When we got to the fourth patient the examiner said: 'Examine this patient's eyes'. We were in a darkened room so I asked whether just to look at the fundi. They said: 'Look at everything'. I asked for the lights to be turned up in order to check acuity, fields, pupils and movements. There was no abnormality found. However, the patient had classic *optic atrophy* in the left eye on fundoscopy. I was asked for a differential diagnosis and the possible significance of the field defect. (Apparently he had a *bitemporal hemianopia* and a *pituitary tumour*.)

For the last patient I was again asked to examine the cardiovascular system. There was a collapsing pulse. I was stopped and asked what the diagnosis was. I said this could be *aortic regurgitation* and listed the findings that I would expect. I finished examining the patient and confirmed the findings of aortic incompetence. We then discussed the Austin Flint murmur.

The examiners were quite rude. Even if my examination technique was not good enough to pass the exam, I do not expect to be grabbed by the back of the suit. The examiners should not use their unfair advantage to behave in a way which would be completely unacceptable in public! (Fail)

Four months later I resat the exam. My first short case was: 'Examine this man's abdomen'. I said I would like to move the bed in order to examine him from the correct side. Their response was: 'Extra marks for moving the bed in Part II!'. When the bed came apart in their hands and I had reassembled it and then moved it, the examiner said: 'Extra marks for knowing how the bed works!'. Eventually, the findings were of *hepatosplenomegaly* and a small amount of *ascites*. There were no stigmata of chronic liver disease or lymphadenopathy. I said that the possible diagnoses were . . .

When we arrived at the second patient the examiner said: 'Examine this patient's hair'. She had a full head of hair and eyebrows but little on her forearms and none in her axillae. I was then allowed to ask if she had ever had hair here, and she said: 'Yes'. She looked mildly cushingoid and the skin was fine and thin. I thought the diagnosis was of *panhypopituitarism* in a patient who had been given steroid replacement. I said: 'The possible causes are . . . and would you like me to check the visual fields?'.

The third patient had proliferative retinopathy and maculopathy.

For the next patient the examiners said: 'This man is breathless. Would you examine him?'. He looked as though he had *ankylosing spondylitis* so I asked him to look up but he could not. I said this was likely to be the diagnosis and described the possible associated features of kyphosis and upper lobe fibrosis with a restrictive deficit. The examiner then asked me to examine his eyes. I found *proptosis* with no lid lag or exophthalmos. He was clinically euthyroid with no goitre and I said the most likely diagnosis was of dysthyroid eye disease. The examiner asked if there was any connection and I said: 'No'.

I was then asked to listen to a patient's heart. I felt the apex and the carotid pulse which I then used to time the murmur at the same time as assessing its character. I found *mitral stenosis* and sinus rhythm. I said that the patient had mitral stenosis because of the loud first heart sound and the mid-diastolic murmur with a presystolic accentuation. There was no evidence of pulmonary hypertension.

I was then taken to a patient with a *skin rash*. I described it and said it did not have the characteristics of psoriasis, eczema or lichen planus, etc. I said I really did not know what it was. The examiners said they did not know either and were going to biopsy it!

The last patient had an asymmetrical oligoarthropathy in the small joints of the hands. The examiners seemed to like the quick routine I had been shown which assessed function of all joints, grip and power, pincer and opposition, and fine finger movements. She was a West Indian girl with patchy depigmentation on the face. I said the differential diagnosis of oligoarthropathy included *systemic lupus erythematosus* which turned out to be the actual diagnosis.

On this occasion the examiners were very pleasant and no one grabbed me by the back of my suit! (Pass)

Downward spirals

'I completely collapsed when one of my short case examiners introduced herself as Dr X.'

244. I had heard the previous day from a colleague who had also been examined at Newham General that he had encountered a woman examiner who had given him a really difficult time. My anxiety about this was increased when someone else reported: 'I hope it isn't Dr X, she fails everyone!' followed by a few other stories. I completely collapsed when one of my short case examiners introduced herself as Dr X.

Short case 1: cardiology – a young West Indian woman. 'Examine the cardiovascular system.' I thought she had mixed *mitral and aortic valve disease*. There was absolutely no feedback from the examiners as to whether this was right or wrong.

Short case 2: neurology – a young Asian man. 'Examine these legs.' There was a *spastic paraparesis* and a *peripheral neuropathy*. I was heavily criticized for attempting to demonstrate cerebellar signs in someone who was obviously very weak but I attempted to defend this. I then became very flustered when asked to list the causes of this combination of signs. I handled all this very badly and even when pushed on the issue of the man's ethnicity and what I should be considering (presumably tuberculosis causing a cord compression), I remained pretty inarticulate. From here on there was a complete loss of confidence and everything was badly handled.

Short case 3: abdomen – an elderly, wasted, ill-looking lady. 'Examine the abdomen.' I found a *hepatic mass* and *1 cm splenomegaly*. There was no ascites. I described the findings as above. The examiner started pushing me on the causes of the mass (which was attached to, but discrete from, the liver). I felt uncomfortable as he had not moved away from the patient's bed and to my horror I ended up saying what I had kept avoiding saying – the word 'tumour' in front of the patient. I knew this was a disaster.

Short case 4: chest – a middle-aged, obese man. 'Examine the respiratory system.' I found *clubbing* as well as very traumatized nails (multiple peripheral splinters). There was poor chest wall movement bilaterally with inspiratory and expiratory crepitations. I suggested *fibrotic lung disease* with an intercurrent infective exacerbation. There was no feedback at all from the examiners. (Fail)

'The examiner was aware I was bluffing and asked for more and more detail.'

245. I was first taken to a gentleman and asked to examine his abdomen. I grabbed for his hand after introducing myself but was told firmly, but politely, to stick to the abdomen. I found a *small spleen* and at this point the examiner stopped me and asked for my findings. He then requested me to ask the patient three questions to elucidate a cause. I asked about alcohol abuse and travel abroad (in particular, malaria) and then I was stumped so I asked a daft question about rheumatoid arthritis (thinking of Felty's syndrome). This was silly because I had already had a look at the gentleman's hands! It annoyed the examiner because it was at the bottom of his differential diagnosis!

I was then led to a fully dressed lady and asked to listen to her aortic area and to decide whether she had aortic incompetence. They did not like it when I tried to take her sweatshirt off to examine her properly. They expected me to examine her around her clothing. I was not sure whether I could hear an aortic incompetent murmur because I had never been convinced by one in the past! So I did a daft thing again and said I thought there was one. He then asked me what other features I would look for on general examination. We went through all of these and of course she did not have any of them. At this point he asked me to look at her generally and it was then that I noticed her malar flush and peripheral oedema. He suggested these were more in keeping with mitral valve disease and asked me to listen for this. I heard a *mitral incompetent murmur*. I was very uptight over my errors from the last case and annoyed because I felt I had been deliberately misled.*

I was then taken to the one case I particularly dread, *diplopia*, and was asked to examine the visual movements. I totally went to pieces and did this very badly. I was unable to establish what the lesion was even after the examiner tried to help. He seemed particularly interested in the *nystagmus* and the direction in which it was maximal. I wondered if I had missed ataxic nystagmus and the diplopia of multiple sclerosis.

I was then taken to a lady and asked to examine her fundi. She had definite *diabetic retinopathy* and after stepping back ready to say this, the examiner said to me that there were no prizes for the diagnosis. It was obviously diabetic retinopathy but could I describe in detail

---

*The examiner would argue that your houseman would not be unfair in asking you to check if a patient had aortic incompetence, even if he had not heard the early diastolic murmur himself. This is, after all, the most missed valvular lesion.

what I saw and where each feature was! I should probably have admitted defeat but instead I strung together what I had seen and made up the position of these relative to the disc. The examiner was aware I was bluffing and asked for more and more detail.

He then took me to a lady and announced that she had had atrial fibrillation and asked me to suggest a cause. I noticed a *thyroidectomy scar* and so offered thyrotoxicosis. I was asked to examine for this and found her clinically euthyroid but with exophthalmos. Presumably, she had had thyrotoxicosis treated in the past. He then asked for another cause so I suggested mitral valve disease and then noticed a mid-sternal scar. He asked me to listen to her mitral valve which I did literally. At this point I got a sarcastic comment: 'Can you pretend this is the MRCP and examine the heart properly?'. By now exasperated, I retorted that he had asked me to listen to the mitral valve and he did concede this. I proceeded to listen to the precordium and heard a *prosthetic valve* but was unable to remember how to distinguish between mitral and aortic prostheses. Again, I bluffed and probably got it wrong. With very little comment I was dismissed.

I was thrown in this attempt by the fact that although the cases were relatively straightforward, either the questions or the approach to each case was not. There seemed to be a deliberate attempt to confuse me and to lead me astray. I found it useful the second time round to think about the different ways a short case could be presented other than the straightforward 'Examine this cardiovascular system'. I also learnt by experience that it is helpful to have some 'answers' ready relating to lists of common causes of, for example, splenomegaly. (Fail)

'I forgot to assess her speech and only knew one way to demonstrate dysdiadochokinesis.'

246. I was taken to the first patient and the examiner said: 'Examine this lady's cardiovascular system'. After I presented my findings of lone *mitral incompetence*, he said: 'Did you hear mitral stenosis?'. My reply was: 'No'. He said: 'Did you hear aortic valve disease?'. Again my reply was: 'No'.

We went to the next patient. The examiner said: 'Examine this lady's *cerebellar signs* from the waist up'. This was the start of the downward spiral syndrome. I forgot to assess her speech and only knew one way to demonstrate dysdiadochokinesis. The examiner was not impressed.

For the third case he said: 'Look at this lady's hands'. She had *rheumatoid arthritis* and I even remembered to

look for, and noticed, the cushingoid facies. However, the follow-up question was a 'killer'. 'Outline your surgical options here.' I was stuffed!

The fourth case was: 'Look at this *fundus*'. I could not see a thing! She was middle-aged and therefore I went for diabetic retinopathy. I still do not know whether I was right or not.

The examiner led me on. 'Look at this lady's hands.' She had *hereditary haemorrhagic telangiectasia*. We talked about inheritance, presentation and management. At last I had a decent case!

The final patient was: 'Examine this man's abdomen'. He had massive *splenomegaly* and *lymphadenopathy*. All my examiner wanted to know was what I knew about *Waldenström's macroglobulinaemia*! (Fail)

'The examiners were very upset and so was I.'

247. I was asked to examine a lady's chest and I hurt her during the examination. The examiners were very upset and so was I. The whole exam went downhill from there onwards. This particular patient, however, had a *right lower lobe fibrosis* from tuberculosis.

The examiners then said to me: 'What does that man have?'. They were pointing to a gentleman who was disappearing through a door at the time. I correctly replied *ankylosing spondylitis*.

I was then taken to another gentleman and asked if he needed treatment. He had a definite *parkinsonian tremor* with rigidity and a little bradykinesia but was walking very well. I said, 'Not at the moment' and explained why.

I was then asked to comment on another patient's rash. It was of fading *erythema nodosum* on the legs of a girl of about 20 years. They asked about the most common cause in this age group. I said Crohn's disease and ulcerative colitis and the examiners replied: 'Good'.

I was then taken to the next patient and asked to examine his eyes. I really muddled this up! I asked to test his visual acuity but he had not brought his reading glasses with him. I then missed a *central scotoma* and *optic atrophy*!

The next patient was an 'Examine this lady's abdomen'. She had a 2 cm liver and a 4 cm spleen. They uncovered her chest and asked the diagnosis. She had multiple spider naevi so I suggested *chronic liver disease*. At last the examiners seemed happy!

I was taken to the next patient. 'Your house officer thinks this man has had a *cerebrovascular accident* (CVA), do you agree?' I thought he had had a CVA affecting the left side but they were not happy that the right side was normal. I did not look for fasciculation and I wondered if he actually had motor neurone disease.

The last patient was a spot diagnosis and I was asked to just look. It was a girl who was covered from her shoulders downwards. She had a positive Corrigan's sign and I said that she probably had *aortic regurgitation*. They asked if she needed surgery so I said: 'Yes', after feeling a collapsing pulse. (Fail)

Anecdotes

The examination setting brings into play its own circumstances and idiosyncrasies which may influence, or even interfere with, the process of the examination. The examiner may wilfully or unknowingly hide a crucial clue and the patient may volunteer a helpful suggestion, all of which enrich the candidate's experience. In this section we present a collection of short anecdotes which reflect the varied and often unexpected scenarios of the exam. The pass/fail conclusion at the end of each anecdote should not be attributed to the anecdote alone; it reflects simply whether the candidate passed or failed the whole exam.

248. A candidate was asked: 'Examine the back of this man's chest'. He found a left thoracotomy scar in a man in his thirties. Even though the examiners were standing in front of it, trying to stop him seeing it, he managed to spot the sputum pot and diagnosed bronchiectasis. (Pass)

249. While examining the fundi, the candidate pressed the wrong button on the new type of ophthalmoscope that he had been given and the batteries fell out! The examiners handed him an older ophthalmoscope with which he was more familiar and he went on to diagnose proliferative diabetic retinopathy with a lot of fibrosis. (Fail)

250. A candidate was asked to examine the abdomen. She started with the hands but was told: 'No, just the abdomen'. There was a 15 cm spleen palpable with an obvious notch and liver just palpable on deep inspiration. After presenting her findings, she was asked why she had auscultated. She said that listening to bowel sounds was part of her normal examination of the abdomen. They asked if it was relevant to the patient in question and she answered: 'No'. They then asked that if she had auscultated over the spleen what might

she have heard? She was then asked about the significance of a splenic rub! The likely diagnosis was discussed although it is not clear whether or not the patient actually had a splenic rub. (Pass)

251. A candidate was asked to feel a patient's abdomen. He found a mass in the left hypochondrium which felt like a polycystic kidney but was dull to percussion, moved medially with respiration and was not ballottable. The examiners asked him what he thought it was. The candidate said that he was unsure and expressed his dilemma, based on the signs he had found. The examiners said: 'If you could ask one question, what would it be?'. The candidate said: 'Does anyone in your family have kidney disease?'. The patient answered: 'Yes'. The candidate then went on to ask 'Is it polycystic kidneys?'. The patient answered: 'Yes'. The candidate turned to the examiners and said: 'I'm sorry, I asked two questions'. The examiners laughed and at that moment the bell went. (Pass)

252. A candidate was asked: 'Examine this young lady's abdomen'. She found a 20–30-year-old woman with obvious abdominal distension who otherwise looked well. There was slight hirsutism, no lymphadenopathy, no mouth signs and a mass arising from the pelvis. There was no spleen on palpation or percussion and no palpable liver or kidneys. The examiners asked: 'What do you think this is?'. The candidate summarized the findings and said she thought that the patient might be pregnant. 'Do you think we would include a pregnant woman in the MRCP exam?' asked the examiners. 'You might,' the candidate replied. The other examiner said: 'Yes, we might, it's an unfair exam! Would you like to re-examine her to see if there is a spleen?'. The candidate demonstrated again that there was not. The candidate reports that she was led away feeling unsure of what she had missed. She later rang the organizing registrar who said that the diagnosis was not known but that she had a pelvic mass and an enlarged spleen on ultrasound. (Pass)

253. A candidate was shown a West Indian lady who had a wig and a Bell's palsy. He got the Bell's palsy and was then asked to look at her head. She had severe, scarring alopecia and he was asked to give some possible causes. He suggested trauma and/or autoimmune disease but was not really sure what the correct diagnosis was. When he got home his mother told him that she believes she would have got that one right – it follows attempts to straighten the hair! (Pass)

254. A candidate was asked to examine the chest of a patient 'from the front only'. She found all the findings compatible with a left, upper zone fibrosis/collapse and suggested that this could be caused by previous tuberculosis. She was then allowed to inspect the patient's back which revealed a thoracoplasty scar. The candidate was told that she was correct. (Pass)

255. A candidate was asked to examine a chest from the back only. He noticed a left lower thoracotomy scar but failed to mention it or to put any of the other clinical signs he found together. He told us the examiners took the opportunity to hang, draw and quarter him! (Fail)

256. A candidate was asked to examine a woman's legs and found erythema ab igne. The examiners then asked for the differential diagnosis of reticular rashes on the legs and for the different skin biopsy appearances! (Pass)

257. A candidate was asked to examine a patient's cardiovascular system. He found several murmurs and suggested patent ductus arteriosus but he is still not sure whether that was correct. He commented that the examiners were irritated because he felt the pulse first. They seemed to want him to go straight to the precordium, even though they had asked for a 'cardiovascular system' examination. (Pass)

258. While giving her findings for a patient with aortic regurgitation, a candidate mentioned Corrigan's pulse. The examiner asked: 'Who was Corrigan?', although she thought he was not too serious when asking this! They then went on to ask her for the causes of aortic regurgitation and they felt that she should have mentioned degenerative valve disease higher up on her list. (Pass)

259. A candidate was asked to examine a patient's eyes and then the neck. He found unilateral proptosis and a goitre and diagnosed thyrotoxicosis. However, he did not notice the proptosis until he looked from above. (Pass)

260. A candidate was asked to examine a lady's left fundus as she had deteriorating vision in the left eye. He started to examine the right eye and the examiner said: 'Actually, I have told you that the problem is in her left eye!'. The diagnosis was a branch retinal artery occlusion. (Fail)

261. A candidate was asked to examine an abdomen. He found a palpable left kidney which he suspected to be either polycystic or hydronephrotic. There was also a mass in the right iliac fossa which he thought was probably a transplanted kidney. (Pass)

262. A candidate was asked to look at a man's hands. He found purple, swollen fingers with no arthritis, nail involvement or evidence of scleroderma but he noted some telangiectasia on his face and lips. He was told that he could ask the patient some questions to determine the cause. He said he thought the patient had Raynaud's disease but wondered retrospectively if this may have been a case of CREST syndrome. He reported: 'The examiners wanted the causes of Raynaud's phenomenon and for me to look for evidence of diseases such as scleroderma, systemic lupus erythematosus, etc. They wanted me to ask the patient if he worked with vibrating tools and what happened to his hands if he put them into cold water'. (Pass)

263. 'Look at this man's abdomen and describe what you see.' The candidate found a distended abdomen in a middle-aged man who had tattoos, an everted umbilicus, reduced body hair and purpura. The examiners asked, 'What else would you look for?'. He said: 'Jaundice, spider naevi, Dupuytren's contractures and leuconychia'. He was then asked to look for these signs which were all present. Then he was requested to examine the man's abdomen. This revealed marked ascites and a tender, two finger-breadths liver but no splenomegaly. As they were walking away, they asked him the likely cause of his signs and he answered, 'Alcohol-related liver disease'. The examiners asked him why he thought this and he replied that the patient was wearing a T-shirt advertising Foster's beer! They smiled! (Pass)

264. A candidate was asked to examine a patient's abdomen. He found hepatosplenomegaly. The examiners then showed him the arteriovenous shunt and asked him to re-examine the abdomen. His diagnosis then became polycystic kidneys! He was sure he had failed outright but tried to keep his head, remembering that it was possible to get by with one disaster! (Pass)

265. A candidate was asked to examine the abdomen of a woman with jaundice and hepatosplenomegaly. The examiners got annoyed when he started with examining her hands. (Pass)

266. A candidate reported that his examiners started 5 min late and he was not given any extra time. He had to undress three of the patients and get them positioned correctly. He also found explaining his findings as he went along difficult as one of the examiners appeared very deaf! (Pass)

267. A candidate was asked to examine the respiratory system of a patient with chronic bronchitis and emphysema. He was asked if there was loss of cardiac dullness. He examined for this and found that there was. (Pass)

268. A candidate was asked: 'Look at this rash in a 16-year-old girl'. There was a maculopapular rash on the limbs but not on the trunk. There was no involvement of the eyes, nails, joints or mouth. He was asked what the diagnosis was and if he would like to ask the patient some questions. The condition had been present for 5 years and the joints were painful. He offered the differential diagnosis of juvenile chronic arthritis or systemic lupus erythematosus. In retrospect, he feels it was the former (Still's disease). (Pass)

269. A candidate was asked to examine the abdomen of a woman who weighed 'about 20 stone'. He found two subcostal masses and diagnosed hepatosplenomegaly. In retrospect, he was sure that they were polycystic kidneys and that arguing the case for hepatosplenomegaly made matters worse and wasted a lot of time. (Fail)

270. The examiner said: 'This gentleman is icteric, please examine his abdomen'. He found hepatomegaly and a mid-line laparotomy scar. He presented these findings. 'Does he have ascites?' He told the examiner that his findings were equivocal and that an ultrasound was needed to define this. 'Does he have splenomegaly?' He replied that he could not feel a spleen but there was a dullness to percussion over the splenic area. He was counselled after he had failed the exam. Apparently the liver that he had felt was a palpable gallbladder. The examiner's comments were: 'He refused to commit himself as to the presence of ascites and hedged on the presence of splenomegaly'. (Fail)

271. A candidate was asked to examine a patient's left eye with the ophthalmoscope provided. He reported that he found optic atrophy, a detached retina, laser photocoagulation scars and aphakia. He suggested that the patient had had a diabetic cataract previously. The examiner asked about primary and secondary optic atrophy and then asked about the refractive error of the patient – covering the head of the ophthalmoscope with his hand as he did so! (Pass)

272. A candidate was asked to look in a patient's eye. He could find no abnormality and said so. He was then informed that he had looked into the left eye, whereas he had actually been asked to look into the right eye! The examiners were both laughing, although the candidate was embarrassed and very apologetic. The right eye showed obvious optic atrophy and he was then asked for a list of possible causes. (Pass)

273. A candidate was asked to examine a patient who had a right pleural effusion – the patient was very deaf and every time he asked him to say '99' he took a deep breath instead! (Pass)

274. A candidate was told: 'Examine this rash but don't rub it'. He found a brownish, macular rash on a young, healthy-looking woman. He had no idea what the diagnosis was. In retrospect, he thinks it must have been mastocytosis. (Fail)

275. A candidate was told that a patient had a chronic cough. On examination, he found right upper lobe consolidation and offered a differential diagnosis of tumour or tuberculosis. He was then shown the patient's chest X-ray which showed a cavity with a crescentic upper border and he diagnosed a mycetoma. (Pass)

276. In his second attempt, a candidate was asked to listen to a heart. He heard a mid-diastolic murmur and came up with the diagnosis of mitral stenosis. The examiner asked him to auscultate again; on doing this, he thought he could also hear an early diastolic murmur. (Fail)

277. A candidate was asked to examine the pulse of a patient and found a right brachial artery aneurysm. He reports that the examiner expected him to find the right radial pulse reduced in volume compared to the left but that he could not confirm this. The possible causes he offered were traumatic, iatrogenic or mycotic and, in retrospect, feels that it was most likely to have been a mycotic aneurysm caused by subacute bacterial endocarditis many years before. (Pass)

278. A candidate was asked to look at a man's face. He found herpes zoster in the left ear and in the distribution of the mandibular division of the trigeminal nerve. He also reported a left facial nerve paralysis and wasting of the left side of the tongue with deviation of the protruded tongue to the left. He diagnosed Ramsay Hunt's syndrome plus herpes affecting the Vth and XIIth cranial nerves. He was asked if such extensive involvement was possible and he answered: 'It appears so!'. (Pass)

279. A candidate was asked to examine the fundus of a patient. He found that the lens had been removed because of a cataract. It was very difficult to see the fundus so he guessed the diagnosis of diabetic retinopathy which he still believes was probably correct. (Pass)

280. After being asked to examine the heart on his first short case, a candidate reported that he found mitral stenosis with an opening snap. The examiners asked him to point out the second left intercostal space. 'That's too high,' said one examiner, 'It's here!' 'No it's not, it's here,' said the second. 'Well, it's a silly landmark anyway,' said the first. 'I agree,' said the second, 'Let's move on!' (Pass)

281. A candidate was asked to examine a man's abdomen. The patient had several of the signs of chronic liver disease and ascites. After much deliberation, the candidate said he could not feel the liver although he expected it to be there. He was criticized for his technique of examining the spleen (which the candidate says had been taught to him by an experienced examiner) and the examiners told him that the cyanosis was not a sign of liver disease. The candidate commented, 'This all proves that examiners are only human'.* (Pass)

282. A candidate was brought to an elderly lady with an obvious left hemiparesis and with a catheter *in situ*. He offered the diagnosis and explained why. He then had to examine the legs neurologically. He found this

---

*The candidate did not give the details of the technique that was criticized. We have known some examiners to get exasperated if a candidate, after having found no large splenomegaly at a preliminary light palpation, starts palpating from the right iliac fossa. They argue that this technique is to look for a spleen that is large enough to cross the mid-line, but it is also large enough for detection on light palpation! The examiners were also right to point out that cyanosis is not a sign of liver disease.

very difficult as she was demented and would not co-operate. However, he managed to demonstrate some findings in keeping with the left hemiparesis. They were about to dismiss him when he commented on the marked tibial bowing (sabre tibia) and volunteered a differential diagnosis. The examiners looked pleased. He felt that by making his comments on the tibia he may have made the difference with regard to passing or failing. (Pass)

Some anecdotes in the first person
283. I was asked: 'Look at this man's hands'. He had clubbing and the examiner asked me the causes. I looked at his feet but could not see any clubbing there. However, I noted abnormalities in the left tibia and diagnosed osteomyelitis. The patient nodded encouragingly but the examiner looked really cross! (Pass)

284. 'This man has some strange feelings in his feet and legs, would you examine them?' The patient was totally bald and was wearing some sort of corset around his waist. He had a peripheral neuropathy but I had expected to find a dermatome pattern because of the corset. I really got into a mess! The examiner told me that the corset was for an incisional hernia following a splenectomy. I suggested he had pernicious anaemia as a cause for the splenomegaly and neuropathy, then possibly that he had diabetes in association with the alopecia. I eventually worked out that he had had vincristine for leukaemia! The examiners were very good-natured throughout all of this. (Fail)

285. 'Please examine this abdomen.' I did so and found definite splenomegaly. 'What is the diagnosis?', the examiner asked. I replied that he most likely had chronic myeloid leukaemia (CML) but the examiner blew a fuse and said that he had just wanted me to say that he had a 'large spleen'! (Fail)

286. 'Ask this lady some questions and find out what the problem is', was the instruction addressed to a candidate. He found a rather garrulous lady with senile dementia. He did not ask her questions very well and the examiner stepped in to help. The diagnosis was discussed and the examiner apparently agreed that it was difficult. Afterwards the candidate was told by the organizing registrar that they had had difficultly finding good cases – otherwise this dementia case would probably not have been included in the examination. (Pass)

287. I was asked to examine the abdomen of a 60-year-old man. I found polycystic kidneys and an enlarged liver and I demonstrated the scars of the dialysis fistula. The examiners laughed when I went on to test for a spleen as they said that to find a patient with polycystic kidneys, liver and spleen was an examiner's dream!* (Pass)

288. I was asked to examine the legs, neurologically, in a 50-year-old man. I was told that he had a burning sensation in his feet but he did not drink. The patient then said that he did drink until he had got diabetes! We all laughed and they then said: 'Show us how you would have proceeded anyway!'. (Pass)

289. The neurological case that I was asked to examine would not initially come out from under the bedclothes! I think that most people would have panicked but, given appropriate coaxing, the patient was eased into a suitable position! (Pass)

290. On arriving for the exam, I encountered an old chap who I thought was a caretaker from the hospital. I said to him: 'I'm fairly nervous. Is there a toilet nearby?'. So he laughed and pointed me in the right direction. I later discovered that he was one of my examiners! However, I felt there was a friendly atmosphere. He asked me to examine a woman's legs neurologically. He said that she had become very weak but was now getting better. The unfortunate lady was totally deaf and I was almost shouting to make her hear my examination requests.† At each point during the examination I was stopped and asked what I had thought, and what I would do next. The sensory testing was an absolute nightmare. She seemed to have a fairly global weakness with absent reflexes and a patchy sensory loss. I thought the diagnosis was probably Guillain–Barré syndrome. The examiner agreed and then held my arm and said that he appreciated that it was very difficult! (Pass)

291. I was asked to look at a man's chest. 'What do you see?' asked the examiner. There was bilateral gynaecomastia. 'If you were in the clinic what would you want to examine next?' 'The liver,' I said. 'Go on then.' I struggled to demonstrate a normal-sized liver. 'What would you examine next?' he said. 'His testes,' I

answered. 'Go on then.' He had bilateral flaccid testes the size of peas. 'What's the diagnosis?' said the examiner. There then followed a nasty discussion about testosterone replacement and its relation to hair, skin texture and gonadal size! (Pass)

292. I was asked to examine a patient's abdomen. I started at the hands but was told to go straight to the abdomen.‡ There was a renal transplant in the left groin and a left radial fistula with tenderness in the left loin, and I thought there was a palpable kidney. I did not palpate too firmly because it was painful and they did not mind this. The patient was also cushingoid. I felt the diagnosis was a left renal transplant with a ?polycystic kidney and that he was cushingoid as a result of the steroids. At this stage the patient put his thumbs up! We then went on to the next patient and I was asked to examine her cranial nerves. It was an elderly lady with a complete right ptosis and her eye was looking down and out. Before I had completed the examination of the IIIrd, IVth and VIth cranial nerves, she started to vomit. Therefore we left her! However, we continued to discuss the causes of a IIIrd nerve palsy. I said that diabetes was the most common cause and they said multiple sclerosis was. We then went through the entire list! They asked for investigations and I offered a blood glucose and a CT scan. (Pass)

293. 'This man has been short of breath recently, could you examine his chest to find out why?' The expansion seemed reduced on the right side but the breath sounds were reduced at the left base. I could not recover from this conflicting information and completed my examination not having a clue what I was going to say. I could not go back over the findings as they were rushing me. I stood up and confidently gave the signs for a left pleural effusion. They said: 'Some people, when they say 'left' really mean 'right', are you sure this is left?'. I realized I had got the wrong side but I could not retract what I had said so I repeated that I had carefully examined the patient and felt the signs were on the left. Then the bell went. The moral of this is that whenever they tell you to speed up – slow down. (Pass)

294. Examiner: 'Feel this woman's pulse and tell me what you find'.

---

*and a patient's nightmare!

†It is often advisable to face the deaf person and lower your voice to a bass tone, because many deaf people can hear bass notes better than higher pitched ones, and many can lip read as well.

‡It is useful when this happens because it indicates that there are no signs in the hands because you would not be stopped if there were. It also reduces the likelihood that the condition is one which might have signs in the hands such as chronic liver disease.

Answer: 'There is atrial fibrillation'.

Examiner: 'and . . . ? This is the MRCP, not finals'.

Answer: 'The pulse is of good volume and possibly collapsing in character'.

Examiner: 'and . . . ?'

Answer: [Long silence – you could hear a penny drop!] 'I did not count the rate'.

Examiner: 'No you didn't, but what is it approximately?'

Answer: '80 beats/min'.

Examiner: 'Now continue to examine the precordium and tell us what you find'.

Answer: 'There are no thrills, nor a palpable heart sound. The apex beat is displaced to the anterior axillary line and there is a loud pansystolic murmur of mitral regurgitation. There are no clinical signs to suggest mitral stenosis but this could be silent so I would arrange for an echocardiogram.' (Pass)

295. The examiner handed me an ophthalmoscope. 'This patient is having trouble with her vision. Would you examine her eyes?' I commented on the cataract and then described hard exudates, both blot and flame haemorrhages, arteriovenous nipping and microaneurysms. I said that the features were consistent with both diabetes mellitus and hypertension. This did not please one of the examiners who said that hypertensive retinopathy should have more superficial flame haemorrhages. I stood my ground and said that she did in fact have quite numerous flame haemorrhages, but otherwise the appearances suggested diabetes. He finally asked me what her refractive index was. When my answer was rather quick at 14 dioptres, he tried to trip me up by saying that I had not included my own refractive error. However, I was able to point out that I had contact lenses and so I was perfectly corrected! (Pass)

296. I was asked to examine a man having been told that he had weak hands. On inspection, he had wasted small muscles bilaterally in a distal rather than a proximal distribution. There was no Horner's syndrome or fasciculation of the tongue and there was no sensory loss. The feet were also involved. There was a discussion then about findings that looked like a pure motor neuropathy. It could have been Charcot–Marie–Tooth but I opted for porphyria as this was Professor Goldberg's unit in Glasgow! The examiners smiled for the one and only time – either in absolute amusement at the ridiculous answer or because I was correct! (Pass)

297. My last case would have been an easy cardiovascular system case except for the patient's stomach which must have been the loudest rumbling stomach in history – audible at 100 paces! I think she had atrial fibrillation, mixed mitral valve disease and aortic regurgitation. It would have been OK if I could have heard the blessed murmurs without the orchestrations from her gut! (Pass)

298. I had to examine a lady with Graves' eye disease who also had a VIth cranial nerve palsy. I found trying to examine her pupils and eye movements rather difficult because she was silhouetted against the backdrop of a bay window – perhaps I should have turned her round. (Pass)

299. I lost the membrane off my stethoscope during my respiratory case. It was a patient with a pleural effusion. I was very puzzled at finding a completely quiet chest – something which I had never seen beforehand. I suspected a pleural effusion from the percussion and vocal resonance. However, I discovered the faulty stethoscope at the very end of the examination. The examiners wanted to hear first what I thought, but did eventually agree to a second listening! (Pass)

300. 'What's the diagnosis?' I was given no history. However, the diagnosis was obvious as there was evidence of psoriatic plaques together with arthropathy and nail changes. I was asked what was atypical about the patient and so I mentioned that the plaques did not have any scales. The examiner asked why and I suggested that it had been treated. The examiner then said something to me in Latin and asked what it meant.* I did not have a clue. The examiners both laughed but said nothing, except that the exam was now over! (Pass)

301. I was asked to examine a patient's fundi. They were very abnormal but goodness knows what the diagnosis was! I said hypertensive retinopathy because no laser burns were present, and I could not imagine someone having such terrible diabetic retinopathy without having had photocoagulation! (Pass)

302. After my first three cases the 'dove' took over. I was taken to a man and told that he recently had a problem with his eyesight but that things were now

*The patient probably had guttate (from Latin for 'spots that resemble drops') psoriasis in which salmon pink plaques with minimal scales appear on the face and trunk.

improving. 'Would you like to examine his fundi?' I did not have a clue what was going on. He seemed to have a mixture of disc swelling and atrophy but I said that I was very unsure about the degree of swelling. The examiner said that if he told me that the disc was definitely swollen, what would be my differential diagnosis? At this point the head of my ophthalmoscope fell off! I said that partially treated benign intracranial hypertension or a tumour treated with radiotherapy would both give this appearance. As we walked to the next patient, the head of my ophthalmoscope fell off again. I said how awful it must be for them to take candidates like me around! (Pass)

303. The short cases went very well. The examiners were extremely pleasant and they even carried my ophthalmoscope box for me! I felt confident and very much in command. However, for my fifth short case I was asked to examine a chest. I could find no physical signs at all and I said so. The examiner said: 'That's very honest'. I was devastated. Whilst walking away the other examiner whispered to me, 'Never mind, we couldn't hear anything either when we listened this morning!'. In fact, it was an upper lobe collapse that had resolved. (I passed the short cases but failed the exam.)

Miscellaneous

304. A candidate was asked to examine the heart. He could find no abnormality and said so because he thought he had to be honest. He has no idea what the diagnosis was. He failed.

305. A candidate was asked to examine a man's abdomen. He could find no abnormality and diagnosed a normal abdomen. In retrospect he is not sure if he missed something. Though he failed the clinical, he felt he had passed the short case section.

Useful tips

Novice candidates preparing for MRCP pick up tips from their tutors, senior colleagues and other candidates who have 'already been there'. Then through their own experiences, they develop their own. Some have been passed to us through our surveys and we present a selection of them here.

306. Practise, again and again, on 'short case patients' and when you think you have done enough – do more!

307. Practise being harassed. Get some 'mock' examiners to put you under stress. Nervousness gets no

credit; the examiner is more likely to think that in a real emergency you would not rise to the challenge.

308. In every spare moment, practise talking short case records (not just reading them) and talking lists (not just writing them). Get the order of lists right – give the common and uncontroversial ones first. Avoid controversial causes completely.

309. Practise presenting cases as much as examining them. If you can present clearly and quickly it is as impressive as examining well.

310. You have got to really practise doing short cases with SpRs, consultants, friends – even the dog or a doll! You have got to be able to examine without thinking and to then come up with sensible diagnoses from your clinical findings.

311. Dress smartly and conservatively.

312. Take to the examination a stethoscope, a pen torch, red-headed hat pin (dip a white-headed one in red paint if necessary), a tape measure, some cotton wool and some orange sticks.*

313. Be polite to the patient and the examiners; say 'Please' and 'Thank you'. The occasional use of 'Sir/Madam' will not do any harm.

314. You will have read the instruction outside the room and, on entering, you will be introduced to the patient. Do not ask the examiners to repeat the instruction but read the instruction carefully – it may contain a clue which you will miss without care. Greet the patient politely and get on with the task in hand.

315. Do not hurt the patient, especially during the abdominal examination. Look at the patient's face during deep palpation.

316. Make sure that during the examination of the patient, you let the examiner see that you are doing the correct things – as one does in a driving test.

317. Do not be put off by any of the examiner's mannerisms.

*Equipment is provided but it is so much easier to use one's own. You may wish to take your own tendon hammer, sterile pins and ophthalmoscope. At least with the latter you know how to use it and you will have put in new batteries and have the lens set for your own lens correction.

318. Think while you are examining. Extend the end of the examination by a few seconds, if necessary, to give you time to put the findings together, and to prepare what you are going to say before you turn to the examiner.

319. Do not panic if you find very few signs in a patient. It is better to miss something subtle than to make up something that is not there.

320. Practise having to comment on your findings as you proceed through any clinical examination of a patient.

321. Do not let your tie or hair dangle in the patient's face. When you have finished, be sure to leave the patient adequately covered up.

322. Present cases to the examiner as if you are speaking to an equal about an easy case.

323. Be confident – but not overconfident. A supercilious attitude is fatal.

324. Look at the examiner rather than at the patient or the floor when answering. Speak clearly and fluently. Do not mumble.

325. Take time to think before opening your mouth.

326. Keep cool, even when interrupted, and have a systematic examination technique to fall back on if you cannot make a spot diagnosis at the start.

327. Be aware that the stress of the examination can cause you to 'blurt out' things you do not really mean. Keep calm and think before you speak.

328. Remember common things are common. Beware of thinking that because it is the MRCP it is likely to be rare, although there will be the rarer cases (the usual suspects) as well.

329. Do not talk while the examiners are talking and be wary of arguing with them. If you say something which is definitely wrong then be prepared to say: 'I withdraw that', rather than trying to defend it. Remind yourself that the examiner is the judge and the jury!

330. Do not try to pull the wool over the examiner's eyes. He or she is eminent and intelligent or he or she

would not be an examiner, and will resent it if you treat him or her as a fool.

331. Do not guess or waffle. Cut your losses and admit if you do not know.

332. Avoid strange mannerisms of speech and action, including using your hands excessively when speaking. Avoid 'ers' in your speech as much as possible.

333. Do not be casual. Say 'myocardial infarction' rather than 'heart attack' or 'MI'. Stand properly without leaning on the bed or putting your hands in your pockets.

334. Avoid using trade names of drugs – always use the proper pharmacological name.

335. Do not mention in your presentation that a physical sign is dubious or 'slight', e.g. starting your presentation on a case of mitral stenosis with: 'The pulse is slightly collapsing'.*

336. At the end say: 'Thank you', in a sincere manner.

337. Be careful in your choice of hotel for the night before the exam. A candidate recalls: 'For my first attempt, I booked a random hotel and ended up with a room in a cheap hotel overlooking a road which was busy all night, with burglar alarms going off. The walls were thin and the televisions and other loud noises of the neighbours could be heard going on throughout most of the night. For subsequent exam visits, I was very careful with my choice of hotel and always rang up to plead for a room in a corner, well away from any roads or other sources of noise, explaining to the hotelier that I had an exam to do. I believe this important strategy is essential.'

Quotations

These quotations are valuable suggestions and remarks derived from candidates' own experiences in the exam, and they have crystallized them in one or two sentences. We have grouped them under suitable headings which

---

*You should know that mitral stenosis does not have a collapsing pulse and if there is aortic incompetence then you would have heard the appropriate additional murmur. If it is not present then do not mention a 'possible collapsing pulse'. Leave out what does not fit. The examiners would tear you to shreds!

highlight their main points. It is no surprise that the chief lessons one learns from them is to practise, adopt good bedside manners and wear a confident and caring countenance. We have put our remarks in the footnotes wherever we felt a comment was warranted.

Adopt good bedside manners

338. The examination is not really very different to the final MB but obviously set at a higher level and with no help or encouragement from the examiners. Your approach to the patient is very important.

339. Do not panic; be kind to the patient and do not let the examiners hassle you.

340. Always introduce yourself by name to the patient and explain what you are going to do (in lay terms). Position the patient correctly and check whether the area to be examined is painful. Do not be afraid to ask the examiner if you can examine another but relevant part of the body if you consider this necessary (he or she can always say 'no').

341. For women, I would suggest that you wear something comfortable which will accommodate your stethoscope and to leave your handbag in a cloakroom. There is enough stress without worrying if your blouse buttons are undone or whether you have left your handbag by the previous patient!

342. Remember to suggest moving away from the patient when having to use words like 'tumour' or 'multiple sclerosis'.

343. Play the game. Introduce yourself to the patients and explain what you are going to do. Always expose the patient fully and then stand back and look at them before starting. There is plenty that can be missed if you do not take the time to 'observe'. It is also said that you always fail the exam if you hurt the patient. In my exam, I grabbed a patient by the hand – it was obviously sore and they shouted out. However, I apologized profusely and got away with it.

344. The short cases went well. However, the lack of feedback was very difficult to cope with. The examiners, though, seemed happy with my simple but confident answers. I think I appeared caring and was polite to the patients. I smiled a lot at the examiners and tried to be relaxed yet professional. It all seemed to work!

Practise clinical examination and presentation

345. Do not try the MRCP too soon. See as much general medicine as possible in a busy job – 'cushy' jobs are not helpful in the end.

346. Be very professional in your presentation. I agree it's an easy exam – it's easy to fail!

347. Senior colleagues and consultants had prepared me for the psychological torture I was about to endure!

348. Go to as many clinical courses for MRCP as possible. Work out the best method for the examination of each system and practise it until it is second nature to you. Be as direct and positive in your answers as possible (even if they are wrong!).

349. I failed badly on the short cases. Do not take the examination unless you can properly prepare for it. I was very anxious and was not thinking while I was examining. I kept imagining that the cases were supposed to be difficult, rare or complex, but on the day they were very straightforward.

350. Talk through as many short cases as possible before the exam with someone who has been through it recently or with someone who is used to teaching. Preferably do this on a one-to-one basis or in a small group.

351. Practising the technique of examination is essential so that it becomes second nature under stress. Persuade colleagues to grill you mercilessly on short cases and with the differential diagnoses. Certain 'favourite' topics seem to recur. Make sure you know these. Also, in the exam, do not make any statements unless you can back them up.

352. The most important point is to look professional, as if you have done it quickly and thoroughly a hundred times before. You do not need to know that much theoretical knowledge. Every clinical station has the necessary equipment but you will probably prefer to take your own as you will be much more familiar with it.

353. Before the examination I spent 6 weeks getting registrars to take me on short cases and then questioning me under examination conditions. Be meticulous about examination technique and do not be fooled by the apparent relaxed nature of the examiners – examine everything properly. Do not listen to tutors saying that one mistake makes a failed exam – it is not true.

354. Get together with someone else doing the exam and practise until you are bored with reciting the appropriate litany. I only just practised enough and wished I had started 2 months earlier. It is the only way, especially if you can get someone senior (and preferably nasty!) to put you through it!

355. The more practice at presenting short cases, the better.

356. I had a lot of practice presenting short cases to a 'hawk' of a senior registrar. This experience was invaluable.

357. Adopt a systematic approach to the examination of all the major systems and have the features of the common clinical conditions at your fingertips, e.g. upper and lower motor neurone lesions, the auscultatory findings of various valvular lesions, etc. A well-integrated, comprehensive system is needed for presenting the findings to examiners. Do not rush the presentation and omit important points.

358. It is important to have a method for examining each system. I do not think the examiners necessarily want you to make a definitive diagnosis in every case but you should be able to describe adequately the physical signs and offer some logical diagnostic possibilities.

Get it right

359. Do not rush a case – the examiners were very keen to stop me once they considered that I had enough information to make a diagnosis.

360. If you are unsure of the diagnosis then describe the findings and give them a differential diagnosis.

361. Do not be afraid to allow a few seconds of silence to pass before answering a question. Use this time to collect and organize your thoughts so that your answer comes in a logical order.

362. Know the diagnosis before you finish examining the patient and then state it confidently. Be prepared for further questions about the physical signs and on the management of the disease.

363. When examining fundi, do not stop until you have finished and have thought of what to say.

364. Do not make comments that cannot be substantiated. Everything will be challenged if you are on the borderline.

365. The examiners already had in their mind what answers they would accept and they kept on until they got the actual wording they wanted.

366. Try not to be obtuse in the short cases or to pick on unimportant details, as the examiners may then draw you into a frustrating and often irrelevant discussion as to what you mean and sidetrack you away from the main issue.

367. If you know the diagnosis from just observing the patient (e.g. scleroderma), there seems to be a ritual series of questions and answers (swallowing, etc.) that you should anticipate and be prepared for.

368. I missed optic atrophy on one of my short cases. The moral is, if the fundus looks normal, to always ask yourself, 'Is there optic atrophy?'.

369. In general, I found that getting the diagnosis right was not as important as I had been led to believe. Examining the patient with a systematic plan in mind and having a good differential diagnosis at each stage was much more important.

370. The examiners were very pleasant all the time and, as I got more cases right, I became more confident – and then I even started to enjoy myself. The examiners did not harass me but seemed concerned to let me get as much right as possible.

371. The short cases went really well. After the first case they did not ask any more aggressive questions. I think I had already satisfied them. Start well and look confident even if you do not know anything!

Listen, obey and do not stray

372. Just stick to what they ask and do not mess around. For example, do not start checking the temperature just because you hear a murmur. It seems to irritate them.

373. Do only what is asked of you. Give positive and concise answers to questions, unless a differential diagnosis is requested.

374. Always do a full examination of the system asked for – show off your technique. Do not be put off by 'dead-pan' examiners. The result comes as a particular shock when you have been sitting exams for many years without failing them.

375. I think I passed because I took the examiner's instructions one step further, e.g. I felt the pulse of someone with a dysphasia. Perhaps that is the secret!

376. Look at the patient as a whole and not just the system you are examining. So much useful information can be obtained by good observation.

377. They may ask you just to listen to the heart so that you cannot get clues from the pulse and palpation. In this case, one just has to do the best one can.

378. I think that they liked the way I examined the first patient, which was a neurological case in which I extended the examination beyond the legs, and then decided that I was probably competent.

379. Perform the physical examination and answer questions as requested. Try asking patients as much as possible; I had to look at a fundus so I asked the patient if he was diabetic and my examiners made no attempt to stop me. I was left with the impression that the exam, although difficult, is fundamentally fair.

One wrong does not make one fail
380. Treat each short case individually and put your apparent disasters behind you.

381. Do not be put off if you get a few things wrong. I made a lot of mistakes (that I know of!) and still passed.

382. Do not be distracted by mistakes made (or imagined) in preceding cases or by an examiner's mannerisms or approach.

383. I was put off right from the beginning after they stopped me during the examination of the first case – a vague, non-specific instruction was given and I had not found enough to be sure of. I was on the downward slope from then on. I might have passed had I pulled myself together and put the experience of that case behind me.

384. At the time and until I received my result, I was convinced I had failed. I think the experience of my previous attempt helped considerably, because I consciously reminded myself to put each bit behind me after I had done it, and not to dwell on my mistakes.

385. Never, never, never give up. I made many mistakes and thought I had had it but I still passed. You do not have to get it all (or even mostly) right if you can appear logical, *caring** and reasonably sensible. The examiners were totally non-committal and obviously trying to see how confident I was. I nearly failed myself!

If you say less they want more
386. After my first case there was a long silence as if they were waiting for me to say more – I went to pieces after this.

387. Be prepared for supplementary questions and for examiners who disagree or argue with your comments, but do not fall into the trap of arguing back. Just try and justify yourself and retract a statement if you know you have said something stupid.

388. Be complete in your examination – examine everything even if it does not seem relevant. For example, all hearts need to be listened to for early diastolic and mid-diastolic murmurs even if you think you already have the diagnosis. Every possible aspect of eyes needs to be looked at if asked to 'examine the eyes', unless something in the instruction suggests otherwise.

389. I was shown a patient with a IIIrd cranial nerve palsy (and possibly a IVth) following transfrontal surgery. I was asked why the eye was down and out.† I was a bit shaky on this – one takes it for granted that the pupil is dilated without asking why! I got really hot under the collar with this one.

Humility is more persuasive than self-righteousness
390. Be kind and confident but humble in the short cases.

391. By far the major problem was keeping my head and holding my ground politely when we disagreed.

---

*Our italics. It is the *raison d'être* of being a doctor.
†Because of the unopposed actions of the lateral rectus (abduction) and superior oblique (depression and abduction) muscles.

392. Learn good examination techniques for all systems. Do not argue with the examiners and be polite to the patients.

393. If you know you have made a glaring error, retract the remark and start again. If you are right (or at least think you are), stick to your answer.

394. The MRCP short cases are not a test of your medical knowledge. Mine is not profound. It is simply a test of whether you are competent at your job. If you think that you are and can convince the examiners of that then you will pass.

Keep cool: agitation generates aggression

395. 'Panic not.' This is greatly helped if you have practised a lot of short cases under stress and seen most things before.

396. A good start is a great help. It is like skating on thin ice – if you keep going and do not fall through, then you make it.

397. The most off-putting aspect of each case is the lack of feedback from the examiners as to whether you are right or wrong. This is much more disconcerting than outright criticism.

398. Stay calm and talk sensibly even when the diagnosis appears unclear (easy to say – difficult to do!).

399. At the end of the exam I was sure I had failed as I did not have a clue what was wrong with one of the patients and did not do very well on another. However, I was wrong in my pass/fail self-assessment. A factor in my pass mark must have been that I did not lose my nerve and I remained calm, even after the mistakes. After all, it is as much a test of your nerve as your knowledge.

400. I did not feel confident enough to think I had passed, but I thought I had a reasonable chance. It is so important to start well, keep calm, score points when you can and treat each case independently. I did not do that in my first attempt and failed as a result; I maintained my concentration (with a supreme effort of will!) in the second attempt and it paid off.

401. Relax – and enjoy what are predominantly easy but beautifully classical signs.

Simple explanations raise simple questions

402. Very simple, straightforward answers seem to prompt straightforward questions.

403. They appear to be satisfied with a good physical examination and interpretation of simple basic signs but I am sure they penalize heavily if obvious signs are missed. They seemed quite happy for me to ask the patient questions.* It is a great relief when the answers are what you want and also gives one time to think while the patient is answering.

404. The examiners seem to be impressed by short definitive answers and not with long lists of differential diagnoses. I think it is best to answer questions as directly as possible and get on to the next patient.

405. Always be honest – it pays in the end.

Think straight, look smart and speak convincingly

406. If the diagnosis is obvious then focus down and elicit all the relevant signs, regardless of the generality of the instruction. If the diagnosis is not immediately obvious, examine the relevant parts systematically and hope for the best. Do not be put off by mistakes or be paranoid about your performance. I was, and suffered for it.

407. Be definite about the positive findings; do not hedge your answer with 'possibly', 'almost', 'perhaps'. If there is no obvious first-choice answer then give a sensible and relevant differential diagnosis.

408. I think I failed because of hesitancy; I gave no impression of confidence and blurted out statements without thinking.

409. You must be quick and comprehensive in your examination; it looks bad if you need to go back to do something which you had forgotten.

410. Do not change your mind half way through – as long as you are sure you are right.

*Asking the relevant but not the forbidden questions ('What is the diagnosis?') may be appreciated by some examiners, as part of developing a good rapport with the patient.

You have seen it all before

411. My cases were more straightforward than I had been led to expect. In fact, nothing was particularly rare.

412. It is easy to be daunted by the feeling that there will be conditions you have never heard of and that the cases will be difficult and rare. After my experience in four attempts, it seems that in most cases the same old conditions keep recurring and they are mostly straight-forward if only you can keep calm.

413. The cases are simple (the ones I saw were!). It is the candidate who makes them difficult and he or she may fail him or herself.

414. This was a much more enjoyable and interesting exam than Part I. With a single-minded approach to passing an exam rather than learning everything about medicine, it is much more straightforward than people think. Remember that the majority of the examiners' knowledge outside their own field is unlikely to be much greater than your own (after revising!) and par-ticularly about details. As long as you can justify your answers it will be difficult to fault you. After all, what more is the exam for than to reassure consultants that they can stay at home while you are looking after their patients!

415. When you come out of the exam you realize that after months and months of hard work and swotting, the amount of knowledge you actually used could be written on a postage stamp!

Use your eyes first and most

416. One of the short cases – pretibial myxoedema – was given away by the eyes. I think, from talking to other people, there is often an obvious 'clue' in the short cases.

417. Spend at least 10–15 seconds just looking at the patient before even attempting an examination. When presenting, speak slowly and clearly and look the exam-iners in the eye.

418. Always look at the patient as a whole as well as the part in question. In one case (skin lesions in a black person) my first impulse was to suspect a tropical disease (?cutaneous leishmaniasis!) but the presence of exophthalmos gave me the diagnosis (pretibial myx-

oedema). Do not be put off by examiners who are (as mine were) totally non-committal.

419. Do exactly what is asked but give yourself a second or two to look at the whole patient from the end of the bed.

420. Remember to look at the bedside for clues – in my case I missed the tablet containers which would have suggested hypertensive retinopathy. When exam-ining fundi, keep looking until you have covered all areas and try not to panic if you think you are taking too long.

Doing and forgetting

421. I examined the patient in an orderly sequence looking for the right things but for some reason, when I came to present the case, I could not recall my findings with regard to the stigmata of chronic liver disease. I could not even remember whether she was jaundiced!

422. The examiners were fair and did not try to unsettle me. I fell down on presenting my findings and should have practised this more. In the heat of the moment, I went through the examination routine and then discovered I could not remember what I had found! I had also had a car crash driving up to the exam so that did not help to steady the nerves! Advice – do not drive there!

Examiners are different

423. The examiners were very pleasant and wanted to see how confident I was when faced with a problem. They could have failed me on many things but appeared to be wanting to see how my mind worked. They like you to be slick, thorough and to present your find-ings precisely without dithering. I am sure they assess you very quickly on the first two cases and decide whether they would like you to be in charge of their patients. Stay relaxed and be honest.

424. I felt that the examiners unnecessarily rushed me. Some patients were not undressed and not on their bed. This seemed to frustrate them as well as myself though I didn't let it show and I tried to take it all in my stride. I had very little indication from their expres-sion as to whether I was saying or doing the right thing. I found the lack of feedback to be very disconcerting but I knew it was to be expected and therefore I did not let it upset me.

425. Some of my examiners were very aggressive and sarcastic in their approach. Also the way they interrupted and corrected me made me feel completely incompetent and stupid.

426. It was very unnerving not getting any feedback and on one or two occasions they said: 'I see', which always sounds very ominous!

427. Do not get flustered. If you say something silly, retract it quickly and continue to talk. The examiners can be aggressive and try to hurry you. Do not let them! Look smart in what you wear and be nice to the patients.

428. Try to be calm and imagine that you are seeing the cases in a clinic and carrying out a routine examination. The examiners made me very nervous, especially with their comments which, in retrospect, I should have tried to ignore. They were only trying to test my knowledge and physiological comprehension of the physical signs I had elicited.

429. There was nothing difficult. The examiners were polite, unobtrusive, to the point and clear about their requirements. They were also amazingly expressionless throughout.

430. I wish the examiners were a little more friendly and did not interrupt every 10–15 seconds!

431. Do not be bullied by the examiners. There is no substitute for experience. You can pass even if you make a mess of one short case.

432. Do not let them rattle you. Never think you have failed until you get the letter.

433. Do not let the examiners rush you as you are then likely to make mistakes and this just surrenders all control to them. They cannot fail you for a methodical clinical examination.

434. The examiners kept asking me if I was sure of my findings as though they were trying to put me off. I wish I was this good always!

Additional comments and quotes from candidates

435. I had no time for my central nervous system examination and I thought that the ethics station was much easier than any practice sessions that I had had on previous courses. I found that on courses the actors were fairly horrible in so far as they cried and shouted. This never happens in the real exam or even in real life.

436. I thought the exam was bizarre but I passed!

437. The few minutes break that is given in between each station is very useful. For example, if you have a bad case or a bad examiner (or both as in my case) it gives you time to compose yourself.

438. Know your basic information really well. Therefore, it is useful to revise material from the written exam. You need to know lists for causes of things and it is important to know them in a logical order.

Appendices

These books exist as they are because of many previous candidates who, over the years, have completed our surveys and given us invaluable insight into the candidate experience. Please give something back by doing the same for the candidates of the future. For all of your sittings, whether they be a triumphant pass or a disastrous fail . . .

Remember to fill in the survey at www.ryder-mrcp.org.uk

THANK YOU

1 | Website links

Resuscitation Council (UK)
www.resus.org.uk

US Centers for Disease Control and Prevention (CDC)
www.cdc.gov/

CDC HIV website
www.cdc.gov/hiv/default.htm

General Medical Council (GMC)
www.gmc-uk.org/

GMC standards of practice
www.gmc-uk.org/guidance/good_medical_practice.asp

Department of Health
www.dh.gov.uk/en/index.htm

GMC guidelines on consent
http://www.gmc-uk.org/guidance/consent_guidance_index.asp

Department of Health guidelines on consent
www.doh.gov.uk/consent/index.htm

Driver and Vehicle Licensing Agency (DVLA)
www.dvla.gov.uk

DVLA at-a-glance guide to current medical standards of the fitness to drive
www.dft.gov.uk/dvla/medical/ataglance.aspx

International Huntington Association
www.huntington-assoc.com/

International Huntington Association guidelines for the molecular genetics predictive test in Huntington disease
www.huntington-assoc.com/guidel.htm

Unrelated Live Transplant Regulatory Authority (ULTRA)
www.dh.gov.uk/en/Publicationsandstatistics/Publications/AnnualReports/ DH_4106493

British Medical Association (BMA)
http://bma.org.uk/

BMA ethics
http://bma.org.uk/practical-support-at-work/ethics

BMA guidelines on withholding and withdrawing life prolonging medical treatment
http://bma.org.uk/practical-support-at-work/ethics/ethics-a-to-z

Royal College of Pathologists
www.rcpath.org/

Royal College of Pathologists guidelines for the retention of tissues and organs at postmortem examination
www.dhsspsni.gov.uk/hoi-pathologists.pdf

Multiple Sclerosis Society (UK)
www.mssociety.org.uk/

Department for Work and Pensions
www.dwp.gov.uk/

Blood Transfusion Service (UK)
www.blood.co.uk/

Department of Health guidelines on hepatitis B-infected healthcare workers
www.dh.gov.uk/en/Publicationsandstatistics/Publications/ PublicationsPolicyAndGuidance/DH_073164

Action on Smoking and Health (ASH)
www.ash.org.uk/

MRSA guidelines for nursing staff
www.nhs.uk/Conditions/MRSA/Documents/RCN%20MRSA%20guidelines.pdf

Medical Defence Union (library of contents)
www.the-mdu.com/section_Hospital_doctors_and_specialists/topnav_advice_ centre_1/index.asp

2 | Abbreviations

5-HT	5-hydroxytryptamine
AAFB	alcohol- and acid-fast bacilli
ABPM	ambulatory blood pressure monitoring
ACE	angiotensin-converting enzyme
AChR	acetylcholine receptor
ACTH	adrenocorticotrophic hormone
AF	atrial fibrillation
AFB	acid-fast bacilli
AIDS	acquired immunodeficiency syndrome
ALT	alanine aminotransferase
ANTI-CCP	anti-cyclic citrullinated peptide
ANCA	antineutrophil cytoplasmic antibody
ARB	angiotensin II receptor blocker
AST	aspartate aminotransferase
ATT	antituberculous treatment
BCG	bacille Calmette–Guérin
BIH	benign intracranial hypertension
BMD	bone mineral density
BMI	Body Mass Index
BP	blood pressure
CABG	coronary artery bypass graft
CBT	cognitive behavioural therapy
CCB	calcium channel blocker
CCDC	consultant in communicable disease control
CFC	chlorofluorocarbon
CFS	chronic fatigue syndrome
CHD	coronary heart disease
CICN	community infection control nurse
CK	creatine kinase
CMV	cytomegalovirus
CNS	central nervous system
COPD	chronic obstructive pulmonary disease
CPAP	continuous positive airway pressure
CPHM	consultant in public health medicine
CPR	cardiopulmonary resuscitation
CRH	corticotrophin-releasing hormone
CRP	C-reactive protein
CSF	cerebrospinal fluid
CT	computed tomography
CVA	cerebrovascular accident

DEXA	dual-energy X-ray absorptiometry
DMARD	disease-modifying antirheumatic drug
DNAR	Do Not Attempt Resuscitation
DoH	Department of Health
DOT	directly observed therapy
DVT	deep vein thrombosis
EBUS	endobronchial ultrasound
EBV	Epstein–Barr virus
ECG	electrocardiogram
EEG	electroencaphalogram
eGFR	estimated glomerular filtration rate
EMG	electromyography
ENT	ear, nose and throat
EPP	exposure-prone procedure
ESR	erythrocyte sedimentation rate
EWTD	European Working Time Directive
FBC	full blood count
FEV_1	forced expiratory volume in 1 sec
FVC	forced vital capacity
GA	general anaesthesia
GABA	γ-amino butyric acid
GCA	giant cell arteritis
GCS	Glasgow Coma Score
GGT	γ-glutamyl transferase
GI	gastrointestinal
GMC	General Medical Council
GP	general practitioner
GPCOG	General Practitioner Assessment of Cognition Score
GTN	glyceryl trinitrate
Hb	haemoglobin
HDL	high-density lipoprotein
HERS	Heart and Estrogen/Progestin Replacement Study
HIV	human immunodeficiency virus
HPA	Health Protection Agency
HRT	hormone replacement therapy
HTA	Human Tissue Authority

IBD	inflammatory irritable bowel disease	**PCT**	primary care trust
IBS	irritable bowel syndrome	**PCWP**	pulmonary capillary wedge pressure
ICAS	Independent Complaints Advocacy Service	**PD**	Parkinson's disease
		PDD	Parkinson's disease-related dementia
ICU	intensive care unit	**PE**	pulmonary embolism
INR	international normalized ratio	**PEFR**	peak expiratory flow rate
ITP	idiopathic thrombocytopenic purpura	**PEG**	percutaneous endoscopic gastrostomy
IV	intravenous	**PEP**	postexposure prophylaxis
IVIG	intravenous immunoglobulin	**PIP**	proximal interphalangeal
		PJP	*Pneumocystis jirovecii* pneumonia
LBD	Lewy body dementia	**PM**	postmortem
LFT	liver function test	**PMBV**	percutaneous mitral balloon valvotomy
LMP	last menstrual period	**PMR**	polymyalgia rheumatica
LMWH	low molecular weight heparin	**PR**	per rectum
LPA	Lasting Power of Attorney	**PTHrP**	parathyroid hormone-related protein
LTOT	long-term oxygen therapy		
		RA	rheumatoid arthritis
MAOI	monoamine oxidase inhibitor	**RBC**	red blood cell
MCA	Mental Capacity Act		
MCP	metacarpophalangeal	**SA**	*Staphylococcus aureus*
MC&S	microscopy, culture and sensitivities	**SBE**	subacute bacterial endocarditis
MCV	mean cell volume	**SHOT**	Serious Hazards of Transfusion
MDI	metered dose inhaler	**SIGN**	Scottish Intercollegiate Guidelines Network
MDR-TB	multidrug-resistant tuberculosis		
MDT	multidisciplinary team	**SLE**	systemic lupus erythematosus
ME	myalgic encephalomyelitis	**SNAP**	sensory nerve action potential
MI	myocardial infarction	**STEMI**	ST elevation myocardial infarction
MMSE	Mini-Mental State Examination	**SVT**	supraventricular tachycardia
MRI	magnetic resonance imaging		
MS	multiple sclerosis	**TB**	tuberculosis
MRSA	methicillin-resistant *Staphylococcus aureus*	**TENS**	transcutaneous electrical nerve stimulation
MSU	mid-stream urine	**TFT**	thyroid function test
		TIA	transient ischaemic attack
NICE	National Institute of Health and Clinical Excellence	**TNF**	tumour necrosis factor
		TSH	thyroid-stimulating hormone
NIV	non-invasive ventilation		
NSAID	non-steroidal anti-inflammatory drug	**U&E**	urea and electrolytes
		UTI	urinary tract infection
OGD	oesophagogastroduodenoscopy		
OGTT	oral glucose tolerance test	**WBC**	white blood cell
OSA	obstructive sleep apnoea	**WCC**	white cell count
		WHI	Women's Health Initiative
PALS	Patient Advisory Liaison Service	**WHO**	World Health Organization
PCI	percutaneous coronary intervention		
PCR	polymerase chain reaction	**XDR-TB**	extensively drug-resistant tuberculosis

Index

MRCP – it teaches more than it tests*

*'When you come out of the exam you realize that after months and months of hard work and swotting, the amount of knowledge you actually used could be written on a postage stamp!' (Section F, Quotation 415)

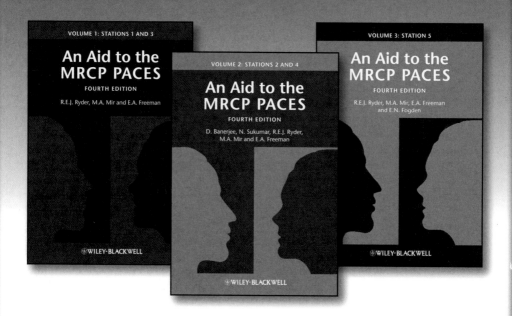